INTERMITTENT

FASTING FOR

WOMEN

OVER 50

|1070+ Tasty & Easy Recipes to Enjoy Fully for Master All the Secrets to Promote Longevity, Detoxify Your Body & Reset Your Metabolism in a Totally Healthy Way (28 Day Plan Included).

Belle Hoyles

2

TABLE OF CONTNTS

4

8

Intermittent fasting (IF) is a type of dieting that involves eating in a stricter way than normal. With intermittent fasting, you would eat your meals within a shorter period of time than normal, as well as fast for extended periods of time. During the times that you aren't eating, your body's fat reserves are used to produce energy. You may also choose to simply eat less overall on this type of diet.

Studies have shown that this type of dieting can also reduce risk factors of chronic diseases, such as high blood pressure and inflammation.

This book will detail the basics of intermittent fasting for women over 50, including what it is, how to determine which type of intermittent fasting schedule would be best for you given your goals or conditions, sample schedules and recipes, common misconceptions about intermittent fasting diets among seniors, as well as many other benefits associated with this unique diet plan.

You can choose many different types of intermittent fasting regimens depending on your goals or health conditions.

1. You may not eat for 16 hours (known as an extended fast), followed by a 24-hour period of normal eating (a modified fast), followed by another 16-hour period of normal eating (a shortened fast).

2. In the fasting periods, you may eat your regular meal amounts during an 8-hour window.

3. You should consume adequate amounts of water during fasting times to help prevent dehydration and increase your metabolic rate.

4. You should avoid all forms of exercise during the fasting periods in order to prevent muscle breakdown.

Intermittent fasting benefits are numerous and include:

1. Weight loss. If you're able to lose weight with this type of diet, then that's a big plus! Studies have found that some intermittent fasting diets can lead to weight loss (particularly among older people).

2. Decreased risk for chronic disease. Studies have shown that intermittent fasting leads to lower, glucose and insulin levels, and a reduction of inflammation markers. All of these changes can help decrease the risk for chronic

diseases such as heart disease and diabetes.

3. Better management of type 2 diabetes and other metabolic conditions. If you already have metabolic conditions such as type 2 diabetes or insulin resistance, then this type of diet can help you manage it better by helping control your blood sugar levels and taking the stress off your endocrine system by fasting periodically throughout the week.

4. Improved mood and mental health. One study found that older women who used intermittent fasting for six months reported significantly improved mood and mental health.

5. Improved cardiovascular health. Intermittent fasting may improve your cardiovascular health by helping you lose weight, reducing chronic inflammation, and creating an environment of "inflammation-free" cells in the body.

Therefore, it is very important to consider your specific health conditions when determining which type of intermittent fasting regimen is best for you. Depending on your primary concern and health condition, you may find that one type of intermittent fasting works best for you while another will not be as effective.

To determine which type of intermittent fasting schedule is best for you:

1. Determine your main health concern. ADF and 5:2 diets are typically considered best for weight loss, while TRF has been shown to help with decreasing chronic disease risk factors like high blood pressure, inflammation, and insulin levels in the body. However, some people have found that ADF and TRF also help them with managing their diabetes better. Ultimately, it can depend on your personal health goals as well as how effectively these dieting protocols work for your particular type of health condition.

2. Choose a schedule that fits your lifestyle. If you can't enjoy your regular meals every day, then don't choose a plan that requires extreme caloric restrictions. For example, if you generally eat three meals per day, having one meal

every other day may not work well for you. Keep in mind that each type of intermittent fasting schedule has slightly different rules (e.g., the time between meals) that you should be aware of as well, as any dietary restrictions (e.g., no artificial sweeteners).

Important Takeaways on Intermittent Fasting

1. You can choose different types of intermittent fasting regimens depending on your personal health goals and risks for chronic disease.

2. ADF may help you lose weight and improve your insulin sensitivity, while TRF may help you lose weight and lower risk factors for chronic disease. Each type of intermittent fasting schedule has slightly different rules you should be aware of.

3. Each type of intermittent fasting program can have slightly different health benefits and risks depending on your personal health goals. It is important to consider the pros and cons of each type of diet before proceeding if it's possible that these negative side effects will influence how well you stick to the diet in the long run.

Women over 50 know that aging brings changes in their bodies, hormones, and metabolism. Oftentimes, these factors can conspire to make it difficult to lose weight.

For many women over 50, intermittent fasting has provided impressive results for both weight loss and overall health. This will give you an overview of this proven approach that has helped so many. You'll also learn the fundamentals of how it works and what you need to get started right away and slim down without feeling cheated!

Intermittent fasting is a type of diet that has been used for many years. It eliminates the guesswork and allows men and women over 50 to enjoy eating a satisfying meal every day without a lot of worry or stress about what they are eating.

The intermittent fasting diet for women over 50 requires an individual to cycle between periods where we consume our normal number of calories daily, followed by higher caloric consumption. This is referred to as a fast, and will typically last anywhere from 12 to 36 hours. During this time, you are 'fasting' and it is important to eat a healthy, nutrient-rich meal that has plenty of protein and healthy fats that will keep you feeling full longer. You should follow the plan so that your fast lasts for 12 hours every day and then consume a larger than normal meal during your eating period.

There are several different ways to structure your intermittent fasting plan when doing it for weight loss for women over 50. Many people opt to have their fasting period on a Monday through Friday schedule with weekends off. Others choose a daily schedule with fasting periods between the hours of 11:00 pm and 7:00 am. This is referred to as the 16/8 fasting schedule.

One thing you should avoid while doing an intermittent fasting plan is eating late at night. You may be tempted to eat some extra calories in the evening if you are doing a daily fast, but this will defeat the purpose of trying it for weight loss.

During your fast, make sure you have plenty of water on hand so you don't feel sick or dizzy when it's time to eat your meal at night. It's important to drink some water 15 minutes before you eat your meal.

Intermittent fasting is highly effective in helping people achieve their goals when done properly. When your metabolism slows down as you age, it can be difficult to keep weight off over time without having the right plan in place.

WHAT IS AN INTERMITTENT DIET?

If you want to lose weight, we have so many diets that we often don't pay attention to how they work or what risks and benefits they present. One of the latest trends in the world of food is intermittent fasting, which is very popular among athletes and is considered by many to be one of the most effective methods for weight loss.

There are several ordinary fasting methods, and the most popular are:

- Scheme 16:8. Also known as the Lean gains method. This scheme divides the day into 2 parts: 8 hours of eating and 16 hours of fasting.
- On alternate days (5:2). This model's idea is that the calorie intake is reduced to a maximum of 500/600 calories 2 days a week. The days need not be consecutive, and on the other days, you can eat whatever you want.
- Eat-Stop-Eat.

On all models, you can drink low-calorie drinks such as coffee and tea without sugar.

BENEFITS OF INTERMITTENT FASTING DIET

The benefits of intermittent fasting are unequivocal, and for those trying to improve their health and lifestyle, it is a must. As many studies have found, intermittent fasting is more effective than long-term caloric restriction in alleviating age-associated diseases.

The following is a list of the most notable benefits of intermittent fasting.

-Improves Brain Function and Memory

Fasting can greatly improve memory and brain functioning, reduce the risk and severity of degenerative conditions such as Alzheimer's disease and help you think more clearly. The reason for this is that during intermittent fasting, your body gets rid of toxins, which it will no longer have to process as food is not consumed. As a result, your brain can function more optimally. Also, by clearing out damaged cells in the hippocampus (which controls learning, memory formation and emotion) it helps prevent their uncontrolled division which leads to mental illnesses like schizophrenia.

-Fights Cancer

Many types of cancer cells have shown to be dependent on glucose for growth and survival. Thus, by reducing the glucose supply (through intermittent fasting) you essentially starve the cancer cells.

-Improves Metabolism

Fasting significantly improves your metabolism by increasing your metabolic flexibility (the body's ability to switch between glucose or fat burning depending on what is required) and insulin sensitivity. As cells become more sensitive to insulin, this will help prevent insulin resistance. Intermittent fasting helps you maintain a healthy weight and can help with weight loss.

-Reduces Inflammation

A growing number of studies have found that intermittent fasting can significantly reduce inflammation in the body by promoting the growth of anti-inflammatory myeloid-derived suppressor cells (MDSCs). These are specific types of white blood cells capable of 'putting out' chronic low-level inflammation. Additionally, intermittent fasting reduces the number of inflammatory markers in the body.

-Can Improve Mood

Many people who suffer from mood disorders such as depression, anxiety or bipolar disorder find that intermittent fasting helps improve their moods and reduce symptoms of their disorders. This is because intermittent fasting helps get rid of excess hormones in your body (which often cause these disorders) and reduces oxidative stress in your brain (which can help alleviate symptoms). In one study, patients with depression found that intermittent fasting was a more effective treatment for them than conventional treatments.

-Lowers Blood Pressure

Blood pressure is lower in people who practice intermittent fasting when compared to those who do not fast regularly. This is because intermittent fasting can reduce high blood pressure and cholesterol levels, which in turn lowers blood pressure.

--Improves Liver Health

Intermittent fasting can have a protective effect on your liver by decreasing bad (LDL) cholesterol and detoxifying the liver of harmful compounds/metabolites which lead to liver disease. This is because the liver will be able to get rid of old or damaged cells during an intermittent fast. Intermittent fasting has also been shown to help treat fatty liver disease.

-Helps Manage Diabetes

A growing number of people suffer from type 1 and type 2 diabetes today, and it is thought that there are more than 382 million people suffering from this disease worldwide. If you suffer from this ailment and want to manage it naturally, then intermittent fasting can help you do this. Intermittent fasting can have a remarkable effect on promoting healthy blood sugar levels, reducing blood sugar spikes and improving insulin sensitivity.

-Fights Depression

Intermittent fasting can help to fight depression. This is because, as mentioned above, it can help improve the levels of inflammatory markers in your body, which may lessen feelings of depression. Additionally, it has been shown that individuals who often suffer from depression have low levels of brain-derived neurotrophic factor (BDNF).

-Reduces Inflammation in Chronic Fatigue Syndrome (CFS)

Chronic fatigue syndrome is a disease that affects approximately 300,000 people in the UK. People suffering from this condition find that their energy levels are very low, their immune response is impaired and they have a great deal of pain and muscle ache. It is thought that a lot of these symptoms occur because of the presence of inflammatory markers in the body, which can lead to chronic inflammation.

-Fights Bacterial Infections

Intermittent fasting helps your immune system to function properly by increasing the number of white blood cells and 'killer T-cells' in your body. By increasing your white blood cell count, you can fight off infections more effectively. Studies have shown that intermittent fasting can be effective at treating a wide range of bacterial infections, including intestinal infections, urinary tract infections and genital infections.

-Fights Viral Infections

As mentioned above, it has been found that intermittent fasting is effective in fighting bacterial infections. However, continuous fasts have also shown to help fight viral infections. This is because this diet helps to increase the number of white blood cells, which can help eradicate viral infections.

-Helps Fight Toxoplasmosis (A Cat Disease)

Intermittent fasting helps your body produce more antibodies against Toxoplasmosis. This is because inter-mitotic fasts can increase the number of B cells and activate (or switch on) the production of antibody-producing cells. By doing this, you will have a greater chance of fighting off an infection.

Helps Fight Ebola

Intermittent fasting has also been shown to be effective in treating Ebola and other hemorrhagic viruses. This is because your immune response is boosted when you are fasting so it will be easier for you to fight off an infection. A study carried out on mice found that intermittent fasts can help protect the brain from Ebola and other hemorrhagic viruses.

-Lowers Risk of Kidney Diseases

Kidney damage is most commonly caused because of high blood pressure, which can lead to kidney disease. Intermittent fasting helps normalize blood pressure and reduce levels of bad (LDL) cholesterol which can help lower your risk of kidney disease.

-Helps Fight Alzheimer's Disease

Studies show that people who suffer from Alzheimer's disease have low levels of brain-derived neurotrophic factor (BDNF), which leads to memory loss and a decrease in other cognitive functions. As explained earlier, BDNF plays a major role in the growth, differentiation and maintenance of neurons in the CNS. When you fast, your body produces more BDNF so your brain will be able to grow and repair itself. This is just one of many benefits fasting has been shown to have on your brain.

-Decreases Risk of Skin Cancer

Cells in the skin are constantly producing free radicals. These free radicals can damage the cells in your body and increase your risk of skin cancer. It has been shown that intermittent fasting can reduce the production of these free radicals so you will have a lowered risk of developing skin cancer.

-Helps Prevent Heart Disease

People who have heart disease often experience damaged blood vessels and inflammation throughout their bodies, which can cause heart disease. Because fasting can lower your levels of bad (LDL) cholesterol, it helps to improve the function of blood vessels and decrease inflammation. This will not only reduce your risk of developing heart disease but it will help to treat the symptoms of heart disease.

-Reduces Blood Pressure

Intermittent fasting can lower both systolic and diastolic blood pressure, which can greatly reduce your risk of developing heart disease. This is because when you fast your body switches from using glucose as its main source of energy to using fat stores — this process is called ketosis. Ketosis is a natural way for your body to use fat as energy while starving, and it causes your blood pressure to drop dramatically.

WHAT CHANGES ARE THERE IN THE BODY?

Intermittent fasting only exceeds the caloric limit. Hormone balance also changes, so the body learns to handle fat stores properly. Here are some of the main improvements that are happening:

Increase insulin sensitivity, especially in combination with exercise. This point is essential for people trying to lose weight because if they have low insulin levels, it is easier to burn fat. Studies show that being overweight can affect insulin's ability to reduce blood sugar levels and consequently release it in larger amounts, further increasing fat accumulation.

Why Choose Intermittent Fasting?

Experts have no doubts about the benefits of this practice. Present in many cultures for centuries—abstinence from food helps the body attack excess fat: the cells put in a stick, will go in search of the stored fat to be used as fuel, giving an incredible acceleration to the metabolism. Running out of energy, our body will be forced to burn fat to meet all its needs.

Intermittent fasting has been a topic of conversation for a lot of time. The first study is about reducing calories to strengthen the body. Reducing energy supply is seen as a "hermetic" stimulus. A small amount of stress can increase cell endurance. Intermittent feeding contributes to the calorie factor, which prolongs fasting status, thus maintaining certain hormones' status for a long time, with very low insulin levels. It seems that scientific evidence shows that this approach can effectively optimize metabolism while slowing down aging.

With intermittent intervals of eating, food intake is isolated for a certain period, and hunger remains for the rest of the time, experts continue. Typically, the so-called 16:8 regime is practiced, that is, 16 hours without food, with food concentrated on the remaining 8 hours. It is generally a matter of skipping dinner or breakfast, depending on your preferences.

It is essential to always remember that no form of abstinence from food can compensate for damage caused by poor nutrition. Therefore, even with intermittent fasting, the hours you eat must be balanced and prefer vegetables, fruits, whole grains, nuts, fish, lean meats, and healthy fats, like extra-virgin olive oil. However, it is wrong to look for performance in the sugar, beverage, and food industries that endanger health. The risk should not be underestimated, especially if you have lots of pounds to lose. But nothing is excessive.

Make Intermittent Fast to Lose Weight

Skipping meals creates a caloric deficit, and hence, weight loss. Of course, as long as you don't balance the fasting period with high sugar or fat foods because this type of diet doesn't say precisely what you can and cannot eat. Studies show that regular fasting, when used correctly, also helps prevent type 2 diabetes, and the body learns to process digested food more efficiently. Other studies also show that a combination of strength training and the 16:8 method allows you to reduce your body fat percentage beyond what is eliminated by exercise alone. So, it seems very useful when combined with regular exercise.

Note, important. This type of diet is not suitable for diabetics or high blood pressure and pregnant women or nursing mothers. It is best before practicing this type of diet to consult with a doctor.

Many women who follow this diet complain of hunger and fatigue, which can quickly occur if they skip meals. But some say that after a critical phase (about 2–3 days), hunger disappears. The average weight loss is around 1.5 kg. a week (3 lbs.), sometimes more, sometimes even less. But it is important to try to stay with the plan, and only in case of need, you can slightly adjust your eating, and lose weight faster. If you are too hungry, you can drink green tea or black coffee so you can hold yourself until the next meal. Regular fasting is not for everyone but is a good way to reduce body fat. However, you need to control your diet and avoid burgers, pizza, and French fries. The goal is to keep eating healthy and eating a balanced diet.

BEST INTERMITTENT FASTING TYPES TO FOLLOW

Are you thinking about intermittent fasting? What a great decision!

Imagine coming home after work feeling too tired and drained to cook dinner or even think about dinner options.

You're tired of that same old meal. You crave something different. You wish you had a variety of recipes to choose from in order to change it up.

There are also a lot of delicious frozen meals if you don't feel like cooking or don't have the time, but they aren't always healthy or high-quality options.

Healthy homemade meals are a good alternative that not only taste better than frozen ones, but they are also more nutritious and save money compared to eating out or buying processed foods.

That's why you learned how to cook in the first place! But it becomes a problem when you are tired and want to get food as quickly as possible, or when you can't find the time.

The average American household has less than an hour of free time per day. It's not because we're watching Netflix all day, it's usually because we have jobs and other responsibilities. Time is precious. That precious time should not be spent cooking dinner if you don't enjoy it.

That's why I love intermittent fasting so much! It really helps me solve all these problems and more:

Intermittent fasting saves me time because I don't have to cook two meals every day. I just have one big meal in the evening and I'm ready for the next day.

Intermittent fasting saves me money because I can replace my favorite pricey fast-food burger with a healthy homemade meal of meat, vegetables and eggs.

Intermittent fasting saves my health from getting worse. Fast food is often high in trans-fatty acids, sugar and salt. Eating too many processed foods can lead to digestive problems, fatigue and eventually put you at risk for developing chronic illnesses like diabetes or heart disease.

Intermittent fasting is not just good for your body, it's also extremely beneficial for your brain. Studies show that fasting makes people smarter, healthier and happier.

Intermittent fasting can also help increase your self-discipline because it gives you a break from food addiction and unhealthy cravings.

Many people lose weight when they start intermittent fasting because they become more aware of ingredients in their meals and stop eating out as often, which saves them money.

And since most people eat the same thing for too long, this makes them sick of it or bored of the food. Introducing variety into your diet is healthy! Not to mention that being bored of the same old food is less likely to happen if you're eating different kinds of foods during your feast window. Variety is key! It keeps things interesting and prevents boredom.

Intermittent fasting is great for making your healthy homemade meals last longer. Imagine going to the store with a list of ingredients made by you and filling up a gallon-sized bag of food.

Then you have to go back home and cook more food—not because it will taste better, but because you're running out! This happens all the time when people eat out all the time. Now imagine if you could just buy what you need without going back home at all. You could go grab your groceries from a shelf instead of standing in line for an hour at the grocery store. You could spend less time standing around and more time doing what you love.

This is what it's like to practice intermittent fasting – everything gets done on the fly with no planning whatsoever. This requires a lot of self-discipline and discipline from others! At first, it may be difficult to schedule your daily activities around food because schedules are sometimes flexible.

5:2

The 5:2 eating routine is another reasonable alternative. This fast encourages you to ordinarily eat for five days during the week and fast for the other two days and only eat about 600 calories. This is at times called the Easy Diet, as well. It's suggested that on these fasting days, individuals will eat around 500 to 600 calories.

You'll ordinarily eat all week long, for instance, and on Monday and Thursdays, you'll have just two little dinners within about 500 calories. You can pick anytime as your fasting days, as long as you don't have them in consecutive order. Pick your two busiest days of the week. What's more, make them your fasting days.

There aren't numerous reports out there about the 5:2 eating regimen, yet it will give the greater part of the advantages you can find with intermittent fasting. You can do it without the need to think the entire day about making dinners.

THE 5:2 DIET

DAY 1	DAY 2	DAY 3	DAY 4	DAY 5	DAY 6	DAY 7
Eats normally	Women: 500 calories Men: 600 calories	Eats normally	Eats normally	Women: 500 calories Men: 600 calories	Eats normally	Eats normally

16/8 Fasting:

THE 16:8 DIET

	DAY 1	DAY 2	DAY 3	DAY 4	DAY 5	DAY 6	DAY 7
MIDNIGHT							
4 AM	FAST	FAST	FAST	FAST	FAST	FAST	FAST
8 AM							
12 PM	First meal	First meal	First meal	First meal	First meal	First meal	First meal
4 PM	Last meal by 8PM	Last meal by 8PM	Last meal by 8PM	Last meal by 8PM	Last meal by 8PM	Last meal by 8PM	Last meal by 8PM
8 PM	FAST	FAST	FAST	FAST	FAST	FAST	FAST
MIDNIGHT							

16/8 intermittent fasting includes restricting the utilization of food sources and calorie-containing drinks to a set window of eight hours out of each day and avoiding nourishment for the remaining 16 hours. This cycle can be rehashed as often as you like — from only a single time or two times a week to consistently, contingent upon your preference. 16/8 intermittent fasting has soared in popularity as of late, particularly among those hoping to get in shape and burn fat. While different weight control plans frequently set severe standards and guidelines, 16/8 regime is not difficult to follow and can give real outcomes with negligible exertion.

It's by and large thought to be not so much prohibitive, but rather more adaptable than numerous other eating regimen models and can undoubtedly find a way into pretty much any way of life. Notwithstanding upgrading weight reduction, 16/8 intermittent fasting is likewise accepted to improve glucose control, help improve brain capacity and lengthen lifespan.

Eat Stop Eat:

EAT-STOP-EAT

DAY 1	DAY 2	DAY 3	DAY 4	DAY 5	DAY 6	DAY 7
Eat normally	24-hour fast	Eat normally	Eat normally	24-hour fast	Eat normally	Eat normally

Eat Stop Eat is an interesting way to deal with intermittent fasting that is portrayed by the consideration of up to two non-back-to-back fasting days out of each week.

For the remaining 5–6 days of the week, you can eat unreservedly. However, it's suggested to settle on reasonable food choices and try not to eat too much. Although it appears to be illogical, you will, in any case, eat something on each scheduled day of the week when using the Eat Stop Eat technique.

For example, in case you're fasting from 9 a.m. Tuesday until 9 a.m. Wednesday, you'll try to eat a supper before 9 a.m. on Tuesday. Your next supper will happen after 9 a.m. on Wednesday. Thusly, you guarantee you're fasting for an entire 24 hours — yet no longer.

Remember that even on fasting and long periods of Eat Stop Eat, legitimate hydration is unequivocally encouraged.

12:12 Intermittent Fasting Protocol:

12 Hr Intermittent Fasting
- Eat normally 12 hours a day
- Fast 12 hours a day

	DAY 1	DAY 2	DAY 3	DAY 4	DAY 5	DAY 6	DAY 7
12 AM							
4 AM							
8 AM							
12 PM			First Meal - 8am				
4 PM			Last Meal - 8pm				
8 PM							
12 PM							

The guidelines for this eating routine are straightforward. You must choose and stick to a 12-hour fasting window consistently. As indicated by certain analysts, fasting for 10–16 hours can make the body transform its fat stores into energy, which discharges ketones into the circulation system. This should energize weight reduction. This kind of intermittent fasting plan might be a decent alternative for novices.

For instance, an individual could decide to fast between 7 p.m. to 7 a.m. They would have to complete their supper before 7 p.m. also, wait until 7 a.m. to have breakfast. However, they would be snoozing for a significant part of the time in the middle.

THE 14:10 INTERMITTENT FASTING PROTOCOL:

THE 14:10 DIET

	DAY 1	DAY 2	DAY 3	DAY 4	DAY 5	DAY 6	DAY 7
MIDNIGHT / 4 AM	FAST	FAST	FAST	FAST	FAST	FAST	FAST
10 AM / 12 PM	First meal	First meal	First meal	First meal	First meal	First meal	First meal
4 PM	Last meal by 8PM	Last meal by 8PM	Last meal by 8PM	Last meal by 8PM	Last meal by 8PM	Last meal by 8PM	Last meal by 8PM
8 PM / MIDNIGHT	FAST	FAST	FAST	FAST	FAST	FAST	FAST

Intermittent fasting 14:10 has an eating segment of 10 hours and a fasting segment of 14 hours. One basic way to deal with doing this is to eat regularly in the hours between 9 a.m. to 7 p.m. The timeframe between 7 p.m. to 9 a.m. the following day is the fasting window.

During the eating period, you can eat your typical suppers and snacks. Moreover, during the fasting window, you are not allowed to eat any calories. In any case, you can drink water and unsweetened espresso or green tea.

20:4 Intermittent Fasting Protocol:

INTERMITTENT FASTING 20:4 PLAN

AYURGO.COM

Time	DAY 1	DAY 2	DAY 3	DAY 4	DAY 5	DAY 6	DAY 7
Midnight	fasting	fasting	fasting	fasting	fasting	fasting	fasting
02:00 PM	Eating	Eating	Eating	Eating	Eating	Eating	Eating
	fasting	fasting	fasting	fasting	fasting	fasting	fasting
06:00 PM	Eating	Eating	Eating	Eating	Eating	Eating	Eating
Midnight	fasting	fasting	fasting	fasting	fasting	fasting	fasting

This eating routine is viewed as a sort of intermittent fasting, an umbrella term for eating models that incorporate times of diminished caloric admission over a described period. The 20:4 is also known as the Warrior Diet, which depends on the eating examples of old heroes, who ate little during the day and afterward ate around evening time. Individuals following this eating regimen undereat for 20 hours out of every day, then devour as much food as they want around evening time.

During the 20-hour fasting period, the practitioners are urged to devour modest quantities of dairy items, hard-boiled eggs, and veggies, and organic foods, as well as a lot of non-calorie liquids.

HOW TO START INTERMITTENT FASTING DIET

Intermittent fasting is not a diet, it's a lifestyle. It's been touted as one of the best ways to lose weight and live healthier. As you know, a healthy lifestyle consists of proper nutrition and exercise, but intermittent fasting has also been shown to have many benefits for your physical and mental health!

This section will take an in-depth look at what intermittent fasting is, the different stages of fasting, what health benefits it has to offer, as well as how to optimize your intermittent fasting for weight loss or overall bettering your life.

In a nutshell, intermittent fasting is the voluntary restriction of caloric intake and/or food intake for a specific period of time.

Your body naturally stores fat just in case there is a famine or food shortage. Your body is excellent at storing and using fat for fuel! This means that when you go through a fast, your body doesn't want to burn muscle for fuel because it would rather store it than burn it.

STEP 1: GET CLEAR ON YOUR GOALS

Having clear goals can take you far in life generally, but don't underestimate the importance of defining your objectives before you begin an IF regimen.

In my case, it was losing the excess weight I had put on during and after pregnancy (this consequently solved a bunch of other health issues for me), improving metabolic health as well as achieving mental sharpness and focus. Broadly speaking, I wanted to experience an overall better health for my own sake, and most importantly, my baby's. However, my research indicated that I needed to define exactly what I wanted out of IF in order to reap its full benefits.

Defining your goals when it comes to IF is critical for a number of reasons. First and foremost, it allows you to pick the most suitable IF method that will effectively take you closer to what you want. For instance, the Alternate-Day IF method is more fitting for those aiming to lose weight while the 16:8 methods are more of a healthy lifestyle change.

Step 2: Choose Your Method

Now that you know exactly what you're seeking from IF, the next step involves picking a suitable IF method that will help you achieve your goals.

You can choose from any of the methods of IF depending on your goals, personal preferences and health conditions.

In addition to your specific goals regarding IF, other factors also go into choosing an IF method that would yield the most benefits for you. These include the length of time you want to fast for, your daily routine, what field of work you're employed in and what a typical workday looks like for you, the specific climatic conditions prevailing in your part of the world, and how often you dine out with friends and family, to name a few.

Once you have chosen an IF method, though, remember that you're not stuck with it forever. It is completely possible to transition from one type of IF to another if you find that your current regimen isn't working for you or if you think you've mastered the moderate forms of IF (think 16:8 method) and want to go pro and explore some relatively challenging routes such as the Alternate-Day fasting.

Besides, it is advisable for a person to give at least one month's serious go to any particular

IF method before quitting or switching it up for good.

Step 3: Identify Your Calorie Needs

Now that you know what you want from IF and how you're going to approach it, the next step involves finding a way to figure out and manage your calories. While IF is naturally designed to create a calorie deficit when you're fasting, this can be quickly turned into a surplus if you're not mindful of the calories you consume during your eating windows.

Some people practicing IF are usually the least concerned about counting and measuring the calories they consume. Although keeping track of our caloric consumption is important to a certain extent (even while fasting intermittently), these folks are of the opinion that their caloric consumption is automatically taken care of as a direct result of fasting intermittently. While this may work out well for someone who doesn't suffer from (or is prone to) an eating disorder such as Anorexia, Orthorexia and Binge eating, it can be detrimental for individuals whose eating disorders may be triggered by IF.

Keeping a track of the number of calories you consume during IF is also important because even if certain methods of IF such as the Alternate-Day fasting do allow for caloric consumption during fasting days, there is a limit to how many of these calories we can consume. Again, this restriction is meant to facilitate the benefits of IF such as weight loss.

Besides, there is a popular opinion that as long as you consume just under 50 calories in the morning, you will be considered to be in the fasted state. This can be critical for those practicing the 16:8 methods by having an early dinner and delayed breakfast in an attempt to reach a 16-hour milestone with their fasting. Such people can drink plain water or have a cup of black coffee (no added sugar!) without the risk of breaking their fast in the mornings.

But, guess what, this also implies that you have to be mindful of the calories you consume in order to make sure that your IF regimen is not put to waste.

All of this leads to one conclusion only: whether you're fasting or feasting, you must keep an eye on your caloric consumption in order to achieve your goals with IF. At least in the beginning.

As you get the hang of doing IF in any shape or form that you think best suits you and your situation, the focus on calorie intake will usually wind-up fading into the background as IF and your new eating habits get ingrained into your schedule. You will find that you do not need to track the calories as much because you know the approximate amounts which you consume on a daily basis.

This is when the much-vaunted benefit of not needing to calorie count comes back straight into play, with a vengeance! Because you have more practice and have already established a fair routine and habit of doing your IF lifestyle, your daily caloric intake is more or less at your fingertips. Consequently, you end up not having to pay too much attention to that, and can carry on with your daily stuff without having to worry about the caloric count.

Step 4: Conduct Meal Planning (Without Overdoing It!)

And no. I'm not about to contradict myself here.

IF is quite liberating in the sense that it allows you to let go of the tedious job of meal planning all the time.

And I'm not going back on my words here.

IF is not a practice meant to put restrictions on someone when it comes to what they eat.

Nonetheless, we all know that a balanced and nutritious diet is critical for maintaining good health, regardless of whether or not you practice IF.

Making unhealthy food choices when you finally sit down to eat in an IF regimen is not only detrimental for your overall health but will also put any and all of your efforts with regards to IF go to waste.

And you don't want that.

This will not help you keep track of your caloric intake (and thereby lose and maintain weight consistently) but also ensure that you have everything you need to cook a healthy, nutritious and delicious meal on hand.

Because let's be honest, we are more susceptible to ordering takeaway food; however, eating unhealthy snacks when prepping a healthy meal at home becomes difficult due to any reason.

Frankly, if you find yourself eating loads of unhealthy food when you aren't fasting, you might as well not fast at all!

Step 5: Begin Your IF Journey with the Pedal to the Metal!

Along with all of my very best wishes, here are a few points that I would like you to keep in mind while you're at it:

Make the calories count in the beginning by keeping the nutritional value of any food you consume insight

Practice moderation, both while fasting and feasting

Take IF as an opportunity to improve your eating habits and food choices. Fewer meals mean more time for preparing healthy food to dine on!

IF isn't a one-size-fits-all approach so keep experimenting to figure out what works best for you!

INTERMITTENT FASTING LIFESTYLE

START THE DAY WITH A GLASS OF WATER

Drink 250ml of more water on an empty stomach. This will help you support your energy level and help you digest well for the day. Don't drink unhealthy juices on an empty stomach. It might give you terrible gas trouble and an enlarged tummy.

MINIMIZE SUGAR INTAKE

Excessive intake of sugar will harm your body in all the ways possible and all your hard work will be in vain. You can eat sweet fruits and vegetables if you have a sweet tooth.

AVOID OILY FOOD

Oily food lowers your cholesterol, especially deep-fried items such as fried eggs, fish, and many more. Eating oily food can give you trouble.

GET ENOUGH SLEEP

Sleep helps your memory and problem-solving skills. It boosts your energy level and mood — even more than coffee! Research also shows that people who lack sleep are more likely to eat junk food and use drugs. Sadly, many teens don't get enough sleep each night. In some cases, that can lead to serious consequences like decreased cognitive function, lower resistance to disease, or even unsafe driving on the road.

Sleep problems are not just a problem for teenagers. Adults can lack sleep too! Sleep issues are more common among adults than you might think. The National Sleep Foundation estimates that one in three adults has trouble sleeping or has fallen asleep during the day because of a sleep disorder, such as obstructive sleep apnea or restless legs syndrome.

STRENGTH TRAIN

Intermittent fasting likely doesn't cause more muscle loss than other weight reduction programs, like counting calories. Adding exercise — particularly strength training — to your intermittent fasting technique can assist you with maintaining your muscles.

KEEP A FOOD JOURNAL

Keeping a food journal will help you with watching your calories. Furthermore, you will see any weight reduction all through your fast. This will help you with coordinating eating affinities and developing a step-by-step plan, as demonstrated by the prerequisites and increase your benefits.

EAT HEALTHILY

Abstain from eating foods bad for you after a fast. Healthy meals should be the center of consideration. They will assist you with getting the vital supplements, for example, nutrients, to give you more energy during the fasting timeframe.

AVOID STRESS

Whenever we begin something new, especially if it is related to our body, we need to consider the possible stress it may cause. Stressing out about it might make it worst. Keep calm, do your thing, and do not stress out. Remember that fasting implies not eating foods for some time. When fasting, be consistent with yourself and try not to eat before the scheduled time. It will guarantee that you lose the greatest amount of weight and get the most benefits from intermittent fasting in solid terms.

INCLUDE EXERCISES IN YOUR DAILY ROUTINE

Here are a few tips on how to include exercises in your daily routine.

- Take the stairs (within reason) instead of using the elevator. You don't have to go up a 10-story building using the stairs! If you have a long way to go up or down, take the stairs a couple of flights and then complete your trip with the elevator.
- When you talk with your family members at home, don't shout from the top floor and bottom floor. Go up or climb down and talk with them.
- Find a sporting activity you thoroughly enjoy and do it as often as is convenient. When you are doing something, you want, you'll hardly think of it as exercise, and you are likely to stay committed.
- If you are at work, instead of sending emails or text messages to coworkers, walk up to them and talk to them face to face.
- If possible, convert your one-on-one meetings to a walking meeting. Hold the meeting while taking a stroll outside.
- Stop 1–2 blocks from your destination and walk the rest of the way. Make walking your preferred mode of transportation.
- Take your dog for walks daily. If you don't have a dog, adopt one. It might seem that you are merely walking your dog, but you are exercising your muscles.
- Take brisk walks as often as possible. Remember to put on comfortable shoes when walking briskly. You can bring your walking shoes with you to make it easy for you to change into them.

FIND SOMETHING TO DO WHEN YOU FAST

It is said that an inactive mind is the devil's showroom. When you fast intermittently and are not busy, food will be the only thing on your mind, compelling you to eat before the fast-breaking time. You can learn a new skill or get a hobby, start reading or research about anything that interests you.

TURBOCHARGING INTERMITTENT FASTING

Intermittent fasting is potent. It is one of the key pieces I recommend for women over 50 years old. But it is not enough to maximize the metabolic potential in risk-prone individuals. In order to turbocharge intermittent fasting, you need to combine it with a healthy diet that extends beyond just food—think of balance (calories in – calories out), sleep (quality and quantity), and activity frequency.

INTERMITTENT FASTING AND EXERCISE WORKING TOGETHER

Think of it as a very powerful medicine for women over 50 years old. It's like an herbal supplement mixed in with the famed Slim-Fast shakes and then topped off with jogging. People who begin intermittent fasting lose more fat than those who only do regular exercise. This is because intermittent fasting activates your body to make new cells that burn fat. That means immediately after you had food, your body uses the time before and during the fast to repair cells and make more of them. After that, it can be converted into fat for fuel instead of muscle

The research on intermittent fasting is still relatively young. Early studies have been done on mice. One of the first studies on humans was conducted in Germany. These researchers found that women who followed a calorie-restricted intermittent fasting diet lost more weight than women who only did regular exercise. However, our bodies cannot be fooled by intermittent fasting for long periods of time. You will still need to continue eating enough in order to prevent malnutrition, but you will not be able to maintain the fasts' effects on your metabolism if you do not make some adjustments to your diet with exercise. Exercise can also help you achieve more because it burns energy that is stored as fat.

INTERVAL TRAINING

You do not need to exercise for several hours a day to burn your fat stores. Intermittent fasting has more impact on your metabolism because when you exercise, you are also burning fat as fuel and then repairing cells at night so that your body can make more cells that burn fat. Everyone, including women over 50 years old, should do at least 30 minutes of interval training per week.

It's easier than you think—like burst training. Burst training is interval training with very short bursts of high-intensity exercise and longer periods of low-intensity activity. It is great for women over 50 years old because when you exercise, your body burns off energy stores. Fortunately, when your body is deprived of carbohydrate fuel during the fast and when you exercise, the energy used to fix your muscles and organs comes from fat instead of muscle.

Burst training is a good way to shed those extra pounds because it burns off more calories than aerobic training while using less time. But the reason I recommend burst training to women over 50 years old is that it also helps them reduce their belly fat, which most women tend to gain after menopause as they lose muscle mass and estrogen levels decline.

WHY YOU SHOULD EXERCISE WHILE INTERMITTENT FASTING

1. For added weight loss

Exercise and intermittent fasting work together to make your body produce more fat-burning cells. Doing both together also puts you in a great position to reduce belly fat and to lose weight.

Exercise also helps increase the levels of leptin, which is a hormone that signals how full you are. This means that if you exercise while intermittent fasting, you can eat more without feeling hungry or gaining weight. Exercise also helps boost your insulin sensitivity, which is the ability of your cells to use glucose for fuel instead of storing it as fat. You will turn those extra pounds into muscle instead of fat because exercise helps your body use the energy it needs for growth and repair instead of storing it as fat.

2. For better health

Exercise helps prevent cardiovascular diseases because it improves your blood flow and normalizes high blood pressure. It also reduces stress and depression, which both make your body hold onto fat stores. Exercise can also help you sleep better at night. You will not only gain muscle mass while you exercise, but you will also have more energy to do more activities during the day. Plus, if you exercise regularly while intermittent fasting, you will burn fat even during rest periods, which means that your metabolism is always active and burning off calories wherever possible. This slows down the aging process, as well as making your body more resilient to disease and fat gain from overeating in the future.

3. For better cognitive function

Exercise also helps to clear your mind so that you will not have as many distractions from food, which can influence your appetite. Since exercise improves your mood and mental clarity, it is a great way to stay focused while you are in the middle of an intermittent fast.

4. For better sleep quality during fasting

Interval training is a great way to burn fat and improve sleep quality during fasting. Interval training targets more than just your muscles and burns more calories than aerobic training because of the short bursts of high-intensity exercise and longer periods of low-intensity activity. It is also easier to recover from than aerobic exercise, which is much more wearisome.

If you want benefits for your heart and a better night's rest, try interval training exercises. This short burst of vigorous activity allows you to get in shape without having to worry about overexerting yourself.

WHAT KIND OF INTERVAL TRAINING WORKS?

Most fitness experts recommend doing 15 rounds of between 30 seconds and 2 minutes on high-intensity sprints with only 1 minute to catch your breath in between rounds. You should do this 3 times per week to get the benefits of exercise and intermittent fasting. You should also try to mix up your exercise routine by alternating between burst and steady-state training. If you prefer, you can also do 2-minute bursts with 1-minute rest periods.

Some of the best exercises for interval training include running, hill sprints, sprints in place, skipping rope, boxing, kettlebell swings or even jumping rope.

CALORIE RESTRICTION IN ADDITION TO INTERMITTENT FASTING

Women over 50 years old who follow a calorie-restricted diet are better protected from age-related diseases. Calorie restriction is a way of eating that can extend your lifespan by up to 15–20 percent. On the other hand, those who eat more calories tend to have less muscle mass and bigger bellies. In contrast, you should practice intermittent fasting combined with calorie restriction because it is more effective in preventing disease than when you restrict your calories alone. One study found that intermittent fasting and a calorie-restricted diet had similar effects on glucose levels, fat mass,

inflammation, and blood pressure compared to when women ate their regular diets.

Calorie restriction helps reduce inflammation because it helps us eat foods low in fat. As a result, our bodies burn less of our own fatty acids and more carbohydrate fuel when they are needed by our cells. That leads to less generation of free radicals that can damage cells, which eventually causes disease. Also, calorie restriction is associated with lower levels of blood glucose. The reason for the reduction in blood glucose is also related to free radical production since high blood sugar levels increase the oxidization of molecules including fats, protein, and DNA. Calorie restriction can also make it easier to prevent obesity because women who eat fewer calories are more likely to absorb food correctly into their cells well and not store it as fat. This is because their gastrointestinal system is more sensitive to the effects of energy—which helps them absorb amino acids—than it is to the effects of calories. Calorie restriction also helps reduce glucose levels and prevent muscle protein breakdown. This is one purpose for which our cells use glucose, so a calorie-restricted diet can help us live longer and be more efficient at using glucose as fuel.

Calorie restriction is also especially important in preventing chronic diseases such as cancer and diabetes. A lot of times when we think of cancer, we think about tumors, but they can be found in other areas as well including blood vessels, lungs, liver, soft tissue and bone marrow. People die of cancer not necessarily because they have cancer (though that is part of the story) but because their bodies go into a state of chronic stress. Our cells need the energy to function, and when our cells are in a state of chronic stress, we are not able to respond appropriately to the damage going on in our body. Chronic inflammation takes a lot of energy, so cancer and other diseases tend to be linked with chronic inflammation. The only way to prevent chronic disease is by reducing the amount of energy we take in through food, which means targeting calories.

Why focus on calories? Because that's the only real thing you can change about yourself, and it's really easy. Calories are everywhere—they are in the grains and beans you eat, in the milk and eggs you use, and even in the fruits and vegetables. The only things that you cannot get calories from are fats, proteins, and fiber. What's more, since they are so pervasive throughout your food supply, it is very easy for calorie-restricted women over 50 years old to get enough calories.

WHY YOU SHOULD COMBINE CALORIE RESTRICTION WITH INTERMITTENT FASTING

1. It lowers the risk of contracting age-related ailments

Research has shown that when you do intermittent fasting and calorie restriction, you can achieve a long lifespan, but that is not the only benefit. Intermittent fasting and calorie restriction are also associated with a lower risk for age-related diseases including heart disease and cancer. First of all, keeping your body in a constant state of hunger allows it to burn off more fat than when you are regularly eating. Calorie restriction also forces your body to use sugar as fuel instead of less efficient fat cells because if it doesn't get enough glucose (sugar) it will break down its own muscle cells for fuel.

Start intermittent fasting and calorie restriction to reduce your risk of heart disease. In addition, it is very important to keep your blood pressure under control because it can lead to heart disease and hypertension. Intermittent fasting helps reduce blood pressure because when you are in a fasted state, you will lose a lot of excess salt—which makes up about 20 percent of your body weight—along with water weight and fat mass. So, if you combine caloric restriction with intermittent fasting, you will be less likely to suffer from chronic diseases later in life.

2. It helps prevent cancer

The major cause of cancer is inflammation caused by free radicals that stay around the body along with damaged cells instead of dying off rapidly after they cause tissue damage. The best way to avoid this by eating foods that reduce inflammation. Women over 50 years old who do intermittent fasting and calorie restriction are less likely to suffer from chronic inflammation.

3. It helps prevent diabetes

People with diabetes have a lot of excess sugar in their blood because an enzyme is missing that normally converts glucose into energy for the body but cannot do so in the case of type 1 diabetes because it cannot produce insulin. On the other hand, people with type 2 diabetes convert glucose into energy too efficiently, and the body fails to respond to insulin in order to use it effectively.

There are many ways for women over 50 years old to prevent diabetes—intermittent fasting and calorie restriction is just one of them.

4. It reduces your risk for Alzheimer's disease

Inflammation increases the production of free radicals that cause damage to the brain. Free radicals make proteins out of their own amino acids; they won't fold properly, creating protein strands that are very unstable, which means that it is an easy place for harmful proteins to get in and cause damage. This is why maintaining a healthy balance between oxygen supply and waste removal can help prevent dementia. When your body is exposed to free radicals, it tries to protect itself by reducing blood flow to the brain as well as making new blood vessels grow inside the brain. However, if blood vessels form in the wrong place or form too many blood vessels, they can cause inflammation. Epileptic seizures, migraines, and Alzheimer's disease are all associated with inflammation.

Since you are likely to be less susceptible to Alzheimer's disease as you get older, aerobic exercise is the best way to maintain brain health and reduce your risk of Alzheimer's disease. The type of stroke that occurs as a result of heart attacks and cardiovascular diseases also increases your risk of developing Alzheimer's disease later in life. Exercise reduces blood pressure and heart rate, which prevent blood vessels from forming inside the brain. Instead of trying to turn your brain off, you should try to prevent free radicals from damaging it.

5. It helps you live longer and have more energy

Women over 50 years old who follow an intermittent fasting plan with calorie restriction are better able to metabolize fats. In addition, calorie restriction helps prevent obesity because it makes women put on weight more slowly, so they can be more efficient at using calories as a fuel source for their cells instead of storing them as fat in their bodies.

The benefits of calorie restriction are not just due to the number of calories you take in but also because it helps you resist disease caused by too much of something else. When you consume foods that cause too many caloric intakes, your body makes a lot of fat and proteins to help you store those excess calories. However, if you don't have enough energy, your body will burn these extra calories and won't make as much energy as it needs in order to keep up with its basic functions such as breathing and brain function.

HOW TO COMBINE CALORIE RESTRICTION WITH INTERMITTENT FASTING

Calorie restriction is an important component of intermittent fasting because it provides women over 50 years old with a way to save up nutrition for the times when they can eat normally.

Women over 50 years old who follow intermittent fasting and calorie restriction should keep track of their calories by using a diet app that tells you exactly how many calories are in each food item and portion size.

There are many ways you can use intermittent fasting and calorie restriction to meet your goals. You need to make sure that you don't go over your daily calorie limit at any time of the day because it is not healthy for your body. First thing in the morning, eat a protein-rich breakfast—ideally, you will follow this with a low-carbohydrate lunch as well—and skip dinner. In addition, try drinking 12–24 oz. of water two hours prior to lunch and dinner to help reduce your appetite.

Alternatively, you can eat a big meal at the start of the day, and try to eat less as the day goes on. You should definitely do this if you have a big lunch or dinner so that you don't feel hungry when you go to bed. In addition, if you notice that you are losing weight very slowly, then it might be a good idea to exercise more while following this diet to make up for any extra calories that aren't being burned off by your body.

A lot of people who practice intermittent fasting see amazing results in losing weight by eating one meal per day and eating high-quality protein and fat in lower quantities than they normally would throughout the rest of the day.

COMBINING INTERMITTENT FASTING WITH CARB CYCLING

Carb cycling is a way to make your body more efficient at metabolizing and using carbohydrates because it prevents you from getting too much of something, which means that your cells are not overworked. You can also benefit from carb cycling if you have a condition like metabolic syndrome—a condition in which diabetes and heart disease are combined—because it makes your body more resistant to insulin.

Carbohydrate metabolism is deregulated in patients with type 2 diabetes, so the best way to reduce insulin resistance while improving overall health is by eating a diet higher in protein like intermittent fasting and calorie restriction. The benefits of carb cycling include building lean muscle mass and boosting blood glucose levels after exercise in order to recover quickly.

When you follow a carb cycling plan, eat carbohydrates in the form of fruits and vegetables, which are rich in antioxidants—nutrients that neutralize free radicals. You can also eat whole grains and legumes because of their high-fiber content, which is important for long-term health. Carb cycling has been shown to reduce hunger and improve the function of mitochondria, which means that your cells can produce more energy with less effort. It also helps the body break down fat into ketones so that it is easier to burn as fuel instead of storing it in our bodies.

The best way to combine carb cycling with intermittent fasting and calorie restriction is to eat a low-carbohydrate breakfast to keep your hunger at bay for several hours, then eat high-carbohydrate foods like fruit or vegetables for your second meal. The third meal of the day should be the largest meal, which means that you should eat a lot of protein, and only have enough carbohydrates to get through the rest of the day.

COMBINING CALORIE RESTRICTION WITH FASTING EVERY OTHER DAY

Many women over 50 years old have trouble losing weight because their bodies start burning fat more slowly. However, intermittent fasting allows women over 50 years old to control blood sugar levels and insulin sensitivity by helping them lose body fat faster than they would otherwise.

When you follow an intermittent fasting program, your body will go into ketosis, which is a state where it cannot get enough glucose to produce energy properly. When it is in this state, ketones are produced by the liver and released into the blood stream while fat stores are broken down to generate energy. The best way to make sure that you don't have too much fat in your body is to combine calorie restriction with fasting every other day. That way you can have more time between meals when your body is burning fat as fuel instead of storing it in its tissues.

Women over 50 years old who combine intermittent fasting and calorie restriction may find that it is easier for them to lose fat in the short term than if they were following an intermittent fasting program on its own. Use this fad diet only if you are not trying to lose weight but rather eating fewer calories than you need so that your body has the energy it needs to function properly. When you combine intermittent fasting with calorie restriction, it is important to eat a diet high in lean protein, low-carbohydrate, and vegetables and fruits because these are the foods that can help you stay full throughout the day.

MISTAKES TO AVOID

FORCING IT ON YOUR SELF

Forcing the body into fasting is yet another error. It is necessary to note that it is not for everybody to start intermittent fasting. It's all right to re-assess if this is the best strategy for you. Yes, some say that our bodies will cope quite frequently with hunger, but that doesn't imply that it's the best choice for everyone to do right now.

Not all bodies are developed for intermittent fasting. Ask yourself this easy question if intermittent fasting seems like a relentless challenge and emotional drain, is the compromised standard of life worth it?

Intermittent fasting has become a huge trend in the fitness community over the last year. It's an easy way to diet, get healthier, and it's been shown to increase significant weight-loss benefits.

Intermittent fasting means eating within a restricted time frame, say from 12 pm until 6 pm for example. You skip breakfast and eat your food during this time period instead. This encourages your body to go into "fasting mode" so that you can burn more fat throughout the day instead of relying on glucose from food sources like carbohydrates or sugars.

One of the main sources of intermittent fasting is also known as the 8-hour Diet. This diet involves only two complete meals for eight hours (breakfast and dinner). The idea is based on the fact that your body uses about 16-24 hours to fully digest a meal. If you eat within these eight hours, you will not be eating anymore and your body will start to break down fat stores.

This method is great for losing weight but what happens if you don't have access to this time frame? Do you need to slow down, or skip a meal in order to fast for an entire day?

RUSHING INTO INTERMITTENT FASTING

You are more likely to get hungry all the time and discouraged if you are regularly eating every 3 to 4 hours and then unexpectedly shrink your mealtime to only 8 hours. According to some experts, individuals will stop intermittent fasting if they start by fasting for many hours without a transition time from a prior eating style. One of the greatest errors you can create is to start dramatically.

You can set yourself up for failure if you dive into IF without easing into it. It may not be easy to move from consuming three regular-sized meals or six tiny meals per day to eating only within 4 hours.

Instead, gradually proceed into fasting. If you are going for the 16/8 technique, progressively increase the period between meals so you can operate inside 12 hours comfortably. Then, add multiple hours a day before you get to the 8-hour window.

There are levels of intermittent fasting. The primary factor most diets don't harvest benefits is their drastic deviation from our usual eating habits. Sometimes, it can seem not easy to sustain. You think about it if someone is new to IF, then they're used to eating every 2 hours, you are going to be very uncomfortable during long hours of fasting. It is normal to have a transition time, but it should feel better.

A remarkably strong communicator is the body itself. If it feels like trouble, it will let you know. And it is a common fact that you will feel like crap to starve yourself out of literally nowhere for 23 hours.

If you are stubborn about the principle of fasting, begin with the 12:12 approach of a beginner: fast for 12 hours a day and feed in the next 12-hour window.

That's pretty similar to what a person is used to doing nowadays, and who knows that it could be the only practical way to pursue it. You should level up to 16:8 once it seems comfortable, where you consume over an 8-hour window and fast during the remainder of the day. The best advantage about IF is its simplicity. Choose a schedule that encourages you to adhere to a time frame without feeling bad. The number of hours we go between meals is slowly extended until hitting a 12-hour feeding time. Then switch to an eating window of 10 hours and decrease by tiny amounts before meeting your target.

EXPECTING INTERMITTENT FASTING TO CHANGE YOUR LIFE

Another error people seem to make is that they make their lives more about fasting than living. Because someone is fasting, they don't need to turn down the dinner request from their mates or a birthday celebration. That is not going to make it less satisfying and can still maintain such a lifestyle. Instead, on days where you have commitments with people, move your day backward or forward by a couple of hours so you can always enjoy socializing.

Note, there is versatility in intermittent fasting.

CHOOSING THE WRONG FASTING PLAN FOR YOURSELF

If you are trying something that would make your lifestyle difficult, it's not the best option. Don't sign yourself up for disappointment: fasting only for few days, then going back to your earlier unhealthy ways won't be good for you. It's about adjusting the lifestyle you can maintain over a long time. Don't try to start the fast at 6 p.m. if you are a night person. If you are a regular gym-goer, then pick a fasting schedule that will suit your style.

Anyone else does not know your lifestyle. The specialist is you. And you have to make changes if you want to stick to the fasting pattern. If you are ready to pursue Intermittent Fasting and look for whole grains and healthy food such as fish, chicken and fruits, vegetables, and nutritious sides such as tofu, legumes, and quinoa for weight loss, then fasting will benefit you. If you haven't picked the right IF strategy, it will not give you success. If you are a committed gym-goer six days each week, the perfect

schedule might not be fast on two of those days.

EATING TOO MUCH IN THE FASTING WINDOW

Most of the time, people want to pursue Intermittent Fasting is because it involves eating fewer calories; it means they also will have less time to eat. In the duration of the fasting window, though, certain individuals will consume their normal number of calories. This will imply you are not going to lose weight. Do not consume the normal intake of calories in the window. Rather, when you break the fast, expect to consume about 1200 to 1500 calories. If it is 4, 6, 8 hours, the number of meals you can consume would depend on the fasting window duration.

If you need to overeat and are in a condition of starvation, reconsider the strategy you want to adopt or relax off the IF for a day to regroup and then get back on board.

NOT PAYING ATTENTION TO THE NUTRIENT QUALITY OF THE FOODS

When following intermittent fasting, people often rely on fast foods to concentrate on what to eat more than what they should consume. We should not anticipate intermittent fasting to achieve our fitness goals if we continue with refined foods. By adopting nutritious foods steadily, aim to adjust your lifestyle along with your meal routine progressively.

Were you aware that most people are eating a diet high in processed foods?

A lot of these processed food items are refined and have lost a lot of their nutrients from processing. These nutrients are the sources of vitamins and minerals that help your body stay healthy.

It may seem like-- if you're consuming more calories than you need in order to function each day--that it won't matter what type of food you eat. But it's important not only to consume quality calories, but also to consume enough calories in order to get the right amount that your body needs for each day.

When you're eating fewer calories than you need in order to function, your body doesn't get the energy it needs for each day. Especially when your body is getting a lot of energy from refined products, which many current diets contain.

Becoming aware of the quality of food is important because you will be able to understand how much nutrition the foods are giving you in order to help your health become better as well!

By cutting out these processed and refined foods from your diet, you'll be able to open up more room for nutritious food choices.

RESTRICTING THE FOOD INTAKE TOO MUCH

Not eating sufficiently and going too far with fasting is not acceptable. You've got to note that fasting isn't for starving. Our bodies need fuel to move around, work properly, think straight, and converse naturally, and that fuel comes from food. It takes a toll on daily life to limit your food consumption so much, and that's not the main concern of what fasting is all about.

"What" is overlooked in favor of the 'when'; IF is a time-centered diet, and most schedules do not include any clear guidelines during the feeding window for the kinds of food to consume. However, this is not an accessible invitation for French fries, beer, and milkshakes to thrive. Fasting isn't magic. In addition to certain minor physiological effects, the main influence on weight reduction is when you minimize the hours of feeding and the number of calories you eat.

If you've already had a pre-workout snack, it can sound alien to exercise when fasting. But when there are no calories, the body has loads of resources left in the body fat to use. As for every diet or workout schedule, consulting with the doctor first is a smart practice, but with intermittent fasting, exercising may be healthy.

Keep up with your normal fitness regimen or do something like cycling, which is low-impact. You should consume a protein-rich meal after that. Always make sure to consult with your doctor first because, as someone over 50, you should not do strenuous exercises while fasting.

Sadly, by selecting the wrong types of foods, you cannot easily reverse the influence. During the feeding hours, change your mindset from a "treating yourself" attitude to one that centers around consuming the most nutrient-packed, nourishing meals you can find. To better fill yourself up and carry you during the fasting process, we suggest making sure any meal or snack contains a mix of fiber, protein, and good fats.

- Cook all the meals at home and try not to eat takeout or in restaurants.
- Pay attention to nutrition labels and make sure to not consume forbidden ingredients like modified palm oil, corn syrup, high fructose.
- Try to consume low sodium and beware of added sugar.
- Do not eat processed foods.
- Add fiber, good fats, fiber, and lean proteins to your plate.

Other Common Mistake:

Fasting is not generally seen as a diet, yet a specific lifestyle and recommended eating schedule. This type of eating plan has increased enormous notoriety as of late, particularly for women over 50. As we have seen, you may fast for 16 hours and eat during an 8-hour window. That is the 16:8 plan and is commonly seen as the standard intermittent fasting plan. A few people follow the alternate day plan, with low-calorie intake on one day and the usual amount the following. Whatever the way you handle it, when your goal is to get in shape, intermittent fasting is famous for one peculiar characteristic: it only works when is done correctly.

There are a few potential health benefits when following intermittent fasting. Among the benefits, we may include the decreased danger of malignant growth, diabetes, and heart disease. Fasting can trigger autophagy, which is known to help with dementia. Regardless of whether you use one or another kind of intermittent fasting, it is critical to avoid the traps that can undermine your endeavors.

LOOKING FOR TOO MANY IMPROVEMENTS TOO FASTLY

You are preparing to begin something new, and you are eager to receive all the rewards as fast as possible. It is expected that you are excited about this new lifestyle and want to dive into it fully. Nevertheless, attempting to get such a large number of improvements too early immediately may disrupt your endeavors.

The key is to begin gradually by including a couple of changes one after another. For instance, if you have chosen to do 2 500-calorie days every week while having a regular number of calories, the other 5, consider beginning with only 1 500-calorie day. After a couple of weeks, you can feel more confident, including the second day into your weekly schedule.

TRYING TO STICK TO THE WRONG PLAN

There are many different approaches to put intermittent fasting into your daily schedule. For instance, if your fasting plan includes not eating from 8 p.m. until early afternoon every day and having a challenging activity that begins right in the first part of the day, this is most likely not the right plan for you.

What works for one person may not necessarily fit in for another one. To get the most intermittent fasting rewards, you should take your time to analyze different types of plans thoroughly. It is all right if it takes a little longer to find out the plan that best works for you.

MISUNDERSTANDING REAL HUNGER SIGNS

Perhaps the best thing that I have learned from my intermittent fasting test is that I found a good pace about appetite shows.

No doubt, your stomach may be growling, and you may desire something yummy.

Yet, you are not hungry.

It may also be wonderful to binge with your family or friends and enjoy the social part of feasting.

Yet, again, you are not hungry.

Intermittent fasting will teach you that if you stand by fasting long enough, more often than not, your "hunger" will generally blur in no more than 5–10 minutes.

It most likely already happened without you noticing or giving it a particular thought.

How many times at work you were planning to go to eat, then, some last-minute rush job showed up, and 1–2 hours passed by, while you overlooked your stomach's protest?

Before looked like the most urgent priority, eating was overshadowed by something new that popped up. And you survived!

In any case, yielding and eating too early is one of the severe mix-ups with intermittent fasting. Think that merely drinking some water and allowing it 10 minutes or so, usually, your appetite will calm down.

Try not to break your intermittent fasting plan before you even begin.

Try not to give in to bogus hunger easily!

USING INTERMITTENT FASTING AS AN EXCUSE TO OVEREAT

One of the most harmful intermittent fasting mistakes is giving in to the temptation to say, "What the heck, I've starved myself throughout all the day, I deserve to reward myself for supper!" and then diving in a crazy feast of junk food bombing yourself with unhealthy stuff.

Please don't be that woman.

You would feel hopeless and most likely put on weight.

We don't want that.

Although intermittent fasting is not a diet because it does not confine what you eat, it is yet critical to settle on healthier food decisions. You want, most of all, to have a healthy relationship with your food and your body.

You can overeat and put on weight even by eating just once per day, in case you are eating a more significant number of calories than your body consumes.

While you don't need to be an absolute stickler and space for adaptability, still be shrewd.

Help yourself out, and don't go crazy during your eating window.

NOT EATING ENOUGH

If you have yet to attempt intermittent fasting, the risk of not eating enough during eating times may appear to be illogical.

Actually, for some people, after not eating for an unusually long period, it is common to become less hungry.

In some cases, fasting can thoroughly kill your appetite.

Unless you are deliberately doing a total fast (not suggested if not under medical control), however, it is anything but a good idea to decide not to eat enough.

If you should not eat sufficiently for too long, you can easily wreck your digestion and unbalance your hormones.

Moreover, you will deny your body of fundamental nutrients, which can help health avoiding issues that are far more important than the loss of a couple of additional pounds.

Consult your physician about a complete, healthy calorie intake that fits weight loss and may help you reach your desired outcomes.

FAILING TO PLAN YOUR MEALS IN ADVANCE

While calorie tallying is not essential (however, honestly, you will show more signs of improvement results if you do it), carefully planning and thinking about what you will eat when your eating period arrives, is an excellent intermittent fasting hack.

That will allow you not to improvise when you are finally going to sit down at the table.

Rather than going like "I'm starving and need to eat now no matter what" and then heading to the closest, cheapest unhealthy junk food, you better learn to tell yourself, "Well, I'm feeling hungry now, but I can wait, I'm not dying, and something healthy and delicious is waiting for me, later."

Using this opportunity to consider what you will eat when you eat and sticking to healthier options will only benefit you over the long term.

You will learn how to eat for effective weight loss while decreasing caloric intake, keeping you satisfied, and boosting your self-confidence.

In case you are fasting for 16 hours, you can easily invest 5 minutes of your time planning what meal will break your fast later.

It is not unreasonably hard and will prepare for a slimmer future!

SUPER FOODS

Avocado

Eating the highest-calorie food when attempting to lose weight can seem strange. Although, because of its high content of unsaturated fat, avocados can make you feel full throughout the day, even during the longest times of fasting. Even when a person doesn't feel full, evidence shows unsaturated fats help make their body feel full. The body sends signals that it has adequate calories and will not move into hunger mode in an emergency. Unsaturated fats hold these signals running for longer, even though you get a little hungry during a fasting time. Another research also showed that it could keep you satisfied for hours. So, you must add this green mushy fruit to your diet during intermittent fasting

Cruciferous Vegetables

Broccoli, cauliflower, and Brussels sprouts are full of the most important nutrition fiber. It's essential to consume fiber-rich foods that keep the body regular and make the gut function smoothly, especially when you eat after intervals. Fiber may also help one to feel full, which might be a positive thing if you can't eat for 16 hours. Cruciferous vegetables may also minimize cancer risk.

Potatoes

As mentioned before, potatoes are one of the heartiest foods to eat that will keep you full, as the main course or snack or in lunch during intermittent fasting. Not all the foods that are white and starchy are bad for you, but French fries and potato chips do not count as healthy options.

Legumes & Beans

In the IF lifestyle, the favorite addition to chili may be your best mate. Food, including carbohydrates, offers energy for physical activity. It is not asked of you to carb-load to insane amounts, but tossing some low-calorie carbohydrates like legumes and beans into the diet plan will certainly not cause any harm. During the fasting hours, this will hold you active, and without calorie limits, foods such as black beans, chickpeas, peas, and lentils are shown to lower body weight.

FOODS TO AVOID DURING INTERMITTENT FASTING

To do intermittent fasting correctly, many products are not healthy to eat. You can stay away from foods that contain huge amounts of salt, sugar, and fat that are calorie-dense. These foods won't fill you up fast, and they might also leave you hungry. They have little or no nutrients, as well.

Avoid these ingredients to sustain a safe intermittent feeding regimen:

- Processed foods
- Snack chips
- Refined grains
- Trans-fat
- Alcoholic beverages
- Sugar-sweetened beverages
- Microwave popcorn.
- Candy bars
- Processed meat

Besides, you must avoid foods which are rich in added sugar. Sugar is devoid of any nutrients and contributes to sweet, hollow calories in the form of refined foods and beverages, which is what you should avoid while you're intermittently fasting. Because the sugar metabolizes super-fast, it will make you even hungrier.

You should avoid these sugar-packed foods if you are trying to do intermittent fasting:

- Frosted Cakes
- Cookies
- Sugar added Fruit juice
- Candies
- Sugary cereals and granola
- Barbecue sauce and ketchup

Foods such as nuts, lean proteins, seeds, fresh vegetables, and fruits should be your main focus during intermittent fasting as they help in weight loss and help keep your stomach full.

For eliminating all the nutritional deficiencies, healthy eating is the key to successful intermittent fasting.

SNACKS AND APPETIZERS

1 CRISPY BACON FAT BOMBS

Preparation Time: 10 minutes
Cooking Time: 3 minutes
Servings: 4
Ingredients:

- 4 thick bacon slices
- 4 oz. cream cheese
- 1 green chile, seeded, chopped
- tsp. onion powder
- Salt and pepper to taste

Directions:

Cook the bacon in a skillet for 3 minutes. Let cool, then crumble. Reserve the bacon fat.

In a bowl, combine the remaining ingredients. Add the bacon fat and mix.

Shape the mixture into 4 fat bombs. Refrigerate for 30 minutes.

Roll the fat bombs in the crumbled bacon. Serve.

Nutrition: Total Carbs: 1.4 g; Net Carbs: 0.5 g; Fat: 12.9 g; Protein: 5.7 g; Calories: 141

2 PIZZA BALLS

Preparation Time: 8 minutes
Cooking Time: 0
Servings: 6
Ingredients:

- 2 oz. fresh mozzarella
- 2 oz. cream cheese
- 2 tbsp. olive oil
- 2 tsp. tomato paste
- 6 large kalamata olives, pitted
- 12 fresh basil leaves

Directions:

In a food processor, mix all ingredients, except basil, until they form a smooth cream, about 30 seconds.

Form mixture into 6 balls.

Place 1 basil leaf on top and bottom of each ball and secure with a toothpick.

Serve or refrigerate for up to 3 days.

Nutrition: Total Carbs: 1 g; Net Carbs: 0 g; Fat: 8 g; Protein: 3 g; Calories: 82.

3 RASPBERRY CREAM FAT BOMBS

Preparation Time: 10 minutes
Cooking Time: 0 minutes
Servings: 2
Ingredients:

- 1 packet raspberry Jell-O (sugar-free)
- 2tsp. gelatin powder
- ½ cup of boiling water
- ½ cup heavy cream

Directions:

Mix Jell-O and gelatin in boiling water in a medium bowl.

Stir in cream slowly and mix it for 1 minute.

Divide this mixture into candy molds. Refrigerate them for 30 minutes. Enjoy.

Nutrition: Calories: 197; Fat: 19.2 g; Cholesterol: 11 mg Sodium: 78 mg.

4 CAULIFLOWER TARTAR BREAD

Preparation Time: 10 minutes
Cooking Time: 50 minutes
Servings: 4
Ingredients:

- 3 cups cauliflower rice
- 10 large eggs, yolks and egg whites separated
- ¼ tsp. cream of tartar
- ¼ cup coconut flour
- ½ tbsp. gluten-free baking powder
- tsp. sea salt - 6 tbsp. butter
- 6 cloves garlic, minced
- 1 tbsp. fresh rosemary, chopped
- 1 tbsp. fresh parsley, chopped

Directions:

Preheat your oven to 350°F. Layer a 9x5-inch pan with wax paper.

Place the cauliflower rice in a suitable bowl and then cover it with plastic wrap.

Heat it for 4 minutes in the microwave. Heat more if the cauliflower isn't soft enough.

Place the cauliflower rice in a kitchen towel and squeeze it to drain excess water.

Transfer drained cauliflower rice to a food processor.

Add coconut flour, sea salt, baking powder, butter, egg yolks, and garlic. Blend until crumbly.

Beat egg whites with cream of tartar in a bowl until foamy.

Add egg white mixture to the cauliflower mixture and stir well with a spatula.

Fold in rosemary and parsley.

Spread this batter in the prepared baking pan evenly.

Bake it for 50 minutes until golden then allow it to cool.

Nutrition: Calories: 104; Fat: 8.9 g; Cholesterol: 57 mg Sodium: 340 mg Carbohydrates: 4.7 g.

5 BUTTERY SKILLET FLATBREAD

Preparation Time: 10 minutes
Cooking Time: 10 minutes
Servings: 4
Ingredients:

- 1 ½ cup almond flour
- 2tbsp. coconut flour
- 1tsp. xanthan gum
- ½ tsp. baking powder
- ½ tsp. salt
- 1 whole egg + 1 egg white
- 3 tbsp. water (if needed)

- 2 tbsp. oil, for frying
- 2 tbsp. melted butter, for brushing

Directions:

Mix xanthan gum with flours, salt, and baking powder in a suitable bowl.

Beat egg and egg white in a separate bowl then stir in the flour mixture.

Mix well until smooth. Add one tablespoon of water if the dough is too thick.

Place a large skillet over medium heat and heat oil.

Nutrition: Calories: 272; Fat: 18; Cholesterol: 6.1.

6 MARINATED EGGS

Preparation Time: 2 hours & 10 minutes
Cooking Time: 7 minutes
Servings: 4
Ingredients:

- 6 eggs
- 1 ¼ cups water
- ¼ cup unsweetened rice vinegar
- 2 tbsp. coconut aminos
- Salt and black pepper to the taste
- 2 garlic cloves, minced
- 2 tsp. stevia
- 4 oz. cream cheese
- 1 tbsp. chives, chopped

Directions:

Put the eggs in a pot, add water to cover and bring to a boil over medium heat. Cover and cook for 7 minutes.

Rinse eggs with cold water and leave them aside to cool down.

In a bowl, mix 1 cup of water with coconut aminos, vinegar, stevia and garlic and whisk well.

Put the eggs in this mix, cover with a kitchen towel and leave them aside for 2 hours, rotating from time to time.

Peel eggs, cut in halves and put egg yolks in a bowl.

Add ¼ cup water, cream cheese, salt, pepper and chives and stir well.

Stuff egg whites with this mix and serve them.

Enjoy!

Nutrition: Calories: 289; Protein: 15.86 g; Fat: 22.62 g; Carbohydrates: 4.52 g; Sodium: 288 mg.

7 TASTY ONION AND CAULIFLOWER DIP

Preparation Time: 20 minutes
Cooking Time: 30 minutes
Servings: 24
Ingredients:

- 2 and ½ cups chicken stock
- 1 cauliflower head, florets separated
- ¼ cup mayonnaise

½ cup yellow onion, chopped
¾ cup cream cheese
½ tsp. chili powder
½ tsp. cumin, ground
½ tsp. garlic powder
Salt and black pepper to the taste

Directions:

Put the stock in a pot, add cauliflower and onion. Heat up over medium heat and cook for 30 minutes.

Add chili powder, salt, pepper, cumin and garlic powder and stir.

Also, add cream cheese and stir a bit until it melts.

Blend using an immersion blender and mix with the mayo.

Transfer to a bowl and keep in the fridge for 2 hours before you serve it.

Enjoy!

Nutrition: Calories: 40; Protein: 1.23 g; Fat: 3.31 g; Carbohydrates: 1.66 g; Sodium: 72 mg.

8 TACO FLAVORED CHEDDAR CRISPS

Preparation Time: 20 minutes
Cooking Time: 5 minutes
Servings: 6
Ingredients:

¾ cup sharp cheddar cheese, finely shredded
¼ cup parmesan cheese, finely shredded
¼ teaspoon chili powder
¼ teaspoon ground cumin

Directions:

Preheat the oven to 400°F.

Line cookie sheet with parchment paper.

In a bowl, toss all ingredients together until well mixed.

Make 12 piles of cheese parchment paper.

Press down the cheese into a thin layer of cheese.

Bake for 5 minutes until cheese is bubby.

Allow to cool on parchment paper.

When completely cool, peel the paper away from the crisps.

These are a good intermittent substitute for chips. They are cheesy and crisp. Enjoy!

Nutrition: Calories: 13; Protein: 1.36 g; Fat: 0.2 g; Carbohydrates: 1.43 g; Sodium: 42 mg.

9 INTERMITTENT SEED CRISPY CRACKERS

Preparation Time: 60 minutes
Cooking Time: 55 minutes
Servings: 30
Ingredients:

⅓ cup almond flour
⅓ cup sunflower seed kernels
⅓ cup pumpkin seed kernels
⅓ cup flaxseed - ⅓ cup chia seeds
1 tbsp. ground psyllium husk powder
½ tsp. salt
¼ cup melted coconut oil
1 cup boiling water

Directions:

Preheat the oven to 300°F.

Stir all dry ingredients together in a medium-sized bowl until thoroughly mixed.

Add coconut oil and boiling water to dry ingredients and stir until all ingredients are mixed well.

On a flat surface, roll the dough between two pieces of parchment paper until approximately ⅛ inch thick.

Slide the dough, still between parchment paper onto a baking sheet.

Remove the top layer of parchment paper and place dough on a baking sheet into the oven.

Bake 40 minutes until golden brown.

Score the top of the dough into cracker sized pieces.

Leave in the oven to cool down.

When the big cracker is cool, break into pieces.

These crackers can be stored in an airtight container after they are completely cool.

Nutrition: Calories: 61; Carbohydrates: 1 g; Protein: .2 g; Fat: .6 g; Sodium: 90 mg.

10 PARMESAN CRACKERS

Preparation Time: 10 minutes
Cooking Time: 5 minutes
Servings: 8
Ingredients:

1 tsp. butter
8 oz. full-fat parmesan, shredded

Directions:

Preheat the oven to 400°F.

Line a baking sheet with parchment paper and lightly grease the paper with butter.

Spoon the parmesan cheese onto the baking sheet in mounds, spread evenly apart.

Spread out the mounds with the back of a spoon until they are flat.

Bake for about 5 minutes, or until the center are still pale, and edges are browned.

Remove, cool, and serve.

Nutrition: Calories: 133; Fat: 11 g; Carb: 1 g; Protein: 11 g; Sodium: 483 mg.

11 DEVILED EGGS

Preparation Time: 15 minutes
Cooking Time: 10 minutes
Servings: 12

Ingredients:

6 large eggs, hardboiled, peeled and halved lengthwise
¼ cup creamy mayonnaise
¼ avocado, chopped
¼ cup Swiss cheese, shredded
½ tsp. Dijon mustard
Ground black pepper
6 bacon slices, cooked and chopped

Directions:

Remove the yolks and place them in a bowl. Place the whites on a plate, hollow-side up.

Mash the yolks with a fork and add Dijon mustard, cheese, avocado, and mayonnaise. Mix well and season the yolk mixture with black pepper.

Spoon the yolk mixture back into the egg white hollows and top each egg half with the chopped bacon.

Serve.

Nutrition: Calories: 85; Fat: 7 g; Carb: 2 g; Protein: 6 g; Sodium: 108 mg.

12 ALMOND GARLIC CRACKERS

Preparation Time: 10 minutes
Cooking Time: 15 minutes
Servings: 4

Ingredients:

½ cup almond flour
½ cup ground flaxseed
⅓ cup shredded Parmesan cheese
1 tsp. garlic powder
½ tsp. salt
Water as needed

Directions:

Line a baking sheet with parchment paper and preheat the oven to 400°F.

In a bowl, mix salt, Parmesan cheese, garlic powder, water, ground flaxseed, and almond meal. Set aside for 3 to 5 minutes.

Put dough on the baking sheet and cover with plastic wrap. Flatten the dough with a rolling pin.

Remove the plastic wrap and score the dough with a knife to make dents.

Bake in the oven for 15 minutes.

Remove, cool, and break into individual crackers.

Nutrition: Calories. 96; Fat. 14 g; Carb. 4 g; Protein: 4 g; Sodium: 446 mg.

13 BACON RANCH FAT BOMBS

Preparation Time: 15 minutes
Cooking Time: 15 minutes
Servings: 4
Ingredients:

8 oz. full-fat cream cheese, softened
1 tbsp. ranch dressing dry mix
8 slices bacon

Directions:

Preheat the oven to 375°F.

Cook the bacon strips on a baking tray for 15 minutes. Let cool, then crumble.

In a bowl, add cream cheese and sprinkle with ranch dressing dry mix. Stir in the bacon. Mix thoroughly.

Form a ball out of 1 tablespoon of the mixture. Repeat to form 3 more bombs. Refrigerate for 2 hours. Serve.

Nutrition: Total Carbs: 9.5 g; Net Carbs: 2.7 g; Fat: 38.9 g; Protein: 11.4 g; Calories: 419.

14 SALMON MASCARPONE BALLS

Preparation Time: 7 minutes
Cooking Time: 0
Servings: 6
Ingredients:

3 oz. smoked salmon, chopped
3 oz. mascarpone
½ tsp maple flavor
½ tsp chives, chopped
3 tbsp hemp hearts

Directions:

In a small food processor, combine salmon, mascarpone, maple flavor, and chives. Pulse a few times until blended together.

Form mixture into 6 balls.

Put hemp hearts on a medium plate and roll individual balls through to coat evenly.

Serve immediately or refrigerate for up to 3 days.

Nutrition: Total Carbs: 1 g; Net Carbs: 0 g; Fat: 5 g; Protein: 3 g; Calories: 65.

15 BRIE CHEESE FAT BOMBS

Preparation Time: 15 minutes
Cooking Time: 3 minutes
Servings: 6
Ingredients:

2 oz. full-fat cream cheese
¼ cup unsalted butter
½ cup Brie cheese, chopped
2 tbsp ghee
1 white onion, diced
4 garlic clove, minced
½ tsp paprika
Salt, pepper to taste
6 lettuce leaves

Directions:

In a food processor, mix the cream cheese and butter. Transfer to a bowl. Mix in the Brie.

In a pan, add onion and garlic and cook 3 minutes over medium heat with ghee. Let cool. Once cooled, combine with the cheese and butter mixture.

Season with the spices and mix. Refrigerate for 30 minutes.

Make 6 fat bombs out of the mixture. Serve on lettuce leaves.

Nutrition: Total Carbs: 1.7 g; Net Carbs: 1.4 g; Fat: 16.2 g; Protein: 3.3 g; Calories: 158.

16 SALTED CARAMEL AND BRIE BALLS

Preparation Time: 5 minutes
Cooking Time: 5 minutes
Servings: 6
Ingredients:

4 oz. Brie, roughly chopped
2 oz. salted macadamia nuts
½ tsp caramel flavor
2 tbsp. butter
1 large apple, chopped

Directions:

In a food processor, mix all ingredients until a coarse mix forms, about 30 seconds.

Form mixture into 6 balls.

In a saucepan, melt the butter, then add the chopped apples. Cook until apples for about 5 minutes.

Spoon the apples over the brie balls. Serve or refrigerate for up to 3 days.

Nutrition: Total Carbs: 1 g; Net Carbs: 0 g; Fat: 12 g; Protein: 5 g; Calories: 130.

17 INTERMITTENT POPCORN CHEESE PUFFS

Preparation Time: 5 minutes
Cooking Time: 5 minutes
Servings: 4
Ingredients:

4 oz. cheddar cheese sliced

Directions:

Cut the cheddar into little ¼-inch squares.

Cover the pan with baking parchment.

Leave the cheddar to dry out for in any event 24 hours.

The following day preheat your oven to 390°F. and heat the cheddar for 3-5 minutes until it is puffed up.

Leave to cool for 10 minutes before serving.

Nutrition: Calories: 114; Fat: 9 g; Carbs: 2.2 g; Protein: 7 g.

18 PARMESAN VEGETABLE CRIPS

Preparation Time: 5 minutes
Cooking Time: 10 minutes
Servings: 4
Ingredients:

¾ cup shredded zucchini
¼ cup shredded carrots
2 cups shredded Parmesan cheese
1 tbsp. olive oil
¼ tsp. black pepper

Directions:

Set the oven to 375°F. Arrange a cookie tray with parchment paper.

Wrap shredded vegetables in a paper towel and remove excess moisture.

Mix all ingredients in a bowl and mix well.

Put tablespoon-sized mounds onto the prepared cookie sheet.

Bake for 7 to 10 minutes until lightly browned.

Let it cool for at least 2 to 3 minutes and serve.

Nutrition: Calories: 206; Fat: 14.1 g; Carbs 3.6 g; Protein 15.8 g.

19 NORI SNACK ROLLS

Preparation Time: 5 minutes
Cooking Time: 10 minutes
Servings: 4
Ingredients:

2 tbsp. almond, cashew, peanut, or another nut butter
2 tbsp. tamari, or soy sauce
4 standard nori sheets
½ mushroom, sliced
1 tbsp. pickled ginger
½ cup grated carrots

Directions:

Set the oven to 350°F.

Combine together the nut butter and tamari until smooth and very thick. Layout a nori sheet, rough side up, the long way.

Spread a thin line of the tamari mixture on the far end of the nori sheet, from side to side. Lay the mushroom slices, ginger, and carrots in a line at the other end (the end closest to you).

Fold the vegetables inside the nori, rolling toward the tahini mixture, which will seal the roll. Repeat to make 4 rolls.

Bring on a baking sheet. Then bake for 8 to 10 minutes, or the rolls are slightly browned and crispy at the ends. Let the rolls cool for a few minutes; then slice each roll into 3 smaller pieces.

Nutrition: Calories: 79; Total fat: 5 g; Carbs: 6 g; Fiber: 2 g; Protein: 4 g.

20 RISOTTO BITES

Preparation Time: 15 minutes
Cooking Time: 20 minutes
Servings: 12
Ingredients:

½ cup bread crumbs
2 tsp. paprika
1 tsp. chipotle powder or ground cayenne pepper
1 ½ cups cold Green Pea Risotto

Nonstick cooking spray

Directions:

Set the oven to 425°F.

Line a baking sheet using parchment paper.

On a large plate, put and combine the panko, paprika, and chipotle powder. Set aside.

Make the 2 tablespoons of the risotto into a ball.

Roll in the bread crumbs, then put on the prepared baking sheet. Repeat to make a total of 12 balls.

Spray the tops of the risotto bites with nonstick cooking spray; then bake for at least 15 to 20 minutes until it starts to brown. Cool it before storing it in a large airtight container in a single layer.

Nutrition: Calories: 100; Fat: 2 g; Protein: 6 g; Carbohydrates: 17 g; Fiber: 5 g; Sugar: 2 g; Sodium: 165 mg.

21 CURRIED TOFU "EGG SALAD" PITAS

Preparation Time: 15 minutes
Cooking Time: 0 minutes
Servings: 4
Ingredients:

1 pound extra-firm tofu, drained and patted dry

½ cup vegan mayonnaise, homemade or store-bought

¼ cup chopped mango chutney, homemade or store-bought

1 tsp. Dijon mustard

1 tbsp. hot or mild curry powder

1tsp. salt

⅛ tsp. ground cayenne

¾ cup shredded carrots

½ cup celery ribs, minced

¼ cup minced red onion

8 small Boston or other soft lettuce leaves

7-inch whole-wheat pita bread, halved

Directions:

Crumble the tofu; then put it in a large bowl. Add the mayonnaise, chutney, mustard, curry powder, salt, and cayenne, and stir well until thoroughly mixed.

Add the carrots, celery, and onion and stir to combine. Refrigerate for 30 minutes to allow the flavors to blend.

Tuck a lettuce leaf inside each pita pocket. Spoon some tofu mixture on top of the lettuce and serve.

Nutrition: Calories: 533; Protein: 26.13 g; Fat: 29.38 g; Carbohydrates: 50.62 g.

22 BLACK SESAME WONTON CHIPS

Preparation Time: 5 minutes
Cooking Time: 5 minutes

Servings: 24
Ingredients:

12 Vegan Wonton Wrappers

Toasted sesame oil

⅓ cup black sesame seeds

Salt

Directions:

Preheat the oven to 450°F. Lightly grease with oil on a baking sheet and set aside. Cut the wonton wrappers in half crosswise, brush them with sesame oil, and arrange them in a single layer on the prepared baking sheet.

Sprinkle wonton wrappers with the sesame seeds and salt to taste. Bake until crisp and golden brown, 5 to 7 minutes. Cool completely before serving.

Nutrition: Calories: 89; Protein: 3.11 g; Fat: 4.32 g; Carbohydrates: 10 g.

23 TAMARI TOASTED ALMONDS

Preparation Time: 2 minutes
Cooking Time: 8 minutes
Servings: 4
Ingredients:

½ cup raw almonds, or sunflower seeds

2 tbsp. tamari, or soy sauce

1 tsp. toasted sesame oil

Directions:

Heat a dry skillet to medium-high heat, then add the almonds, stirring very frequently to keep them from burning. Once the almonds are toasted, 7 to 8 minutes for almonds, or 3 to 4 minutes for sunflower seeds, pour the tamari and sesame oil into the hot skillet and stir to coat.

You can turn off the heat, and as the almonds cool, the tamari mixture will stick to and dry on the nuts.

Nutrition: Calories: 89; Total fat: 8 g; Carbs: 3 g; Fiber: 2 g; Protein: 4 g.

24 TEMPEH-PIMIENTO CHEEZE BALL

Preparation Time: 5 minutes
Cooking Time: 30 minutes
Servings: 8
Ingredients:

8 oz. tempeh, cut into ½inch

1 (2 oz.) jar chopped pimientos, drained

¼ cup nutritional yeast

¼ cup vegan mayonnaise, homemade or store-bought

1 tbsp. soy sauce

¾ cup chopped pecans

Directions:

In a medium saucepan with simmering water, cook the tempeh for at least 30 minutes. Set aside to cool. In a food processor,

combine the cooled tempeh, pimientos, nutritional yeast, mayo, and soy sauce. Process until smooth.

Transfer the tempeh mixture to a bowl and refrigerate until firm and chilled, at least 2 hours or overnight.

In a dry skillet, toast the pecans at medium heat until lightly toasted, about 5 minutes. Set aside to cool.

Form the tempeh mixture into a ball, and roll it in the pecans, pressing the nuts slightly into the tempeh mixture, so they stick. Place in the fridge for at least 1 hour before serving.

Nutrition: Calories: 304; Protein: 17.59 g; Fat: 21.09 g; Carbohydrates: 13.26 g.

25 PEPPERS AND HUMMUS

Preparation Time: 15 minutes
Cooking Time: 0 minutes
Servings: 4
Ingredients:

1 (15-oz.) can chickpeas, drained and rinsed

juice of 1 lemon or 1 tbsp. prepared lemon juice

¼ cup tahini

3 tbsp. olive oil

½ tsp. ground cumin

1 tbsp. water

¼ tsp. paprika

red bell pepper, sliced

green bell pepper, sliced

orange bell pepper, sliced

Directions:

In a food processor, combine chickpeas, lemon juice, tahini, 2 tablespoons of olive oil, cumin, and water.

Process on high speed until blended, about 30 seconds. Scoop the hummus into a bowl and drizzle with the remaining 1 tablespoon of olive oil. Sprinkle with paprika and serve with sliced bell peppers.

Nutrition: Calories: 364; Protein: 12.41 g; Fat: 22.53 g; Carbohydrates: 31.65 g.

26 DECONSTRUCTED HUMMUS PITAS

Preparation Time: 15 minutes
Cooking Time: 0 minutes
Servings: 4
Ingredients:

2 garlic clove, crushed

¾ cup tahini (sesame paste

2 tbsp. fresh lemon juice

1 tsp. salt

⅛ tsp. ground cayenne

¼ cup water

1 ½ cups cooked or 1 (15.5 oz. can) chickpeas, rinsed and drained
medium carrots, grated (about 1 cup)
1 (7-inch) pita bread, preferably whole wheat, halved
1 large ripe tomato, cut into ¼ inch slices
2 cups fresh baby spinach

Directions:

In a blender or food processor, mince the garlic. Add the tahini, lemon juice, salt, cayenne, and water. Process until smooth.

Take the chickpeas in a bowl and crush slightly with a fork. Add the carrots and the reserved tahini sauce and toss to combine. Set aside.

Spoon 2 or 3 tablespoons of the chickpea mixture into each pita half. Tuck a tomato slice and a few spinach leaves into each pocket and serve.

Nutrition: Calories: 885; Protein: 39.5 g; Fat: 36.19 g; Carbohydrates: 109.52 g.

27 REFRIED BEAN AND SALSA QUESADILLAS

Preparation Time: 5 minutes
Cooking Time: 6 minutes
Servings: 4
Ingredients:

1 tbsp. canola oil, plus for frying
1 ½ cups cooked or 1 (15.5 oz. can) pinto beans, drained and mashed
1 tsp. chili powder
4 (10-inch whole-wheat flour tortillas)
1 cup tomato salsa, homemade or store-bought
½ cup minced red onion (optional)

Directions:

In a medium saucepan, heat the oil at medium flame. Put the mashed beans and chili powder and cook, stirring, until hot, about 5 minutes. Set aside.

Put 1 tortilla on a work surface and scoop at least ¼ cup of the beans across the bottom.

Put on the top the beans with the salsa and onion, if using.

Fold the top half of the tortilla on the filling and press slightly.

In a large skillet, warm a thin layer of oil over medium heat. Place the folded quesadillas, 1 or 2 at a time, into the hot skillet and heat until hot, turning once, about 1 minute per side.

Cut the quesadillas into 3 or 4; then set it on plates.

Serve immediately.

Nutrition: Calories: 940; Protein: 55.58 g; Fat: 12.07 g; Carbohydrates: 158.5 g.

28 TEMPEH TANTRUM BURGERS

Preparation Time: 15 minutes
Cooking Time: 40 minutes
Servings: 4
Ingredients:

8 oz. tempeh, cut into ½inch dice
¾ cup chopped onion
2 garlic cloves, chopped
¾ cup chopped walnuts
½ cup old-fashioned or quick-cooking oats
1 tbsp. minced fresh parsley
½ tsp. dried oregano
½ tsp. dried thyme
½ tsp. salt
¼ tsp. freshly ground black pepper
1 tbsp. olive oil
Dijon mustard
whole-grain burger rolls
Sliced red onion, tomato, lettuce, and avocado

Directions:

In a medium saucepan with simmering water, cook the tempeh for 30 minutes. Drain and set aside to cool.

In a food processor, combine together the onion and garlic and process until minced.

Put the cooled tempeh, walnuts, oats, parsley, oregano, thyme, salt, and pepper. Process until well blended. Shape the mixture into 4 equal patties.

In a huge skillet, warm the oil at medium heat. Put the burgers and cook until cooked thoroughly and browned on both sides, about 7 minutes per side.

Spread the desired amount of mustard onto each half of the rolls and layer each roll with lettuce, tomato, red onion, and avocado, as desired. Serve immediately.

Nutrition: Calories: 372; Protein: 16.3 g; Fat: 28.49 g; Carbohydrates: 17.4 g.

29 MACADAMIA-CASHEW PATTIES

Preparation Time: 10 minutes
Cooking Time: 10 minutes
Servings: 4
Ingredients:

¾ cup chopped macadamia nuts
¾ cup chopped cashews
1 medium carrot, grated
1 small onion, chopped
2 garlic clove, minced
1 jalapeño or another green chile, seeded and minced
¾ cup old-fashioned oats - ¾ cup dry unseasoned bread crumbs
2 tbsp. minced fresh cilantro
½ tsp. ground coriander

Salt and freshly ground black pepper to taste
2 tsp. fresh lime juice
2 tsp Canola or grapeseed oil, for frying
4 sandwich rolls
Lettuce leaves and condiment of choice

Directions:

In a food processor, combine together the macadamia nuts, cashews, carrot, onion, garlic, chile, oats, bread crumbs, cilantro, coriander, and salt and pepper to taste. Process until well mixed. Add the lime juice and process until well blended. Taste, adjusting seasonings if necessary. Shape the mixture into 4 equal patties.

In a huge skillet, warm a thin layer of oil on medium heat. Put the patties and cook until golden brown on both sides, turning once about 10 minutes total. Serve on sandwich rolls with lettuce and condiments of choice.

Nutrition: Calories: 748; Protein: 19.71 g; Fat: 49.96 g; Carbohydrates: 68.9 g.

30 TURMERIC PEPPERS PLATTER

Preparation Time: 10 minutes
Cooking Time: 20 minutes
Servings: 4
Ingredients:

2 green bell peppers, cut into wedges
2 red bell peppers, cut into wedges
2 yellow bell peppers, cut into wedges
2 tbsp. avocado oil
2 garlic cloves, minced
bunch basil, chopped
A pinch of salt and black pepper
1 tbsp. balsamic vinegar

Directions:

Warm a pan with the oil on medium heat, add the garlic and the vinegar and cook for 2 minutes.

Add the peppers and the other ingredients, toss, cook over medium heat for 18 minutes, arrange them on a platter and serve as an appetizer.

Nutrition: Calories: 120; Fat: 8.2 Fiber: 2 Carbs: 4 Protein 2.3

31 MUSHROOM CAKES

Preparation Time: 10 minutes
Cooking Time: 12 minutes
Servings: 6
Ingredients:

cup shallots, chopped
1 tbsp. olive oil
garlic cloves, minced
pound mushrooms, minced
1 tbsp. almond flour
¼ cup coconut cream
1 tbsp. flaxseed with 2 tbsp. water

¼ cup parsley, chopped

Directions:

In a bowl, combine the shallots with the garlic, the mushrooms, and the other ingredients, except for the oil. Stir well and shape medium cakes out of this mix.

Heat a pan with the oil over medium heat. Add the mushroom cakes and cook for 6 minutes on each side. Arrange them on a platter and serve as an appetizer.

Nutrition: Calories: 222; Fat: 4; Fiber: 3; Carbs: 8; Protein: 10.

32 CABBAGE STICKS

Preparation Time: 10 minutes
Cooking Time: 30 minutes
Servings: 4
Ingredients:

1 pound cabbage, leaves separated and cut into thick strips
2 tbsp. olive oil
2 tbsp. balsamic vinegar
1 tsp. ginger, grated
1 tsp. hot paprika
A pinch of salt and black pepper

Directions:

Spread the cabbage strips on a baking sheet lined with parchment paper. Add the oil, the vinegar, and the other ingredients. Toss and cook at 400°F for 30 minutes.

Divide the cabbage strips into bowls and serve as a snack.

Nutrition: Calories: 300; Fat: 4; Fiber: 7; Carbs: 18; Protein: 6.

33 CAULIFLOWER POPCORNS

Preparation Time: 10 minutes
Cooking Time: 25-30 minutes
Servings: 4
Ingredients:

4 cups large cauliflower florets
2 tsp. butter, melted
Salt, as required
3 tbsp. parmesan cheese, shredded

Directions:

Set the oven to 450°F. Grease a roasting pan.

Put all together with the ingredients, except for Parmesan, in a large bowl and toss to coat well.

Place the cauliflower florets into a prepared roasting pan and spread in an even layer.

Roast for about 25-30 minutes.

Remove from oven and transfer the cauliflower popcorns onto a platter.

Sprinkle with the Parmesan cheese and serve.

Nutrition: Calories: 80; Protein: 4.74 g; Fat: 4.79 g; Carbohydrates: 5.84 g.

34 WALNUT BARK

Preparation Time: 10 minutes
Cooking Time: 4 minutes
Servings: 4
Ingredients:
For Bark:

¼ cup coconut oil
¼ cup natural peanut butter
1 tsp. organic vanilla extract
8 drops liquid vanilla stevia
1 cup walnuts, chopped
Pinch of salt

For Chocolate Drizzle:

oz. 70% dark chocolate, chopped
tsp. coconut oil

Directions:
For bark:

Line 2, large plates with parchment paper.

Set the coconut oil and peanut butter in a microwave-safe bowl and microwave on High for about 30-40 seconds.

Remove the bowl from the microwave and stir in the remaining ingredients.

Divide the mixture evenly onto each plate.

For the drizzle:

In a microwave-safe bowl, add the chocolate and coconut oil and microwave on High for about 1 minute.

Drizzle chocolate mixture over the bark and freeze for about 30 minutes or until set completely before serving.

Serve.

Nutrition: Calories: 418; Protein: 9.86 g; Fat: 38.45 g; Carbohydrates: 12.55 g.

35 ALMOND BRITTLES

Preparation Time: 10 minutes
Cooking Time: 15 minutes
Servings: 4
Ingredients:

1 cup almonds
¼ cup butter
½ cup Swerve
1 tsp. organic vanilla extract
¼ tsp. salt
⅛ tsp. coarse salt

Directions:

Line a 9x9-inch cake pan using parchment paper.

Add the butter, Swerve, vanilla, and ¼ teaspoon of salt in an 8-inch nonstick skillet over medium heat and cook until well combined, stirring continuously.

Stir in the almonds and bring to a boil, stirring continuously.

Cook for about 2-3 minutes, stirring continuously.

Remove the skillet from heat and place the mixture evenly into the prepared pan.

With the back of a spoon, stir to spread the almonds and sprinkle with salt.

Set aside for about 1 hour or until cooled completely.

Break into pieces and serve.

Nutrition: Calories: 130; Protein: 1.79 g; Fat: 13.18 g; Carbohydrates: 0.34 g.

36 TROPICAL COCONUT BALLS

Preparation Time: 15 minutes
Cooking Time: 30 minutes
Servings: 2
Ingredients:

1 cup shredded coconut (unsweetened)
6 tbsp. coconut milk (full-fat)
2 tbsp. melted coconut oil
¼ cup almond flour
2 tbsp. lemon juice
2 tbsp. ground chia seeds - Zest of 1 lemon
10 drops stevia (alcohol-free)
⅛ tsp. sea salt

Directions:

Preheat the oven to 250°F.

Place the shredded coconut in a large bowl and pour the coconut milk into it.

Add the almond flour, ground chia, sea salt, coconut oil, lemon zest and lemon juice to the bowl.

Mix everything together until well combined.

Take 1 tablespoon of the mixture and form a ball out of it. Repeat with the remaining mixture.

Line a baking tray using parchment paper and place the small balls on it.

If you find the mixture too dry while making the balls, add one tablespoon (extra) of coconut oil to the mixture.

Bake the coconut balls for 30 minutes and remove them from the oven.

Let it cool completely at room temperature.

Transfer the balls into another container carefully and refrigerate it for 30 minutes.

Serve chilled and enjoy!

Nutrition: Calories 134; Fat: 13.1 g; Protein: 2.2 g; Net carb: 1.1 g.

37 JICAMA FRIES

Preparation Time: 5 minutes
Cooking Time: 10 minutes
Servings: 2
Ingredients:

> 2 Jicama (sliced into thin strips)
> ½ tsp. onion powder
> 1 tbsp. avocado oil
> Cayenne pepper (pinch)
> tsp. paprika
> Sea salt, to taste

Directions:

> Dry roast the jicama strips in a non-stick frying pan (or you can also grease the pan with a bit of avocado oil)
> Place the roasted jicama fries into a large bowl and add the onion powder, cayenne pepper, paprika, and sea salt.
> Drizzle over the avocado oil and toss the contents until the flavors are incorporated well.
> Serve immediately and enjoy!

Nutrition: Calories 92; Fat: 7 g; Protein: 1 g; Net carb: 2 g.

38 WALNUT PARMESAN BITES

Preparation Time: 10 minutes
Cooking Time: 10 minutes
Servings: 10
Ingredients:

> 6 oz. freshly grated Parmesan cheese
> 2 tbsp. chopped walnuts
> 1 tbsp. unsalted butter
> ½ tbsp. chopped fresh thyme

Directions:

> Set the oven to 350°F. Line two large rimmed baking sheets with baking paper and set aside.
> In a food processor, combine the Parmesan cheese and butter. Blend until combined.
> Pour in the walnuts and pulse until crushed and combined with the mixture.
> Using a tablespoon, scoop the mixture onto the prepared baking sheets. Then top with chopped thyme.
> Bake for at least 8 minutes, or until golden brown.
> Transfer to a cooling rack and let sit for about 30 minutes. Serve and enjoy!

Nutrition: Calories: 80; Fat: 3 g; Carbs: 7 g; Protein: 7 g.

39 CINNAMON BUTTER

Preparation Time: 10 minutes + 1 hour chilling
Cooking Time: 0 minutes
Servings: 8
Ingredients:

> ½ cup butter, at room temperature
> 5 drops liquid stevia
> ½ tsp. Pure vanilla extract
> ½ tsp. ground cinnamon
> ⅛ tsp. sea salt

Directions:

> Combine the butter, vanilla, cinnamon, salt, and stevia in a large bowl. Mix well until smooth.
> Line a baking sheet using a wax paper then spread the cinnamon butter mixture on top. Roll the paper to seal the butter mixture, then seal the ends.
> Refrigerate the butter for 1 hour before using it. Store in the refrigerator for up to 2 weeks. Best served on the Intermittent Bread or with celery sticks.

Nutrition: Calories: 103; Fat: 12 g; Carbs: 0.1 g; Protein: 0.1 g.

40 MIXED BERRIES CRISP

Preparation Time: 10 minutes
Cooking Time: 12 minutes
Serves 4
Ingredients:

> ½ cup fresh blueberries
> ½ cup chopped fresh strawberries
> ⅓ cup frozen raspberries, thawed
> 1 tbsp. honey
> 1 tbsp. freshly squeezed lemon juice
> ⅔ cup whole-wheat pastry flour
> 3 tbsp. packed brown sugar
> 2 tbsp. unsalted butter, melted

Directions:

> Place the strawberries, blueberries, and raspberries in a baking pan and drizzle the honey and lemon juice over the top.
> Combine the pastry flour and brown sugar in a small mixing bowl.
> Add the butter and whisk until the mixture is crumbly. Scatter the flour mixture on top of the fruit.
> Place the pan on the bake position.
> Set time to 12 minutes.
> When cooking is complete, the fruit should be bubbly and the topping should be golden brown.

Nutrition: Calories: 170; Carbs: 8 g; Fat: 6 g; Protein: 16 g.

41 CRISPY SQUASH

Preparation Time: 5 minutes
Cooking Time: 20 minutes
Servings: 4
Ingredients:

> 2 cups butternut squash, cubed
> 2 tbsp. olive oil
> Salt and black pepper to taste
> ¼ tsp. dried thyme
> 1 tbsp. fresh parsley, finely chopped

Directions:

> In a bowl, add squash, olive oil, salt, pepper, thyme, and toss to coat.
> Place the squash in the air fryer and Air Fry for 14 minutes at 360°F, shaking once or twice. Serve sprinkled with fresh parsley.

Nutrition: Calories: 100; Carbs: 5 g; Fat: 2 g; Protein: 3 g.

42 CLASSIC FRENCH FRIES

Preparation Time: 5 minutes
Cooking Time: 30 minutes
Servings: 4
Ingredients: (2 servings)

> 2 russet potatoes, cut into strips
> 2 tbsp. olive oil
> Kosher salt and black pepper to taste
> ½ cup aioli

Directions:

> Preheat the fryer to 400°F. Grease the air fryer basket with cooking spray.
> In a bowl, brush the strips with olive oil and season with salt and black pepper. Put it in the air fryer and cook for 20-22 minutes, turning once halfway through, until crispy. Serve with garlic aioli.

Nutrition: Calories: 120; Carbs: 7 g; Fat: 4 g; Protein: 6 g.

43 INTERMITTENT BACON BURGER BOMBS

Preparation Time: 10 minutes
Cooking Time: 60 minutes
Servings: 12
Ingredients:

> 12 slices bacon
> 12 cubes smoked cheddar cheese, (1-inch)
> 12 rounds sausage patties, raw, (1-oz.)

To Taste:

> Cumin, onion powder, salt, pepper

Directions:

> Preheat oven to 350°F. Layout sausage rounds on a cookie sheet lined with parchment paper.
> Dust sausage with cumin, onion powder, salt, and pepper.
> Place a piece of cheese in the middle of the sausage rounds.
> Form a ball around the cheese with the sausage. Roll it in your hands to make a good circle shape.
> Wrap bacon around the sausage balls.
> Bake at 350°F for an hour.
> Enjoy with your favorite burger condiments!

Nutrition: Calories: 249; Fat: 20.4 g; Carbs: 1.3 g; Protein: 14.4 g.

44 AVOCADO AND TEMPEH BACON WRAPS

Preparation Time: 10 minutes
Cooking Time: 8 minutes
Servings: 4
Ingredients:

- 2 tbsp. olive oil
- 8 oz. tempeh bacon, homemade or store-bought
- 4 (10-inch) soft flour tortillas or lavash flatbread
- ¼ cup vegan mayonnaise, homemade or store-bought
- 4 large lettuce leaves
- 2 ripe Hass avocados, pitted, peeled, and cut into ¼ inch slices
- large ripe tomato, cut into ¼ inch slices

Directions:

In a huge skillet, warm the oil to medium heat temperature. Put the tempeh bacon and cook until browned on both sides, about 8 minutes. Remove from the heat and set aside.

Place 1 tortilla on a work surface. Spread with some of the mayonnaise and one-fourth of the lettuce and tomatoes.

Peel and pit then thinly slice the avocado and place the slices on top of the tomato. Add the reserved tempeh bacon and roll up tightly. Repeat with remaining ingredients and serve.

Nutrition: Calories: 788; Protein: 28.25 g; Fat: 52.02 g; Carbohydrates: 62.36 g.

45 BACON, ARTICHOKE & ONION FAT BOMBS

Preparation Time: 15 minutes
Cooking Time: 8 minutes
Servings: 4
Ingredients:

- 2 bacon slices
- 2 tbsp ghee
- ½ large onion, peeled, diced
- garlic clove, minced
- ⅓ cup canned artichoke hearts, sliced
- ¼ cup sour cream
- ¼ cup mayonnaise
- 1 tbsp. lemon juice
- ¼ cup Swiss cheese, grated
- Salt, pepper to taste
- 4 avocado halves, pitted

Directions:

In a hot skillet, fry the bacon for 5 minutes. Let cool, then crumble.

Cook the onion and garlic using ghee for 3 minutes.

Combine the onion and garlic with the bacon and the remaining ingredients. Mix well. Season with salt and pepper. Refrigerate for

30 minutes. Fill the avocado halves with the mixture and serve.

Nutrition: Total Carbs: 10 g; Net Carbs: 4 g; Fat: 39.6 g; Protein: 6.6 g; Calories: 408.

46 BACON-WRAPPED CHICKEN BOMBS

Preparation Time: 15 minutes
Cooking Time: 35-45 minutes
Servings: 6
Ingredients:

- 2 lb. (about 3) boneless, skinless, chicken breasts
- 10 oz. frozen spinach
- 4 oz. cream cheese, softened
- ½ cup full-fat ricotta
- Salt and pepper to taste
- 12 slices bacon

Directions:

Thaw the spinach out, then wring with water.

Set the oven to 375°F.

Mix the spinach in the cream cheese and ricotta.

Season with salt and pepper to taste.

Chop the chicken breasts in half. You want them to be still thick enough to cut pouches into.

Cut pockets into 1 of the ends of every piece of chicken. Stuff the pockets with the cheese filling.

Wrap 2 slices of bacon around per piece of chicken. Seal the open end and any holes where filling might seep out.

Sear the bacon-wrapped chicken in a hot skillet. You do not have to brown all the sides equally because they will be finished off in the oven.

Set the pieces of chicken into an oven-safe dish while you finish the others.

Bake for at least 35-45 minutes until the bacon is well-crisped, and the chicken is cooked all the way through. The chicken is completely cooked when it reaches 165°F.

Nutrition: Calories: 384.8; Fat: 20.5 g; Carbs: 2.3 g; Protein: 44.8g.

47 SPICY BACON AND AVOCADO BALLS

Preparation Time: 45 minutes
Cooking Time: 8 minutes
Servings: 6
Ingredients:

- 4 slices bacon
- 1 medium avocado
- 1 tbsp. coconut oil
- 1 tbsp. bacon fat
- 1 tbsp. green onions, finely chopped
- 1 tbsp. cilantro, finely chopped

- 1 small jalapeño pepper, seeded, finely chopped
- ¼ tsp sea salt

Directions:

Over medium heat, cook bacon until golden, about 4 minutes on each side.

Drain bacon on a paper towel. Save bacon fat for later.

Once the bacon is cool, chop 2 slices into crumbles.

Cut remaining 2 slices into 3 pieces each.

Smash avocado with a fork in a small bowl.

Add coconut oil and cooled bacon fat to avocado.

Add onion, cilantro, jalapeño, salt, and bacon crumbles. Blend well.

Refrigerate for 30 minutes.

Form mixture into 6 balls.

Place the remaining 6 bacon pieces on a plate, then top each with an avocado ball.

Serve or refrigerate for up to 3 days.

Nutrition: Total Carbs: 3 g; Net Carbs: 1 g; Fat: 18 g; Protein: 3 g; Calories: 181.

48 BBQ CHICKEN

Preparation Time: 5 minutes
Cooking Time: 30 minutes
Servings: 4
Ingredients:

- 1 whole small chicken, cut into pieces
- 1 tsp. salt
- 1 tsp. smoked paprika
- 1 tsp. garlic powder
- 1 cup BBQ sauce

Directions:

Mix salt, paprika, and garlic powder and coat the chicken pieces. Place in the air fryer basket and bake for 18 minutes at 400°F. Remove to a plate and brush with barbecue sauce.

Wipe the fryer clean from the chicken fat. Return the chicken to the fryer, skin-side up, and bake for 5 more minutes at 340°F.

Nutrition: Calories: 230; Carbs: 12 g; Fat: 9 g; Protein: 23 g.

49 BACON-WRAPPED MOZZARELLA STICKS

Preparation Time: 5 minutes
Cooking Time: 5 minutes
Servings: 2
Ingredients:

- 2 slices thick bacon
- 2 Frigo® Cheese Heads String Cheese sticks
- Coconut oil – for frying

For Dipping:

- Low-sugar pizza sauce

Directions:

> Warm the oil to 350° F in a deep fryer.
> Slice the cheese stick in half. Wrap it with the bacon and close it using the toothpick.
> Cook the sticks in the hot fryer for 2 to 3 minutes
> Drain on a towel and cool. Serve with your sauce.

Nutrition: Protein: 7 g; Total Fat: 9 g; Net Carbohydrates: 1 g; Calories: 103.

50 DUCK FAT ROASTED RED POTATOES

Preparation Time: 5 minutes
Cooking Time: 25 minutes
Servings: 4
Ingredients:

> 4 red potatoes, cut into wedges
> 1 tbsp. garlic powder
> 2 tbsp. thyme, chopped
> 3 tbsp. duck fat, melted

Directions:

> Preheat the air fryer to 380°F. In a bowl, mix duck fat, garlic powder, salt, and pepper. Add the potatoes and shake to coat.
> Place in the basket and bake for 12 minutes. Remove the basket, shake and continue cooking for another 8-10 minutes until golden brown. Serve warm topped with thyme.

Nutrition: Calories: 110 Carbs: 8 g; Fat: 5 g; Protein: 7 g.

51 BACON PICKLE FRIES

Preparation Time: 10 minutes
Cooking Time: 15 minutes
Servings: 12
Ingredients:

> 12 slices bacon
> 12 Pickle spears
> ¼ cup Intermittent-friendly-Ranch dressing

Directions:

> Set the oven at 425° F.
> Prepare a baking tin using a layer of parchment baking paper.
> Wrap each of the pickles using a piece of bacon and arrange on the prepared baking tray.
> Bake until crispy (12 to 15 minutes). Turn after about halfway through the cycle (7 minutes).
> Serve with your favorite ranch or other dressing.

Nutrition: Protein: 2 g; Total Fat: 16 g; Net Carbohydrates: 1.2 g; Calories: 159.

52 CHICKEN POPCORNS

Preparation Time: 15 minutes
Cooking Time: 20-25 minutes
Servings: 4

Ingredients:

> ½-pound grass-fed chicken thigh, cut into bite-sized pieces
> 7 oz. unsweetened coconut milk
> 1 tsp. ground turmeric
> Salt and ground black pepper, as required
> 1 tbsp. coconut flour
> 1 tbsp. desiccated coconut
> 1 . coconut oil, melted

Directions:

> Place the chicken, coconut milk, turmeric, salt, and black pepper in a large bowl and mix well.
> Cover the bowl; then place it in the refrigerator to marinate overnight.
> Preheat the oven to 390°F.
> Place the coconut flour and desiccated coconut in a shallow dish and mix well.
> Coat the chicken pieces evenly with coconut mixture.
> Arrange the chicken piece onto a baking sheet and drizzle with oil.
> Bake for about 20-25 minutes.
> Take off the baking sheet from the oven and transfer the chicken popcorn onto a platter.
> Set aside to cool slightly.
> Serve warm.

Nutrition: Calories: 179; Protein: 13.4 g; Fat: 12.32 g; Carbohydrates: 4.1 g.

53 CHICKEN WINGS WITH ALFREDO SAUCE

Preparation Time: 5 minutes
Cooking Time: 20 minutes
Servings: 4
Ingredients:

> 1 ½ lb. chicken wings, pat-dried
> Salt to taste
> ½ cup Alfredo sauce

Directions:

> Season the wings with salt. Arrange them in the greased air fryer basket, without touching and Air Fry for 12 minutes until no longer pink in the center. Work in batches if needed. Flip them, increase the heat to 390°F and cook for 5 more minutes. Plate the wings and drizzle with Alfredo sauce to serve.

Nutrition: Calories: 150; Carbs: 7 g; Fat: 5 g; Protein: 14 g.

54 TURKEY MEATBALLS WITH SPAGHETTI SQUASH

Preparation Time: 15 minutes
Cooking Time: 35 minutes
Servings: 4
Ingredients:

> 1 lb. lean ground turkey
> 1 lb. spaghetti squash, halved and seeds removed
> 2 egg whites
> ⅓ cup green onions, diced fine
> ¼ cup onion, diced fine
> 2 ½ tbsp. flat-leaf parsley, diced fine
> 1 tbsp. fresh basil, diced fine

What you'll need from the store cupboard:

> 14 oz. can no-salt-added tomatoes, crushed
> ⅓ cup soft whole wheat bread crumbs
> ¼ cup low sodium chicken broth
> 1 tsp garlic powder
> 1 tsp thyme
> 1 tsp oregano
> ½ tsp red pepper flakes
> ½ tsp whole fennel seeds

Directions:

> In a small bowl, combine bread crumbs, onion, garlic, parsley, pepper flakes, thyme, and fennel.
> In a large bowl, combine turkey and egg whites. Add bread crumb mixture and mix well. Cover and chill for 10 minutes. Heat the oven to broil.
> Place the squash, cut side down, in a glass baking dish. Add 3-4 tablespoons of water and microwave on high 10-12 minutes, or until fork tender.
> Make 20 meatballs from the turkey mixture and place on a baking sheet. Broil 4-5 minutes. Turn and cook 4 more minutes.
> In a large skillet, combine tomatoes and broth and bring to a simmer over low heat. Add meatballs, oregano, basil, and green onions. Cook, stirring occasionally, 10 minutes or until heated through.
> Use a fork to scrape the squash into "strands" and arrange on a serving platter. Top with meatballs and sauce and serve.

Nutrition: Calories 253; Total Carbs: 15 g; Net Carbs: 13 g; Protein: 27 g; Fat: 9 g; Sugar: 4 g; Fiber: 2 g.

55 HAM 'N' CHEESE PUFFS

Preparation Time: 15 minutes
Cooking Time: 30 minutes
Servings: 8
Ingredients:

> 6 large eggs
> 10 oz. sliced deli ham, diced
> ½ cup shredded cheddar cheese
> ¾ cup mayonnaise
> ⅓ cup coconut flour
> ⅓ cup coconut oil
> ⅓ tsp. baking powder
> ⅓ tsp. baking soda
> Nonstick cooking spray

Directions:

- Set the oven to 350°F. Lightly coat rimmed baking sheet using nonstick cooking spray and set aside.
- In a bowl, put together the eggs, coconut oil, and mayonnaise then mix. Set aside.
- In a separate bowl, combine the baking soda, baking powder, and coconut flour. Add the dry ingredients to the wet ingredients and mix well until smooth.
- Fold the ham and cheddar cheese into the mixture and set aside.
- Cut the dough into 18 small pieces; then arrange on the prepared baking sheet.
- Bake for 30 minutes, or until the puffs are golden brown and set.
- Arrange the puffs on a cooling rack and allow to cool slightly.
- Keep in a sealed container for up to 5 days. If desired, reheat in the microwave before serving.

Nutrition: Calories: 249; Fat: 20 g; Carbs: 3 g; Protein: 15 g.

56 CHOCOLATE DIPPED CANDIED BACON

Preparation Time: 20 minutes
Cooking Time: 1 hour & 15 minutes
Servings: 6
Ingredients:

- ½ tsp. cinnamon
- 2 tbsp. brown sugar alternative – ex. surkin gold
- 16 thin-cut slices bacon
- ½ oz. cacao butter or coconut oil
- 3 oz. 85% dark chocolate
- 1 tsp. sugar-free maple extract

Directions:

- Whisk the Surkin Gold and cinnamon together.
- Arrange the bacon strips on a parchment paper-lined tray and sprinkle using half of the mixture. Do the other side with the rest of the seasoning mixture.
- Set the oven to reach 275° Fahrenheit. Bake until caramelized and crispy (approximately 1 hour and 15 minutes).
- Heat a skillet to melt the cocoa butter and chocolate. Pour the maple syrup into the mixture and stir well. Set aside until it reaches room temperature.
- Arrange the bacon on a platter to cool thoroughly before dipping into the chocolate.
- Dip half of each strip of the bacon into the chocolate.

- Arrange on a tray for the chocolate to solidify. Either place it in the refrigerator or on the countertop.

Nutrition: Protein: 3 g; Total Fat: 4.1 g; Net Carbohydrates: 1.1 g; Calories: 54.

57 TURKEY & MUSHROOM CASSEROLE

Preparation Time: 15 minutes
Cooking Time: 50 minutes
Servings: 8
Ingredients:

- 1 lb. cremini mushrooms, washed and sliced
- 1 onion, diced
- 6 cup cauliflower, grated
- 4 cup turkey, cooked and cut in bite-size pieces
- 2 cup reduced-fat Mozzarella, grated, divided
- 1 cup fat-free sour cream
- ½ cup lite mayonnaise
- ¼ cup reduced-fat parmesan cheese
- 2 tbsp. olive oil, divided
- 2 tbsp. Dijon mustard
- 1 ½ tsp thyme
- 1 ½ tsp poultry seasoning

Directions:

- Heat oven to 375°F. Grease a 9x13-inch baking dish with cooking spray.
- In a medium bowl, stir together sour cream, mayonnaise, mustard, ½ teaspoon of each thyme and poultry seasoning, 1 cup of the mozzarella, and parmesan cheese.
- Heat 2 teaspoons of oil in a large skillet over med-high flame. Add mushrooms and sauté until they start to brown and all liquid is evaporated. Transfer them to the prepared baking dish.
- Add 2 more teaspoons of oil to the skillet along with the onion and sauté until soft and they start to brown. Add the onions to the mushrooms.
- Add another 2 teaspoons of oil to the skillet with the cauliflower. Cook, stirring frequently, until it starts to get soft, about 3-4 minutes. Add the remaining thyme and poultry seasoning and cook 1 more minute.
- Season with salt and pepper and add to baking dish. Place the turkey over the vegetables and stir everything together.
- Spread the sauce mixture over the top and stir to combine. Sprinkle the remaining mozzarella over the top and bake for 40 minutes, or until bubbly and cheese is golden

brown. Let cool for 5 minutes, then cut and serve.

Nutrition: Calories: 351; Total Carbs: 13 g; Net Carbs: 10 g; Protein: 37 g; Fat: 16 g; Sugar: 5 g; Fiber: 3 g.

58 CARAMELIZED BACON KNOTS

Preparation Time: 10 minutes
Cooking Time: 15 minutes
Servings: 4
Ingredients:

- 8 sliced portions of bacon
- 1 tbsp. black pepper
- tbsp. low-carb sweetener - your preference

Directions:

- Mix the pepper and sweetener in a small bowl (ex. erythritol or xylitol). Set aside.
- Slice each bacon in half. Tie each half into a knot.
- Press the bacon knots into the pepper mixture, turning them over to coat as much as possible. Place the dipped knots onto a wire rack placed on a baking tin.
- Place the bacon knots under a hot broiler and cook until they're to your liking (5-7 minutes. per side).
- Cool on a layer of paper towels to remove excess grease as needed.
- Serve as soon as they're ready.

Nutrition: Protein: 5 g; Total Fat: 17 g; Net Carbohydrates: 1 g; Calories: 187.

59 BROILED BACON WRAPS WITH DATES

Preparation Time: 10 minutes
Cooking Time: 15-20 minutes
Servings: 6
Ingredients:

- 1 lb. sliced bacon
- 8 oz. pitted dates

Directions:

- Warm up the oven to reach 425°F.
- Use a ½ slice of bacon and wrap each of the dates. Close with a toothpick.
- Put the wraps on a baking tray and bake them for 15-20 minutes. Serve hot.

Nutrition: Protein: 19 g; Total Fat: 10 g; Net Carbohydrates: 5 g; Calories: 203.

60 COCONUT SHRIMP

Preparation Time: 15 minutes
Cooking Time: 8 minutes
Servings: 3
Ingredients:

- ¼ cup almond flour
- ½ tsp. garlic powder, divided
- ½ tsp. paprika, divided

Salt and freshly ground black pepper, to taste

2 large eggs, beaten

1 tbsp. unsweetened almond milk

½ cup unsweetened flaked coconut

¼ cup pork rinds, crushed

½-pound large shrimp, peeled and deveined

Nonstick cooking spray

Directions:

Place the flour, half the spices, salt, and black pepper in a shallow dish and blend well.

Place the eggs and almond milk in a second shallow dish and beat well.

Place the coconut, pork rinds, remaining spices, salt, and black pepper and blend well.

Coat shrimp with flour mixture, then the egg mixture and eventually coat with the coconut mixture.

Again, dip in the egg mixture and coat with the coconut mixture.

Turn the "Temperature Knob" of PowerXL Air Fryer Grill to line the temperature to 380°F.

Turn the "Function Knob" to settle on "Air Fry."

Turn the "Timer Knob" to line the Time for 8 minutes.

After preheating, arrange the shrimp into the greased air fry basket.

Insert the air fry basket at position 2 of the Air Fryer Grill.

Flip the shrimp once halfway through.

When the cooking time is over, transfer the shrimp onto a platter.

Serve immediately.

Nutrition: Calories: 234; Fat: 13.8 g; Carb: 5.9 g; Protein: 20 g.

61 FISH STICKS

Preparation Time: 15 minutes
Cooking Time: 15 minutes
Servings: 8
Ingredients:

16 oz. tilapia fillets, sliced into strips

1 cup all-purpose flour

2 eggs

1 ½ cups breadcrumbs

Salt to taste

Directions:

Dip fish strips in flour and then in eggs.

Mix breadcrumbs and salt.

Coat fish strips with breadcrumbs.

Add fish strips to a crisper plate.

Place crisper plate inside the basket.

Choose air fry setting.

Cook fish strips at 390°F for 12 to 15 minutes, flipping once halfway through.

Nutrition: Calories: 324; Fat: 21.5 g; Saturated Fat: 4 g; Trans Fat: 0 g;

Carbohydrates: 7.5 g; Fiber: 2 g; Sodium: 274 mg; Protein: 20 g.

62 RICE BITES

Preparation Time: 10 minutes
Cooking Time: 10 minutes
Servings: 4
Ingredients:

3 cups cooked risotto

⅓ cup Parmesan cheese, grated

1 egg, beaten

3 oz. mozzarella cheese, cubed

¾ cup breadcrumbs

Directions:

In a bowl, mix the risotto, Parmesan cheese, and egg.

Make 20 equal-sized balls from the mixture.

Insert a mozzarella cube in the center of every ball.

With your fingers, smooth the risotto mixture to hide the mozzarella.

In a shallow dish, add the breadcrumbs.

Coat the balls with breadcrumbs.

Turn the "Temperature Knob" of PowerXL Air Fryer Grill to line the temperature to 390°F.

Turn the "Function Knob" to settle on "Air Fry."

Turn the "Timer Knob" to line the Time for 10 minutes.

After preheating, arrange the balls in the air fryer basket in a single layer.

Insert the air fryer basket at position 2 of the Air Fryer Grill.

When the cooking time is over, transfer the balls onto a platter.

Serve warm.

Nutrition: Calories: 241; Fat: 5.2 g; Carb, 36.9 g; Protein: 10 g.

63 GRILLED TOMATO SALSA

Preparation Time: 15 minutes
Cooking Time: 10 minutes
Servings: 4 to 8
Ingredients:

1 onion, sliced

1 jalapeño pepper, sliced in half

5 tomatoes, sliced

2 tbsp. oil

Salt and pepper to taste

1 cup cilantro, trimmed and sliced

1 tbsp. lime juice

1 tsp. lime zest

2 tbsp. ground cumin

3 cloves garlic, peeled and sliced

Directions:

Coat onion, jalapeño pepper and tomatoes with oil.

Season with salt and pepper.

Add grill grate to your Power XL Grill.

Press grill setting.

Choose max temperature and set it to 10 minutes.

Press starts to preheat.

Add vegetables to the grill.

Cook for 5 minutes per side.

Transfer to a plate and let cool.

Add vegetable mixture to a food processor.

Stir in remaining ingredients. Pulse until smooth.

Nutrition: Calories: 369; Fat: 16 g; Carbohydrates: 37 g; Fiber: 5 g; Protein: 14 g.

64 PARMESAN FRENCH FRIES

Preparation Time: 15 minutes
Cooking Time: 40 minutes
Servings: 6
Ingredients:

1 lb. French fries

½ cup mayonnaise

2 cloves garlic, minced

1 tbsp. oil

Salt and pepper to taste

1 tsp. garlic powder

½ cup Parmesan cheese, grated

1 tsp. lemon juice

Directions:

Add a crisper basket to your Power XL Grill.

Select the air fry function.

Set it to 375°F for 22 minutes.

Press starts to preheat.

Add fries to the basket.

Cook for 10 minutes.

Shake and cook for another 5 minutes.

Toss in oil and sprinkle with Parmesan cheese.

Mix the remaining ingredients in a bowl.

Serve fries with this sauce.

Nutrition: Calories: 445; Fat: 27 g; Carbohydrates: 25 g; Fiber: 2 g; Protein: 20 g.

65 HOMEMADE FRIES

Preparation Time: 15 minutes
Cooking Time: 45 minutes
Servings: 6
Ingredients:

1 lb. large potatoes, sliced into strips

2 tbsp. vegetable oil

Salt to taste

Directions:

Toss potato strips in oil.

Add crisper plate to the air fryer basket inside the Power XL Grill.

Choose air fry function. Set it to 390°F for 3 minutes.

Press Start to preheat.

Add potato strips to the crisper plate.

Cook for 25 minutes.

Stir and cook for another 20 minutes.

Nutrition: Calories: 183; Fat: 7.4 g; Carbohydrates: 5.4 g; Fiber: 1 g; Protein: 22.3 g.

66 FRIED GARLIC PICKLES

Preparation Time: 20 minutes
Cooking Time: 15 minutes
Servings: 6
Ingredients:
- ¼ cup all-purpose flour
- Pinch baking powder
- 2 tbsp. water
- Salt to taste
- 20 dill pickle slices
- 2 tbsp. cornstarch
- 1 ½ cups panko bread crumbs
- 2 tsp. garlic powder
- 2 tbsp. canola oil

Directions:
- In a bowl, combine flour, baking powder, water and salt.
- Add more water if the batter is too thick.
- Put the cornstarch in a second bowl, and mix breadcrumbs and garlic powder in a third bowl.
- Dip pickles in cornstarch, then in the batter and finally dredge with breadcrumb mixture.
- Add crisper plate to the air fryer basket inside the Power XL Grill.
- Press Air Fry setting.
- Set it to 360°F for 3 minutes.
- Press Start to preheat.
- Add pickles to the crisper plate.
- Brush with oil.
- Air fry for 10 minutes.
- Flip, brush with oil and cook for another 5 minutes.

Nutrition: Calories: 112; Fat: 4.6 g; Carbohydrates: 18.6 g; Fiber: 2 g; Protein: 1.7 g.

67 ZUCCHINI STRIPS WITH MARINARA DIP

Preparation Time: 1 hour & 10 minutes
Cooking Time: 30 minutes
Servings: 8
Ingredients:
- 2 zucchinis, sliced into strips
- Salt to taste
- 1 ½ cups all-purpose flour
- 2 eggs, beaten
- 2 cups bread crumbs
- 2 tsp. onion powder
- 1 tbsp. garlic powder
- ¼ cup Parmesan cheese, grated
- ½ cup marinara sauce

Directions:
- Season zucchini with salt. Let sit for 15 minutes.
- Pat dry with paper towels. Add flour to a bowl.
- Add eggs to another bowl.
- Mix remaining ingredients, except for marinara sauce, in a third bowl.
- Dip zucchini strips in the first, second and third bowls.
- Cover with foil and freeze for 45 minutes.
- Add crisper plate to the air fryer basket inside the Power XL Grill.
- Select the air fry function.
- Preheat to 360°F for 3 minutes. Add zucchini strips to the crisper plate.
- Air fry for 20 minutes. Flip and cook for another 10 minutes.
- Serve with marinara dip.

Nutrition: Calories: 364; Fat: 35 g; Saturated Fat: 17 g; Trans Fat: 0 g; Carbohydrates: 8 g; Fiber: 1.5 g; Sodium: 291 mg; Protein: 8 g.

68 GREEK POTATOES

Preparation Time: 20 minutes
Cooking Time: 30 minutes
Servings: 4
Ingredients:
- 1 lb. potatoes, sliced into wedges
- 2 tbsp. olive oil
- 1 tsp. paprika
- 2 tsp. dried oregano
- Salt and pepper to taste
- ¼ cup onion, diced
- 2 tbsp. lemon juice
- 1 tomato, diced
- ¼ cup black olives, sliced
- ½ cup feta cheese, crumbled

Directions:
- Add crisper plate to the air fryer basket inside the Power XL Grill.
- Choose Air Fry setting. Set it to 390°F.
- Preheat for 3 minutes.
- While preheating, toss potatoes in oil.
- Sprinkle with paprika, oregano, salt and pepper.
- Add potatoes to the crisper plate.
- Air fry for 18 minutes. Toss and cook for another 5 minutes.
- Add onion and cook for 5 minutes.
- Transfer to a bowl.
- Stir in the rest of the ingredients.

Nutrition: Calories: 368; Fat: 24.2 g; Carbohydrates: 21 g; Fiber: 4.1 g; Protein: 17.6 g.

69 RANCH CHICKEN FINGERS

Preparation Time: 15 minutes
Cooking Time: 20 minutes
Servings: 4
Ingredients:
- 2 lb. chicken breast fillet, sliced into strips
- 1 tbsp. olive oil
- 1 oz. ranch dressing seasoning mix
- 4 cups breadcrumbs
- Salt to taste

Directions:
- Coat chicken strips with olive oil.
- Sprinkle all sides with ranch seasoning.
- Cover with foil and refrigerate for 1 to 2 hours.
- In a bowl, mix breadcrumbs and salt.
- Dredge the chicken strips with seasoned breadcrumbs.
- Add crisper plate to the air fryer basket inside the Power XL Grill.
- Choose air fry setting.
- Set it to 390°F. Preheat for 3 minutes.
- Add chicken strips to the crisper plate.
- Cook for 15 to 20 minutes, flipping halfway through.

Nutrition: Calories: 188; Fat: 3.2 g; Carbohydrates: 28.5 g; Fiber: 6.2 g; Protein: 29.4g.

70 PROSCIUTTO-WRAPPED ASPARAGUS

Preparation Time: 10 minutes
Cooking Time: 12 minutes
Servings: 6
Ingredients:
- 12 spears asparagus, trimmed
- 2 tsp. olive oil
- Salt and freshly ground black pepper, to taste
- 12 prosciutto slices

Directions:
- Drizzle the asparagus spears with oil and ten, sprinkle with salt and black pepper.
- Wrap one prosciutto slice around each asparagus spear from top to bottom.
- Turn the "Temperature Knob" of PowerXL Air Fryer Grill to line the temperature to 300°F.
- Turn the "Function Knob" to settle on "Air Fry."
- Turn the "Timer Knob" to line the Time for 10 minutes.
- After preheating, arrange the asparagus spears into the greased air fry basket.
- Insert the air fry basket at position 2 of the Air Fryer Grill.
- Flip the asparagus spears once halfway through.
- When the cooking time is over, transfer the asparagus spears onto a platter.
- Serve hot.

Nutrition: Calories: 144; Fat: 8.7 g; Carb: 1.9 g; Protein: 16 g.

71 BACON BELL PEPPERS

Preparation Time: 10 minutes
Cooking Time: 5 minutes
Servings: 16
Ingredients:
- 1 pack bacon slices
- 12 bell peppers, sliced in half
- 8 oz. cream cheese

Directions:

Stuff bell pepper halves with cream cheese.

Wrap with bacon slices.

Preheat Power XL Grill to 500°F.

Add bell peppers to the grill.

Grill for 3 to 5 minutes.

Nutrition: Calories: 482; Fat: 42 g; Carbohydrates: 14 g; Fiber: 5 g; Protein: 28 g.

72 BACON AND ASPARAGUS SPEARS

Preparation Time: 15 minutes
Cooking Time: 8 minutes
Servings: 4
Ingredients:

20 spears asparagus
4 bacon slices
1 tbsp. olive oil
1 tbsp. sesame oil
1 garlic clove, crushed

Directions:

Warm your Air Fryer to 380°F.

Take a small bowl and add oil, crushed garlic, and mix.

Separate asparagus into four bunches and wrap them in bacon.

Brush wraps with oil and garlic mix. Transfer to your Air Fryer basket.

Cook for 8 minutes.

Serve and enjoy!

Nutrition: Calories: 175; Fat: 15 g; Carbohydrates: 6 g; Protein: 5 g.

73 CRUNCHY PARMESAN ASPARAGUS

Preparation Time: 10 minutes
Cooking Time: 10 minutes
Servings: 4
Ingredients:

¼ cup all-purpose flour
Salt to taste
2 eggs, beaten
¼ cup Parmesan cheese, grated
½ cup breadcrumbs
1 cup asparagus, trimmed
Cooking spray

Directions:

Mix flour and salt in a bowl.

Add eggs to a second bowl.

Combine Parmesan cheese and breadcrumbs in a third bowl.

Dip asparagus spears in the first, second and third bowls.

Spray with oil.

Add crisper plate to the air fryer basket inside the Power XL Grill.

Set it to air fry.

Preheat at 390°F for 3 minutes.

Add asparagus to the plate.

Air fry for 5 minutes per side.

Nutrition: Calories: 243; Fat: 10.5 g; Saturated Fat: 3 g; Trans Fat: 0 g; Carbohydrates: 10 g; Fiber: 3 g; Sodium: 824 mg; Protein: 35 g.

74 CORN & CARROT FRITTERS

Preparation Time: 8 to 10 minutes
Cooking Time: 12 minutes
Servings: 4 to 5
Ingredients:

4 oz. canned sweet corn kernels, drained
1 tsp. sea salt flakes
1 tbsp. cilantro, chopped
1 carrot, grated
1 yellow onion, finely chopped
1 medium-sized egg, whisked
¼ cup of self-rising flour
⅓ tsp. baking powder
2 tbsp. milk
1 cup Parmesan cheese, grated
⅓ tsp. brown sugar

Directions:

Place your Air Fryer on a flat kitchen surface; plug it and turn it on. Set temperature to 350°F and let it preheat for 4-5 minutes.

Press the carrot in the colander to remove excess liquid. Arrange the carrot between several sheets of kitchen towels and pat it dry.

Then, mix the carrots with the remaining ingredients in a big bowl. Make small balls from the mixture.

Gently flatten them with your hand. Spitz the balls with nonstick cooking oil.

Add the in balls to the basket.

Push the air-frying basket in the air fryer. Cook for 8-10 minutes.

Slide-out the basket; serve warm!

Nutrition: Calories: 274; Fat: 8.3 g; Carbohydrates: 38.8 g; Fiber: 2.3 g; Protein: 15.6 g.

75 BUTTER BAKED NUTS

Preparation Time: 10 minutes
Cooking Time: 15 minutes
Servings: 4
Ingredients:

1 cup raw almonds or pistachios
1 cup raw peanuts
1 tbsp. butter, melted
½ cup raw cashew nuts
Salt to taste

Directions:

Take Power XL multi-cooker, arrange it over a cooking platform, and open the top lid.

In the pot, arrange a reversible rack and place the Crisping Basket over the rack.

In the basket, add the nuts.

Seal the multi-cooker by locking it with the crisping lid; ensure to keep the pressure release valve locked/sealed.

Select the "AIR CRISP" mode and adjust the 350°F temperature level. Then, set Timer to 10 minutes and press "STOP/START"; it will start the cooking process by building up inside pressure.

When the Timer goes off, quick release pressure by adjusting the pressure valve to the VENT.

After pressure gets released, open the pressure lid.

Add the butter on top and season with some salt; shake well.

Seal the multi-cooker by locking it with the crisping lid; ensure to keep the pressure release valve locked/sealed.

Select "BAKE/ROAST" mode and adjust the 350°F temperature level. Then, set Timer to 5 minutes and press "STOP/START"; it will start the cooking process by building up inside pressure.

When the timer goes off, quick release pressure by adjusting the pressure valve to the VENT. After pressure gets released, open the pressure lid.

Serve warm and enjoy!

Nutrition: Calories: 192; Fat: 16 g; Saturated Fat: 2 g; Trans Fat: 0 g; Carbohydrates: 6.5 g; Fiber: 3 g; Sodium: 64 mg; Protein: 7.5 g.

76 EGGS SPINACH SIDE

Preparation Time: 5 minutes
Cooking Time: 12 minutes
Servings: 2 to 3
Ingredients:

1 medium-sized tomato, chopped
1 tsp. lemon juice
½ tsp. coarse salt
2 tbsp. olive oil
4 eggs, whisked
5 oz. spinach, chopped
½ tsp. black pepper
½ cup basil, roughly chopped

Directions:

Place your air fryer on a flat kitchen surface; plug it and turn it on. Set temperature to 280°F and let it preheat for 4-5 minutes.

Take out the air-frying basket and gently coat it using olive oil.

In a bowl of medium size, thoroughly mix the ingredients except for the basil leaves.

Add the mixture to the basket. Push the air-frying basket in the air fryer. Cook for 10-12 minutes.

Slide-out the basket; top with basil and serve warm with sour cream!

Nutrition: Calories: 272; Fat: 23 g; Carbohydrates: 5.4 g; Fiber: 2 g; Protein: 13.2 g.

77 SQUASH AND CUMIN CHILI

Preparation Time: 10 minutes
Cooking Time: 25 minutes
Servings: 4
Ingredients:

- 1 medium butternut squash
- 1 tsp. cumin seed
- 1 large pinch of chili flakes
- 1 tbsp. olive oil
- 1 ½ oz. pine nuts
- 1 small bunch of fresh coriander, chopped

Directions:

- Take the squash and slice it.
- Remove seeds and cut into smaller chunks.
- Take a bowl and add chunked squash, spice, and oil.
- Mix well.
- Preheat your Fryer to 360°F and add the squash to the cooking basket.
- Roast for 20 minutes. Ensure to shake the basket from time to time to avoid burning.
- Take a pan and place it over medium heat. Add pine nuts to the pan, and dry toast for 2 minutes.
- Sprinkle nuts on top of the squash and serve.
- Enjoy!

Nutrition: Calories: 414; Fat: 15 g; Carbohydrates: 10 g; Protein: 16g.

78 FRIED UP AVOCADOS

Preparation Time: 10 minutes
Cooking Time: 20 minutes
Servings: 6
Ingredients:

- ½ cup almond meal
- ½ tsp. salt
- 1 Hass avocado, peeled, pitted, and sliced
- Aquafaba from one bean can (bean liquid)

Directions:

- Take a shallow bowl and add almond meal, salt.
- Pour Aquafaba in another bowl, dredge avocado slices in Aquafaba and then into the crumbs to get a nice coating.
- Assemble them in a single layer in your Air Fryer cooking basket; don't overlap.
- Cook for 10 minutes at 390°F. Give the basket a shake and cook for 5 minutes more.
- Serve and enjoy!

Nutrition: Calories: 356; Fat: 14 g; Carbohydrates: 8 g; Protein: 23 g.

79 HEARTY GREEN BEANS

Preparation Time: 5 minutes
Cooking Time: 10 to 15 minutes
Servings: 6
Ingredients:

- 1-pound green beans washed and de-stemmed
- 1 lemon
- Pinch of salt
- ¼ tsp. oil

Directions:

- Add beans to your Air Fryer cooking basket.
- Squeeze a few drops of lemon.
- Season with salt and pepper.
- Drizzle olive oil on top.
- Cook for 10-12 minutes at 400°F.
- Once done, serve and enjoy!

Nutrition: Calories: 84; Fat: 5 g; Carbohydrates: 7 g; Protein: 2 g.

80 PARMESAN CABBAGE WEDGES

Preparation Time: 5 minutes
Cooking Time: 20 minutes
Servings: 4
Ingredients:

- ½ head cabbage
- 2 cups parmesan
- 4 tbsp. melted butter
- Salt and pepper to taste

Directions:

- Preheat your Air Fryer to 380°F.
- Take a container and add melted butter, and season with salt and pepper.
- Cover cabbages with your melted butter.
- Coat cabbages with parmesan.
- Transfer the coated cabbages to your Air Fryer and bake for 20 minutes.
- Serve with cheesy sauce and enjoy!

Nutrition: Calories: 108; Fat: 7 g; Carbohydrates: 11 g; Protein: 2 g.

81 EXTREME ZUCCHINI FRIES

Preparation Time: 10 minutes
Cooking Time: 15 to 20 minutes
Servings: 4
Ingredients:

- 3 medium zucchinis, sliced
- 2 egg whites
- ½ cup seasoned almond meal
- 2 tbsp. grated parmesan cheese
- ¼ tsp. garlic powder

Directions:

- Preheat your Fryer to 425°F.
- Take the Air Fryer cooking basket and place a cooling rack.
- Coat the rack with cooking spray.
- Take a bowl, add egg whites, beat it well, and season with some pepper and salt.

Take another bowl and add garlic powder, cheese, and almond meal.

- Take the Zucchini sticks and dredge them in the egg and finally breadcrumbs.
- Transfer the Zucchini to your cooking basket and spray a bit of oil.
- Bake for 20 minutes and serve with Ranch sauce.
- Enjoy!

Nutrition: Calories: 367; Fat: 28 g; Carbohydrates: 5 g; Protein: 4 g.

82 EASY FRIED TOMATOES

Preparation Time: 5 minutes
Cooking Time: 10 minutes
Servings: 3
Ingredients:

- 1 green tomato
- ¼ tbsp. Creole seasoning
- Salt and pepper to taste
- ¼ cup almond flour
- ½ cup buttermilk

Directions:

- Add flour to your plate and take another plate and add buttermilk.
- Cut tomatoes and season with salt and pepper.
- Make a mix of creole seasoning and crumbs.
- Take tomato slice and cover with flour, place in buttermilk and then into crumbs.
- Repeat with all tomatoes.
- Preheat your fryer to 400°F.
- Cook the tomato slices for 5 minutes.
- Serve with basil and enjoy!

Nutrition: Calories: 166; Fat: 12 g; Carbohydrates: 11 g; Protein: 3 g.

83 ROASTED UP BRUSSELS

Preparation Time: 10 minutes
Cooking Time: 15 minutes
Servings: 4
Ingredients:

- 1 block Brussels sprouts
- ½ tsp. garlic
- 2 tsp. olive oil
- ½ tsp. pepper
- Salt as needed

Directions:

- Preheat your Fryer to 390°F.
- Remove leaves off the chokes, leaving only the head.
- Wash and dry the sprouts well.
- Make a mixture of olive oil, salt, and pepper with garlic.
- Cover sprouts with the marinade and let them rest for 5 minutes.
- Transfer coated sprouts to Air Fryer and cook for 15 minutes.
- Serve and enjoy!

Nutrition: Calories: 43; Fat: 2 g; Carbohydrates: 5 g; Protein: 2 g.

84 ROASTED BRUSSELS AND PINE NUTS

Preparation Time: 10 minutes
Cooking Time: 35 minutes
Servings: 6
Ingredients:

 15 oz. Brussels sprouts
 1 tbsp. olive oil
 1 ¼ oz. raisins, drained
 Juice of 1 orange
 1 ¼ oz. toasted pine nuts

Directions:

 Take a pot of boiling water, then add sprouts and boil them for 4 minutes.
 Transfer the sprouts to cold water and drain them well.
 Place them in a freezer and cool them.
 Take your raisins and soak them in orange juice for 20 minutes.
 Warm your Air Fryer to a temperature of 392°F.
 Take a pan and pour oil, and stir the sprouts.
 Take the sprouts and transfer them to your Air Fryer.
 Roast for 15 minutes.
 Serve the sprouts with pine nuts, orange juice, and raisins!

Nutrition: Calories: 260; Fat: 20 g; Carbohydrates: 10 g; Protein: 7g.

85 LOW-CALORIE BEETS DISH

Preparation Time: 10 minutes
Cooking Time: 10 minutes
Servings: 2
Ingredients:

 4 whole beets
 1 tbsp. balsamic vinegar
 1 tbsp. olive oil
 Salt and pepper to taste
 2 springs rosemary

Directions:

 Wash your beets and peel them.
 Cut beets into cubes.
 Take a bowl and mix in rosemary, pepper, salt, vinegar.
 Cover beets with the prepared sauce.
 Coat the beets with olive oil.
 Preheat your Fryer to 400°F.
 Transfer beets to Air Fryer cooking basket and cook for 10 minutes.
 Serve with your cheese sauce and enjoy!

Nutrition: Calories: 149; Fat: 1 g; Carbohydrates: 5 g; Protein: 30 g.

86 BROCCOLI AND PARMESAN DISH

Preparation Time: 5 minutes
Cooking Time: 20 minutes
Servings: 4
Ingredients:

 1 fresh head broccoli
 1 tbsp. olive oil
 1 lemon, juiced
 Salt and pepper to taste
 1-oz. parmesan cheese, grated

Directions:

 Wash broccoli thoroughly and cut them into florets.
 Add the listed ingredients to your broccoli and mix well.
 Preheat your fryer to 365°F.
 Air fry broccoli for 20 minutes.
 Serve and enjoy!

Nutrition: Calories: 114; Fat: 6 g; Carbohydrates: 10 g; Protein: 7 g.

87 HEALTHY LOW CARB FISH NUGGET

Preparation Time: 5 minutes
Cooking Time: 10 minutes
Servings: 4
Ingredients:

 1-pound fresh cod
 2 tbsp. olive oil
 ½ cup almond flour
 2 larges finely beaten eggs
 1-2 cups almond meal

Directions:

 Preheat your Air Fryer to 388°F.
 Take a food processor and add olive oil, almond meal, salt, and blend.
 Take three bowls and add almond flour, almond meal, beaten eggs individually.
 Take cods and cut them into slices of 1-inch thickness and 2-inch length.
 Dredge slices into flour, eggs, and crumbs.
 Transfer nuggets to Air Fryer cooking basket and cook for 10 minutes until golden.
 Serve and enjoy!

Nutrition: Calories: 196; Fat: 14 g; Carbohydrates: 6 g; Protein: 14 g.

88 FRIED UP PUMPKIN SEEDS

Preparation Time: 10 minutes
Cooking Time: 60 minutes
Servings: 2
Ingredients:

 1 ½ cups pumpkin seeds
 Olive oil as needed
 1 ½ tsp. salt
 1 tsp. smoked paprika

Directions:

 Cut pumpkin and scrape out seeds and flesh.
 Separate flesh from seeds and rinse the seeds under cold water.
 Bring two-quarter of salted water to boil and add seeds, boil for 10 minutes.

 Drain seeds and spread them on a kitchen towel.
 Dry for 20 minutes.
 Preheat your fryer to 350°F.
 Take a bowl and add seeds, smoked paprika, and olive oil.
 Season with salt and transfer to your Air Fryer cooking basket.
 Cook for 35 minutes, enjoy it!

Nutrition: Calories: 237; Fat: 21 g; Carbohydrates: 4 g; Protein: 12 g.

89 DECISIVE TIGER SHRIMP PLATTER

Preparation Time: 5 minutes
Cooking Time: 10 minutes
Servings: 6
Ingredients:

 1 ¼ pound tiger shrimp, or a count of about 16 to 20
 ¼ tsp. cayenne pepper
 ½ tsp. old bay seasoning
 ¼ tsp. smoked paprika
 1 tbsp. olive oil

Directions:

 Preheat your Fryer to 390°F.
 Take a bowl and add the listed ingredients.
 Mix well.
 Transfer the shrimp to your fryer cooking basket and cook for 5 minutes.
 Remove and serve the shrimp over cauliflower rice if preferred.
 Enjoy!

Nutrition: Calories: 251; Carbohydrate: 3 g; Protein: 17 g; Fat: 19 g.

90 AIR FRIED OLIVES

Preparation Time: 5 minutes
Cooking Time: 8 minutes
Servings: 4
Ingredients:

 1 (5 ½-oz. / 156-g;) jar pitted green olives
 ½ cup all-purpose flour
 Salt and pepper, to taste
 ½ cup bread crumbs
 1 egg

Directions:

 Preheat the air fryer oven to 400°F (204°C).
 Take away the olives from the jar and dry thoroughly with paper towels.
 In a small bowl, combine the flour with salt and pepper to taste. Place the bread crumbs in another small container. In a third small bowl, beat the egg.
 Grease the basket with cooking spray.
 Drench the olives in the flour, then the egg, and then the bread crumbs.
 Place the breaded olives in the air fryer basket. It is okay to stack them.

Coat the olives with cooking spray.

Place the air fryer basket onto the warming pan.

Slide into Rack Position 2.

Select Air Fry and set the Time to 6 minutes.

Flip the olives and air fry for an additional 2 minutes, or until brown and crisp.

Cool for 5 minutes before serving.

Nutrition: Calories: 188; Fat: 6.8 g; Carbs: 1.9 g; Protein: 30.3 g.

91 BACON-WRAPPED DATES

Preparation Time: 10 minutes
Cooking Time: 6 minutes
Servings: 6
Ingredients:

12 dates, pitted

6 slices of high-quality bacon, cut in half

Cooking spray

Directions:

Preheat the air fryer oven to 360°F (182°C).

Cover each date with half a bacon slice and secure with a toothpick.

Grease the air fryer basket with cooking spray. Then place bacon-wrapped dates in the basket.

Place the air fryer basket onto the baking pan.

Slide into Rack Position 2, select Air Fry, set Time to 6 minutes, or wait until the bacon is crispy.

Remove the dates and allow them to cool on a wire rack for 5 minutes before serving.

Nutrition: Calories: 246; Protein: 14.4 g; Fiber: 0.6 g; Net Carbohydrates: 2.0 g; Fat: 17.9 g; Sodium: 625 mg; Carbohydrates: 2.6 g.

92 BACON-WRAPPED SHRIMP AND JALAPEÑO

Preparation Time: 20 minutes
Cooking Time: 13 minutes
Servings: 8
Ingredients:

24 large shrimp, peeled and deveined, about ¾ pound (340 g)

5 tbsp. barbecue sauce, divided

12 strips bacon, cut in half

24 small pickled jalapeño slices

Directions:

Toss together the shrimp and three tablespoons of the barbecue sauce. Let stand for 15 minutes. Soak 24 wooden toothpicks in water for 10 minutes. Wrap 1-piece bacon around the shrimp and jalapeño slice, then secure with a toothpick.

Preheat the air fryer oven to 350°F (177°C).

Put the shrimp in the air fryer basket, spacing them ½ inch apart.

Place the air fryer basket onto the baking pan.

Slide into Rack Position 2, select Air Fry, and set Time to 10 minutes.

Turn shrimp over with tongs and air fry for 3 minutes more, or until bacon is golden brown and shrimp are cooked through.

Brush with the remaining barbecue sauce and serve.

Nutrition: Calories: 246; Protein: 14.4 g; Fiber: 0.6 g; Net Carbohydrates: 2.0 g; Fat: 17.9 g; Sodium: 625 mg; Carbohydrates: 2.6 g.

93 BREADED ARTICHOKE HEARTS

Preparation Time: 5 minutes
Cooking Time: 8 minutes
Servings: 14
Ingredients:

14 whole artichoke hearts, packed in water

1 egg

½ cup all-purpose flour

⅓ cup panko bread crumbs

1 tsp. Italian seasoning

Directions:

Preheat the air fryer oven to 380°F (193C).

Squeeze excess water from the artichoke hearts and place them on paper towels to dry.

In a small bowl, beat the egg.

In another small bowl, place the flour.

In a third small bowl, blend the bread crumbs and Italian seasoning, and stir.

Spritz the air fryer basket by means of cooking spray.

Drench the artichoke hearts in the flour, then the egg, and then the bread crumb mixture.

Place the breaded artichoke hearts in the air fryer basket. Coat them with cooking spray.

Place the air fryer basket onto the baking pan.

Slide into Rack Position 2, select Air Fry, and set Time to 8 minutes. You may wait until the artichoke hearts have browned and are crisp. Flip once halfway through the cooking time.

Let cool for 5 minutes before serving.

Nutrition: Calories: 149; Fat: 1 g; Carbohydrates: 5 g; Protein: 30 g.

94 BRUSCHETTA WITH BASIL PESTO

Preparation Time: 10 minutes
Cooking Time: 5 to 7 minutes
Servings: 4
Ingredients:

8 slices French bread, ½ inch thick

2 tbsp. softened butter

1 cup shredded Mozzarella cheese

½ cup basil pesto

1 cup chopped grape tomatoes

Directions:

Preheat the air fryer oven to 350°F (177°C).

Spread the bread with the butter and position butter-side up in a baking pan.

Slide the baking pan into Rack Position 1 and select Convection Bake. Set Time to 4 minutes, or wait until the bread is light golden brown.

Remove the bread from the oven and top each piece with some of the cheese.

Back to the oven and bake for 1 to 3 minutes more, or until the cheese melts.

In the meantime, combine the pesto, tomatoes, and green onions in a small bowl.

When the cheese has melted, remove the bread from the oven and put it on a serving platter. Top each slice utilizing some of the pesto mixtures and serve.

Nutrition: Calories: 251; Carbohydrate: 3 g; Protein: 17 g; Fat: 19 g.

95 CAJUN ZUCCHINI CHIPS

Preparation Time: 5 minutes
Cooking Time: 16 minutes
Servings: 4
Ingredients:

2 large zucchinis, cut into ⅛-inch-thick slices

2 tsp. Cajun seasoning

Cooking spray

Directions:

Preheat the air fryer oven to 370°F (188°C).

Spray the air fryer basket lightly with cooking spray.

Put the zucchini slices in a medium bowl and spray them generously with cooking spray.

Sprinkle the Cajun seasoning over the zucchini and stir to make sure they are evenly coated with oil and seasoning.

Put the slices in a single layer in the air fryer basket, making sure not to overcrowd.

Place the air fryer basket onto the baking pan.

Slide into Rack Position 2.

Select Air Fry and set the Time to 8 minutes.

Flip the slices over and air fry for an additional 7 to 8 minutes, or until they are as crunchy and brown as you prefer.

Serve immediately.

Nutrition: Calories: 367; Fat: 28 g; Carbohydrates: 5 g; Protein: 4 g.

96 CHEESY APPLE ROLL-UPS

Preparation Time: 5 minutes
Cooking Time: 5 minutes
Servings: 8
Ingredients:

8 slices whole wheat sandwich bread
4 oz. (113-g.) Colby Jack cheese, grated
½ small apple, chopped
2 tbsp. butter, melted

Directions:

Preheat the air fryer oven to 390°F (199°C).

Take away the crusts from the bread and flatten the slices with a rolling pin. Don't be gentle. Press hard so that the bread will be fragile.

Top bread slices with cheese and chopped apple, dividing the ingredients evenly.

Roll up each slice tightly and secure each with one or two toothpicks.

Brush outside of rolls with melted butter. Place them in the air fryer basket.

Place the air fryer basket onto the baking pan.

Slide into Rack Position 2, select Air Fry, and set Time to 5 minutes. You may also wait until the outside is crisp and nicely browned.

Serve hot.

Nutrition: Calories: 147; Fat: 9.5 g; Carbohydrates: 13.8 g; Sugar: 2.1 g; Protein: 1.9 g; Sodium: 62 mg.

97 CHEESY JALAPEÑO POPPERS

Preparation Time: 5 minutes
Cooking Time: 10 minutes
Servings: 4
Ingredients:

8 jalapeño peppers
½ cup whipped cream cheese
¼ cup shredded Cheddar cheese

Directions:

Preheat the air fryer oven to 360°F (182°C).

Practice a paring knife to carefully cut off the jalapeño tops; then scoop out the ribs and seeds. Set aside.

In a medium bowl, combine the whipped cream cheese and shredded Cheddar cheese. Place the mixture in a sealable plastic bag, and using a pair of scissors, cut off one corner from the bag. Gently squeeze some cream cheese mixture into each pepper until almost full.

Place a piece of parchment paper on the bottom of the air fryer basket and place the poppers on top, distributing evenly.

Place the air fryer basket onto the baking pan.

Slide into Rack Position 2, select Air Fry, and set Time to 10 minutes.

Allow the poppers to cool for 5 to 10 minutes before serving.

Nutrition: Calories: 456; Fat: 60 g; Carbohydrates: 7 g; Protein: 15 g.

98 CHEESY STEAK FRIES

Preparation Time: 5 minutes
Cooking Time: 20 minutes
Servings: 5
Ingredients:

1 (28-oz. / 794-g.) bag frozen steak fries
Cooking spray
½ cup beef gravy
1 cup shredded Mozzarella cheese
2 scallions, green parts only, chopped

Directions:

Preheat the air fryer oven to 400°F (204°C).

Place the frozen steak fries in the air fryer basket.

Place the air fryer basket onto the baking pan.

Slide into Rack Position 2, select Air Fry, and set Time to 10 minutes.

Shake the basket and spritz the fries with cooking spray. Sprinkle with salt and pepper. Air fry for an additional 8 minutes.

Pour the beef gravy into a medium, microwave-safe bowl—microwave for 30 seconds, or until the sauce is warm.

Sprinkle the fries with the cheese. Air fry for an additional 2 minutes until the cheese is melted.

Transfer the fries to a serving dish. Drizzle the fries with gravy and sprinkle the scallions on top for a green garnish. Serve warm.

Nutrition: Calories 1536; Fat 123.7 g; Protein 103.4 g.

99 CRISPY BREADED BEEF CUBES

Preparation Time: 10 minutes
Cooking Time: 8 minutes
Servings: 4
Ingredients:

1-pound (454-g.) sirloin tip, cut into 1-inch cubes
1 cup cheese pasta sauce
1 ½ cups soft bread crumbs
2 tbsp. olive oil
½ tsp. dried marjoram

Directions:

Preheat the air fryer oven to 360°F (182°C).

In a medium container, toss the beef with the pasta sauce to coat.

In a shallow bowl, blend the bread crumbs, oil, and marjoram, and stir completely. Put the beef cubes, one at a Time, into the bread crumb mixture to coat methodically. Transfer the beef to the air fryer basket.

Place the air fryer basket onto the baking pan.

Slide into Rack Position 2, select Air Fry, set Time to 8 minutes, or until the beef is at least 145°F (63°C), and the outside is crisp and brown. Shake the basket once during cooking time.

Serve hot.

Nutrition: Calories: 262; Total Fat: 9.4 g; Carbs: 8.2 g; Protein: 16.2 g.

100 CORIANDER ARTICHOKES

Preparation Time: 5 minutes
Cooking Time: 20 minutes
Servings: 4
Ingredients:

12 oz. artichoke hearts
1 tbsp. lemon juice
1 tsp. coriander, ground
½ tsp. cumin seeds
½ tsp. olive oil

Directions:

Mix all the ingredients, toss.

Introduce the pan in the fryer and cook at 370°F for 15 minutes.

Divide the mix between plates and serve as a side dish.

Nutrition: Calories: 200; Fat: 7 g; Fiber: 2 g; Carbs: 5 g; Protein: 8 g.

101 SPINACH AND ARTICHOKES SAUTÉ

Preparation Time: 5 minutes
Cooking Time: 15 minutes
Servings: 4
Ingredients:

10 oz. artichoke hearts; halved
2 cups baby spinach
3 garlic cloves
¼ cup veggie stock
2 tsp. lime juice
Salt and black pepper to taste.

Directions:

Mix all the ingredients, toss, introduce in the fryer and cook at 370°F for 15 minutes.

Divide between plates and serve.

Nutrition: Calories: 209; Fat: 6 g; Fiber: 2 g; Carbs: 4 g; Protein: 8 g.

102 GREEN BEANS

Preparation Time: 5 minutes
Cooking Time: 20 minutes
Servings: 4
Ingredients:

- 6 cups green beans; trimmed
- 1 tbsp. hot paprika
- 2 tbsp. olive oil
- A pinch of salt and black pepper

Directions:

Take a bowl and mix the green beans with the other ingredients, toss, put them in the air fryer's basket and cook at 370°F for 20 minutes.

Divide among plates and serve as a side dish.

Nutrition: Calories: 120; Fat: 5 g; Fiber: 1 g; Carbs: 4 g; Protein: 2 g.

103 BOK CHOY AND BUTTER SAUCE

Preparation Time: 5 minutes
Cooking Time: 15 minutes
Servings: 4
Ingredients:

- 2 bok choy heads; trimmed and cut into strips
- 1 tbsp. butter; melted
- 2 tbsp. chicken stock
- 1 tsp. lemon juice
- 1 tbsp. olive oil

Directions:

Mix all the ingredients, toss and introduce the pan to the air fryer. Then cook at 380°F for 15 minutes.

Split between plates and serve as a side dish.

Nutrition: Calories: 141; Fat: 3 g; Fiber: 2 g; Carbs: 4 g; Protein: 3 g.

104 TURMERIC MUSHROOM

Preparation Time: 5 minutes
Cooking Time: 15 minutes
Servings: 4
Ingredients:

- 1 lb. brown mushrooms
- 4 garlic cloves; minced
- ¼ tsp. cinnamon powder
- 1 tsp. olive oil
- ½ tsp. turmeric powder

Directions:

Mix all the fixings and toss.

Put the mushrooms in your air fryer's basket and cook at 370°F for 15 minutes.

Divide the mix between plates and serve as a side dish.

Nutrition: Calories: 208; Fat: 7 g; Fiber: 3 g; Carbs: 5 g; Protein: 7 g.

105 CREAMY FENNEL

Preparation Time: 5 minutes

Cooking Time: 12 minutes
Servings: 4
Ingredients:

- 2 big fennel bulbs; sliced
- ½ cup coconut cream
- 2 tbsp. butter; melted
- Salt and black pepper to taste.

Directions:

In a pan that fits the air fryer, combine all the ingredients, toss, introduce in the machine and cook at 370°F for 12 minutes.

Divide between plates and serve as a side dish.

Nutrition: Calories: 151; Fat: 3 g; Fiber: 2 g; Carbs: 4 g; Protein: 6 g.

106 AIR FRIED GREEN TOMATOES

Preparation Time: 5 minutes
Cooking Time: 17 minutes
Servings: 4
Ingredients:

- 2 medium green tomatoes
- ⅓ cup grated Parmesan cheese.
- ¼ cup blanched finely ground almond flour.
- 1 large egg

Directions:

Slice tomatoes into ½-inch-thick slices. Take a medium bowl, whisk the egg. Take a large bowl, mix the almond flour and Parmesan.

Dip each tomato slice into the egg, then scour in the almond flour mixture. Put the slices into the air fryer basket.

Adjust the temperature to 400°F and set the timer for 7 minutes. Flip the slices midway over the cooking time. Serve immediately.

Nutrition: Calories: 106; Protein: 6.2 g; Fiber: 1.4 g; Fat: 6.7 g; Carbs: 5.9 g.

107 SEASONED POTATO WEDGES

Preparation Time: 10 minutes
Cooking Time: 20 minutes
Servings: 4
Ingredients:

- 4 russet potatoes
- 1 tbsp. bacon fat
- 1 tsp. paprika
- 1 tsp. chili powder
- 1 tsp. salt

Directions:

Wash potatoes and portion into eight slices.

Warm bacon fat in the microwave for 10 seconds.

Combine all of your dry seasonings in a bowl and toss to mix.

Add bacon fat to the bowl and stir.

Toss the wedges in the bowl and transfer to the basket.

Cook at the preset chicken setting, tossing halfway through.

Nutrition: Calories: 171; Sodium: 684 mg; Dietary Fiber: 5.6 g; Fat: 1.9 g; Carbs: 34.3 g; Protein: 5.1 g.

108 HONEY ROASTED CARROTS

Preparation Time: 5 minutes
Cooking Time: 10 minutes
Servings: 4
Ingredients:

- 1 tbsp. olive oil
- 3 cups baby carrots
- 1 tbsp. honey
- salt and pepper to taste

Directions:

In a container, put the carrots; then, drizzle with oil and honey.

Sprinkle on salt and pepper. Blend it entirely using a wooden spoon.

Put the carrots in the basket and cook at 400°for 10 minutes.

For best results, serve immediately.

Nutrition: Calories: 83; Sodium: 74 mg; Dietary Fiber: 2.5 g; Fat: 3.5 g; Carbs: 13 g; Protein: 1.3 g.

109 ONION RINGS

Preparation Time: 7 minutes
Cooking Time: 7 minutes
Servings: 4
Ingredients:

- 1 tsp. baking powder
- 1 cup panko breadcrumbs
- 2 eggs
- 1 large Vidalia onion
- 1 cup all-purpose flour

Directions:

Peel, core, and cut the onion into rings.

Combine the flour, salt, and baking powder in a bag and shake well to combine.

Add the onions to the bag and toss to coat.

Beat the eggs in a shallow bowl.

Spread the panko crumbs over a plate.

Remove one ring at a time. Shake off any extra flour and dip in the egg. Then dredge through the bread crumb.

Add 5 to 7 rings to the fryer and cook at 400°F for 7 minutes.

Flip the rings halfway through and serve hot.

Nutrition: Calories: 186; Sodium: 615 mg; Dietary Fiber: 1.8 g; Fat: 2.6 g; Carbs: 33.3 g; Protein: 7.1 g.

110 CHICKEN KEBAB

Preparation Time: 15 minutes
Cooking Time: 15 minutes
Servings: 6
Ingredients:

- 1.5 lb. boneless chicken breast, cut into large, bite-sized pc
- ½ tsp. smoked paprika
- 1 tsp. turmeric
- ½ tsp. ground black pepper
- ¼ cup plain Greek yogurt

Directions:

- Place chicken into a large bowl.
- Put Greek yogurt, smoked paprika, black pepper, and turmeric in a small blender container and process till you get a smooth mixture.
- Pour the blend over the chicken and coat it evenly.
- Allow chicken to marinate for 15 minutes.
- Put the chicken inside the basket of the air fryer.
- Set the air fryer to 370°F and cook for 15 minutes.
- After 8 minutes, flip the chicken over and continue cooking.
- Once done, allow them to sit for several minutes and serve.

Nutrition: Calories: 150; Fats: 2 g; Protein: 20 g; Carbs: 0.5 g.

111 ITALIAN BREAKFAST SAUSAGE WITH BABY POTATOES AND VEGETABLES

Preparation Time: 15 minutes
Cooking Time: 30 minutes
Servings: 4
Ingredients:

- 1 lb. sweet Italian sausage links, sliced on the bias (diagonal)
- 2 cups baby potatoes, halved
- 2 cups broccoli florets
- 1 cup onions cut into 1-inch chunks
- 2 cups small mushrooms -half or quarter the large ones for uniform size
- 1 cup baby carrots
- 2 tbsp. olive oil
- ½ tsp. garlic powder
- ½ tsp. Italian seasoning
- 1 tsp. salt
- ½ tsp. pepper

Directions:

- Preheat the oven to 400°F.
- In a large bowl, add the baby potatoes, broccoli florets, onions, small mushrooms, and baby carrots.
- Add in the olive oil, salt, pepper, garlic powder and Italian seasoning and toss to evenly coat. Spread the vegetables onto a sheet pan in one even layer.
- Arrange the sausage slices on the pan over the vegetables. Bake for 30 minutes – make sure to sake halfway through to prevent sticking. Allow to cool.
- Distribute the Italian sausages and vegetables among the containers and store in the fridge for 2-3 days

Nutrition: Calories: 321; Fat: 16 g; Carbs: 23 g; Protein: 22 g.

112 CAULIFLOWER FRITTERS WITH HUMMUS

Preparation Time: 15 minutes
Cooking Time: 15 minutes
Servings: 4
Ingredients:

- 2 (15-oz.) cans chickpeas, divided
- 2 ½ tbsp. olive oil, divided, plus more for frying
- 1 cup onion, chopped, about ½ a small onion
- 2 tbsp. garlic, minced
- 2 cups cauliflower, cut into small pieces, about ½ a large head
- ½ tsp. salt
- black pepper

Topping:

- Hummus, of choice
- Green onion, diced

Directions:

- Preheat oven to 400°F. Rinse and drain 1 can of the chickpeas. Place them on a paper towel to dry off well.
- Then put the chickpeas into a large bowl, removing the loose skins that come off, and toss with 1 tablespoon of olive oil, spread the chickpeas onto a large pan and sprinkle with salt and pepper.
- Bake for 20 minutes. Stir and then bake an additional 5-10 minutes until very crispy.
- Once the chickpeas are roasted, transfer them to a large food processor and process until broken down and crumble - Don't over process them and turn it into flour, as you need to have some texture. Place the mixture into a small bowl, set aside.
- In a large pan over medium-high heat, add the remaining 1 ½ tablespoon of olive oil. Once heated, add in the onion and garlic, cook until lightly golden brown, about 2 minutes.
- Then add in the chopped cauliflower, cook for an additional 2 minutes, until the cauliflower is golden.

Turn the heat down to low and cover the pan, cook until the cauliflower is fork tender and the onions are golden brown and caramelized, stirring often, about 3-5 minutes.

- Transfer the cauliflower mixture to the food processor. Drain and rinse the remaining can of chickpeas and add them into the food processor, along with the salt and a pinch of pepper.
- Blend until smooth, and the mixture starts to ball. Stop to scrape down the sides as needed.
- Transfer the cauliflower mixture into a large bowl and add in ½ cup of the roasted chickpea crumbs, stir until well combined.
- In a large bowl over medium heat, add in enough oil to lightly cover the bottom of a large pan. Working in batches, cook the patties until golden brown, about 2-3 minutes, flip and cook again. Serve.

Nutrition: Calories: 333; Carbohydrates: 45 g; Fat: 13 g; Protein: 14 g.

113 OVERNIGHT BERRY CHIA OATS

Preparation Time: 15 minutes
Cooking Time: 5 minutes
Servings: 1
Ingredients:

- ½ cup Quaker Oats rolled oats
- ¼ cup chia seeds
- 1 cup milk or water
- Pinch of salt and cinnamon
- maple syrup, or a different sweetener, to taste
- 1 cup frozen berries of choice or smoothie leftovers

Toppings:

- Yogurt
- Berries

Directions:

- In a jar with a lid, add the oats, seeds, milk, salt, and cinnamon, refrigerate overnight. On serving day, puree the berries in a blender.
- Stir the oats, add in the berry puree and top with yogurt and more berries, nuts, honey, or garnish of your choice. Enjoy!

Nutrition: Calories: 405; Carbs: 65 g; Fat: 11 g; Protein: 17 g.

114 RASPBERRY VANILLA SMOOTHIE

Preparation Time: 5 minutes
Cooking Time: 5 minutes
Servings: 2 cups
Ingredients:

- 1 cup frozen raspberries
- 6-oz. container of vanilla Greek yogurt
- ½ cup of unsweetened vanilla almond milk

Directions:

Take all of your ingredients and place them in a blender. Process until smooth and liquified.

Nutrition: Calories: 155; Protein: 7 g; Fat: 2 g; Carbohydrates: 30 g.

115 BLUEBERRY BANANA PROTEIN SMOOTHIE

Preparation Time: 5 minutes
Cooking Time: 5 minutes
Servings: 1
Ingredients:

- ½ cup frozen and unsweetened blueberries
- ½ banana slices up
- ¼ cup plain nonfat Greek yogurt
- ¼ cup unsweetened vanilla almond milk
- 2 cups of ice cubes

Directions:

Add all of the ingredients into a blender. Blend until smooth.

Nutrition: Calories: 230; Protein: 19.1 g; Fat: 2.6 g; Carbohydrates: 32.9 g.

116 CHOCOLATE BANANA SMOOTHIE

Preparation Time: 5 minutes
Cooking Time: 0 minutes
Servings: 2
Ingredients:

- 2 bananas, peeled
- 1 cup unsweetened almond milk, or skim milk
- 1 cup crushed ice
- 3 tbsp. unsweetened cocoa powder
- 3 tbsp. honey

Directions:

In a blender, combine the bananas, almond milk, ice, cocoa powder, and honey. Blend until smooth.

Nutrition: Calories: 219; Protein: 2 g; Carbohydrates: 57 g; Fat: 2 g.

117 MOROCCAN AVOCADO SMOOTHIE

Preparation Time: 5 minutes
Cooking Time: 0 minutes
Servings: 4
Ingredients:

- 1 ripe avocado, peeled and pitted
- 1 overripe banana
- 1 cup almond milk, unsweetened
- 1 cup of ice

Directions:

Place the avocado, banana, milk, and ice into your blender. Blend until smooth with no pieces of avocado remaining.

Nutrition: Calories: 100; Protein: 1 g; Fat: 6 g; Carbohydrates: 11 g.

118 GREEK YOGURT WITH FRESH BERRIES, HONEY AND NUTS

Preparation Time: 5 minutes
Cooking Time: 0 minutes
Servings: 1
Ingredients:

- 6 oz. nonfat plain Greek yogurt
- ½ cup fresh berries of your choice
- 1 tbsp. (.25-oz.) crushed walnuts
- 1 tbsp. honey

Directions:

In a jar with a lid, add the yogurt. Top with berries and a drizzle of honey. Top with the lid and store in the fridge for 2-3 days.

Nutrition: Calories: 250; Carbs: 35 Fat: 4 g; Protein: 19 g.

119 MEDITERRANEAN EGG MUFFINS WITH HAM

Preparation Time: 15 minutes
Cooking Time: 15 minutes
Servings: 6
Ingredients:

- 9 Slices of thin cut deli ham
- ½ cup canned roasted red pepper, sliced + additional for garnish
- ⅓ cup fresh spinach, minced
- ¼ cup feta cheese, crumbled
- 5 large eggs
- Pinch of salt
- Pinch of pepper
- 1 ½ tbsp. Pesto sauce
- Fresh basil for garnish

Directions:

Preheat oven to 400°F. Coat a muffin tin with cooking spray, generously. Line each of the muffin tin with 1 ½ pieces of ham — making sure there aren't any holes for the egg mixture to come out.

Place some of the roasted red pepper in the bottom of each muffin tin. Place 1 tablespoon of minced spinach on top of each red pepper. Top the pepper and spinach off with a large ½ tbsp of crumbled feta cheese.

In a medium bowl, whisk together the eggs salt and pepper, divide the egg mixture evenly among the 6 muffin tins.

Bake for 15 to 17 minutes until the eggs are puffy and set. Remove each cup from the muffin tin. Allow to cool completely

Distribute the muffins among the containers, store in the fridge for 2 - 3days or in the freezer for 3 months.

Nutrition: Calories: 109; Carbs: 2 g; Fat: 6 g; Protein: 9 g.

120 QUINOA BAKE WITH BANANA

Preparation Time: 15 minutes
Cooking Time: 1 hour & 10 minutes
Servings: 8
Ingredients:

- 3 cups medium over-ripe bananas, mashed
- ¼ cup molasses
- ¼ cup pure maple syrup
- 1 tbsp. cinnamon
- 2 tsp. raw vanilla extract
- 1 tsp. ground ginger
- 1 tsp. ground cloves
- ½ tsp. ground allspice
- ½ tsp. salt
- 1 cup quinoa, uncooked
- 2 ½ cups unsweetened vanilla almond milk
- ¼ cup slivered almonds

Directions:

In the bottom of a 2 ½-3-quart casserole dish. Mix together the mashed banana, maple syrup, cinnamon, vanilla extract, ginger, cloves, allspice, molasses, and salt until well mixed.

Add in the quinoa, stir until the quinoa is evenly in the banana mixture. Whisk in the almond milk, mix until well combined, cover and refrigerate overnight or bake immediately.

Heat oven to 350°F. Whisk the quinoa mixture making sure it doesn't settle to the bottom.

Cover the pan with tinfoil and bake until the liquid is absorbed, and the top of the quinoa is set, about 1 hour to 1 hour and 15 minutes.

Turn the oven to high broil, uncover the pan, sprinkle with sliced almonds, and lightly press them into the quinoa.

Broil until the almonds just turn golden brown, about 2-4 minutes, watching closely, as they burn quickly. Allow to cool for 10 minutes then slice the quinoa bake.

Distribute the quinoa bake among the containers, store in the fridge for 3-4 days.

Nutrition: Calories: 213; Carbs: 41 g; Fat: 4 g; Protein: 5 g.

121 SUN-DRIED TOMATOES, DILL AND FETA OMELET CASSEROLE

Preparation Time: 15 minutes
Cooking Time: 40 minutes
Servings: 6
Ingredients:

    12 large eggs
    2 cups whole milk
    8 oz. fresh spinach
    2 cloves garlic, minced
    12 oz. artichoke salad with olives and peppers, drained and chopped
    5 oz. sun-dried tomato
    feta cheese, crumbled
    1 tbsp. fresh chopped dill or 1 tsp dried dill
    1 tsp. dried oregano
    1 tsp. lemon pepper
    1 tsp. salt
    4 tsp. olive oil, divided

Directions:

    Preheat oven to 375°F. Chop the fresh herbs and artichoke salad. In a skillet over medium heat, add 1 tablespoon of olive oil.
    Sauté the spinach and garlic until wilted, about 3 minutes. Oil a 9x13 inch baking dish, layer the spinach and artichoke salad evenly in the dish.
    In a medium bowl, whisk together the eggs, milk, herbs, salt and lemon pepper. Pour the egg mixture over vegetables, sprinkle with feta cheese.
    Bake in the center of the oven for 35-40 minutes until firm in the center. Allow to cool. Slice and distribute among the storage containers. Store for 2-3 days or freeze for 3 months.

Nutrition: Calories: 196; Carbohydrates: 5 g; Fat: 12 g; Protein: 10 g.

122 BREAKFAST TACO SCRAMBLE

Preparation Time: 15 minutes
Cooking Time: 1 hour & 25 minutes
Servings: 4
Ingredients:

    8 large eggs, beaten
    ¼ tsp. seasoning salt
    1 lb. 99% lean ground turkey
    2 tbsp. Greek seasoning
    ½ small onion, minced
    2 tbsp. bell pepper, minced
    4 oz. can tomato sauce
    ¼ cup water

¼ cup chopped scallions or cilantro, for topping

For the potatoes:
    12 (1 lb.) baby gold or red potatoes, quartered
    4 tsp. olive oil
    ¾ tsp. salt
    ½ tsp. garlic powder
    fresh black pepper, to taste

Directions:

    In a large bowl, beat the eggs and add with seasoning salt. Preheat the oven to 425°F. Spray a 9x12 or large oval casserole dish with cooking oil.
    Add the potatoes, 1 tablespoon of oil, ¾ teaspoons of salt, garlic powder and black pepper and toss to coat. Bake for 45 minutes to 1 hour, tossing every 15 minutes.
    In the meantime, brown the turkey in a large skillet over medium heat, breaking it up while it cooks. Once no longer pink, add in the Greek seasoning.
    Add in the bell pepper, onion, tomato sauce and water, stir and cover, simmer on low for about 20 minutes. Spray a different skillet with nonstick spray over medium heat.
    Once heated, add in the eggs seasoned with ¼ teaspoon of salt and scramble for 2–3 minutes, or cook until it sets.
    Distribute ¾ cup of turkey and ⅔ cup of eggs and divide the potatoes in each storage container, store for 3-4 days.

Nutrition: Calories: 450; Fat: 19 g; Carbs: 24.5 g; Protein: 46 g.

123 GREEK BEANS TORTILLAS

Preparation Time: 5 minutes
Cooking Time: 20 minutes
Servings: 4
Ingredients:

    1 red onion, chopped
    2 garlic cloves, minced
    1 tbsp. olive oil
    1 green bell pepper, sliced
    3 cups canned pinto beans, drained and rinsed
    2 red chili peppers, chopped
    4 tbsp. parsleys, chopped
    1 tsp. cumin, ground
    A pinch of salt and black pepper
    4 whole wheat Greek tortillas
    1 cup cheddar cheese, shredded

Directions:

    Heat up a pan with the oil over medium heat. Add the onion and sauté for 5 minutes.

Add the rest of the ingredients, except the tortillas and the cheese, stir and cook for 15 minutes.
Divide the beans mix on each Greek tortilla; also divide the cheese, roll the tortillas and serve for breakfast.

Nutrition: Calories: 673; Fat: 14.9; Fiber: 23.7; Carbs: 75.4; Protein: 39.

124 BAKED CAULIFLOWER HASH

Preparation Time: 10 minutes
Cooking Time: 25 minutes
Servings: 4
Ingredients:

    4 cups cauliflower florets
    1 tbsp. olive oil
    2 cups white mushrooms, sliced
    1 cup cherry tomatoes, halved
    1 yellow onion, chopped
    2 garlic cloves, minced
    ¼ tsp. garlic powder
    3 tbsp. basil, chopped
    3 tbsp. mint, chopped
    1 tbsp. dill, chopped

Directions:

    Spread the cauliflower florets on a baking sheet lined with parchment paper. Add the rest of the ingredients, introduce to the oven at 350°F and bake for 25 minutes.
    Divide the hash between plates and serve for breakfast.

Nutrition: Calories: 367; Fat: 14.3; Fiber: 3.5; Carbs: 16.8; Protein: 12.2.

125 EGGS, MINT AND TOMATOES

Preparation Time: 10 minutes
Cooking Time: 15 minutes
Servings: 2
Ingredients:

    2 eggs, whisked
    2 tomatoes, cubed
    2 tsp. olive oil
    1 tbsp. mint, chopped
    1 tbsp. chives, chopped
    Salt and black pepper to the taste

Directions:

    Heat up a pan with the oil over medium heat. Add the tomatoes and the rest of the ingredients except the eggs, stir and cook for 5 minutes.
    Add the eggs, toss, cook for 10 minutes more, divide between plates and serve.

Nutrition: Calories: 300; Fat: 15.3; Fiber: 4.5; Carbs: 17.7; Protein: 11.

126 BACON, SPINACH AND TOMATO SANDWICH

Preparation Time: 5 minutes
Cooking Time: 0 minutes
Servings: 1
Ingredients:

- 2 whole-wheat bread slices, toasted
- 1 tbsp. Dijon mustard
- 3 bacon slices
- Salt and black pepper to the taste
- 2 tomato slices
- ¼ cup baby spinach

Directions:

- Spread the mustard on each bread slice, divide the bacon and the rest of the ingredients on one slice, top with the other one, cut in half and serve for breakfast.

Nutrition: Calories: 246; Fat: 11.2; Fiber: 4.5; Carbs: 17.5; Protein: 8.3.

127 COTTAGE CHEESE AND BERRIES OMELET

Preparation Time: 5 minutes
Cooking Time: 4 minutes
Servings: 1
Ingredients:

- 1 egg, whisked
- ½ tsp. olive oil
- 1 tsp. cinnamon powder
- 1 tbsp. almond milk
- 3 oz. cottage cheese
- 4 oz. blueberries

Directions:

- In a bowl, mix the egg with the rest of the ingredients, except the oil and toss.
- Heat up a pan with the oil over medium heat. Add the eggs mix, spread, cook for 2 minutes on each side. Transfer to a plate and serve.

Nutrition: Calories: 219; Protein: 2 g; Carbohydrates: 57 g; Fat: 2 g.

128 SALMON FRITTATA

Preparation Time: 5 minutes
Cooking Time: 27 minutes
Servings: 4
Ingredients:

- 1-pound gold potatoes, roughly cubed
- 1 tbsp. olive oil
- Cooking spray
- 2 salmon fillets, skinless and boneless
- 8 eggs, whisked
- 1 tsp. mint, chopped
- A pinch of salt and black pepper

Directions:

- Put the potatoes in a pot and add water to cover. Bring to a boil over medium heat, cook for 12 minutes, drain and transfer to a bowl.
- Arrange the salmon on a baking sheet lined with parchment paper. Grease with cooking spray and broil over medium-high heat for 5 minutes on each side. Cool down, flake and put in a separate bowl.
- Heat up a pan with the oil over medium heat. Add the potatoes, salmon, and the rest of the ingredients, except the eggs and toss.
- Add the eggs on top. Put the lid on and cook over medium heat for 10 minutes.
- Divide the salmon between plates and serve.

Nutrition: Calories: 220 ; Protein: 4 g; Carbohydrates: 47 g; Fat: 2 g.

129 CORIANDER MUSHROOM SALAD

Preparation Time: 5 minutes
Cooking Time: 7 minutes
Servings: 6
Ingredients:

- ½ pounds white mushrooms, sliced
- 1 tbsp. olive oil
- 3 garlic cloves, minced
- Salt and black pepper to the taste
- 1 tomato, diced
- 1 avocado, peeled, pitted and cubed
- 3 tbsp. lime juice
- ½ cup chicken stock
- 2 tbsp. coriander, chopped

Directions:

- Heat up a pan with the oil over medium heat. Add the mushrooms and sauté them for 4 minutes.
- Add the rest of the ingredients. Toss, cook for 3-4 minutes more, divide into bowls and serve for breakfast.

Nutrition: 119; Protein: 2 g; Carbohydrates: 52 g; Fat: 11 g.

130 CINNAMON APPLE AND LENTILS PORRIDGE

Preparation Time: 5 minutes
Cooking Time: 10 minutes
Servings: 4
Ingredients:

- ½ cup walnuts, chopped
- 2 green apples, cored, peeled and cubed
- 3 tbsp. maple syrup
- 3 cups almond milk
- ½ cup red lentils
- ½ tsp. cinnamon powder
- ½ cup cranberries, dried
- 1 tsp. vanilla extract

Directions:

- Put the milk in a pot and heat it up over medium heat. Add the walnuts, apples, maple syrup and the rest of the ingredients. Toss, simmer for 10 minutes, divide into bowls and serve.

Nutrition: Calories: 150; Fat: 2; Fiber: 1; Carbs: 3; Protein: 5.

131 LENTILS AND CHEDDAR FRITTATA

Preparation Time: 10 minutes
Cooking Time: 15 minutes
Servings: 4
Ingredients:

- 1 red onion, chopped
- 2 tbsp. olive oil
- 1 cup sweet potatoes, boiled and chopped
- ¾ cup ham, chopped
- 4 eggs, whisked
- ¾ cup lentils, cooked
- 2 tbsp. Greek yogurt
- Salt and black pepper to the taste
- ½ cup cherry tomatoes, halved
- ¼ cup cheddar cheese, grated

Directions:

- Heat up a pan with the oil over medium heat. Add the onion, stir and sauté for 2 minutes.
- Add the rest of the ingredients, except the eggs and the cheese. Toss and cook for 3 minutes more.
- Add the eggs. Sprinkle the cheese on top, cover the pan and cook for 10 minutes more.
- Slice the frittata, divide between plates and serve.

Nutrition: Calories: 219; Protein: 2 g; Carbohydrates: 57 g; Fat: 2 g.

132 SEEDS AND LENTILS OATS

Preparation Time: 10 minutes
Cooking Time: 50 minutes
Servings: 4
Ingredients:

- ½ cup red lentils
- ¼ cup pumpkin seeds, toasted
- 2 tsp. olive oil
- ¼ cup rolled oats
- ¼ cup coconut flesh, shredded
- 1 tbsp. honey
- 1 tbsp. orange zest, grated
- 1 cup Greek yogurt
- 1 cup blackberries

Directions:

- Spread the lentils on a baking sheet lined with parchment paper. Introduce to the oven and roast at 370°F for 30 minutes.
- Add the rest of the ingredients except the yogurt and the berries. Toss and bake at 370°F for 20 minutes more.
- Transfer this to a bowl, add the rest of the ingredients. Toss, divide into

smaller bowls and serve for breakfast.

Nutrition: Calories: 204; Fat: 7.1; Fiber: 10.4; Carbs: 27.6; Protein: 9.5.

133 ORZO AND VEGGIE BOWLS

Preparation Time: 10 minutes
Cooking Time: 0 minutes
Servings: 4
Ingredients:

2 ½ cups whole-wheat orzo, cooked
14 oz. canned cannellini beans, drained and rinsed
1 yellow bell pepper, cubed
1 green bell pepper, cubed
A pinch of salt and black pepper
3 tomatoes, cubed
1 red onion, chopped
1 cup mint, chopped
2 cups feta cheese, crumbled
2 tbsp. olive oil
¼ cup lemon juice
1 tbsp. lemon zest, grated
1 cucumber, cubed
1 ¼ cup kalamata olives, pitted and sliced
3 garlic cloves, minced

Directions:

In a salad bowl, combine the orzo with the beans, bell peppers and the rest of the ingredients. Toss, divide the mix between plates and serve for breakfast.

Nutrition: Calories: 411; Fat: 17; Fiber: 13; Carbs: 51; Protein: 14.

134 LEMON PEAS QUINOA MIX

Preparation Time: 10 minutes
Cooking Time: 20 minutes
Servings: 4
Ingredients:

1 ½ cups quinoa, rinsed
1-pound asparagus, steamed and chopped
3 cups water
2 tbsp. parsley, chopped
2 tbsp. lemon juice
1 tsp. lemon zest, grated
½ pound sugar snap peas, steamed
½ pound green beans, trimmed and halved
A pinch of salt and black pepper
3 tbsp. pumpkin seeds
1 cup cherry tomatoes, halved
2 tbsp. olive oil

Directions:

Put the water in a pot and bring to a boil over medium heat. Add the quinoa, stir and simmer for 20 minutes.
Stir the quinoa, add the parsley, lemon juice and the rest of the ingredients. Toss, divide between plates and serve for breakfast.

Nutrition: Calories: 417; Fat: 15; Fiber: 9; Carbs: 58; Protein: 16.

135 WALNUTS YOGURT MIX

Preparation Time: 10 minutes
Cooking Time: 0 minutes
Servings: 6
Ingredients:

2 ½ cups Greek yogurt
1 ½ cups walnuts, chopped
1 tsp. vanilla extract
¾ cup honey
2 tsp. cinnamon powder

Directions:

In a bowl, combine the yogurt with the walnuts and the rest of the ingredients. Toss, divide into smaller bowls and keep in the fridge for 10 minutes before serving for breakfast.

Nutrition: Calories: 388; Fat: 24.6; Fiber: 2.9; Carbs: 39.1; Protein: 10.2.

136 STUFFED PITA BREADS

Preparation Time: 5 minutes
Cooking Time: 15 minutes
Servings: 4
Ingredients:

1 ½ tbsp. olive oil
1 tomato, cubed
1 garlic clove, minced
1 red onion, chopped
¼ cup parsley, chopped
15 oz. canned fava beans, drained and rinsed
¼ cup lemon juice
Salt and black pepper to the taste
4 whole-wheat pita bread pockets

Directions:

Heat up a pan with the oil over medium heat. Add the onion, stir and sauté for 5 minutes.
Add the rest of the ingredients. Stir and cook for 10 minutes more.
Stuff the pita pockets with this mix and serve for breakfast.

Nutrition: Calories: 382; Fat: 1.8; Fiber: 27.6; Carbs: 66; Protein: 28.5.

137 FARRO SALAD

Preparation Time: 5 minutes
Cooking Time: 4 minutes
Servings: 2
Ingredients:

1 tbsp. olive oil
A pinch of salt and black pepper
1 bunch baby spinach, chopped
1 avocado, pitted, peeled and chopped
1 garlic clove, minced
2 cups farro, already cooked
½ cup cherry tomatoes, cubed

Directions:

Heat up a pan with the oil over medium heat. Add the spinach, and the rest of the ingredients. Toss, cook for 4 minutes, divide into bowls and serve.

Nutrition: Calories: 157; Fat: 13.7; Fiber: 5.5; Carbs: 8.6; Protein: 3.6.

138 CRANBERRY AND DATES SQUARES

Preparation Time: 30 minutes
Cooking Time: 0 minutes
Servings: 10
Ingredients:

12 dates, pitted and chopped
1 tsp. vanilla extract
¼ cup honey
½ cup rolled oats
¾ cup cranberries, dried
¼ cup almond avocado oil, melted
1 cup walnuts, roasted and chopped
¼ cup pumpkin seeds

Directions:

In a bowl, mix the dates with the vanilla, honey and the rest of the ingredients. Stir well and press everything on a baking sheet lined with parchment paper.
Keep in the freezer for 30 minutes. Cut into 10 squares and serve for breakfast.

Nutrition: Calories: 263; Fat: 13.4; Fiber: 4.7; Carbs: 14.3; Protein: 3.5.

139 CHEESY EGGS RAMEKINS

Preparation Time: 10 minutes
Cooking Time: 10 minutes
Servings: 2
Ingredients:

1 tbsp. chives, chopped
1 tbsp. dill, chopped
A pinch of salt and black pepper
2 tbsp. cheddar cheese, grated
1 tomato, chopped
2 eggs, whisked
Cooking spray

Directions:

In a bowl, mix the eggs with the tomato and the rest of the ingredients, except the cooking spray, and whisk well.
Grease 2 ramekins with the cooking spray. Divide the mix into each ramekin, bake at 400°F for 10 minutes and serve.

Nutrition: Calories: 104; Fat: 7.1; Fiber: 0.6; Carbs: 2.6; Protein: 7.9.

140 LEEKS AND EGGS MUFFINS

Preparation Time: 10 minutes
Cooking Time: 20 minutes
Servings: 2
Ingredients:

3 eggs, whisked

¼ cup baby spinach
2 tbsp. leeks, chopped
4 tbsp. parmesan, grated
2 tbsp. almond milk
Cooking spray
1 small red bell pepper, chopped
Salt and black pepper to the taste
1 tomato, cubed
2 tbsp. cheddar cheese, grated

Directions:

In a bowl, combine the eggs with the milk, salt, pepper and the rest of the ingredients, except the cooking spray, and whisk well.

Grease a muffin tin with the cooking spray and divide the eggs mixture in each muffin mold.

Bake at 380°F for 20 minutes and serve them for breakfast.

Nutrition: Calories: 308; Fat: 19.4; Fiber: 1.7; Carbs: 8.7; Protein: 24.4.

141 ARTICHOKES AND CHEESE OMELET

Preparation Time: 10 minutes
Cooking Time: 8 minutes
Servings: 1
Ingredients:

1 tsp. avocado oil
1 tbsp. almond milk
2 eggs, whisked
A pinch of salt and black pepper
2 tbsp. tomato, cubed
2 tbsp. kalamata olives, pitted and sliced
1 artichoke heart, chopped
1 tbsp. tomato sauce
1 tbsp. feta cheese, crumbled

Directions:

In a bowl, combine the eggs with the milk, salt, pepper and the rest of the ingredients, except the avocado oil, and whisk well.

Heat up a pan with the avocado oil over medium-high heat. Add the omelet mix and spread into the pan. Cook for 4 minutes and flip. Cook for 4 minutes more, transfer to a plate and serve.

Nutrition: Calories: 303; Fat: 17.7; Fiber: 9.9; Carbs: 21.9; Protein: 18.2.

142 QUINOA AND EGGS SALAD

Preparation Time: 5 minutes
Cooking Time: 0 minutes
Servings: 4
Ingredients:

4 eggs, soft boiled, peeled and cut into wedges
2 cups baby arugula
2 cups cherry tomatoes, halved
1 cucumber, sliced
1 cup quinoa, cooked
1 cup almonds, chopped
1 avocado, peeled, pitted and sliced
1 tbsp. olive oil
½ cup mixed dill and mint, chopped
A pinch of salt and black pepper
Juice of 1 lemon

Directions:

In a large salad bowl, combine the eggs with the arugula and the rest of the ingredients. Toss, divide between plates and serve for breakfast.

Nutrition: Calories: 519; Fat: 32.4; Fiber: 11; Carbs: 43.3; Protein: 19.1.

143 CORN AND SHRIMP SALAD

Preparation Time: 10 minutes
Cooking Time: 10 minutes
Servings: 4
Ingredients:

4 ears of sweet corn, husked
1 avocado, peeled, pitted and chopped
½ cup basil, chopped
A pinch of salt and black pepper
1-pound shrimp, peeled and deveined
1 ½ cups cherry tomatoes, halved
¼ cup olive oil

Directions:

Put the corn in a pot. Add water to cover, bring to a boil over medium heat and cook for 6 minutes. Drain, cool down, cut corn from the cob and put it in a bowl.

Thread the shrimp onto skewers and brush with some of the oil.

Place the skewers on the preheated grill. Cook over medium heat for 2 minutes on each side, remove from skewers and add over the corn.

Add the rest of the ingredients to the bowl. Toss, divide between plates and serve for breakfast.

Nutrition: Calories: 371; Fat: 22; Fiber: 5; Carbs: 25; Protein: 23.

144 TOMATO AND LENTILS SALAD

Preparation Time: 10 minutes
Cooking Time: 35 minutes
Servings: 4
Ingredients:

2 yellow onions, chopped
4 garlic cloves, minced
2 cups brown lentils
1 tbsp. olive oil
A pinch of salt and black pepper
½ tsp. sweet paprika
½ tsp. ginger, grated
3 cups water
¼ cup lemon juice
¾ cup Greek yogurt
3 tbsp. tomato paste

Directions:

Heat up a pot with the oil over medium-high heat. Add the onions and sauté for 2 minutes.

Add the garlic and the lentils. Stir and cook for 1 minute more.

Add the water, bring to a simmer and cook covered for 30 minutes.

Add the lemon juice and the remaining ingredients, except for the yogurt. toss, divide the mix into bowls. Top with the yogurt and serve.

Nutrition: Calories: 294; Fat: 3; Fiber: 8; Carbs: 49; Protein: 21.

145 COUSCOUS AND CHICKPEAS BOWLS

Preparation Time: 10 minutes
Cooking Time: 6 minutes
Servings: 4
Ingredients:

¾ cup whole-wheat couscous
1 yellow onion, chopped
1 tbsp. olive oil
1 cup water
2 garlic cloves, minced
15 oz. canned chickpeas, drained and rinsed
A pinch of salt and black pepper
15 oz. canned tomatoes, chopped
14 oz. canned artichokes, drained and chopped
½ cup Greek olives, pitted and chopped
½ tsp. oregano, dried
1 tbsp. lemon juice

Directions:

Put the water in a pot. Bring to a boil over medium heat. Add the couscous, stir and take off the heat. Cover the pan, leave aside for 10 minutes and fluff with a fork.

Heat up a pan with the oil over medium-high heat. Add the onion and sauté for 2 minutes.

Add the rest of the ingredients. Toss and cook for 4 minutes more.

Add the couscous. Toss, divide into bowls and serve for breakfast.

Nutrition: Calories: 340; Fat: 10; Fiber: 9; Carbs: 51; Protein: 11.

146 ZUCCHINI AND QUINOA PAN

Preparation Time: 10 minutes
Cooking Time: 20 minutes
Servings: 4
Ingredients:

1 tbsp. olive oil
2 garlic cloves, minced
1 cup quinoa
1 zucchini, roughly cubed
2 tbsp. basil, chopped
¼ cup green olives, pitted and chopped
1 tomato, cubed

½ cup feta cheese, crumbled

2 cups water

1 cup canned garbanzo beans, drained and rinsed

A pinch of salt and black pepper

Directions:

Heat up a pan with the oil over medium-high heat. Add the garlic and quinoa and brown for 3 minutes.

Add the water, zucchinis, salt and pepper. Toss, bring to a simmer and cook for 15 minutes.

Add the rest of the ingredients. Toss, divide everything between plates and serve for breakfast.

Nutrition: Calories: 310; Fat: 11; Fiber: 6; Carbs: 42; Protein: 11.

147 CHEESY YOGURT

Preparation Time: 4 hours & 5 minutes

Cooking Time: 0 minutes

Servings: 4

Ingredients:

1 cup Greek yogurt

1 tbsp. honey

½ cup feta cheese, crumbled

Directions:

In a blender, combine the yogurt with the honey and the cheese and pulse well.

Divide into bowls and freeze for 4 hours before serving for breakfast.

Nutrition: Calories: 161; Fat: 10; Fiber: 0; Carbs: 11.8; Protein: 6.6.

148 BAKED OMELET MIX

Preparation Time: 10 minutes

Cooking Time: 45 minutes

Servings: 12

Ingredients:

12 eggs, whisked

8 oz. spinach, chopped

2 cups almond milk

12 oz. canned artichokes, chopped

2 garlic cloves, minced

5 oz. feta cheese, crumbled

1 tbsp. dill, chopped

1 tsp. oregano, dried

1 tsp. lemon pepper

A pinch of salt

4 tsp. olive oil

Directions:

Heat up a pan with the oil over medium-high heat. Add the garlic and the spinach and sauté for 3 minutes.

In a baking dish, combine the eggs with the artichokes and the rest of the ingredients.

Add the spinach mix as well. Toss a bit and bake the mix at 375°F for 40

minutes. Divide between plates and serve for breakfast.

Nutrition: Calories: 186; Fat: 13; Fiber: 1; Carbs: 5; Protein: 10.

149 STUFFED SWEET POTATO

Preparation Time: 10 minutes

Cooking Time: 40 minutes

Servings: 8

Ingredients:

8 sweet potatoes, pierced with a fork

14 oz. canned chickpeas, drained and rinsed

1 small red bell pepper, chopped

1 tbsp. lemon zest, grated

2 tbsp. lemon juice

3 tbsp. olive oil

1 tsp. garlic, minced

1 tbsp. oregano, chopped

2 tbsp. parsley, chopped

A pinch of salt and black pepper

1 avocado, peeled, pitted and mashed

¼ cup water

¼ cup tahini paste

Directions:

Arrange the potatoes on a baking sheet lined with parchment paper. Bake them at 400°F for 40 minutes. Cool them down and cut a slit down the middle in each.

In a bowl, combine the chickpeas with the bell pepper, lemon zest, half of the lemon juice, half of the oil, half of the garlic, oregano, half of the parsley, salt and pepper. Toss and stuff the potatoes with this mix.

In another bowl, mix the avocado with the water, tahini, the rest of the lemon juice, oil, garlic and parsley. Whisk well and spread over the potatoes.

Serve cold for breakfast.

Nutrition: Calories: 308; Fat: 2; Fiber: 8; Carbs: 38; Protein: 7.

150 CAULIFLOWER FRITTERS

Preparation Time: 10 minutes

Cooking Time: 50 minutes

Servings: 4

Ingredients:

30 oz. canned chickpeas, drained and rinsed

2 ½ tbsp. olive oil

1 small yellow onion, chopped

2 cups cauliflower florets chopped

2 tbsp. garlic, minced

A pinch of salt and black pepper

Directions:

Spread half of the chickpeas on a baking sheet lined with parchment pepper. Add 1 tablespoon of oil, season with salt

and pepper, toss and bake at 400°F for 30 minutes.

Transfer the chickpeas to a food processor. Pulse well and put the mix into a bowl.

Heat up a pan with ½ tablespoon of oil over medium-high heat. Add the garlic and the onion and sauté for 3 minutes.

Add the cauliflower. Cook for 6 minutes more and transfer this to a blender. Add the rest of the chickpeas. Pulse, pour over the crispy chickpeas mix from the bowl, stir and shape medium fritters out of this mix.

Heat up a pan with the rest of the oil over medium-high heat. Add the fritters, cook them for 3 minutes on each side and serve for breakfast.

Nutrition: Calories: 333; Fat: 12.6; Fiber: 12.8; Carbs: 44.7; Protein: 13.6.

151 VEGGIE QUICHE

Preparation Time: 6 minutes

Cooking Time: 55 minutes

Servings: 8

Ingredients:

½ cup sun-dried tomatoes, chopped

1 prepared pie crust

2 tbsp. avocado oil

1 yellow onion, chopped

2 garlic cloves, minced

2 cups spinach, chopped

1 red bell pepper, chopped

¼ cup kalamata olives, pitted and sliced

1 tsp. parsley flakes

1 tsp. oregano, dried

⅓ cup feta cheese, crumbled

4 eggs, whisked

1 ½ cups almond milk

1 cup cheddar cheese, shredded

Salt and black pepper to the taste

Directions:

Heat up a pan with the oil over medium-high heat. Add the garlic and onion and sauté for 3 minutes.

Add the bell pepper and sauté for 3 minutes more.

Add the olives, parsley, spinach, oregano, salt and pepper, and cook everything for 5 minutes.

Add tomatoes and the cheese. Toss and take off the heat.

Arrange the pie crust in a pie plate. Pour the spinach and tomatoes mix inside and spread.

In a bowl, mix the eggs with salt, pepper, milk and half of the cheese. Whisk and pour over the mixture in the pie crust.

Sprinkle the remaining cheese on top and bake at 375°F for 40 minutes. Cool the quiche down. Slice and serve for breakfast.

Nutrition: Calories: 211; Fat: 14.4; Fiber: 1.4; Carbs: 12.5; Protein: 8.6.

152 POTATO HASH

Preparation Time: 10 minutes
Cooking Time: 15 minutes
Servings: 4
Ingredients:

A drizzle of olive oil
2 gold potatoes, cubed
2 garlic cloves, minced
1 yellow onion, chopped
1 cup canned chickpeas, drained
Salt and black pepper to the taste
1 ½ tsp. allspice, ground
1-pound baby asparagus, trimmed and chopped
1 tsp. sweet paprika
1 tsp. oregano, dried
1 tsp. coriander, ground
2 tomatoes, cubed
1 cup parsley, chopped
½ cup feta cheese, crumbled

Directions:

Heat up a pan with a drizzle of oil over medium-high heat. Add the potatoes, onion, garlic, salt and pepper and cook for 7 minutes.
Add the rest of the ingredients, except the tomatoes, parsley and cheese. Toss, cook for 7 more minutes and transfer to a bowl.
Add the remaining ingredients. Toss and serve for breakfast.

Nutrition: Calories: 535; Fat: 20.8; Fiber: 6.6; Carbs: 34.5; Protein: 26.6.

153 SCRAMBLED EGGS

Preparation Time: 10 minutes
Cooking Time: 10 minutes
Servings: 2
Ingredients:

1 yellow bell pepper, chopped
8 cherry tomatoes, cubed
2 spring onions, chopped
1 tbsp. olive oil
1 tbsp. capers, drained
2 tbsp. black olives, pitted and sliced
4 eggs
A pinch of salt and black pepper
¼ tsp. oregano, dried
1 tbsp. parsley, chopped

Directions:

Heat up a pan with the oil over medium-high heat. Add the bell pepper and spring onions and sauté for 3 minutes.
Add the tomatoes, capers and the olives and sauté for 2 minutes more.
Crack the eggs into the pan. Add salt, pepper and oregano, and scramble for 5 minutes more.
Divide the scramble between plates. Sprinkle the parsley on top and serve.

Nutrition: Calories: 249; Fat: 17; Fiber: 3.2; Carbs: 13.3; Protein: 13.5.

154 WATERMELON "PIZZA"

Preparation Time: 10 minutes
Cooking Time: 0 minutes
Servings: 4
Ingredients:

1 watermelon slice cut 1-inch thick and then from the center cut into 4 wedges resembling pizza slices
6 kalamata olives, pitted and sliced
1-oz. feta cheese, crumbled
½ tbsp. balsamic vinegar
1 tsp. mint, chopped

Directions:

Arrange the watermelon "pizza" on a plate; sprinkle the olives and the rest of the ingredients on each slice and serve right away for breakfast.

Nutrition: Calories: 90; Fat: 3; Fiber: 1; Carbs: 14; Protein: 2.

155 HAM MUFFINS

Preparation Time: 10 minutes
Cooking Time: 15 minutes
Servings: 6
Ingredients:

9 ham slices
5 eggs, whisked
⅓ cup spinach, chopped
¼ cup feta cheese, crumbled
½ cup roasted red peppers, chopped
A pinch of salt and black pepper
1 ½ tbsp. basil pesto
Cooking spray

Directions:

Grease a muffin tin with cooking spray and line each muffin mold with 1 and ½ ham slices.
Divide the peppers and the rest of the ingredients, except the eggs, pesto, salt and pepper into the ham cups.
In a bowl, mix the eggs with the pesto, salt and pepper. Whisk and pour over the peppers mix.
Bake the muffins in the oven at 400°F for 15 minutes and serve for breakfast.

Nutrition: Calories: 109; Fat: 6.7; Fiber: 1.8; Carbs: 1.8; Protein: 9.3.

156 AVOCADO CHICKPEA PIZZA

Preparation Time: 20 minutes
Cooking Time: 20 minutes
Servings: 2
Ingredients:

1 ¼ cups chickpea flour
A pinch of salt and black pepper
1 ¼ cups water
2 tbsp. olive oil
1 tsp. onion powder
1 tsp. garlic, minced
1 tomato, sliced
1 avocado, peeled, pitted and sliced
2 oz. gouda, sliced
¼ cup tomato sauce
2 tbsp. green onions, chopped

Directions:

In a bowl, mix the chickpea flour with salt, pepper, water, oil, onion powder and garlic. Stir well until you obtain a dough. Knead a bit, put in a bowl, cover and leave aside for 20 minutes.
Transfer the dough to a working surface. Shape a bit circle, transfer it to a baking sheet lined with parchment paper and bake at 425°F for 10 minutes.
Spread the tomato sauce over the pizza. Spread the rest of the ingredients and bake at 400°F for 10 minutes more.
Cut and serve for breakfast.

Nutrition: Calories: 416; Fat: 24.5; Fiber: 9.6; Carbs: 36.6; Protein: 15.4.

157 BANANA AND QUINOA CASSEROLE

Preparation Time: 10 minutes
Cooking Time: 1 hour & 20 minutes
Servings: 8
Ingredients:

3 cups bananas, peeled and mashed
¼ cup pure maple syrup
¼ cup molasses
1 tbsp. cinnamon powder
2 tsp. vanilla extract
1 tsp. cloves, ground
1 tsp. ginger, ground
½ tsp. allspice, ground
1 cup quinoa
¼ cup almonds, chopped
2 ½ cups almond milk

Directions:

In a baking dish, combine the bananas with the maple syrup, molasses and the rest of the ingredients. Toss and bake at 350°F for 1 hour and 20 minutes.
Divide the mix between plates and serve for breakfast.

Nutrition: Calories: 213; Fat: 4.1; Fiber: 4; Carbs: 41; Protein: 4.5.

158 AVOCADO SPREAD

Preparation Time: 5 minutes
Cooking Time: 0 minutes
Servings: 8
Ingredients:

- 2 avocados, peeled, pitted and roughly chopped
- 1 tbsp. sun-dried tomatoes, chopped
- 2 tbsp. lemon juice
- 3 tbsp. cherry tomatoes, chopped
- ¼ cup red onion, chopped
- 1 tsp. oregano, dried
- 2 tbsp. parsley, chopped
- 4 kalamata olives, pitted and chopped
- A pinch of salt and black pepper

Directions:

Put the avocados in a bowl and mash with a fork.

Add the rest of the ingredients. Stir to combine and serve as a morning spread.

Nutrition: Calories: 110; Fat: 10; Fiber: 3.8; Carbs: 5.7; Protein: 1.2.

159 AVOCADO TOAST

Preparation Time: 10 minutes
Cooking Time: 0 minutes
Servings: 2
Ingredients:

- 1 tbsp. goat cheese, crumbled
- 1 avocado, peeled, pitted and mashed
- A pinch of salt and black pepper
- 2 whole-wheat bread slices, toasted
- ½ tsp. lime juice
- 1 persimmon, thinly sliced
- 1 fennel bulb, thinly sliced
- 2 tsp. honey
- 2 tbsp. pomegranate seeds

Directions:

In a bowl, combine the avocado flesh with salt, pepper, lime juice and the cheese and whisk.

Spread this onto toasted bread slices. Top each slice with the remaining ingredients and serve for breakfast.

Nutrition: Calories: 348; Fat: 20.8; Fiber: 12.3; Carbs: 38.7; Protein: 7.1.

160 MINI FRITTATAS

Preparation Time: 5 minutes
Cooking Time: 15 minutes
Servings: 12
Ingredients:

- 1 yellow onion, chopped
- 1 cup parmesan, grated
- 1 yellow bell pepper, chopped
- 1 red bell pepper, chopped
- 1 zucchini, chopped
- Salt and black pepper to the taste
- 8 eggs, whisked
- A drizzle of olive oil
- 2 tbsp. chives, chopped

Directions:

Heat up a pan with the oil over medium-high heat. Add the onion, the zucchini and the rest of the ingredients except the eggs and chives and sauté for 5 minutes, stirring often.

Divide this mix on the bottom of a muffin pan. Pour the eggs mixture on top, sprinkle salt, pepper and chives. Bake at 350°F for 10 minutes.

Serve the mini frittatas for breakfast right away.

Nutrition: Calories: 55; Fat: 3; Fiber: 0.7; Carbs: 3.2; Protein: 4.2.

161 BERRY OATS

Preparation Time: 5 minutes
Cooking Time: 0 minutes
Servings: 2
Ingredients:

- ½ cup rolled oats
- 1 cup almond milk
- ¼ cup chia seeds
- A pinch of cinnamon powder
- 2 tsp. honey
- 1 cup berries, pureed
- 1 tbsp. yogurt

Directions:

In a bowl, combine the oats with the milk and the rest of the ingredients except the yogurt. Toss, divide into bowls, top with the yogurt and serve cold for breakfast.

Nutrition: Calories: 420; Fat: 30.3; Fiber: 7.2; Carbs: 35.3; Protein: 6.4.

162 SUN-DRIED TOMATOES OATMEAL

Preparation Time: 10 minutes
Cooking Time: 25 minutes
Servings: 4
Ingredients:

- 3 cups water
- 1 cup almond milk
- 1 tbsp. olive oil
- 1 cup steel-cut oats
- ¼ cup sun-dried tomatoes, chopped
- A pinch of red pepper flakes

Directions:

In a pan, mix the water with the milk. Bring to a boil over medium heat.

Meanwhile, heat up a pan with the oil over medium-high heat. Add the oats, cook them for about 2 minutes and transfer to the pan with the milk.

Stir the oats. Add the tomatoes and simmer over medium heat for 23 minutes.

Divide the mix into bowls. Sprinkle the red pepper flakes on top and serve for breakfast.

Nutrition: Calories: 170; Fat: 17.8; Fiber: 1.5; Carbs: 3.8; Protein: 1.5.

163 QUINOA MUFFINS

Preparation Time: 10 minutes
Cooking Time: 30 minutes
Servings: 12
Ingredients:

- 1 cup quinoa, cooked
- 6 eggs, whisked
- Salt and black pepper to the taste
- 1 cup Swiss cheese, grated
- 1 small yellow onion, chopped
- 1 cup white mushrooms, sliced
- ½ cup sun-dried tomatoes, chopped

Directions:

In a bowl, combine the eggs with salt, pepper and the rest of the ingredients and whisk well.

Divide this into a silicone muffin pan. Bake at 350°F for 30 minutes and serve for breakfast.

Nutrition: Calories: 123; Fat: 5.6; Fiber: 1.3; Carbs: 10.8; Protein: 7.5.

164 QUINOA AND EGGS PAN

Preparation Time: 10 minutes
Cooking Time: 23 minutes
Servings: 4
Ingredients:

- 4 bacon slices, cooked and crumbled
- A drizzle of olive oil
- 1 small red onion, chopped
- 1 red bell pepper, chopped
- 1 sweet potato, grated
- 1 green bell pepper, chopped
- 2 garlic cloves, minced
- 1 cup white mushrooms, sliced
- ½ cup quinoa
- 1 cup chicken stock
- 4 eggs, fried
- Salt and black pepper to the taste

Directions:

Heat up a pan with the oil over medium-low heat. Add the onion, garlic, bell peppers, sweet potato and mushrooms. Toss and sauté for 5 minutes.

Add the quinoa; toss and cook for 1 more minute.

Add the stock, salt and pepper, stir and cook for 15 minutes.

Divide the mix between plates. Top each serving with a fried egg. Sprinkle some salt, pepper and crumbled bacon, and serve for breakfast.

Nutrition: Calories: 304; Fat: 14; Fiber: 3.8; Carbs: 27.5; Protein: 17.8.

165 STUFFED TOMATOES

Preparation Time: 10 minutes
Cooking Time: 15 minutes
Servings: 4
Ingredients:

- 2 tbsp. olive oil
- 8 tomatoes, insides scooped
- ¼ cup almond milk
- 8 eggs
- ¼ cup parmesan, grated
- Salt and black pepper to the taste
- 4 tbsp. rosemary, chopped

Directions:

- Grease a pan with the oil and arrange the tomatoes inside.
- Crack an egg in each tomato. Divide the milk and the rest of the ingredients and introduce the pan in the oven. Bake at 375°F for 15 minutes.
- Serve for breakfast right away.

Nutrition: Calories: 276; Fat: 20.3; Fiber: 4.7; Carbs: 13.2; Protein: 13.7.

166 SUNNY-SIDE UP BAKED EGGS WITH SWISS CHARD, FETA, AND BASIL

Preparation Time: 15 minutes
Cooking Time: 10 minutes
Servings: 4
Ingredients:

- 4 bell peppers, any color
- 1 tbsp. extra-virgin olive oil
- 8 large eggs
- ¾ tsp. kosher salt, divided
- ¼ tsp. freshly ground black pepper, divided
- 1 avocado, peeled, pitted, and diced
- ¼ cup red onion, diced
- ¼ cup fresh basil, chopped
- Juice of ½ lime

Directions:

- Stem and seed the bell peppers. Cut 2 (2-inch-thick) rings from each pepper. Chop the remaining bell pepper into small dice and set aside.
- Heat the olive oil in a large skillet over medium heat. Add 4 bell pepper rings, then crack 1 egg in the middle of each ring.
- Season with ¼ teaspoon of salt and ⅛ teaspoon of black pepper. Cook until the egg whites are mostly set, but the yolks are still runny for 2 to 3 minutes.
- Gently flip and cook for 1 additional minute for an over easy. Move the egg–bell pepper rings to a platter or onto plates and repeats with the remaining 4 bell pepper rings.

In a medium bowl, combine the avocado, onion, basil, lime juice, reserved diced bell pepper, the remaining ¼ teaspoon of kosher salt, and the remaining ⅛ teaspoon of black pepper. Divide among the 4 plates.

Nutrition: Calories: 270; Protein: 15 g; Fat: 19 g; Carbs: 12 g.

167 POLENTA WITH SAUTÉED CHARD AND FRIED EGGS

Preparation Time: 5 minutes
Cooking Time: 20 minutes
Servings: 4
Ingredients:

- 2 ½ cups water
- ½ tsp. kosher salt
- ¾ cups whole-grain cornmeal
- ¼ tsp. freshly ground black pepper
- 2 tbsp. grated Parmesan cheese
- 1 tbsp. extra-virgin olive oil
- 1 bunch (about 6-oz.) Swiss chard, leaves and stems chopped and separated
- 2 garlic cloves, sliced
- ¼ tsp. kosher salt
- ⅛ tsp. freshly ground black pepper
- Lemon juice (optional)
- 1 tbsp. extra-virgin olive oil
- 4 large eggs

Directions:

- For the polenta, bring the water and salt to a boil in a medium saucepan over high heat. Slowly add the cornmeal, whisking constantly.
- Decrease the heat to low. Cover, and cook for 10 to 15 minutes, stirring often to avoid lumps. Stir in the pepper and Parmesan and divide among 4 bowls.
- For the chard, heat the oil in a large skillet over medium heat. Add the chard stems, garlic, salt, and pepper; sauté for 2 minutes. Add the chard leaves and cook until wilted, about 3 to 5 minutes.
- Add a spritz of lemon juice (if desired), toss together, and divide evenly on top of the polenta.
- For the eggs, heat the oil in the same large skillet over medium-high heat. Crack each egg into the skillet, taking care not to crowd the skillet and leaving space between the eggs.
- Cook until the whites are set and golden around the edges, about 2 to 3 minutes. Serve sunny-side up or flip the eggs over carefully and cook 1 minute longer for over easy. Place one egg on top of the polenta and chard in each bowl.

Nutrition: Calories: 310; Protein: 17 g; Fat: 18 g; Carbs: 21 g.

168 SMOKED SALMON EGG SCRAMBLE WITH DILL AND CHIVES

Preparation Time: 5 minutes
Cooking Time: 5 minutes
Servings: 2
Ingredients:

- 4 large eggs
- 1 tbsp. milk
- 1 tbsp. fresh chives, minced
- 1 tbsp. fresh dill, minced
- ¼ tsp. kosher salt
- ⅛ tsp. freshly ground black pepper
- 2 tsp. extra-virgin olive oil
- 2 oz. smoked salmon, thinly sliced

Directions:

- In a large bowl, whisk together the eggs, milk, chives, dill, salt, and pepper. Heat the olive oil in a medium skillet or sauté pan over medium flame.
- Add the egg mixture and cook for about 3 minutes, stirring occasionally. Add the salmon and cook until the eggs are set but moist for about 1 minute.

Nutrition: Calories: 325; Protein: 23 g; Fat: 26 g; Carbs: 1 g.

169 BANANA OATS

Preparation Time: 10 minutes
Cooking Time: 0 minutes
Servings: 2
Ingredients:

- 1 banana, peeled and sliced
- ¾ cup almond milk
- ½ cup cold-brewed coffee
- 2 dates, pitted
- 2 tbsp. cocoa powder
- 1 cup rolled oats
- 1 ½ tbsp. chia seeds

Directions:

- In a blender, combine the banana with the milk and the rest of the ingredients. Pulse, divide into bowls and serve for breakfast.

Nutrition: Calories: 451; Protein: 9 g; Fat: 25 g; Carbs: 55 g.

170 SLOW-COOKED PEPPERS FRITTATA

Preparation Time: 10 minutes
Cooking Time: 3 hours
Servings: 6
Ingredients:

- ½ cup almond milk
- 8 eggs, whisked
- Salt and black pepper to the taste
- 1 tsp. oregano, dried
- 1 ½ cups roasted peppers, chopped
- ½ cup red onion, chopped
- 4 cups baby arugula

1 cup goat cheese, crumbled
Cooking spray

Directions:

In a bowl, combine the eggs with salt, pepper, and oregano and whisk. Grease your slow cooker with the cooking spray, arrange the peppers and the remaining ingredients inside and pour the egg mixture over them.

Put the lid on and cook on Low for 3 hours. Divide the frittata between plates and serve.

Nutrition: Calories: 259; Protein: 16 g; Fat: 20 g; Carbs: 4.4 g.

171 AVOCADO AND APPLE SMOOTHIE

Preparation Time: 5 minutes
Cooking Time: 0 minutes
Servings: 2
Ingredients:

3 cups spinach
1 green apple, cored and chopped
1 avocado, peeled, pitted and chopped
3 tbsp. chia seeds
1 tsp. honey
1 banana, frozen and peeled
2 cups coconut water

Directions:

In your blender, combine the spinach with the apple and the rest of the ingredients. Pulse, divide into glasses and serve.

Nutrition: Calories 168; Fat 10.1; Fiber: 6; Carbs 21; Protein 2.1.

172 GREEK QUINOA BREAKFAST BOWL

Preparation Time: 15 minutes
Cooking Time: 20 minutes
Servings: 6
Ingredients:

12 eggs
¼ cup plain Greek yogurt
1 tsp onion powder
1 tsp granulated garlic
½ tsp salt
½ tsp pepper
1 tsp olive oil
1 (5-oz.) bag baby spinach
1-pint cherry tomatoes, halved
1 cup feta cheese
2 cups cooked quinoa

Directions:

In a large bowl whisk together eggs, Greek yogurt, onion powder, granulated garlic, salt, and pepper. Set aside.

In a large skillet, heat olive oil and add spinach. Cook the spinach until it is slightly wilted, about 3-4 minutes.

Add in cherry tomatoes and cook until tomatoes are softened, 3-4 minutes. Stir in egg mixture and cook until the eggs are set, about 7-9 minutes. Stir in the eggs as they cook to scramble.

Once the eggs have set stir in the feta and quinoa, cook until heated through. Distribute evenly among the containers, store for 2-3 days.

Nutrition: Calories: 357; Carbohydrates: 8 g; Fat: 20 g; Protein: 23 g.

173 MUSHROOM GOAT CHEESE FRITTATA

Preparation Time: 15 minutes
Cooking Time: 35 minutes
Servings: 4
Ingredients:

1 tbsp. olive oil
1 small onion, diced
10 oz. cremini or your favorite mushrooms, sliced
1 garlic clove, minced
10 eggs
⅔ cup half and half
¼ cup fresh chives, minced
2 tsp. fresh thyme, minced
½ tsp. kosher salt
½ tsp. black pepper
4 oz. goat cheese

Directions:

Preheat the oven to 375°F. In an oven-safe skillet or cast-iron pan over medium heat, add olive oil. Add in the onion and sauté for 3-5 minutes until golden.

Add in the sliced mushrooms and garlic. Continue cooking until mushrooms are golden brown, about 10-12 minutes.

In a large bowl, whisk together the eggs, half and half, chives, thyme, salt and pepper. Place the goat cheese over the mushroom mixture and pour the egg mixture over the top.

Stir the MIXTURE in the pan and cook over medium heat until the edges are set but the center is still loose, about 8-10 minutes

Put the pan in the oven and finish cooking for an additional 8-10 minutes or until set. Allow to cool completely before slicing.

Nutrition: Calories: 243; Carbohydrates: 5 g; Fat: 17 g; Protein: 15 g.

174 MEDITERRANEAN FRITTATA

Preparation Time: 8 minutes
Cooking Time: 6 minutes
Servings: 4

Ingredients:

2 tsp. of olive oil
¼ cup of baby spinach, packed
2 green onions
4 egg whites, large
6 large eggs
⅓ cup of crumbled feta cheese, (1.3 oz.) along with sun-dried tomatoes and basil
2 tsp. of salt-free Greek seasoning
¼ tsp. of salt

Directions:

Take a boiler and preheat it. Take a ten-inch ovenproof skillet and pour the oil into it and keep the skillet on a medium flame.

While the oil gets heated, chop the spinach roughly and the onions. Put the eggs, egg whites, Greek seasoning, cheese, as well as salt in a large mixing bowl and mix it thoroughly using a whisker.

Add the chopped spinach and onions into the mixing bowl and stir well.

Pour the mixture into the pan and cook it for 2 minutes or more until the edges of the mixture set well.

Lift the edges of the mixture gently and tilt the pan so that the uncooked portion can get underneath it. Cook for another two minutes so that the whole mixture gets cooked properly.

Broil for two to three minutes till the center gets set. Your Frittata is now ready. Serve it hot by cutting it into four wedges.

Nutrition: Calories: 178; Protein: 16 g; Fat: 12 g; Carbs: 2.2 g.

175 HONEY-CARAMELIZED FIGS WITH GREEK YOGURT

Preparation Time: 5 minutes
Cooking Time: 5 minutes
Servings: 4
Ingredients:

4 fresh halved figs
2 tbsp. melted butter, 30ml
2 tbsp. brown sugar, 30ml
2 cups Greek yogurt 500ml
¼ cup honey, 60ml

Directions:

Take a non-stick skillet and preheat it over a medium flame. Put the butter on the pan and toss the figs into it. Sprinkle in some brown sugar over it.

Put the figs on the pan and cut off the side of the figs. Cook them on a medium flame for 2-3 minutes until they turn golden brown.

Turn over the figs and cook them for 2-3 minutes again. Remove the figs from the pan and let it cool down a little.

Take a plate and put a scoop of Greek yogurt on it. Put the cooked figs over the yogurts and drizzle the honey over it

Nutrition: Calories: 350; Protein: 6 g; Fat: 19 g; Carbs: 40 g.

176 SAVORY QUINOA EGG MUFFINS WITH SPINACH

Preparation Time: 15 minutes
Cooking Time: 20 minutes
Servings: 2
Ingredients:

- 1 cup quinoa
- 2 cups water/ vegetable broth)
- 4 oz. spinach which is about one cup
- ½ chopped onion
- 2 whole eggs
- ¼ cup grated cheese
- ½ tsp. oregano or thyme
- ½ tsp. garlic powder
- ½ tsp. salt

Directions:

Take a medium saucepan and put water in it. Add the quinoa to the water and bring the whole thing to a simmer.

Cover the pan and cook it for 10 minutes till the water gets absorbed by the quinoa. Remove the saucepan from the heat and let it cool down.

Take a nonstick pan and heat the onions till they turn soft and then add spinach. Cook all of them together till the spinach gets a little wilted and then remove it from the heat.

Preheat the oven to 176°C. Take a muffin pan and grease it lightly.

Take a large bowl and add the cooked quinoa along with the cooked onions, spinach, and add cheese, eggs, thyme or oregano, salt, garlic powder, pepper and mix them together.

Put a spoonful of the mixture into a muffin tin. Make sure it is ¼ of a cup. In the preheated pan, bake it for around 20 minutes.

Nutrition: Calories: 61; Protein: 4 g; Fat: 3 g; Carbs: 6 g.

177 AVOCADO TOMATO GOUDA SOCCA PIZZA

Preparation Time: 20 minutes
Cooking Time: 20 minutes
Servings: 2
Ingredients:

- 1 ¼ cups of chickpea or garbanzo bean flour
- 1 ¼ cups of cold water
- ¼ tsp. pepper and sea salt each
- 2 tsp. avocado or olive oil + 1 tsp. extra for heating the pan
- 1 tsp. minced garlic which will be around two cloves
- 1 tsp. onion powder/other herb seasoning powder
- 10 to 12-inch cast iron pan
- 1 sliced tomato
- ½ avocado
- 2 oz. thinly sliced Gouda
- ¼-⅓ cup tomato sauce
- 2 or 3 tsp. chopped green scallion/onion
- Sprouted greens for green
- Extra pepper/salt for sprinkling on top of the pizza
- Red pepper flakes

Directions:

Mix the flour with two teaspoons of olive oil, herbs, water, and whisk it until a smooth mixture forms. Keep it at room temperature for around 15-20 minutes to let the batter settle.

In the meantime, preheat the oven and place the pan inside. Let it heat for around 10 minutes. When the pan gets preheated, chop up the vegetables into fine slices.

Remove the pan after ten minutes using oven mitts. Put one teaspoon of oil and swirl it all around to coat the pan.

Pour the batter into the pan and tilt the pan so that the batter spreads evenly. Lower the oven to 425F and place it back the pan for 5-8 minutes.

Remove the pan from the oven and add the sliced avocado, tomato and, on top of that, add the gouda slices and the onion slices.

Put the pizza back into the oven and wait till the cheese gets melted or the sides of the bread get crusty and brown.

Remove the pizza from the pan and add the microgreens on top, along with the toppings.

Nutrition: Calories: 416; Protein: 15 g; Fat: 10 g; Carbs: 37 g.

178 SHAKSHUKA WITH FETA

Preparation Time: 15 minutes
Cooking Time: 41 minutes
Servings: 4-6
Ingredients:

- 6 large eggs
- 3 tbsp. extra-virgin olive oil
- 1 large onion, halved and thinly sliced
- 1 large red bell pepper, seeded and thinly sliced
- 3 garlic cloves, thinly sliced
- 1 tsp. ground cumin
- 1 tsp. sweet paprika
- ⅛ tsp. cayenne, or to taste
- 1 (28-oz.) can whole plum tomatoes with juices, coarsely chopped
- ¾ tsp. salt, more as needed
- ¼ tsp. black pepper, more as needed
- 5 oz. feta cheese, crumbled, about 1 ¼ cups

To Serve:

- Chopped cilantro
- Hot sauce

Directions:

Preheat oven to 375°F. In a large skillet over medium-low heat, add the oil. Once heated, add the onion and bell pepper, cook gently until very soft, about 20 minutes.

Add in the garlic and cook until tender, 1 to 2 minutes, then stir in cumin, paprika and cayenne. Cook for 1 minute.

Pour in tomatoes, season with ¾ teaspoon of salt and ¼ teaspoon of pepper. Simmer until tomatoes have thickened, about 10 minutes. Then stir in crumbled feta.

Gently crack eggs into skillet over tomatoes and season with salt and pepper. Transfer skillet to oven. Bake until eggs have just set, 7 to 10 minutes. Serve.

Nutrition: Calories: 337; Carbs: 17 g; Fat: 25 g; Protein: 12 g.

179 PEANUT BUTTER BANANA GREEK YOGURT

Preparation Time: 15 minutes
Cooking Time: 0 minutes
Servings: 4
Ingredients:

- 3 cups vanilla Greek yogurt
- 2 medium bananas sliced
- ¼ cup creamy natural peanut butter
- ¼ cup flaxseed meal
- 1 tsp. nutmeg

Directions:

Divide yogurt between four jars with lids. Top with banana slices.

In a bowl, melt the peanut butter in a microwave-safe bowl for 30-40 seconds and drizzle one tbsp on each bowl on top of the bananas. Store in the fridge for up to 3 days.

When ready to serve, sprinkle with flaxseed meal and ground nutmeg. Enjoy!

Nutrition: Calories: 370; Carbs: 47 g; Fat: 10 g; Protein: 22 g.

180 VEGGIE MEDITERRANEAN QUICHE

Preparation Time: 15 minutes
Cooking Time: 55 minutes
Servings: 8
Ingredients:

½ cup sundried tomatoes - dry or in olive oil
Boiling water
1 prepared pie crust
2 tbsp. vegan butter
1 onion, diced
2 cloves garlic, minced
1 red pepper, diced
¼ cup sliced Kalamata olives
1 tsp. dried oregano
1 tsp. dried parsley
⅓ cup crumbled feta cheese
4 large eggs
1 ¼ cup milk
2 cups fresh spinach or ½ cup frozen spinach, thawed and squeezed dry
Salt, to taste
Pepper, to taste
1 cup shredded cheddar cheese, divided

Directions:

If you're using dry sundried tomatoes, in a measuring cup, add the sundried tomatoes and pour the boiling water over until just covered. Allow to sit for 5 minutes or until the tomatoes are soft. Drain and chop tomatoes, set aside.

Preheat oven to 375°F. Fit a 9-inch pie plate with the prepared pie crust, then flute edges, and set aside. In a skillet over medium-high heat, melt the butter.

Add in the onion and garlic, and cook until fragrant and tender, about 3 minutes. Add in the red pepper, cook for an additional 3 minutes, or until the peppers are just tender.

Add in the spinach, olives, oregano, and parsley. Cook until the spinach is wilted (if you're using fresh) or heated through (if you're using frozen), about 5 minutes.

Remove the pan from heat. Stir in the feta cheese and tomatoes. Spoon the mixture into the prepared pie crust, spreading out evenly. Set aside.

In a medium-sized mixing bowl, whisk together the eggs, ½ cup of the cheddar cheese, milk, salt, and pepper. Pour this egg and cheese mixture evenly over the spinach mixture in the pie crust.

Sprinkle top with the remaining cheddar cheese. Bake for 50-55 minutes, or until the crust is golden brown and the egg is set.

Allow to cool completely before slicing.

Nutrition: Calories: 239; Carbs: 19 g; Fat: 15 g; Protein: 7 g.

181 SPINACH, FETA AND EGG BREAKFAST QUESADILLAS

Preparation Time: 15 minutes
Cooking Time: 15 minutes
Servings: 5

Ingredients:

8 eggs (optional)
2 tsp. olive oil
1 red bell pepper
½ red onion
¼ cup milk
4 handfuls of spinach leaves
1 ½ cup mozzarella cheese
5 sun-dried tomato tortillas
½ cup feta
¼ tsp. salt
¼ tsp. pepper
Spray oil

Directions:

In a large non-stick pan over medium heat, add the olive oil. Once heated, add the bell pepper and onion, cook for 4-5 minutes until soft.

In the meantime, whisk together the eggs, milk, salt and pepper in a bowl. Add in the egg/milk mixture into the pan with peppers and onions, stirring frequently, until eggs are almost cooked through.

Add in the spinach and feta, fold into the eggs, stirring until spinach is wilted and eggs are cooked through. Remove the eggs from heat and plate.

Grease a separate large non-stick pan with spray oil, and place over medium heat. Add the tortilla, on one half of the tortilla, spread about ½ cup of the egg mixture. Top the eggs with around ⅓ cup of shredded mozzarella cheese. Fold the second half of the tortilla over, then cook for 2 minutes, or until golden brown.

Flip and cook for another minute until golden brown. Allow the quesadilla to cool completely. Divide among the containers, store for 2 days or wrap in plastic wrap and foil, and freeze for up to 2 months.

Nutrition: Calories: 213; Fat: 11 g; Carbs: 15 g; Protein: 15 g.

182 MEDITERRANEAN QUINOA AND FETA EGG MUFFINS

Preparation Time: 15 minutes
Cooking Time: 30 minutes
Servings: 12
Ingredients:

8 eggs
1 cup cooked quinoa
1 cup crumbled feta cheese
¼ tsp. salt
2 cups baby spinach finely chopped
½ cup finely chopped onion
1 cup chopped or sliced tomatoes, cherry or grape tomatoes
½ cup chopped and pitted Kalamata olives
1 tbsp. chopped fresh oregano
2 tsp. high oleic sunflower oil plus optional extra for greasing muffin tins

Directions:

Preheat oven to 350°F. Prepare 12 silicone muffin holders on a baking sheet or grease a 12-cup muffin tin with oil. Set aside.

In a skillet over medium heat, add the vegetable oil and onions, sauté for 2 minutes. Add tomatoes, sauté for another minute; then add spinach and sauté until wilted, about 1 minute.

Remove from heat and stir in olives and oregano; set aside. Place the eggs in a blender or mixing bowl and blend or mix until well combined.

Pour the eggs in to a mixing bowl (if you used a blender) then add quinoa, feta cheese, veggie mixture, and salt. Stir until well combined.

Pour mixture in to silicone cups or greased muffin tins, dividing equally, and bake for 30 minutes, or until eggs have set and muffins are a light golden brown. Allow to cool completely.

Nutrition: Calories: 113; Carbohydrates: 5 g; Fat: 7 g; Protein: 6 g.

183 GREEN SHAKSHUKA

Preparation Time: 15 minutes
Cooking Time: 15 minutes
Servings: 2
Ingredients:

1 tbsp. olive oil
1 onion, peeled and diced
1 clove garlic, peeled and finely minced
3 cups broccoli rabe, chopped
3 cups baby spinach leaves
2 tbsp. whole milk or cream
1 tsp. ground cumin
¼ tsp. black pepper
¼ tsp. salt (or to taste)
4 eggs

Garnish:

1 pinch sea salt
1 pinch red pepper flakes

Directions:

Preheat the oven to 350°F. Add the broccoli rabe to a large pot of boiling water. Cook for 2 minutes, drain and set aside.

In a large oven-proof skillet or cast-iron pan over medium heat, add in the tablespoon of olive oil along with the diced onions. Cook for about 10 minutes or until the onions become translucent.

Add the minced garlic and continue cooking for about another minute. Cut the par-cooked broccoli rabe into small pieces and stir into the onion and garlic mixture.

Cook for a couple of minutes, then stir in the baby spinach leaves. Continue cooking for a couple more minutes, stirring often, until the spinach begins to wilt. Stir in the ground cumin, salt, ground black pepper, and milk.

Make four wells in the mixture and crack an egg into each well – be careful not to break the yolks. Also, note that it's easier to crack each egg into a small bowl and then transfer them to the pan.

Place the pan with the eggs into the pre-heated oven. Cook for 10 to 15 minutes until the eggs are set to preference. Sprinkle the cooked eggs with a dash of sea salt and a pinch of red pepper flakes.

Nutrition: Calories: 278; Carbs: 18 g; Fat: 16 g; Protein: 16 g.

184 APPLE QUINOA BREAKFAST BARS

Preparation Time: 15 minutes
Cooking Time: 40 minutes
Servings: 12
Ingredients:

2 eggs
1 apple peeled and chopped into ½ inch chunks
1 cup unsweetened apple sauce
1 ½ cups cooked and cooled quinoa
1 ½ cups rolled oats
¼ cup peanut butter
1 tsp. vanilla
½ tsp. cinnamon
¼ cup coconut oil
½ tsp. baking powder

Directions:

Heat oven to 350°F. Spray an 8x8 inch baking dish with oil and set aside. In a large bowl, stir together the apple sauce, cinnamon, coconut oil, peanut butter, vanilla and eggs.

Add in the cooked quinoa, rolled oats and baking powder. Mix until completely incorporated. Fold in the apple chunks.

Spread the mixture into the prepared baking dish, spreading it to each corner. Bake for 40 minutes, or until a toothpick comes out clean. Allow to cool before slicing.

Nutrition: Calories: 230; Fat: 10 g; Carbs: 31 g; Protein: 7 g.

185 BLUEBERRIES QUINOA

Preparation Time: 5 minutes
Cooking Time: 0 minutes
Servings: 4
Ingredients:

2 cups almond milk
2 cups quinoa, already cooked
½ tsp. cinnamon powder
1 tbsp. honey
1 cup blueberries
¼ cup walnuts, chopped

Directions:

In a bowl, mix the quinoa with the milk and the rest of the ingredients. Toss, divide into smaller bowls and serve for breakfast.

Nutrition: Calories: 284; Fat: 14.3 g; Carbs: 15.4 g; Protein: 4.4 g.

186 ENDIVES, FENNEL AND ORANGE SALAD

Preparation Time: 5 minutes
Cooking Time: 0 minutes
Servings: 4
Ingredients:

1 tbsp. balsamic vinegar
2 garlic cloves, minced
1 tsp. Dijon mustard
2 tbsp. olive oil
1 tbsp. lemon juice
Sea salt and black pepper to taste
½ cup black olives, pitted and chopped
1 tbsp. parsley, chopped
7 cups baby spinach
2 endives, shredded
3 medium navel oranges, peeled and cut into segments
2 bulbs fennel, shredded

Directions:

In a salad bowl, combine the spinach with the endives, oranges, fennel, and the rest of the ingredients. Toss and serve for breakfast.

Nutrition: Calories: 97; Fat: 9.1 g; Carbs: 3.7 g; Protein: 1.9 g.

187 HOMEMADE MUESLI

Preparation Time: 15 minutes
Cooking Time: 20 minutes
Servings: 8
Ingredients:

3 ½ cups rolled oats
½ cup wheat bran
½ tsp kosher salt
½ tsp ground cinnamon
½ cup sliced almonds
¼ cup raw pecans, coarsely chopped
¼ cup raw pepitas (shelled pumpkin seeds)
½ cup unsweetened coconut flakes
¼ cup dried apricots, coarsely chopped
¼ cup dried cherries

Directions:

Take a medium bowl and combine the oats, wheat bran, salt, and cinnamon. Stir well. Place the mixture onto a baking sheet.

Next, place the almonds, pecans, and pepitas onto another baking sheet and toss. Pop both trays into the oven and heat to 350°F. Bake for 10-12 minutes. Remove from the oven and pop to one side.

Leave the nuts to cool but take the one with the oats, sprinkle with the coconut, and pop back into the oven for 5 minutes more. Remove and leave to cool.

Find a large bowl and combine the contents of both trays then stir well to combine. Throw in the apricots and cherries and stir well. Pop into an airtight container until required.

Nutrition: Calories: 250; Fat: 10 g; Carbs: 36 g; Protein: 7 g.

188 TANGERINE AND POMEGRANATE BREAKFAST FRUIT SALAD

Preparation Time: 15 minutes
Cooking Time: 20 minutes
Servings: 5
Ingredients:
For the grains:

1 cup pearl or hulled barley
3 cups water
3 tbsp. olive oil, divided
½ tsp kosher salt

For the fruit:

½ large pineapple, peeled and cut into 1 ½" chunks
6 tangerines
1 ¼ cups pomegranate seeds
1 small bunch of fresh mint

For the dressing:

⅓ cup honey
Juice and finely grated zest of 1 lemon
Juice and finely grated zest of 2 limes
½ tsp kosher salt
¼ cup olive oil
¼ cup toasted hazelnut oil (olive oil is fine too)

Directions:

Place the grain into a strainer and rinse well. Grab 2 baking sheets, line with paper, and add the grain. Spread well to cover then leave to dry.

Next, place the water into a saucepan and pop over medium heat. Place a skillet over medium heat, add 2 tablespoons of the oil then add the barley. Toast for 2 minutes.

Add the water and salt and bring to a boil. Reduce to simmer and cook for 40 minutes until most of the liquid has been absorbed. Turn off the heat and leave to stand for 10 minutes to steam cook the rest.

Meanwhile, grab a medium bowl and add the honey, juices, zest, and salt. Stir well. Add the olive oil then nut oil and stir again. Pop until the fridge until needed.

Remove the lid from the barley; then place it onto another prepared baking sheet and leave to cool. Drizzle with oil and leave to cool completely. Then pop into the fridge.

When ready to serve, divide the grains, pineapple, orange, pomegranate, and mint between the bowls. Drizzle with the dressing then serve and enjoy.

Nutrition: Calories: 400; Fat: 23 g; Carbs: 50 g; Protein: 3 g.

189 HUMMUS AND TOMATO BREAKFAST PITTAS

Preparation Time: 5 minutes
Cooking Time: 10 minutes
Servings: 4
Ingredients:

4 large eggs, at room temperature
Salt, to taste
2 whole-wheat pita breads with pockets, cut in half
½ cup hummus
1 medium cucumber, thinly sliced into rounds
2 medium tomatoes, large dice
A handful of fresh parsley leaves, coarsely chopped
Freshly ground black pepper
Hot sauce (optional)

Directions:

Grab a large saucepan, fill with water, and pop over medium heat until it boils. Add the eggs and cook for 7 minutes.

Immediately drain the water and place the eggs under cool water until they cool down. Pop to one side

until you can handle them comfortably.

Peel the eggs and cut them into ¼" slices. Sprinkle with salt, and pop to one side.

Grab a pitta pocket and spread with hummus. Fill with cucumber and tomato, season well then add an egg. Sprinkle with parsley and hot sauce then serve and enjoy.

Nutrition: Calories: 377; Fat: 31 g; Carbs: 17 g; Protein: 11 g.

190 BAKED RICOTTA & PEARS

Preparation Time: 15 minutes
Cooking Time: 30 minutes
Servings: 4
Ingredients:

¼ cup white whole wheat flour
1 tbsp. sugar
¼ tsp. nutmeg
Ricotta cheese
16 oz. container whole-milk
2 large eggs
1 diced pear
2 tbsp. water
1 tsp. vanilla extract
1 tbsp. honey

Also Needed:

4 - 6 oz. ramekins

Directions:

Warm the oven to 400°F. Lightly spritz the ramekins with a cooking oil spray. Whisk the flour, nutmeg, sugar, vanilla, eggs, and ricotta together in a large mixing container.

Spoon the fixings into the dishes. Bake them for 20 to 25 minutes or until they're firm and set. Transfer them to the countertop and wait for them to cool.

In a saucepan, using the medium temperature setting, toss the cored and diced pear into the water for about ten minutes until it's slightly softened.

Take the pan from the burner and stir in the honey. Serve the ricotta ramekins with the warm pear when it's ready.

Nutrition: Calories: 312; Protein: 17 g; Carbs: 0 g; Fat: 17 g.

191 CRUMBLED FETA AND SCALLIONS

Preparation Time: 5 minutes
Cooking Time: 15 minutes
Servings: 12
Ingredients:

2 tbsp. unsalted butter (replace with canola oil for full effect)
½ cup chopped up scallions

1 cup crumbled feta cheese
8 large-sized eggs
⅔ cup milk
½ tsp. dried Italian seasoning
Salt as needed
Freshly ground black pepper as needed
Cooking oil spray

Directions:

Preheat your oven to 400°F. Take a 3-4-oz. muffin pan and grease with cooking oil. Take a non-stick pan and place it over medium heat.

Add butter and allow the butter to melt. Add half of the scallions and stir fry. Keep them to the side. Take a medium-sized bowl; add eggs, Italian seasoning and milk and whisk well.

Add the stir-fried scallions and feta cheese and mix. Season with pepper and salt. Pour the mix into the muffin tin. Transfer the muffin tin to your oven and bake for 15 minutes. Serve with a sprinkle of scallions.

Nutrition: Calories: 106; Fat: 8 g; Carbohydrates: 2 g; Protein: 7 g.

192 SPICY EARLY MORNING SEAFOOD RISOTTO

Preparation Time: 5 minutes
Cooking Time: 15 minutes
Servings: 4
Ingredients:

3 cups clam juice
2 cups water
2 tbsp. olive oil
1 medium-sized chopped up onion
2 minced cloves garlic
1 ½ cups Arborio Rice
½ cup dry white wine
1 tsp. saffron
½ tsp. ground cumin
½ tsp. paprika
1 pound marinara seafood mix
Salt as needed
Ground pepper as needed

Directions:

Place a saucepan over high heat and pour in your clam juice with water and bring the mixture to a boil. Remove the heat.

Take a heavy-bottomed saucepan and stir fry your garlic and onion in oil over medium heat until a nice fragrance comes off.

Add in the rice and keep stirring for 2-3 minutes until the rice has been fully covered with the oil. Pour the wine and then add the saffron.

Keep stirring constantly until it is fully absorbed. Add in the cumin, clam juice and paprika mixture 1 cup at a time, making sure to keep stirring it from time to time.

Cook the rice for 20 minutes until perfect. Finally, add the seafood marinara mix and cook for another 5-7 minutes.

Season with some pepper and salt. Transfer the meal to a serving dish. Serve hot.

Nutrition: Calories: 386; Fat: 7 g; Carbohydrates: 55 g; Protein: 21 g.

193 ROCKET TOMATOES AND MUSHROOM FRITTATA

Preparation Time: 5 minutes
Cooking Time: 15 minutes
Servings: 4
Ingredients:

2 tbsp. butter (replace with canola oil for full effect)
1 chopped up medium-sized onion
2 minced cloves garlic
1 cup coarsely chopped baby rocket tomato
1 cup sliced button mushrooms
6 large pieces eggs
½ cup skim milk
1 tsp. dried rosemary
Salt as needed
Ground black pepper as needed

Directions:

Preheat your oven to 400°F. Take a large oven-proof pan and place it over medium-heat. Heat up some oil.

Stir fry your garlic, onion for about 2 minutes. Add the mushroom, rosemary and rockets and cook for 3 minutes. Take a medium-sized bowl and beat your eggs alongside the milk.

Season it with some salt and pepper. Pour the egg mixture into your pan with the vegetables and sprinkle some Parmesan.

Reduce the heat to low and cover with the lid. Let it cook for 3 minutes. Transfer the pan into your oven and bake for 10 minutes until fully settled.

Reduce the heat to low and cover with your lid. Let it cook for 3 minutes. Transfer the pan into your oven and then bake for another 10 minutes. Serve hot.

Nutrition: Calories: 189; Fat: 13 g; Carbohydrates: 6 g; Protein: 12 g.

194 CHEESY OLIVES BREAD

Preparation Time: 1 hour & 40 minutes
Cooking Time: 30 minutes
Servings: 10

Ingredients:

4 cups whole-wheat flour
3 tbsp. oregano, chopped
2 tsp. dry yeast
¼ cup olive oil
1 ½ cups black olives, pitted and sliced
1 cup water
½ cup feta cheese, crumbled

Directions:

In a bowl, mix the flour with the water, the yeast, and the oil. Stir and knead your dough very well. Put the dough in a bowl, cover with plastic wrap, and keep in a warm place for 1 hour.

Divide the dough into 2 bowls and stretch each ball well. Add the rest of the ingredients to each ball and tuck them inside. Knead the dough well again.

Flatten the balls a bit and leave them aside for 40 minutes more. Transfer the balls to a baking sheet lined with parchment paper, make a small slit in each, and bake at 425F for 30 minutes.

Serve the bread as a Mediterranean breakfast.

Nutrition: Calories: 251; Fat: 7.3 g; Carbs: 39.7 g; Protein: 6.7 g.

195 SWEET POTATO TART

Preparation Time: 10 minutes
Cooking Time: 1 hour & 10 minutes
Servings: 8
Ingredients:

2 pounds sweet potatoes, peeled and cubed
¼ cup olive oil + a drizzle
7 oz. feta cheese, crumbled
1 yellow onion, chopped
2 eggs, whisked
¼ cup almond milk
1 tbsp. herbs de Provence
A pinch of salt and black pepper
6 phyllo sheets
1 tbsp. parmesan, grated

Directions:

In a bowl, combine the potatoes with half of the oil, salt, and pepper. Toss, spread on a baking sheet lined with parchment paper, and roast at 400°F for 25 minutes.

Meanwhile, heat a pan with half of the remaining oil over medium heat. Add the onion, and sauté for 5 minutes.

In a bowl, combine the eggs with the milk, feta, herbs, salt, pepper, onion, sweet potatoes, and the rest of the oil and toss.

Arrange the phyllo sheets in a tart pan and brush them with a drizzle of

oil. Add the sweet potato mix and spread it well into the pan.

Sprinkle the parmesan on top and bake covered with tin foil at 350°F for 20 minutes. Remove the tin foil and bake the tart for 20 minutes more. Cool it down, slice, and serve for breakfast.

Nutrition: Calories: 476; Fat: 16.8 g; Carbs: 68.8 g; Protein: 13.9 g.

196 FULL EGGS IN A SQUASH

Preparation Time: 15 minutes
Cooking Time: 20 minutes
Servings: 5
Ingredients:

2 acorn squash
6 whole eggs
2 tbsp. extra virgin olive oil
Salt and pepper as needed
5-6 pitted dates
8 walnut halves
A fresh bunch of parsley

Directions:

Preheat your oven to 375°F. Slice squash crosswise and prepare 3 slices with holes. While slicing the squash, make sure that each slice measures ¾ inch thick.

Remove the seeds from the slices. Take a baking sheet and line it with parchment paper. Transfer the slices to your baking sheet and season them with salt and pepper.

Bake in your oven for 20 minutes. Chop the walnuts and dates on your cutting board. Take the baking dish out of the oven and drizzle slices with olive oil.

Crack an egg into each of the holes in the slices and season with pepper and salt. Sprinkle the chopped walnuts on top. Bake for 10 minutes more. Garnish with parsley and add maple syrup.

Nutrition: Calories: 198; Fat: 12 g; Carbohydrates: 17 g; Protein: 8 g.

197 BARLEY PORRIDGE

Preparation Time: 5 minutes
Cooking Time: 25 minutes
Servings: 4
Ingredients:

1 cup barley
1 cup wheat berries
2 cups unsweetened almond milk
2 cups water
½ cup blueberries
½ cup pomegranate seeds
½ cup hazelnuts, toasted and chopped
¼ cup honey

Directions:

Take a medium saucepan and place it over medium-high heat. Place barley, almond milk, wheat berries, water and bring to a boil. Reduce the heat to low and simmer for 25 minutes.

Divide amongst serving bowls and top each serving with 2 tablespoons of blueberries, 2 tablespoons of pomegranate seeds, 2 tablespoons of hazelnuts and 1 tablespoon of honey. Serve and enjoy!

Nutrition: Calories: 295; Fat: 8 g; Carbohydrates: 56 g; Protein: 6 g.

198 TOMATO AND DILL FRITTATA

Preparation Time: 5 minutes
Cooking Time: 10 minutes
Servings: 4
Ingredients:

2 tbsp. olive oil
1 medium onion, chopped
1 tsp. garlic, minced
2 medium tomatoes, chopped
6 large eggs
½ cup half and half
½ cup feta cheese, crumbled
¼ cup dill weed
Salt as needed
Ground black pepper as needed

Directions:

Preheat your oven to a temperature of 400°F. Take a large-sized ovenproof pan and heat up your olive oil over medium-high fire. Toss in the onion, garlic, tomatoes and stir fry them for 4 minutes.

While they are being cooked, take a bowl and beat together your eggs, half and half cream and season the mix with some pepper and salt.

Pour the mixture into the pan with your vegetables and top it with crumbled feta cheese and dill weed. Cover it with the lid and let it cook for 3 minutes.

Place the pan inside your oven and let it bake for 10 minutes. Serve hot.

Nutrition: Calories: 191; Fat: 15 g; Carbohydrates: 6 g; Protein: 9 g.

199 GNOCCHI HAM OLIVES

Preparation Time: 5 minutes
Cooking Time: 15 minutes
Servings: 4
Ingredients:

2 tbsp. olive oil
1 medium-sized onion chopped up
3 minced cloves of garlic
1 medium-sized red pepper completely deseeded and finely chopped
1 cup tomato puree
2 tbsp. tomato paste

1 pound gnocchi
1 cup coarsely chopped turkey ham
½ cup sliced pitted olives
1 tsp. Italian seasoning
Salt as needed
Freshly ground black pepper
Bunch fresh basil leaves

Directions:

Take a medium-sized sauce pan and place over medium-high heat. Pour some olive oil and heat it up. Toss in the bell pepper, onion and garlic and sauté for 2 minutes.

Pour in the tomato puree, gnocchi, tomato paste and add the turkey ham, Italian seasoning and olives. Simmer the whole mix for 15 minutes, making sure to stir from time to time.

Season the mix with some pepper and salt. Once done, transfer the mix to a dish and garnish with some basil leaves. Serve hot and have fun.

Nutrition: Calories: 335; Fat: 12 g; Carbohydrates: 45 g; Protein: 15 g.

200 FETA & QUINOA EGG MUFFINS

Preparation Time: 20 minutes
Cooking Time: 45-50 minutes
Servings: 12
Ingredients:

1 cup cooked quinoa
2 cups baby spinach, chopped
½ cup Kalamata olives
1 cup tomatoes
½ cup white onion
1 tbsp. fresh oregano
½ tsp. salt
2 tsp.+ more for coating pans olive oil
8 eggs
1 cup crumbled feta cheese
Also Needed: 12-cup muffin tin

Directions:

Heat the oven to reach 350°F. Lightly grease the muffin tray cups with a spritz of cooking oil.

Prepare a skillet using the medium temperature setting and add the oil. When it's hot, toss in the onions to sauté for two minutes.

Dump the tomatoes into the skillet and sauté for one minute. Fold in the spinach and continue cooking until the leaves have wilted (1 minute).

Transfer the pot to the countertop and add the oregano and olives. Set it aside.

Crack the eggs into a mixing bowl, using an immersion stick blender to mix them thoroughly. Add the

cooked veggies in with the rest of the fixings.

Stir until it's combined and scoop the mixture into the greased muffin cups. Set the timer to bake the muffins for 30 minutes until browned, and the muffins are set. Cool for about ten minutes. Serve.

Nutrition: Calories: 295; Carbs: 3 g; Fat: 23 g; Protein: 19 g.

201 TRIPLE BERRY BANANA SMOOTHIE

Preparation Time: 5 minutes
Cooking Time: 0 minutes
Servings: 2
Ingredients:

½ cup strawberries
2 tbsp. agave syrup
½ cup raspberries
1 burro banana, peeled
½ cup blueberries
1 cup spring water

Directions:

Plug in a high-speed food processor or blender and add all the ingredients to its jar.

Cover the blender jar with its lid and then pulse for 40 to 60 seconds until smooth.

Divide the drink between two glasses and then serve.

Nutrition: Calories: 130; Fats: 1.5 g;5 g; Protein: 26 g; Carbohydrates: 4 g; Fiber:

202 RASPBERRY, PEACH AND WALNUTS SMOOTHIE

Preparation Time: 5 minutes
Cooking Time: 0 minutes
Servings: 2
Ingredients:

½ of peach
½ cup raspberries
1 ½ tbsp. walnuts
2 tbsp. agave syrup
½ tbsp. Bromide Plus Powder
2 cups spring water

Extra:

¼ tsp. salt
⅛ tsp. cayenne pepper

Directions:

Plug in a high-speed food processor or blender and add all the ingredients to its jar.

Cover the blender jar with its lid and then pulse for 40 to 60 seconds until smooth.

Divide the drink between two glasses and then serve.

Nutrition: Calories: 165; Fats: 0.3 g; Protein: 12 g; Carbohydrates: 18.7 g; Fiber: 2.5 g.

203 SMOOTHIE WITH STRAWBERRIES AND COCONUT

Preparation Time: 5 minutes
Cooking Time: 10 minutes
Servings: 2
Ingredients:

1 ½ cup Dr. Sebi's Herbal Tea
¼ cup soft-jelly coconut, shredded
½ cup strawberries
2 tbsp. agave syrup

Directions:

Plug in a high-speed food processor or blender and add all the ingredients to its jar.
Cover the blender jar with its lid and then pulse for 40 to 60 seconds until smooth.
Divide the drink between two glasses and then serve.

Nutrition: Calories: 168; Fats: 2.5 g; Protein: 2 g; Carbohydrates: 38 g; Fiber: 4.5 g.

204 PEAR AND MANGO SMOOTHIE

Preparation Time: 5 minutes
Cooking Time: 0 minutes
Servings: 1
Ingredients:

1 ripe mango, cored and chopped
½ mango, peeled, pitted and chopped
1 cup kale, chopped
½ cup plain Greek yogurt
2 ice cubes

Directions:

Add pear, mango, yogurt, kale, and mango to a blender and puree. Add ice and blend until you have a smooth texture. Serve and enjoy!

Nutrition: Calories: 293; Fat: 8 g; Carbohydrates: 53 g; Protein: 8 g.

205 NUTTY DATE PAPAYA SMOOTHIE

Preparation Time: 5 minutes
Cooking Time: 0 minutes
Servings: 2
Ingredients:

1 papaya, deseeded
3 dates, pitted
1 burro banana, peeled
¼ of key lime, juiced
1 tbsp. Bromide Plus Powder

Extra:

1 cup spring water

Directions:

Plug in a high-speed food processor or blender and add all the ingredients to its jar.
Cover the blender jar with its lid and then pulse for 40 to 60 seconds until smooth.

Divide the drink between two glasses and then serve.

Nutrition: Calories: 152; Fats: 3.6 g; Protein: 2.4 g; Carbohydrates: 33 g; Fiber: 5 g.

206 CUCUMBER AND COCONUT SMOOTHIE

Preparation Time: 5 minutes
Cooking Time: 0 minutes
Servings: 2
Ingredients:

1 burro banana, peeled
½ of cucumber, deseeded
½ tsp. Bromide Plus Powder
½ cup soft-jelly coconut water
½ cup Dr. Sebi's Herbal Tea

Directions:

Plug in a high-speed food processor or blender and add all the ingredients to its jar.
Cover the blender jar with its lid and then pulse for 40 to 60 seconds until smooth.
Divide the drink between two glasses and then serve.

Nutrition: Calories: 138; Fats: 5 g; Protein: 3 g; Carbohydrates: 22 g; Fiber: 3 g.

207 STRAWBERRY AND RHUBARB SMOOTHIE

Preparation Time: 5 minutes
Cooking Time: 3 minutes
Servings: 1
Ingredients:

1 rhubarb stalk, chopped
1 cup fresh strawberries, sliced
½ cup plain Greek strawberries
Pinch of ground cinnamon
3 ice cubes

Directions:

Take a small saucepan and fill with water over high heat. Bring to boil and add rhubarb, boil for 3 minutes. Drain and transfer to the blender.
Add strawberries, honey, yogurt, cinnamon and pulse mixture until smooth. Add ice cubes and blend until thick with no lumps. Pour into glass and enjoy chilled.

Nutrition: Calories: 295; Fat: 8 g; Carbohydrates: 56 g; Protein: 6 g.

208 TAMARIND AND CUCUMBER BREAKFAST DRINK

Preparation Time: 5 minutes
Cooking Time: 0 minutes
Servings: 2
Ingredients:

2 cups Dr. Sebi's Herbal Tea
1 tbsp. tamarind pulp
1 cucumber, deseeded
2 oz. arugula
1 key lime, juiced

Extra:

¼ tsp. salt
⅛ tsp. cayenne pepper

Directions:

Plug in a high-speed food processor or blender and add all the ingredients to its jar.
Cover the blender jar with its lid and then pulse for 40 to 60 seconds until smooth.
Divide the drink between two glasses and then serve.

Nutrition: Calories: 110; Fats: 0.5 g; Protein: 2 g; Carbohydrates: 30.5 g; Fiber: 6.5 g.

209 HEARTY BERRY SMOOTHIE

Preparation Time: 5 minutes
Cooking Time: 0 minutes
Servings: 2
Ingredients:

¼ cup strawberries
¼ cup blueberries
¼ cup blackberries
¼ cup raspberries
2 tbsp. walnuts

Extra:

1 tbsp. Bromide Plus Powder
⅔ cup spring water

Directions:

Plug in a high-speed food processor or blender and add all the ingredients to its jar.
Cover the blender jar with its lid and then pulse for 40 to 60 seconds until smooth.
Divide the drink between two glasses and then serve.

Nutrition: Calories: 180; Fats: 8 g; Protein: 4 g; Carbohydrates: 25 g; Fiber: 5 g.

210 DANDELION GREEN SMOOTHIE

Preparation Time: 5 minutes
Cooking Time: 0 minutes
Servings: 2
Ingredients:

1 cup dandelion greens
½ of cucumber, deseeded
1 apple, cored, deseeded
1 burro banana, peeled
½ tbsp. walnuts

Extra:

½ tsp. Bromide Plus Powder
1 cup soft-jelly coconut milk

Directions:

Plug in a high-speed food processor or blender and add all the ingredients to its jar.
Cover the blender jar with its lid and then pulse for 40 to 60 seconds until smooth.
Divide the drink between two glasses and then serve.

Nutrition: Calories: 317; Fats: 11 g; Protein: 10 g; Carbohydrates: 42 g; Fiber: 7 g.

211 CANTALOUPE SMOOTHIE

Preparation Time: 5 minutes
Cooking Time: 0 minutes
Servings: 2
Ingredients:

1 cantaloupe, peeled, deseeded, sliced
½ cup Dr. Sebi Herbal Tea
½ of burro banana, peeled
½ cup soft-jelly coconut water

Directions:

Plug in a high-speed food processor or blender and add all the ingredients to its jar.

Cover the blender jar with its lid and then pulse for 40 to 60 seconds until smooth.

Divide the drink between two glasses and then serve.

Nutrition: Calories: 114.7; Fats: 0.6 g; Protein: 1.8 g; Carbohydrates: 27.8 g; Fiber: 1 g.

212 WATERMELON REFRESHER

Preparation Time: 5 minutes
Cooking Time: 0 minutes
Servings: 2
Ingredients:

1 watermelon, peeled, deseeded, cubed
1 tbsp. date
½ of key lime, juiced, zest
2 cups soft-jelly coconut water

Directions:

Place watermelon pieces in a high-speed food processor or blender. Add lime zest and juice.

Add date and then pulse until smooth.

Take two tall glasses, fill them with watermelon mixture until two-third full, and then pour in coconut water.

Stir until mixed and then serve.

Nutrition: Calories: 55; Fats: 1.3 g; Protein: 0.9 g; Carbohydrates: 9.9 g; Fiber: 7 g.

213 SMOOTHIE SNACK

Preparation Time: 5 minutes
Cooking Time: 0 minutes
Servings: 2
Ingredients:

1 burro banana, peeled
1 ½ cup mixed berries
1 mango, peeled, destoned, chopped
2 tbsp. walnut milk, homemade
1 tbsp. walnut butter, homemade

Extra:

2 tbsp. agave syrup

Directions:

Plug in a high-speed food processor or blender. Add burro banana and berries, and then pulse at low speed until small pieces of fruits remain in the jar.

Add milk, butter, and agave syrup. Pulse until combined, and then divide the mixture evenly between two bowls.

Top evenly with mango slices and some more berries and then serve.

Nutrition: Calories: 338; Fats: 9.6 g; Protein: 8.6 g; Carbohydrates: 64.3 g; Fiber: 12.1 g.

214 SMOOTHIE WITH NUTS

Preparation Time: 5 minutes
Cooking Time: 0 minutes
Servings: 2
Ingredients:

½ of burro banana, peeled
½ cup figs
2 strawberries
¼ cup Brazil nuts
1 cup spring water

Directions:

Plug in a high-speed food processor or blender and add all the ingredients to its jar.

Cover the blender jar with its lid and then pulse for 40 to 60 seconds until smooth.

Divide the drink between two glasses and then serve.

Nutrition: Calories: 234; Fats: 2 g; Protein: 6.1 g; Carbohydrates: 53.1 g; Fiber: 5.8 g.

215 WATERCRESS DETOX SMOOTHIE

Preparation Time: 5 minutes
Cooking Time: 0 minutes
Servings: 2
Ingredients:

½ cup watercress
½ of avocado, peeled, pitted
1 key lime, juiced
1 cup soft-jelly coconut milk, homemade
1 tsp. Bromide Plus Powder

Directions:

Plug in a high-speed food processor or blender and add all the ingredients to its jar.

Cover the blender jar with its lid and then pulse for 40 to 60 seconds until smooth.

Divide the drink between two glasses and then serve.

Nutrition: Calories: 146; Fats: 10.5 g; Protein: 7 g; Carbohydrates: 7.5 g; Fiber: 2.5 g.

216 MANGO AND ORANGE SMOOTHIE

Preparation Time: 5 minutes
Cooking Time: 0 minutes
Servings: 2
Ingredients:

½ of a large mango, peeled, destoned, cubed
1 key lime, juiced
1 orange, peeled
1 tbsp. agave syrup
1 tbsp. grapeseed oil

Extra:

1 cup herbal tea

Directions:

Plug in a high-speed food processor or blender and add all the ingredients to its jar.

Cover the blender jar with its lid and then pulse for 40 to 60 seconds until smooth.

Divide the drink between two glasses and then serve.

Nutrition: Calories: 163; Fats: 3.4 g; Protein: 1 g; Carbohydrates: 32 g; Fiber: 6 g.

217 GREEN SMOOTHIE WITH APPLE AND BLUEBERRIES

Preparation Time: 5 minutes
Cooking Time: 0 minutes
Ingredients:

1 cup blueberries
1 apple, cored
1 cup turnip greens
¼ cup Brazil nuts
½ tbsp. agave syrup

Extra:

1 cup walnut milk, homemade

Directions:

Plug in a high-speed food processor or blender and add all the ingredients to its jar.

Cover the blender jar with its lid and then pulse for 40 to 60 seconds until smooth.

Divide the drink between two glasses and then serve.

Nutrition: Calories: 215; Fats: 1.1 g; Protein: 2.3 g; Carbohydrates: 48 g; Fiber: 8.3 g.

218 NUTTY SEA MOSS SMOOTHIE

Preparation Time: 10 minutes
Cooking Time: 0 minutes
Servings: 2
Ingredients:

33 g, sea moss, rinsed
1 tbsp. coconut nectar
2 cups spring water, warmed
1 cup walnut milk, unsweetened

Extra:

¼ cup dates

Directions:

Place rinsed seaweed in a medium bowl, pour in the water and let it soak for a minimum of 4 hours until thickened slightly.

Drain the soaked sea moss and transfer into a food processor. Pulse until the smooth paste comes together, and then refrigerate until required.

When ready to drink, transfer 8 tablespoons of sea moss paste into a food processor. Add remaining ingredients and then pulse until smooth.

Divide the drink evenly between two glasses and then serve.

Nutrition: Calories: 100.5; Fats: 0.1 g; Protein: 1.7 g; Carbohydrates: 22.5 g; Fiber: 3.5 g.

219 ZUCCHINI AND AVOCADO SMOOTHIE

Preparation Time: 5 minutes
Cooking Time: 0 minutes
Servings: 2
Ingredients:

3 tbsp. hemp seeds
⅓ cup diced zucchini
1 cup dandelion greens
¼ of a large avocado, peeled, pitted
1 ¼ cup walnut milk, homemade

Directions:

Plug in a high-speed food processor or blender and add all the ingredients to its jar.

Cover the blender jar with its lid and then pulse for 40 to 60 seconds until smooth.

Divide the drink between two glasses and then serve.

Nutrition: Calories: 165; Fats: 6.8 g; Protein: 8.5 g; Carbohydrates: 17.3 g; Fiber: 5.5 g.

220 BLUEBERRY-PIE SMOOTHIE

Preparation Time: 5 minutes
Cooking Time: 0 minutes
Servings: 2
Ingredients:

¼ cup cooked amaranth
1 cup blueberries
1 tsp. Bromide Plus Powder
1 burro banana, peeled
1 tbsp. walnut butter, homemade

Extra:

2 tbsp. date
2 cups soft-jelly coconut milk, homemade

Directions:

Plug in a high-speed food processor or blender and add all the ingredients to its jar.

Cover the blender jar with its lid and then pulse for 40 to 60 seconds until smooth.

Divide the drink between two glasses and then serve.

Nutrition: Calories: 302; Fats: 3 g; Protein: 11 g; Carbohydrates: 60 g; Fiber: 7 g.

221 CUCUMBER AND BASIL CLEANSING DRINK

Preparation Time: 5 minutes
Cooking Time: 0 minutes

Servings: 2
Ingredients:

4 cucumbers, deseeded
1 bunch of basil leaves
2 key limes, juiced
½ tsp. Bromide Plus Powder
2 cups soft-jelly coconut water

Directions:

Plug in a high-speed food processor or blender and add all the ingredients to its jar.

Cover the blender jar with its lid and then pulse for 40 to 60 seconds until smooth.

Divide the drink between two glasses and then serve.

Nutrition: Calories: 56.1; Fats: 0.5 g; Protein: 0.9 g; Carbohydrates: 12 g; Fiber: 2 g.

222 BANANA, PEAR AND COCONUT SMOOTHIE

Preparation Time: 5 minutes
Cooking Time: 0 minutes
Servings: 2
Ingredients:

1 burro banana, peeled
2 cups chopped kale
1 pear, diced
1 cup of soft-jelly coconut water

Directions:

Plug in a high-speed food processor or blender and add all the ingredients to its jar.

Cover the blender jar with its lid and then pulse for 40 to 60 seconds until smooth.

Divide the drink between two glasses and then serve.

Nutrition: Calories: 90; Fats: 0 g; Protein: 1 g; Carbohydrates: 24 g; Fiber: 3 g.

223 WATERMELON AND RASPBERRIES SMOOTHIE

Preparation Time: 5 minutes
Cooking Time: 0 minutes
Servings: 2
Ingredients:

1 cup watermelon chunks
½ cup raspberries
1 key lime, juiced
¼ cup cucumber, deseeded, diced
½ cup soft-jelly coconut water

Directions:

Plug in a high-speed food processor or blender and add all the ingredients to its jar.

Cover the blender jar with its lid and then pulse for 40 to 60 seconds until smooth.

Divide the drink between two glasses and then serve.

Nutrition: Calories110; Fats: 1 g; Protein: 3.4 g; Carbohydrates: 26 g; Fiber: 7 g.

224 PAPAYA AND QUINOA SMOOTHIE

Preparation Time: 5 minutes
Cooking Time: 10 minutes
Servings: 2
Ingredients:

2 cups papaya cubes
2 tbsp. date
1 cup cooked quinoa or amaranth
2 tsp. Bromide Plus Powder
2 cups hemp milk, homemade

Directions:

Plug in a high-speed food processor or blender and add all the ingredients to its jar.

Cover the blender jar with its lid and then pulse for 40 to 60 seconds until smooth.

Divide the drink between two glasses and then serve.

Nutrition: Calories: 224.6; Fats: 7.7 g; Protein: 7 g; Carbohydrates: 33.7 g; Fiber: 3.5 g.

225 AVOCADO AND CUCUMBER SMOOTHIE

Preparation Time: 5 minutes
Cooking Time: 0 minutes
Servings: 2
Ingredients:

1 burro banana, peeled
¼ of an avocado
¼ of a cucumber
1 tbsp. agave syrup
½ cup herbal tea

Extra:

1 tbsp. chopped walnuts
1 cup soft-jelly coconut milk, homemade

Directions:

Plug in a high-speed food processor or blender and add all the ingredients to its jar.

Cover the blender jar with its lid and then pulse for 40 to 60 seconds until smooth.

Divide the drink between two glasses and then serve.

Nutrition: Calories: 103; Fats: 4.5 g; Protein: 1.6 g; Carbohydrates: 16.2 g; Fiber: 2.5 g.

226 ORANGE AND BANANA DRINK

Preparation Time: 5 minutes
Cooking Time: 0 minutes
Servings: 2
Ingredients:

½ of a burro banana, peeled
3 oranges, peeled
1 ½ tbsp. Date
½ tsp. Bromide Plus Powder
1 cup of soft-jelly coconut water

Directions:

Plug in a high-speed food processor or blender and add all the ingredients to its jar.

Cover the blender jar with its lid and then pulse for 40 to 60 seconds until smooth.

Divide the drink between two glasses and then serve.

Nutrition: Calories: 138.5; Fats: 0.6 g; Protein: 1.5 g; Carbohydrates: 35.1 g; Fiber: 4.7 g.

227 LETTUCE, BANANA AND BERRIES SMOOTHIE

Preparation Time: 5 minutes
Cooking Time: 0 minutes
Servings: 2
Ingredients:

½ of a burro banana
¼ cup blueberries
1 cup Romaine lettuce
2 tbsp. key lime juice
½ cup soft jelly coconut water

Directions:

Plug in a high-speed food processor or blender and add all the ingredients to its jar.

Cover the blender jar with its lid and then pulse for 40 to 60 seconds until smooth.

Divide the drink between two glasses and then serve.

Nutrition: Calories: 147; Fats: 0.8; Protein: 3.3 g; Carbohydrates: 36; Fiber: 4 g.

228 APPLE, QUINOA AND FIG SMOOTHIE

Preparation Time: 5 minutes
Cooking Time: 0 minutes
Servings: 2
Ingredients:

½ cup cooked quinoa
½ of a large red apple, cored
1 cup amaranth greens
1 fig
1 tsp. Bromide Plus Powder

Extra:

1 tbsp. raisins
1 tbsp. date
1 cup hemp seed milk, homemade

Directions:

Plug in a high-speed food processor or blender and add all the ingredients to its jar.

Cover the blender jar with its lid and then pulse for 40 to 60 seconds until smooth.

Divide the drink between two glasses and then serve.

Nutrition: Calories: 153; Fats: 1 g; Protein: 3 g; Carbohydrates: 28 g; Fiber: 3 g.

229 STRAWBERRY SHAKE

Preparation Time: 5 minutes

Cooking Time: 0 minutes
Servings: 2
Ingredients:

1 cup strawberries
½ cup Brazil nuts, soaked
1 tbsp. agave syrup
⅓ cup Irish Moss gel
1 ½ cups spring water

Directions:

Plug in a high-speed food processor or blender and add all the ingredients to its jar.

Cover the blender jar with its lid and then pulse for 40 to 60 seconds until smooth.

Divide the drink between two glasses and then serve.

Nutrition: Calories: 137; Fats: 5 g; Protein: 1 g; Carbohydrates: 22 g; Fiber: 2 g.

230 SWEET SUNRISE SMOOTHIE

Preparation Time: 5 minutes
Cooking Time: 0 minutes
Servings: 2
Ingredients:

1 cup mango chunks
1 cup raspberries
½ of a burro banana
1 orange, peeled
1 cup spring water

Directions:

Plug in a high-speed food processor or blender and add all the ingredients to its jar.

Cover the blender jar with its lid and then pulse for 40 to 60 seconds until smooth.

Divide the drink between two glasses and then serve.

Nutrition: Calories: 130; Fats: 0 g; Protein: 0 g; Carbohydrates: 30 g; Fiber: 3 g.

231 GREEN SEA MOSS DRINK

Preparation Time: 5 minutes
Cooking Time: 0 minutes
Servings: 2
Ingredients:

1 apple, cored, diced
2 cups kale
1 cup cucumber chunks
2 cups of coconut water

Extra:

1 key lime, juiced
1 tbsp. of sea moss gel

Directions:

Plug in a high-speed food processor or blender and add all the ingredients to its jar.

Cover the blender jar with its lid and then pulse for 40 to 60 seconds until smooth.

Divide the drink between two glasses and then serve.

Nutrition: Calories: 156; Fats: 1.8 g; Protein: 9.4 g; Carbohydrates: 32.8 g; Fiber: 10.2 g.

232 3 INGREDIENT BANANA HERBAL DRINK

Preparation Time: 5 minutes
Cooking Time: 0 minutes
Servings: 2
Ingredients:

2 burro bananas, peeled
1 cup herbal tea
1 tbsp. agave syrup

Directions:

Plug in a high-speed food processor or blender and add all the ingredients to its jar.

Cover the blender jar with its lid and then pulse for 40 to 60 seconds until smooth.

Divide the drink between two glasses and then serve.

Nutrition: Calories: 177; Fats: 1 g; Protein: 2 g; Carbohydrates: 40 g; Fiber: 4 g.

233 WATERMELON, CANTALOUPE AND MANGO SMOOTHIE

Preparation Time: 5 minutes
Cooking Time: 0 minutes
Servings: 2
Ingredients:

½ of a large mango, peeled
½ of burro banana, peeled
½ cup cantaloupe, peeled
½ cup amaranth greens
½ cup watermelon chunks

Extra:

1 cup soft jelly coconut water

Directions:

Plug in a high-speed food processor or blender and add all the ingredients to its jar.

Cover the blender jar with its lid and then pulse for 40 to 60 seconds until smooth.

Divide the drink between two glasses and then serve.

Nutrition: Calories: 132; Fats: 1 g; Protein: 3.5 g; Carbohydrates: 30.1 g; Fiber: 3.2 g.

234 BLACKBERRY & BANANA SMOOTHIE

Preparation Time: 5 minutes
Cooking Time: 0 minutes
Servings: 2
Ingredients:

1 burro banana, peeled
½ cup blackberries
2 dates, pitted
1 cup mango chunks
¼ cup walnut milk, unsweetened

Extra:

¼ cup coconut water

Directions:

Plug in a high-speed food processor or blender and add all the ingredients to its jar.

Cover the blender jar with its lid and then pulse for 40 to 60 seconds until smooth.

Divide the drink between two glasses and then serve.

Nutrition: Calories: 147.7; Fats: 0.7 g; Protein: 5 g; Carbohydrates: 34 g; Fiber: 4.1 g.

235 GREEN SMOOTHIE WITH RASPBERRIES

Preparation Time: 5 minutes
Cooking Time: 0 minutes
Servings: 2
Ingredients:

1 cup raspberries
1 cup kale leaves
1 tbsp. sea moss
2 tbsp. key lime juice
1 cup soft-jelly coconut milk

Directions:

Plug in a high-speed food processor or blender and add all the ingredients to its jar.

Cover the blender jar with its lid and then pulse for 40 to 60 seconds until smooth.

Divide the drink between two glasses and then serve.

Nutrition: Calories: 151; Fats: 1.2 g; Protein: 3 g; Carbohydrates: 37 g; Fiber: 8 g.

236 VEGGIE-FUL SMOOTHIE

Preparation Time: 5 minutes
Cooking Time: 0 minutes
Servings: 2
Ingredients:

1 pear, cored, deseeded
½ cup watercress
¼ of avocado, peeled
½ cup Romaine lettuce
½ of cucumber, peeled, deseeded

Extra:

1 tbsp. date
½ cup spring water

Directions:

Plug in a high-speed food processor or blender and add all the ingredients to its jar.

Cover the blender jar with its lid and then pulse for 40 to 60 seconds until smooth.

Divide the drink between two glasses and then serve.

Nutrition: Calories: 145; Fats: 6 g; Protein: 1 g; Carbohydrates: 25 g; Fiber: 6 g.

237 APPLE PIE SMOOTHIE

Preparation Time: 5 minutes
Cooking Time: 0 minutes
Servings: 2
Ingredients:

½ of a large apple, deseeded
¼ cup walnuts
2 figs
1 tsp. Bromide Plus Powder

Extra:

1 tbsp. date

Directions:

Plug in a high-speed food processor or blender and add all the ingredients to its jar.

Cover the blender jar with its lid and then pulse for 40 to 60 seconds until smooth.

Divide the drink between two glasses and then serve.

Nutrition: Calories: 170; Fats: 8 g; Protein: 2 g; Carbohydrates: 26 g; Fiber: 8 g.

238 ORANGE AND LETTUCE SMOOTHIE

Preparation Time: 5 minutes
Cooking Time: 0 minutes
Servings: 2
Ingredients:

2 oranges, peeled, sliced
1 cup shredded lettuce, rinsed
2 apples, cored, sliced
1 cup spring water

Directions:

Plug in a high-speed food processor or blender and add all the ingredients to its jar.

Cover the blender jar with its lid and then pulse for 40 to 60 seconds until smooth.

Divide the drink between two glasses and then serve.

Nutrition: Calories: 140; Fats: 0.9 g; Protein: 1.3 g; Carbohydrates: 31.8 g; Fiber: 3 g.

239 GREEN TEA AND LETTUCE DETOX SMOOTHIE

Preparation Time: 5 minutes
Cooking Time: 0 minutes
Servings: 2
Ingredients:

½ of burro banana
¼ cup blueberries, fresh
1 cup Romaine lettuce
3 tbsp. key lime juice

Extra:

½ cup soft jelly coconut water

Directions:

Plug in a high-speed food processor or blender and add all the ingredients to its jar.

Cover the blender jar with its lid and then pulse for 40 to 60 seconds until smooth.

Divide the drink between two glasses and then serve.

Nutrition: Calories: 134; Fats: 4.5 g; Protein: 4.6 g; Carbohydrates: 20 g; Fiber: 3.7 g.

240 CHAMOMILE DELIGHT SMOOTHIE

Preparation Time: 5 minutes
Cooking Time: 0 minutes
Servings: 2
Ingredients:

2 burro bananas, peeled
½ cup chamomile tea
1 tbsp. date
½ cup walnut milk, homemade

Directions:

Plug in a high-speed food processor or blender and add all the ingredients to its jar.

Cover the blender jar with its lid and then pulse for 40 to 60 seconds until smooth.

Divide the drink between two glasses and then serve.

Nutrition: Calories: 142; Fats: 5 g; Protein: 3.5 g; Carbohydrates: 25 g; Fiber: 8.5 g.

241 HONEY DEW AND ARUGULA SMOOTHIE

Preparation Time: 5 minutes
Cooking Time: 0 minutes
Servings: 2
Ingredients:

1 large bunch Calaloo
1 cup cucumber, deseeded
1 large bunch arugulas
¼ cup honeydew pieces
1 pear, diced

Extra:

6 dates, pitted
1 tbsp. sea moss gel
¼ cup key lime juice
2 cups soft-jelly coconut water

Directions:

Plug in a high-speed food processor or blender and add all the ingredients to its jar.

Cover the blender jar with its lid and then pulse for 40 to 60 seconds until smooth.

Divide the drink between two glasses and then serve.

Nutrition: Calories: 189.5; Fats: 2.5 g; Protein: 1.5 g; Carbohydrates: 42.6 g; Fiber: 6.6 g.

242 WATERMELON AND STRAWBERRIES DRINK

Preparation Time: 5 minutes
Cooking Time: 0 minutes
Servings: 2
Ingredients:

1 cup strawberries
1 cup watermelon, chunks
1 tsp. date
1 cup soft jelly coconut water

Directions:

Plug in a high-speed food processor or blender and add all the ingredients to its jar.

Cover the blender jar with its lid and then pulse for 40 to 60 seconds until smooth.

Divide the drink between two glasses and then serve.

Nutrition: Calories: 110; Fats: 0 g; Protein: 0 g; Carbohydrates: 28 g; Fiber: 6 g.

243 SWEET GREEN DRINK

Preparation Time: 5 minutes
Cooking Time: 0 minutes
Servings: 2
Ingredients:

1 cup greens
1 cucumber, peeled, deseeded
1 key lime, peeled
2 dates, pitted

Extra:

2 cups of soft-jelly coconut water

Directions:

Plug in a high-speed food processor or blender and add all the ingredients to its jar.

Cover the blender jar with its lid and then pulse for 40 to 60 seconds until smooth.

Divide the drink between two glasses and then serve.

Nutrition: Calories: 112; Fats: 0.1 g; Protein: 0.3 g; Carbohydrates: 27 g; Fiber: 5 g.

244 BANANA SEA MOSS SMOOTHIE

Preparation Time: 5 minutes
Cooking Time: 0 minutes
Servings: 2
Ingredients:

1 cup kale
½ apple, cored, sliced
1 tsp. sea moss
½ of a burro banana

Extra:

1 tsp. Bromide Plus Powder

Directions:

Plug in a high-speed food processor or blender and add all the ingredients to its jar.

Cover the blender jar with its lid and then pulse for 40 to 60 seconds until smooth.

Divide the drink between two glasses and then serve.

Nutrition: Calories: 115; Fats: 0.5 g; Protein: 2 g; Carbohydrates: 28 g; Fiber: 2 g.

245 BANANA AND WALNUT SMOOTHIE

Preparation Time: 5 minutes
Cooking Time: 0 minutes
Servings: 2
Ingredients:

1 burro banana, peeled

4 dates, pitted, chopped
1 cup walnut milk, homemade
6 tbsp. walnut
1 cup of soft-jelly coconut water

Directions:

Plug in a high-speed food processor or blender and add all the ingredients to its jar.

Cover the blender jar with its lid and then pulse for 40 to 60 seconds until smooth.

Divide the drink between two glasses and then serve.

Nutrition: Calories: 199; Fats: 5 g; Protein: 6 g; Carbohydrates: 34.7 g; Fiber: 3.5 g.

246 LIME AND KALE SMOOTHIE

Preparation Time: 5 minutes
Cooking Time: 0 minutes
Servings: 2
Ingredients:

1 apple, peeled, cored, chopped
2 cups kale leaves
1 tsp. key lime juice
1 ¼ cups orange juice

Extra:

1/16 tsp. cayenne pepper

Directions:

Plug in a high-speed food processor or blender and add all the ingredients to its jar.

Cover the blender jar with its lid and then pulse for 40 to 60 seconds until smooth.

Divide the drink between two glasses and then serve.

Nutrition: Calories: 188; Fats: 1 g; Protein: 4.4 g; Carbohydrates: 50 g; Fiber: 14 g.

247 SOOTHING ARUGULA & APPLE SMOOTHIE

Preparation Time: 5 minutes
Cooking Time: 0 minutes
Servings: 2
Ingredients:

2 cups arugula
1 burro banana, peeled
2 apples, cored
2 cups of soft-jelly coconut water

Extra:

4 tbsp. key lime juice

Directions:

Plug in a high-speed food processor or blender and add all the ingredients to its jar.

Cover the blender jar with its lid and then pulse for 40 to 60 seconds until smooth.

Divide the drink between two glasses and then serve.

Nutrition: Calories: 180; Fats: 0 g; Protein: 0 g; Carbohydrates: 45 g; Fiber: 8 g.

248 BREAKFAST BOOST WITH APPLE AND BERRIES

Preparation Time: 5 minutes
Cooking Time: 0 minutes
Servings: 2
Ingredients:

2 cups greens
1 cup mixed berries
1 apple, cored, diced
1 cup hemp milk, homemade

Directions:

Plug in a high-speed food processor or blender and add all the ingredients to its jar.

Cover the blender jar with its lid and then pulse for 40 to 60 seconds until smooth.

Divide the drink between two glasses and then serve.

Nutrition: Calories: 136.5; Fats: 2.9 g; Protein: 7.1 g; Carbohydrates: 23.4 g; Fiber: 8.1 g.

249 ARU-AVOCADO DETOX SMOOTHIE

Preparation Time: 5 minutes
Cooking Time: 0 minutes
Servings: 2
Ingredients:

2 cups arugula
¼ cup cranberries
½ of avocado, peeled, pitted
1 apple, cored
1 kiwifruit

Extra:

1 tbsp. key lime juice
½ cup spring water

Directions:

Plug in a high-speed food processor or blender and add all the ingredients to its jar.

Cover the blender jar with its lid and then pulse for 40 to 60 seconds until smooth.

Divide the drink between two glasses and then serve.

Nutrition: Calories: 192; Fats: 9.4 g; Protein: 6 g; Carbohydrates: 22 g; Fiber: 4 g.

250 REVITALIZER KALE SMOOTHIE

Preparation Time: 5 minutes
Cooking Time: 0 minutes
Servings: 2
Ingredients:

1 burro banana, peeled
2 cups chopped kale
1 mango, peeled, destoned, diced
1 cup of coconut water

Directions:

Plug in a high-speed food processor or blender and add all the ingredients to its jar.

Cover the blender jar with its lid and then pulse for 40 to 60 seconds until smooth.

Divide the drink between two glasses and then serve.

Nutrition: Calories: 145; Fats: 0.5 g; Protein: 2 g; Carbohydrates: 36.5 g; Fiber: 4.5 g.

251 CLEANSING APPLE AND AVOCADO SMOOTHIE

Preparation Time: 5 minutes
Cooking Time: 0 minutes
Servings: 2
Ingredients:

1 cup of soft-jelly coconut water
1 cup strawberries
1 apple, cored, diced
½ of avocado, peeled, pitted
1 cup Kale

Extra:

1 tbsp. key lime juice
⅛ tsp. cayenne pepper

Directions:

Plug in a high-speed food processor or blender and add all the ingredients to its jar.

Cover the blender jar with its lid and then pulse for 40 to 60 seconds until smooth.

Divide the drink between two glasses and then serve.

Nutrition: Calories: 215; Fats: 7.2 g; Protein: 2.8 g; Carbohydrates: 39.3 g; Fiber: 5.3 g.

252 KALE GREEN SMOOTHIE

Preparation Time: 5 minutes
Cooking Time: 0 minutes
Servings: 2
Ingredients:

2 cups kale leaves
1 cup mango cubes
2 key limes, juiced
1 cup peaches

Extra:

1 ½ cups spring water
1 tbsp. agave syrup

Directions:

Plug in a high-speed food processor or blender and add all the ingredients to its jar.

Cover the blender jar with its lid and then pulse for 40 to 60 seconds until smooth.

Divide the drink between two glasses and then serve.

Nutrition: Calories: 117; Fats: 0.8 g; Protein: 2.5 g; Carbohydrates: 26.4 g; Fiber: 3.5 g.

253 THE GREEN DETOX SMOOTHIE

Preparation Time: 5 minutes
Cooking Time: 0 minutes
Servings: 2

Ingredients:

1 cup kale leaves
1 orange, peeled
2 cups kale leaves
1 burro banana, peeled
⅔ cup spring water

Directions:

Plug in a high-speed food processor or blender and add all the ingredients to its jar.

Cover the blender jar with its lid and then pulse for 40 to 60 seconds until smooth.

Divide the drink between two glasses and then serve.

Nutrition: Calories: 154; Fats: 0.2 g; Protein: 0 g; Carbohydrates: 37.7 g; Fiber: 6.8 g.

254 DANDELION REVITALIZING SMOOTHIE

Preparation Time: 5 minutes
Cooking Time: 0 minutes
Servings: 2
Ingredients:

¼ cup blueberries
½ of a large bunch of dandelion greens
2 baby burro bananas, peeled
½ cup watercress

Extra:

3 dates, pitted
1 tbsp. Bromide Plus powder
1 cup of soft-jelly coconut water
2 tbsp. lime juice

Directions:

Plug in a high-speed food processor or blender and add all the ingredients to its jar.

Cover the blender jar with its lid and then pulse for 40 to 60 seconds until smooth.

Divide the drink between two glasses and then serve.

Nutrition: Calories: 142.5; Fats: 5.1 g; Protein: 5.3 g; Carbohydrates: 26.8 g; Fiber: 9.6 g.

255 POWER BURST BANANA GREEN SMOOTHIE

Preparation Time: 5 minutes
Cooking Time: 0 minutes
Servings: 2
Ingredients:

1 burro banana, peeled
2 cups kale leaves
1 tbsp. walnut butter, homemade
2 cups soft-jelly coconut water

Directions:

Plug in a high-speed food processor or blender and add all the ingredients to its jar.

Cover the blender jar with its lid and then pulse for 40 to 60 seconds until smooth.

Divide the drink between two glasses and then serve.

Nutrition: Calories: 271.1; Fats: 4.3 g; Protein: 1.5 g; Carbohydrates: 56.6 g; Fiber: 10.1 g.

256 MANGO AND ARUGULA SMOOTHIE

Preparation Time: 5 minutes
Cooking Time: 0 minutes
Servings: 2
Ingredients:

1 cup mango chunks
2 cups arugula
¼ cup soft-jelly coconut, shreds
½ of a medium avocado, peeled, pitted
¾ cup of soft-jelly coconut water

Extra:

½ of key lime, zested, juice

Directions:

Plug in a high-speed food processor or blender and add all the ingredients to its jar.

Cover the blender jar with its lid and then pulse for 40 to 60 seconds until smooth.

Divide the drink between two glasses and then serve.

Nutrition: Calories: 220; Fats: 18 g; Protein: 3 g; Carbohydrates: 25 g; Fiber: 7 g.

257 BLUE-GREEN DETOX SMOOTHIE

Preparation Time: 5 minutes
Cooking Time: 0 minutes
Servings: 2
Ingredients:

1 burro banana, peeled
½ cup blueberries
2 cups kale leaves
1 tbsp. agave syrup

Extra:

1 cup walnut milk, unsweetened

Directions:

Plug in a high-speed food processor or blender and add all the ingredients to its jar.

Cover the blender jar with its lid and then pulse for 40 to 60 seconds until smooth.

Divide the drink between two glasses and then serve.

Nutrition: Calories: 220; Fats: 7 g; Protein: 8 g; Carbohydrates: 30 g; Fiber: 4.5 g.

258 PEACHY HEMP SEED SMOOTHIE

Preparation Time: 5 minutes
Cooking Time: 0 minutes
Servings: 2
Ingredients:

2 burro bananas, peeled
2 tbsp. walnut butter, homemade
1 cup peach slices
1 tbsp. hemp seeds
2 cups spring water

Directions:

Plug in a high-speed food processor or blender and add all the ingredients to its jar.

Cover the blender jar with its lid and then pulse for 40 to 60 seconds until smooth.

Divide the drink between two glasses and then serve.

Nutrition: Calories: 250.4; Fats: 12 g; Protein: 5.4 g; Carbohydrates: 35 g; Fiber: 4 g.

259 APPLE AND AVOCADO SMOOTHIE

Preparation Time: 5 minutes
Cooking Time: 0 minutes
Servings: 2
Ingredients:

2 apples, peeled, cored, diced
4 cups kale leaves
1 avocado, peeled, pitted
1 burro banana, peeled
2 tsp. agave syrup

Extra:

1 cup walnut milk, unsweetened

Directions:

Plug in a high-speed food processor or blender and add all the ingredients to its jar.

Cover the blender jar with its lid and then pulse for 40 to 60 seconds until smooth.

Divide the drink between two glasses and then serve.

Nutrition: Calories: 216.4; Fats: 7.5 g; Protein: 2.9 g; Carbohydrates: 39.3 g; Fiber: 7.7 g.

260 KEY LIME TEA

Preparation Time: 5 minutes
Cooking Time: 10 minutes
Servings: 2
Ingredients:

1 sprig of dill weed
1/16 tsp. cayenne pepper
1 tbsp. key lime juice
2 cups spring water

Directions:

Take a medium saucepan, place it over medium-high heat, pour in water, and then bring it to a boil.

Boil for 5 minutes, and then strain the tea into a bowl.

Add lime juice stir until mixed and then stir in cayenne pepper.

Divide tea between two mugs and then serve.

Nutrition: Calories: 2.4; Fats: 0 g; Protein: 0 g; Carbohydrates: 0.5 g; Fiber: 0 g.

261 KALE AND APPLE SMOOTHIE

Preparation Time: 5 minutes
Cooking Time: 0 minutes

Servings: 2
Ingredients:

2 cups kale leaves
2 tbsp. agave syrup
2 small apples, peeled, cored, diced
2 tbsp. key lime juice
1 cup walnut milk, homemade

Directions:

Plug in a high-speed food processor or blender and add all the ingredients to its jar.

Cover the blender jar with its lid and then pulse for 40 to 60 seconds until smooth.

Divide the drink between two glasses and then serve.

Nutrition: Calories: 121; Fats: 3.4 g; Protein: 4.2 g; Carbohydrates: 22 g; Fiber: 6 g.

262 THE 3 INGREDIENT GREEN SMOOTHIE

Preparation Time: 5 minutes
Cooking Time: 0 minutes
Servings: 2
Ingredients:

2 burro bananas, peeled
½ cup lettuce
1 cup spring water
2 cups orange juice, fresh

Directions:

Plug in a high-speed food processor or blender and add all the ingredients to its jar.

Cover the blender jar with its lid and then pulse for 40 to 60 seconds until smooth.

Divide the drink between two glasses and then serve.

Nutrition: Calories: 160; Fats: 0.3 g; Protein: 1.7 g; Carbohydrates: 39.7 g; Fiber: 7.7 g.

263 AMAZING SEA MOSS GREEN DRINK

Preparation Time: 5 minutes
Cooking Time: 0 minutes
Servings: 2
Ingredients:

4 tbsp. sea moss gel
4 cups mixed greens
2 burro bananas, peeled

Directions:

Plug in a high-speed food processor or blender and add all the ingredients to its jar.

Cover the blender jar with its lid and then pulse for 40 to 60 seconds until smooth.

Divide the drink between two glasses and then serve.

Nutrition: Calories: 120; Fats: 0.1 g; Protein: 3.4 g; Carbohydrates: 26 g; Fiber: 3.4 g.

264 KI-KI MANGO & BANANA SMOOTHIE

Preparation Time: 5 minutes
Cooking Time: 0 minutes
Servings: 2
Ingredients:

2 cups mango pieces
2 burro bananas, peeled
2 oranges, peeled
2 tsp. agave syrup
⅓ cup walnut milk, homemade

Directions:

Plug in a high-speed food processor or blender and add all the ingredients to its jar.

Cover the blender jar with its lid and then pulse for 40 to 60 seconds until smooth.

Divide the drink between two glasses and then serve.

Nutrition: Calories: 157; Fats: 2 g; Protein: 3 g; Carbohydrates: 35.5 g; Fiber: 3.5 g.

265 APPLE JUICE MIX

Preparation Time: 5 minutes
Cooking Time: 0 minutes
Servings: 2
Ingredients:

2 cups kale leaves
½ of avocado, peeled, pitted, diced
1 apple, peeled, cored, diced
1 ½ cups apple juice

Directions:

Plug in a high-speed food processor or blender and add all the ingredients to its jar.

Cover the blender jar with its lid and then pulse for 40 to 60 seconds until smooth.

Divide the drink between two glasses and then serve.

Nutrition: Calories: 152; Fats: 8.2 g; Protein: 2.7 g; Carbohydrates: 16.7 g; Fiber: 7.7 g.

266 SMOOTHIE BOWL

Preparation Time: 5 minutes
Cooking Time: 0 minutes
Servings: 2
Ingredients:

1 burro banana, peeled
1 ½ cup mixed berries
1 mango, peeled, destoned, chopped
2 tbsp. walnut milk, homemade
1 tbsp. walnut butter, homemade

Extra:

2 tbsp. agave syrup

Directions:

Plug in a high-speed food processor or blender, add banana and berries and then pulse at low speed until small pieces of fruits remain in the jar.

Add milk, butter, and agave syrup, pulse until combined, and then divide the mixture evenly between two bowls.

Top evenly with mango slices and some more berries and then serve.
Storage instructions:
Divide drink between two jars or bottles, cover with a lid and then store the containers in the refrigerator for up to 3 days.

Nutrition: Calories: 338; Fats: 9.6 g; Protein: 8.6 g; Carbohydrates: 64.3 g; Fiber: 12.1 g.

267 REFRESHING SMOOTHIE WITH NUTS

Preparation Time: 5 minutes
Cooking Time: 0 minutes
Servings: 2
Ingredients:

½ of burro banana, peeled
½ cup figs
2 strawberries
¼ cup Brazil nuts
1 cup spring water

Directions:

Plug in a high-speed food processor or blender and add all the ingredients to its jar.
Cover the blender jar with its lid and then pulse for 40 to 60 seconds until smooth.
Divide the drink between two glasses and then serve.
Storage instructions:
Divide drink between two jars or bottles, cover with a lid and then store the containers in the refrigerator for up to 3 days.

Nutrition: Calories: 234; Fats: 2 g; Protein: 6.1 g; Carbohydrates: 53.1 g; Fiber: 5.8 g.

268 CANTALOUPE SMOOTHIE TEA

Preparation Time: 5 minutes
Cooking Time: 0 minutes
Servings: 2
Ingredients:

1 cantaloupe, peeled, deseeded, sliced
½ cup Dr. Sebi Herbal Tea
½ of burro banana, peeled
½ cup soft-jelly coconut water

Directions:

Plug in a high-speed food processor or blender and add all the ingredients to its jar.
Cover the blender jar with its lid and then pulse for 40 to 60 seconds until smooth.
Divide the drink between two glasses and then serve.
Storage instructions:
Divide drink between two jars or bottles, cover with a lid and then store the containers in the refrigerator for up to 3 days.

Nutrition: Calories: 114.7; Fats: 0.6 g; Protein: 1.8 g; Carbohydrates: 27.8 g; Fiber: 1 g.

269 WATERMELON JUICE

Preparation Time: 5 minutes
Cooking Time: 0 minutes
Servings: 2
Ingredients:

1 watermelon, peeled, deseeded, cubed
1 tbsp. date sugar
½ of key lime, juiced, zest
2 cups soft-jelly coconut water

Directions:

Place watermelon pieces in a high-speed food processor or blender, add lime zest and juice, add date sugar and then pulse until smooth.
Take two tall glasses, fill them with watermelon mixture until two-third full, and then pour in coconut water.
Stir until mixed and then serve.
Storage instructions:
Divide drink between two jars or bottles, cover with a lid and then store the containers in the refrigerator for up to 3 days.

Nutrition: Calories: 55; Fats: 1.3 g; Protein: 0.9 g; Carbohydrates: 9.9 g; Fiber: 7 g.

270 GREEN SMOOTHIE

Preparation Time: 5 minutes
Cooking Time: 0 minutes
Servings: 2
Ingredients:

1 cup dandelion greens
½ of cucumber, deseeded
1 apple, cored, deseeded
1 burro banana, peeled
½ tbsp. walnuts

Extra:

½ tsp. Bromide Plus Powder
1 cup soft-jelly coconut milk

Directions:

Plug in a high-speed food processor or blender and add all the ingredients to its jar.
Cover the blender jar with its lid and then pulse for 40 to 60 seconds until smooth.
Divide the drink between two glasses and then serve.
Storage instructions:
Divide drink between two bottles or jars, cover with their lids and then store the containers in the refrigerator for up to 3 days.

Nutrition: Calories: 317; Fats: 11 g; Protein: 10 g; Carbohydrates: 42 g; Fiber: 7 g.

271 MINERAL SMOOTHIE

Preparation Time: 5 minutes
Cooking Time: 0 minutes
Servings: 2

Ingredients:

1 papaya, deseeded
3 dates, pitted
1 burro banana, peeled
¼ of key lime, juiced
1 tbsp. Bromide Plus Powder

Extra:

1 cup spring water

Directions:

Plug in a high-speed food processor or blender and add all the ingredients to its jar.
Cover the blender jar with its lid and then pulse for 40 to 60 seconds until smooth.
Divide the drink between two glasses and then serve.
Storage instructions:
Divide drink between two jars or bottles, cover with a lid and then store the containers in the refrigerator for up to 3 days.

Nutrition: Calories: 152; Fats: 3.6 g; Protein: 2.4 g; Carbohydrates: 33 g; Fiber: 5 g.

272 TRIPLE BERRY SMOOTHIE

Preparation Time: 5 minutes
Cooking Time: 0 minutes
Servings: 2
Ingredients:

½ cup strawberries
2 tbsp. agave syrup
½ cup raspberries
1 burro banana, peeled
½ cup blueberries
1 cup spring water

Directions:

Plug in a high-speed food processor or blender and add all the ingredients to its jar.
Cover the blender jar with its lid and then pulse for 40 to 60 seconds until smooth.
Divide the drink between two glasses and then serve.

Storage instructions:

Divide drink between two jars or bottles, cover with a lid and then store the containers in the refrigerator for up to 3 days.

Nutrition: Calories: 130; Fats: 1.5 g; Protein: 5 g; Carbohydrates: 26 g; Fiber: 4 g.

273 MANGO SMOOTHIE

Preparation Time: 10 minutes
Cooking Time: 10 minutes
Servings: 4
Ingredients:

1 medium mango; peeled, pitted, and chopped
4 burro bananas, peeled and sliced
½ cup walnuts, chopped
3 cups unsweetened hemp milk
1 cup ice cubes

Directions:

In a high-powered blender, put all ingredients and pulse until creamy.

Place the smoothie into four serving glasses and serve.

Nutrition: Calories: 312; Fats: 1.1 g; Cholesterol: 0 mg; Carbohydrates: 41.8 g; Fiber: 5.6 g; Protein: 7.2 g.

274 PAPAYA SMOOTHIE

Preparation Time: 10 minutes
Cooking Time: 10 minutes
Servings: 2
Ingredients:

½ of medium papaya, peeled and chopped roughly
2 burro bananas, peeled and sliced
1 tbsp. fresh key lime juice
1 ½ cups homemade walnut milk
½ cup ice cubes, crushed

Directions:

In a high-powered blender, put all ingredients and pulse until creamy.

Place the smoothie into two serving glasses and serve.

Nutrition: Calories: 170; Fats: 0.4 g; Cholesterol: 0 mg; Carbohydrates: 37 g; Fiber: 5.2 g; Protein: 2.4 g.

275 KALE & AVOCADO SMOOTHIE

Preparation Time: 10 minutes
Cooking Time: 10 minutes
Servings: 2
Ingredients:

2 cups fresh baby kale
½ avocado; peeled, pitted, and chopped
2 tbsp. agave nectar
½ tsp. ground cinnamon
1 tbsp. hemp seeds, shelled
2 cups chilled spring water

Directions:

In a high-powered blender, put all ingredients and pulse until creamy.

Place the smoothie into two serving glasses and serve.

Nutrition: Calories: 239; Fats: 0 g; Cholesterol: 32 mg; Carbohydrates: 27.8 g; Fiber: 6.5 g; Protein: 5.5 g.

276 CUCUMBER & GREENS SMOOTHIE

Preparation Time: 10 minutes
Cooking Time: 10 minutes
Servings: 2
Ingredients:

1 small seedless cucumber, peeled and chopped roughly
2 cups fresh dandelion greens, chopped
2 tbsp. date
½ tbsp. fresh key lime juice

1 ½ cups spring water
¼ cup ice cubes, crushed

Directions:

In a high-powered blender, put all ingredients and pulse until creamy.

Place the smoothie into two serving glasses and serve.

Nutrition: Calories: 81; Fats: 0.2 g; Cholesterol: 0 mg; Carbohydrates: 19.6 g; Fiber: 2.7 g; Protein: 2.5 g.

277 ORANGE JUICE

Preparation Time: 10 minutes
Cooking Time: 10 minutes
Servings: 2
Ingredients:

6 medium oranges; peeled, seeded, and divided

Directions:

In a juicer, add orange pieces and extract the juice according to the manufacturer's directions.

Transfer into two glasses and serve immediately.

Nutrition: Calories: 259; Fats: 0.1 g; Cholesterol: 0 mg; Carbohydrates: 64.9 g; Fiber: 13.3 g; Protein: 5.3 g.

278 STRAWBERRY JUICE

Preparation Time: 10 minutes
Cooking Time: 10 minutes
Servings: 2
Ingredients:

2 cups fresh strawberries, hulled
1 tsp. fresh key lime juice
2 cups chilled spring water

Directions:

In a high-powered blender, put all ingredients and pulse well.

Through a strainer, strain the juice and transfer into 2 glasses.

Serve immediately.

Nutrition: Calories: 46; Fats: 0 g; Cholesterol: 0 mg; Carbohydrates: 11.1 g; Fiber: 2.9 g; Protein: 1 g.

279 GRAPE JUICE

Preparation Time: 10 minutes
Cooking Time: 10 minutes
Servings: 2
Ingredients:

2 cups seedless red grapes
½ lime
2 cups spring water

Directions:

In a blender, put all ingredients and pulse well.

Through a strainer, strain the juice and transfer into 2 glasses.

Serve immediately.

Nutrition: Calories: 63; Fats: 0.1 g; Cholesterol: 0 mg; Carbohydrates: 16.2 g; Fiber: 0.9 g; Protein: 0.6 g.

280 MANGO JUICE

Preparation Time: 10 minutes
Cooking Time: 10 minutes
Servings: 4
Ingredients:

4 cups mangoes; peeled, pitted, and chopped
2 cups spring water

Directions:

In a blender, put all ingredients and pulse well.

Through a strainer, strain the juice and transfer into 4 glasses.

Serve immediately.

Nutrition: Calories: 99; Fats: 0.2 g; Cholesterol: 0 mg; Carbohydrates: 24.7 g; Fiber: 2.6 g; Protein: 1.4 g.

281 APPLE & KALE JUICE

Preparation Time: 10 minutes
Cooking Time: 10 minutes
Servings: 2
Ingredients:

2 large green apples, cored and sliced
4 cups fresh kale leaves
¼ cup fresh parsley leaves
1 tbsp. fresh ginger, peeled
1 key lime, peeled and seeded
1 cup chilled spring water

Directions:

In a blender, put all ingredients and pulse well.

Through a strainer, strain the juice and transfer into 2 glasses.

Serve immediately.

Nutrition: Calories: 196; Fats: 0.1 g; Cholesterol: 0 mg; Carbohydrates: 47.9 g; Fiber: 8.2 g; Protein: 5.2 g.

282 BLUEBERRY SMOOTHIE

Preparation Time: 5 minutes
Cooking Time: 0 minutes
Servings: 2
Ingredients:

½ cup blueberries
1 burro banana, peeled
¼ cup cooked quinoa
2 tbsp. date sugar
1 cup walnut milk, homemade

Directions:

Plug in a high-speed food processor or blender and add all the ingredients to its jar.

Cover the blender jar with its lid and then pulse for 40 to 60 seconds until smooth.

Divide the drink between two glasses and then serve.

Storage instructions:

Divide drink between two jars or bottles, cover with a lid and then store the containers in the refrigerator for up to 3 days.

Nutrition: Calories: 194; Fats: 5 g; Protein: 5 g; Carbohydrates: 34 g; Fiber: 2 g.

283 SMOOTHIE WITH STRAWBERRIES

Preparation Time: 5 minutes
Cooking Time: 10 minutes
Servings: 2
Ingredients:
- 1 ½ cup Dr. Sebi's Herbal Tea
- ¼ cup soft-jelly coconut, shredded
- ½ cup strawberries
- 2 tbsp. agave syrup

Directions:
Plug in a high-speed food processor or blender and add all the ingredients to its jar.
Cover the blender jar with its lid and then pulse for 40 to 60 seconds until smooth.
Divide the drink between two glasses and then serve.

Storage instructions:
Divide drink between two jars, cover and then store the containers in the refrigerator for up to 3 days.
Nutrition: Calories: 168; Fats: 2.5 g; Protein: 2 g; Carbohydrates: 38 g; Fiber: 4.5 g.

284 BERRY SMOOTHIE

Preparation Time: 5 minutes
Cooking Time: 0 minutes
Servings: 2
Ingredients:
- ¼ cup strawberries
- ¼ cup blueberries
- ¼ cup blackberries
- ¼ cup raspberries
- 2 tbsp. walnuts

Extra:
- 1 tbsp. of Bromide Plus Powder
- ⅔ cup spring water

Directions:
Plug in a high-speed food processor or blender and add all the ingredients to its jar.
Cover the blender jar with its lid and then pulse for 40 to 60 seconds until smooth.
Divide the drink between two glasses and then serve.

Storage instructions:
Divide drink between two jars or bottles, cover with a lid and then store the containers in the refrigerator for up to 3 days.
Nutrition: Calories: 180; Fats: 8 g; Protein: 4 g; Carbohydrates: 25 g; Fiber: 5 g.

285 LIVER-KIDNEY CLEANSING TEA

Preparation Time: 5 minutes
Cooking Time: 0 minutes

Ingredients:
- 1 tsp. dandelion root powder
- 1 tsp. burdock root powder
- 1 cup spring water

Directions:
Place all ingredients in a tea kettle
Boil for 10 minutes, remove from heat, cover and leave for an additional 10 minutes.
Drain and serve
Nutrition: Calories: 120; Fats: 1.4 g; Protein: 6 g; Carbohydrates: 28 g; Fiber: 5 g.

286 REFRESHING KIDNEY CLEANSING TEA

Preparation Time: 5 minutes
Cooking Time: 10 minutes
Servings: 1
Ingredients:
- 1 tsp. Prodigiosa powder
- 1 tsp. burdock root powder
- 1 cup spring water

Directions:
Place all ingredients in a tea kettle
Boil for 10 minutes, remove from heat. Cover and leave for an additional 10 minutes.
Drain and serve
Nutrition: Calories: 132; Fats: 1.6 g; Protein: 4 g; Carbohydrates: 27 g; Fiber: 3 g.

287 MUCUS LIVER CLEANSING TEA

Preparation Time: 5 minutes
Cooking Time: 10 minutes
Servings: 1
Ingredients:
- 1 tsp. dandelion root powder
- 1 tsp. Prodigiosa powder
- 1 cup spring water

Directions:
Place all ingredients in a tea kettle
Boil for 10 minutes. Remove from heat, cover and leave for an additional 10 minutes.
Drain and serve
Nutrition: Calories: 140; Fats: 1.5 g; Protein: 4 g; Carbohydrates: 16 g; Fiber: 6 g.

288 COLON-GALLBLADDER CLEANSING TEA

Preparation Time: 5 minutes
Cooking Time: 10 minutes
Servings: 1
Ingredients:
- 1 tsp. Cascara powder
- 1 tsp. Rhubarb root powder
- 1 cup spring water

Directions:
Place all ingredients in a tea kettle
Boil for 10 minutes. Remove from heat, cover and leave for an additional 10 minutes.
Drain and serve

Nutrition: Calories: 113; Fats: 1.5 g; Protein: 6 g; Carbohydrates: 22 g; Fiber: 3 g.

289 COLON-GALLBLADDER TEA

Preparation Time: 5 minutes
Cooking Time: 10 minutes
Servings: 2
Ingredients:
- 1 tsp. Cascara powder
- 1 tsp. Cahparral
- 1 cup spring water

Directions:
Place all ingredients in a tea kettle
Boil for 10 minutes, remove from heat, cover and leave for an additional 10 minutes.
Drain and serve.
Nutrition: Calories: 130; Fats: 2.5 g; Protein: 5 g; Carbohydrates: 24 g; Fiber: 4 g.

290 RESPIRATORY MUCUS CLEANSING TEA

Preparation Time: 5 minutes
Cooking Time: 10 minutes
Servings: 1
Ingredients:
- 1 tsp. guaco herb
- 1 tsp. mullein
- 1 cup spring water

Directions:
Place all ingredients in a tea kettle
Boil for 10 minutes, remove from heat, cover and leave for an additional 10 minutes.
Drain and serve.
Nutrition: Calories: 142; Fats: 1.8 g; Protein: 4 g; Carbohydrates: 28 g; Fiber: 6 g.

291 RESPIRATORY AND MUCUS SYRUP (ELDERBERRY SYRUP)

Preparation Time: 5 minutes
Cooking Time: 5 minutes
Servings: 1
Ingredients:
- 1 tsp. Elderberry fruit
- 1 cup spring water

Directions:
Place all ingredients in a tea kettle
Boil for 5 minutes. Remove from heat, cover and leave for an additional 10 minutes.
Drain and serve.
Nutrition: Calories: 124; Fats: 1.8 g; Protein: 5 g; Carbohydrates: 19 g; Fiber: 5 g.

292 IMMUNE BOOSTING TEA

Preparation Time: 5 minutes
Cooking Time: 10 minutes
Servings: 1
Ingredients:
- 1 tsp. linden powder
- 1 cup spring water

Directions:
Place all ingredients in a tea kettle

Boil for 5 minutes. Remove from heat, cover and leave for an additional 10 minutes.

Drain and serve.

Nutrition: Calories: 123; Fats: 1.5 g; Protein: 4 g; Carbohydrates: 17 g; Fiber: 4 g.

293 BROMIDE PLUS CLEANSING DRINK

Preparation Time: 5 minutes
Cooking Time: 10 minutes
Servings: 1
Ingredients:

1 tsp. bromide plus powder
1 tsp. dandelion root powder
1 cup spring water

Directions:

Place all ingredients in a tea kettle
Boil for 10 minutes, remove from heat, cover and leave for an additional 10 minutes.

Drain and serve.

Nutrition: Calories: 130; Fats: 1.4 g; Protein: 5 g; Carbohydrates: 27 g; Fiber: 4 g.

294 BROMIDE PLUS REVITALIZING TEA

Preparation Time: 5 minutes
Cooking Time: 5 minutes
Servings: 1
Ingredients:

1 tsp. bromide plus powder
Handful chamomile flowers
1 cup spring water

Directions:

Place flowers and water into a kettle.
Boil for 5 minutes, remove from heat, cover and leave for an additional 10 minutes.

Drain and add bromide powder.
Serve

Nutrition: Calories: 120; Fats: 2.5 g; Protein: 6 g; Carbohydrates: 27 g; Fiber: 5 g.

295 RESPIRATORY POWER BOOST

Preparation Time: 5 minutes
Cooking Time: 10 minutes
Servings: 1
Ingredients:

1 tsp. guaco herb
1 tsp. mullein
1 cup spring water

Directions:

Place all ingredients in a tea kettle
Boil for 10 minutes, remove from heat, cover and leave for an additional 10 minutes.

Drain and serve.

Nutrition: Calories: 110; Fats: 1.2 g; Protein: 5 g; Carbohydrates: 16 g; Fiber: 3 g.

296 CHAMOMILE HERBAL TEA

Preparation Time: 5 minutes

Cooking Time: 5 minutes
Servings: 2
Ingredients:

2 thin apple slices
2 cups boiling spring water
2 tbsp. fresh chamomile flowers, rinsed
1–2 tsp. agave nectar

Directions:

Rinse the teapot with boiling water.
In the warm pot, place the apple slices and with a wooden spoon, mash them.

Add the chamomile flowers and top with boiling water.

Cover the pot and steep for 3–5 minutes.

Strain the tea into two serving cups and stir in the agave nectar.

Serve immediately.

Nutrition: Calories 68; Fat: 0g Cholesterol: 0 mg; Carbohydrates 18.1 g; Fiber 2.9 g; Protein 0.3 g.

297 BURDOCK HERBAL TEA

Preparation Time: 5 minutes
Cooking Time: 5 minutes
Servings: 2
Ingredients:

2 tsp. dried burdock root
2 cups boiling spring water

Directions:

In a teapot, add the burdock root and top with the boiling water.

Cover the pot and steep for 3–5 minutes.

Strain the tea into two serving cups and serve immediately.

Nutrition: Calories: 2; Fat: 0 g; Cholesterol: 0 mg; Carbohydrates: 0.4 g; Fiber: 0.1 g; Protein: 0 g.

298 ELDERBERRY HERBAL TEA

Preparation Time: 10 minutes
Cooking Time: 20 minutes
Servings: 2
Ingredients:

16 oz. spring water
2 tbsp. dried elderberries
½ tsp. ground turmeric
¼ tsp. ground cinnamon
1 tsp. agave nectar

Directions:

In a small saucepan, place water and elderberries, turmeric and cinnamon over medium-high heat and bring to a boil.

Now, adjust the heat to low and simmer for about 15 minutes.

Remove from heat and set aside to cool for about 5 minutes.

Through a fine mesh strainer, strain the tea into serving cups and stir in the agave nectar.

Serve immediately.

Nutrition: Calories: 19; Fat: 0 g; Cholesterol: 0 mg; Carbohydrates: 4.9 g; Fiber: 1.1 g; Protein: 0.1 g.

299 FENNEL HERBAL TEA

Preparation Time: 5 minutes
Cooking Time: 5 minutes
Servings: 2
Ingredients:

2–4 tsp. fennel seeds, crushed freshly
2 cups boiling spring water

Directions:

In a teapot, add the fennel seeds and top with the boiling water.

Cover the pot and steep for 5–10 minutes.

Strain the tea into two serving cups and serve immediately.

Nutrition: Calories: 7; Fat: 0 g; Cholesterol: 0 mg; Carbohydrates: 1.1 g; Fiber: 0.8 g; Protein: 0.3 g.

300 FENNEL & GINGER HERBAL TEA

Preparation Time: 10 minutes
Cooking Time: 5 minutes
Servings: 2
Ingredients:

2 cups spring water
1 tbsp. fennel seeds, crushed slightly
1 (½-inch) piece fresh ginger, peeled and crushed slightly
2 tsp. agave nectar

Directions:

In a small saucepan, add water over medium heat and bring to a rolling boil.

Stir in the fennel seeds and ginger and remove from the heat.

Strain the tea into two serving cups and stir in the agave nectar.

Serve immediately.

Nutrition: Calories: 33; Fat: 0 g; Cholesterol: 0 mg; Carbohydrates: 7.5 g; Fiber: 1.6 g; Protein: 0.5 g.

301 GINGER & CINNAMON HERBAL TEA

Preparation Time: 10 minutes
Cooking Time: 5 minutes
Servings: 1
Ingredients:

1 cup spring water
1 (1-inch) piece fresh ginger, cut into pieces
1 cinnamon stick
1 tsp. agave nectar

Directions:

In a saucepan, add water, ginger, and cinnamon over high heat and bring to a boil.

Now, adjust the heat to low and simmer for about 5 minutes.

Remove the saucepan of tea from the and strain into a serving cup.

Stir in the agave nectar and serve immediately.

Nutrition: Calories: 40; Fat: 0.1 g; Cholesterol: 0 mg; Carbohydrates: 9.6 g; Fiber: 1.3 g; Protein: 0.5 g.

302 GINGER & LIME HERBAL TEA

Preparation Time: 10 minutes
Cooking Time: 10 minutes
Servings: 2
Ingredients:

2 cups spring water
2 tbsp. fresh ginger root, cut into slices
1 tbsp. fresh key lime juice
1 tbsp. agave nectar

Directions:

In a saucepan, add water, ginger, and cinnamon over high heat and bring to a boil.

Now, adjust the heat to low and simmer for about 10 minutes.

Remove the saucepan of tea from the and strain into serving cups.

In the cups, stir in the lime juice and agave nectar and serve immediately.

Nutrition: Calories: 34; Fat: 0 g; Cholesterol: 0 mg; Carbohydrates: 8.6 g; Fiber: 0.6 g; Protein: 0.1 g.

303 LINDEN HERBAL TEA

Preparation Time: 5 minutes
Cooking Time: 10 minutes
Servings: 1
Ingredients:

2 tsp. fresh linden flowers
1 cup spring water
1 tsp. agave nectar

Directions:

In a saucepan, add water over medium heat and bring to a boil.

Stir in the linden flowers and cook for about 1 minute.

Remove from the heat and set aside, covered for about 10 minutes.

Strain the tea into a serving cup and stir in the agave nectar.

Serve immediately.

Nutrition: Calories: 20; Fat: 0 g; Cholesterol: 0 mg; Carbohydrates: 5.3 g; Fiber: 0.3 g; Protein: 0 g.

304 RASPBERRY HERBAL TEA

Preparation Time: 5 minutes
Cooking Time: 5 minutes
Servings: 1
Ingredients:

1–2 tsp. red raspberry leaf tea
1 cup boiling spring water
1 tsp. agave nectar

Directions:

In the teapot, place the raspberry leaf tea and top with boiling water.

Cover the pot and steep for 3–5 minutes.

Strain the tea into two serving cups and stir in the agave nectar.

Serve immediately.

Nutrition: Calories: 20; Fat: 0 g; Cholesterol: 0 mg; Carbohydrates: 5.3 g; Fiber: 0.3 g; Protein: 0 g.

305 ANISE & CINNAMON HERBAL TEA

Preparation Time: 5 minutes
Cooking Time: 15 minutes
Servings: 2

Ingredients:

7-star anise
1 (2-inch) cinnamon stick
2–3 cups water

Directions:

In a saucepan, add water over medium heat and bring to a rolling boil.

Add star anise and cinnamon stick and boil for about 10 minutes.

Remove from heat and steep, covered for about 3 minutes.

Strain the tea into two serving cups and stir in the agave nectar.

Serve immediately.

Nutrition: Calories: 20; Fat: 0 g; Cholesterol: 0 mg; Carbohydrates: 4.4 g; Fiber: 2.3 g; Protein: 0.7 g.

306 LEMON ROOIBOS ICED TEA

Preparation Time: 10 minutes
Cooking Time: 0 minutes
Servings: 4
Ingredients:

4 bags natural, unflavored rooibos tea
4 cups boiling water
3 tbsp. freshly squeezed lemon juice
30–40 drops liquid stevia

Directions:

Put the tea bags into a tea pot and pour the boiling water over the bags.

Set aside to room temperature, then refrigerate the tea until it is ice-cold.

Remove the tea bags. Squeeze them gently.

Add the lemon juice and liquid stevia to taste and stir until well mixed.

Serve immediately, preferably with ice cubes and some nice garnishes, like lemon wedges.

Nutrition: Calories: 70; Carbohydrates: 16 g; Protein: 1 g.

307 LEMON LAVENDER ICED TEA

Preparation Time: 15 minutes
Cooking Time: 0 minutes
Servings: 4

Ingredients:

2 bags natural, unflavored rooibos tea
2 oz. lemon chunks without peel and pith, seeds removed
1 tsp. dried lavender blossoms placed in a tea ball
4 cups water, at room temperature
20–40 drops liquid stevia

Directions:

Place the tea bags, lemon chunks and the tightly-closed tea ball with the lavender blossoms in a 1.5 qt (1.5 l) pitcher.

Pour in the water.

Refrigerate overnight.

Remove the tea bags, lemon chunks and the tea ball with the lavender on the next day. Squeeze the tea bags gently to save as much liquid as possible.

Add liquid stevia to taste and stir until well mixed.

Serve immediately with ice cubes and lemon wedges.

Nutrition: Calories: 81; Carbohydrates: 12 g; Protein: 3 g.

308 CHERRY VANILLA ICED TEA

Preparation Time: 12 minutes
Cooking Time: 0 minutes
Servings: 4
Ingredients:

4 bags natural, unflavored rooibos tea
4 cups boiling water
2 tbsp. freshly squeezed lime juice
1–2 tbsp. cherry flavoring
30–40 drops (or to taste) liquid vanilla stevia

Directions:

Place tea bags into a tea pot and pour the boiling water over the bags.

Put aside the tea cool down first, then refrigerate the tea until it is ice-cold.

Remove the tea bags. Squeeze them lightly.

Add the lime juice, cherry flavoring and vanilla stevia and stir until well mixed.

Serve immediately, preferably with ice cubes and some nice garnishes like lime wedges and fresh cherries.

Nutrition: Calories: 89; Carbohydrates: 14 g; Protein: 2 g.

309 ELEGANT BLUEBERRY ROSE WATER ICED TEA

Preparation Time: 12 minutes
Cooking Time: 0 minutes
Servings: 4
Ingredients:

2 bags herbal blueberry tea
4 cups boiling water

20 drops liquid stevia

1 tbsp. rose water

Directions:

Position tea bags into a tea pot and pour the boiling water over the bags.

Allow tea cool down first, then refrigerate the tea until it is ice-cold.

Remove the tea bags. Press them gently.

Add the liquid stevia and the rose water and stir until well mixed.

Serve immediately, preferably with ice cubes and some nice garnishes, like fresh blueberries or natural rose petals

Nutrition: Calories: 75; Carbohydrates: 10 g; Protein: 2 g.

310 MELBA ICED TEA

Preparation Time: 10 minutes

Cooking Time: 0 minutes

Servings: 4

Ingredients:

1 bag herbal raspberry tea

1 bag herbal peach tea

4 cups boiling water

10 drops liquid peach stevia

20–40 drops (or to taste) liquid vanilla stevia

Directions:

Pour the boiling water over the tea bags.

Leave tea cool down at room temperature, then refrigerate the tea until it is ice-cold.

Remove the tea bags. Press lightly.

Add the peach stevia and stir until well mixed.

Add vanilla stevia to taste and stir until well mixed.

Serve immediately, preferably with ice cubes and some nice garnishes, like vanilla bean, fresh raspberries or peach slices.

Nutrition: Calories: 81; Carbohydrates: 14 g; Protein: 4 g.

311 MERRY RASPBERRY CHERRY ICED TEA

Preparation Time: 11 minutes

Cooking Time: 0 minutes

Servings: 4

Ingredients:

2 bags herbal raspberry tea

4 cups boiling water

1 tsp. stevia-sweetened cherry-flavored drink mix

1 tsp. freshly squeezed lime juice

10–20 drops (or to taste) liquid stevia

Directions:

Put the tea bags into a tea pot and fill in boiling water over the bags.

Let the tea cool down first to room temperature, then chill until it is ice-cold.

Discard tea bags. Squeeze them.

Add the cherry-flavored drink mix and the lime juice and stir until the drink mix is dissolved.

Add liquid stevia to taste and stir until well mixed.

Serve immediately, preferably with ice cubes or crushed ice and some nice garnishes, like fresh raspberries and cherries.

Nutrition: Calories: 82; Carbohydrates: 11 g; Protein: 4 g.

312 VANILLA KISSED PEACH ICED TEA

Preparation Time: 13 minutes

Cooking Time: 0 minutes

Servings: 4

Ingredients:

2 bags herbal peach tea

4 cups boiling water

1 tsp. vanilla extract

1 tsp. freshly squeezed lemon juice

30–40 drops (or to taste) liquid stevia

Directions:

Soak tea bags over boiling water.

Allow to cool down at room temperature, then refrigerate the tea until it is ice-cold.

Remove and press tea bags.

Add the vanilla extract and the lemon juice and stir until well mixed.

Add liquid stevia to taste and stir until well mixed.

Serve immediately, preferably with ice cubes and some nice garnishes, like peach slices.

Nutrition: Calories: 88; Carbohydrates: 14 g; Protein: 3 g.

313 XTREME BERRIED ICED TEA

Preparation Time: 10 minutes

Cooking Time: 0 minutes

Servings: 4

Ingredients:

2 bags herbal wild berry tea

4 cups (950 ml) boiling water

2 tsp. freshly squeezed lime juice

40 drops berry-flavored liquid stevia

10 drops (or to taste) liquid stevia

Directions:

Submerge tea bags into boiling water.

Set aside to cool down, then refrigerate the tea until it is ice-cold.

Pull out tea bags. Squeeze.

Add the lime juice and the berry stevia and stir until well mixed.

Add liquid stevia to taste and stir until well mixed.

Serve immediately.

Nutrition: Calories: 76; Carbohydrates: 14 g; Protein: 4 g.

314 REFRESHINGLY PEPPERMINT ICED TEA

Preparation Time: 15 minutes

Cooking Time: 0 minutes

Servings: 5

Ingredients:

4 bags peppermint tea

4 cups = 950 ml boiling water

2 tsp. stevia-sweetened lime-flavored drink mix

1 cup = 240 ml ice-cold sparkling water

Directions:

Immerse tea bags in boiling water.

Set aside before cooling until it is ice-cold.

Take out tea bags then press.

Add the lime-flavored drink mix and stir until it is properly dissolved.

Add the sparkling water and stir very gently.

Serve immediately, preferably with ice cubes, mint leaves and lime wedges.

Nutrition: Calories: 78; Carbohydrates: 17 g; Protein: 4 g.

315 LEMONGRASS MINT ICED TEA

Preparation Time: 12 minutes

Cooking Time: 0 minutes

Servings: 4

Ingredients:

1 stalk lemongrass, chopped in 1-inch

½ cup chopped, loosely packed mint sprigs

4 cups boiling water

Directions:

Put the lemongrass and the mint into a tea pot and pour the boiling water over them.

Let cool down first to room temperature, then refrigerate until the tea is ice-cold.

Filter out the lemongrass and the mint.

Add liquid vanilla stevia to taste if you prefer some sweetness and stir until well mixed.

Serve immediately, preferably with ice cubes and some nice garnishes, like mint sprigs and lemongrass stalks.

Nutrition: Calories: 89; Carbohydrates: 17 g; Protein: 5 g.

316 SPICED TEA

Preparation Time: 8 minutes

Cooking Time: 0 minutes

Servings: 4

Ingredients:

2 bags Bengal Spice tea

2 tsp. freshly squeezed lemon juice

1 packet zero-carb vanilla stevia

1 packet zero-carb stevia
4 cups boiling water

Directions:

Put the tea bags, lemon juice and both stevia into a tea pot.

Pour in the boiling water.

Put aside to cool over room temperature, then refrigerate.

Pull away tea bags then squeeze it.

Stir gently.

Serve immediately, preferably with ice cubes or crushed ice and some lemon wedges or slices.

Nutrition: Calories: 91; Carbohydrates: 16 g; Protein: 1 g.

317 INFUSED PUMPKIN SPICE LATTE

Preparation Time: 11 minutes
Cooking Time: 0 minutes
Servings: 2
Ingredients:

2 cups almond milk
¼ cup coconut cream
2 tsp. cannabis coconut oil
¼ cup pure pumpkin, canned
½ tsp. vanilla extract
1 ½ tsp. pumpkin spice
½ cup coconut whipped cream
1 pinch of salt

Directions:

Place all ingredients, except the coconut whipped cream, in the pan over a medium-low heat stove.

Whisk well and allow to simmer but don't boil!

Simmer for about 5 minutes.

Pour into mugs and serve.

Nutrition: Calories: 94; Carbohydrates: 17 g; Protein: 3 g.

318 INFUSED TURMERIC-GINGER TEA

Preparation Time: 9 minutes
Cooking Time: 5 minutes
Servings: 1
Ingredients:

1 cup water
½ cup coconut milk
1 tsp. cannabis oil
½ tsp. ground turmeric
¼ cup fresh ginger root, sliced
1 pinch Stevia or maple syrup, to taste

Directions:

Combine all ingredients in a small saucepan over medium heat.

Heat until simmer and turn heat low.

Take the pan off the heat after 2 minutes

Let it cool, strain mixture into cup or mug.

Nutrition: Calories: 98; Carbohydrates: 14 g; Protein: 2 g.

319 INFUSED LONDON FOG

Preparation Time: 17 minutes
Cooking Time: 0 minutes
Servings: 2
Ingredients:

1 cup hot water
1 Earl Grey teabag
1 tsp. cannabis coconut oil
¼ cup almond milk
¼ tsp. vanilla extract
1 pinch Stevia or sugar, to taste

Directions:

Fill up half a mug with boiling water.

Add tea bag; if you prefer your tea strong, add two.

Add cannabis oil and stir well.

Add almond milk to fill your mug and stir through with the vanilla extract

Use Stevia or sugar to sweeten your Earl Grey to taste.

Nutrition: Calories: 76; Carbohydrates: 14 g; Protein: 2 g.

320 INFUSED CRANBERRY-APPLE SNUG

Preparation Time: 10 minutes
Cooking Time: 0 minutes
Servings: 1
Ingredients:

½ cup fresh cranberry juice
½ cup fresh apple juice, cloudy
½ stick cinnamon
2 whole cloves
¼ lemon, sliced
1 pinch of Stevia or sugar, to taste
Cranberries for garnish (optional)

Directions:

Combine all ingredients in a small saucepan over medium heat.

Heat until simmer and turn heat low.

Let it cool, strain the mixture into a mug.

Serve with cinnamon stick and cranberries in a mug.

Nutrition: Calories: 85; Carbohydrates: 15 g; Protein: 3 g.

321 MANGO PEAR SMOOTHIE

Preparation Time: 5 minutes
Cooking Time: 0 minutes
Servings: 1
Ingredients:

2 ice cubes
½ cup Greek yogurt, plain
½ mango, peeled, pitted & chopped
1 cup kale, chopped
1 pear, ripe, cored & chopped

Directions:

Take all ingredients and place them in your blender. Blend together until thick and smooth. Serve.

Nutrition: Calories 350; Protein 40 g; Fat: 12 g; Carbohydrates: 11 g.

322 MEDITERRANEAN SMOOTHIE

Preparation Time: 5 minutes
Cooking Time: 0 minutes
Servings: 2
Ingredients:

2 cups of baby spinach
1 tsp. fresh ginger root
1 frozen banana, pre-sliced
1 small mango
½ cup beet juice
½ cup of skim milk
4-6 ice cubes

Directions:

Take all ingredients and place them in your blender. Blend together until thick and smooth. Serve.

Nutrition: Calories: 168; Protein: 4 g; Fat: 1 g; Carbohydrates: 39 g.

323 FRUIT SMOOTHIE

Preparation Time: 5 minutes
Cooking Time: 0 minutes
Servings: 2
Ingredients:

2 cups blueberries (or any fresh or frozen fruit, cut into pieces if the fruit is large)
2 cups unsweetened almond milk
1 cup crushed ice
½ tsp. ground ginger (or other dried ground spice such as turmeric, cinnamon, or nutmeg)

Directions:

In a blender, combine the blueberries, almond milk, ice, and ginger. Blend until smooth.

Nutrition: Calories: 125; Protein: 2 g; Carbohydrates: 23 g; Fat: 4 g.

324 STRAWBERRY-RHUBARB SMOOTHIE

Preparation Time: 5 minutes
Cooking Time: 3 minutes
Servings: 1
Ingredients:

1 rhubarb stalk, chopped
1 cup sliced fresh strawberries
½ cup plain Greek yogurt
2 tbsp. honey
Pinch of ground cinnamon
3 ice cubes

Directions:

Place a small saucepan filled with water over high heat and bring to a boil. Add the rhubarb and boil for 3 minutes. Drain and transfer the rhubarb to a blender.

Add the strawberries, yogurt, honey, and cinnamon and pulse the mixture until it is smooth. Add the ice and blend until thick, with no ice lumps remaining. Pour the smoothie into a glass and enjoy cold.

Nutrition: Calories: 295; Fat: 8 g; Carbohydrates: 56 g; Protein: 6 g.

325 CHIA-POMEGRANATE SMOOTHIE

Preparation Time: 5 minutes
Cooking Time: 0 minutes
Servings: 2

Ingredients:
 1 cup pure pomegranate juice (no sugar added)
 1 cup frozen berries
 1 cup coarsely chopped kale
 2 tbsp. chia seeds
 3 Medjool dates, pitted and coarsely chopped
 Pinch of ground cinnamon

Directions:
 In a blender, combine the pomegranate juice, berries, kale, chia seeds, dates, and cinnamon; pulse until smooth. Pour into glasses and serve.

Nutrition: Calories: 275; Fat: 5 g; Carbohydrates: 59 g; Protein: 5 g.

326 KALE SMOOTHIE

Preparation Time: 5 minutes
Cooking Time: 0 minutes
Servings: 2

Ingredients:
 2 cups chopped kale leaves
 1 banana, peeled
 1 cup frozen strawberries
 1 cup unsweetened almond milk
 4 Medjool dates, pitted and chopped

Directions:
 Put all the ingredients in a food processor, then blitz until glossy and smooth.
 Serve immediately or chill in the refrigerator for an hour before serving.

Nutrition: Calories: 663; Fat: 10.0g; Carbs: 142.5g; Fiber: 19.0g; Proteins: 17.4 g.

327 HOT TROPICAL SMOOTHIE

Preparation Time: 5 minutes
Cooking Time: 0 minutes
Servings: 4

Ingredients:
 1 cup frozen mango chunks
 1 cup frozen pineapple chunks
 1 small tangerine, peeled and pitted
 2 cups spinach leaves
 1 cup coconut water
 ¼ tsp. cayenne pepper, optional

Directions:
 Add all the ingredients to a food processor, then blitz until the mixture is smooth and combine well.
 Serve immediately or chill in the refrigerator for an hour before serving.

Nutrition: Calories: 283; Fat: 1.9 g; Carbs: 67.9 g; Fiber: 10.4 g; Proteins: 6.4 g.

328 CRANBERRY AND BANANA SMOOTHIE

Preparation Time: 5 minutes
Cooking Time: 0 minutes
Servings: 4

Ingredients:
 1 cup frozen cranberries
 1 large banana, peeled
 4 Medjool dates, pitted and chopped
 1 ½ cups unsweetened almond milk

Directions:
 Add all the ingredients to a food processor, then process until the mixture is glossy and well mixed.
 Serve immediately or chill in the refrigerator for an hour before serving.

Nutrition: Calories: 616; Fat: 8.0 g; Carbs: 132.8 g; Fiber: 14.6 g; Proteins: 15.7 g.

329 PUMPKIN SMOOTHIE

Preparation Time: 5 minutes
Cooking Time: 0 minutes
Servings: 5

Ingredients:
 ½ cup pumpkin purée
 4 Medjool dates, pitted and chopped
 1 cup unsweetened almond milk
 ¼ tsp. vanilla extract
 ¼ tsp. ground cinnamon
 ½ cup ice
 Pinch of ground nutmeg

Directions:
 Add all the ingredients to a blender, then process until the mixture is glossy and well mixed.
 Serve immediately.

Nutrition: Calories: 417; Fat: 3.0 g; Carbs: 94.9 g; Fiber: 10.4 g; Proteins: 11.4 g.

330 SUPER SMOOTHIE

Preparation Time: 5 minutes
Cooking Time: 0 minutes
Servings: 4

Ingredients:
 1 banana, peeled
 1 cup chopped mango
 1 cup raspberries
 ¼ cup rolled oats
 1 carrot, peeled
 1 cup chopped fresh kale
 2 tbsp. chopped fresh parsley
 1 tbsp. flaxseeds
 1 tbsp. grated fresh ginger
 ½ cup unsweetened soy milk
 1 cup water

Directions:
 Put all the ingredients in a food processor, then blitz until glossy and smooth.
 Serve immediately or chill in the refrigerator for an hour before serving.

Nutrition: Calories: 550; Fat: 39.0 g; Carbs: 31.0 g; Fiber: 15.0 g; Proteins: 13.0 g.

331 KIWI AND STRAWBERRY SMOOTHIE

Preparation Time: 5 minutes
Cooking Time: 0 minutes
Servings: 3

Ingredients:
 1 kiwi, peeled
 5 medium strawberries
 ½ frozen banana
 1 cup unsweetened almond milk
 2 tbsp. hemp seeds
 2 tbsp. peanut butter
 1 to 2 tsp. maple syrup
 ½ cup spinach leaves
 Handful broccoli sprouts

Directions:
 Put all the ingredients in a food processor, then blitz until creamy and smooth.
 Serve immediately or chill in the refrigerator for an hour before serving.

Nutrition: Calories: 562; Fat: 28.6 g; Carbs: 63.6 g; Fiber: 15.1 g; Proteins: 23.3 g.

332 BANANA AND CHAI CHIA SMOOTHIE

Preparation Time: 5 minutes
Cooking Time: 0 minutes
Servings: 3

Ingredients:
 1 banana
 1 cup alfalfa sprouts
 1 tbsp. chia seeds
 ½ cup unsweetened coconut milk
 1 to 2 soft Medjool dates, pitted
 ¼ tsp. ground cinnamon
 1 tbsp. grated fresh ginger
 1 cup water
 Pinch of ground cardamom

Directions:
 Add all the ingredients to a blender, then process until the mixture is smooth and creamy. Add water or coconut milk if necessary.
 Serve immediately.

Nutrition: Calories: 477; Fat: 41.0 g; Carbs: 31.0 g; Fiber: 14.0 g; Proteins: 8.0 g.

333 CHOCOLATE AND PEANUT BUTTER SMOOTHIE

Preparation Time: 5 minutes
Cooking Time: 0 minutes
Servings: 4
Ingredients:

- 1 tbsp. unsweetened cocoa powder
- 1 tbsp. peanut butter
- 1 banana
- 1 tsp. maca powder
- ½ cup unsweetened soy milk
- ¼ cup rolled oats
- 1 tbsp. flaxseeds
- 1 tbsp. maple syrup
- 1 cup water

Directions:

Add all the ingredients to a blender, then process until the mixture is smooth and creamy. Add water or soy milk if necessary.

Serve immediately.

Nutrition: Calories: 474; Fat: 16.0 g; Carbs: 27.0 g; Fiber: 18.0 g; Proteins: 13.0 g.

334 GOLDEN MILK

Preparation Time: 5 minutes
Cooking Time: 5 minutes
Servings: 4
Ingredients:

- ¼ tsp. ground cinnamon
- ½ tsp. ground turmeric
- ½ tsp. grated fresh ginger
- 1 tsp. maple syrup
- 1 cup unsweetened coconut milk
- Ground black pepper, to taste
- 2 tbsp. waters

Directions:

Combine all the ingredients in a saucepan. Stir to mix well.

Heat over medium heat for 5 minutes. Keep stirring during the heating.

Allow to cool for 5 minutes, then pour the mixture into a blender. Pulse until creamy and smooth. Serve immediately.

Nutrition: Calories: 577; Fat: 57.3 g; Carbs: 19.7 g; Fiber: 6.1 g; Proteins: 5.7 g.

335 MANGO AGUA FRESCA

Preparation Time: 5 minutes
Cooking Time: 0 minutes
Servings: 2
Ingredients:

- 2 fresh mangoes, diced
- 1 ½ cups water
- 1 tsp. fresh lime juice
- Maple syrup, to taste
- 2 cups ice
- 2 slices fresh lime, for garnish
- 2 fresh mint sprigs, for garnish

Directions:

Put the mangoes, lime juice, maple syrup, and water in a blender. Process until creamy and smooth.

Divide the beverage into two glasses, then garnish each glass with ice, lime slice, and mint sprig before serving.

Nutrition: Calories: 230; Fat: 1.3 g; Carbs: 57.7 g; Fiber: 5.4 g; Proteins: 2.8 g.

336 LIGHT GINGER TEA

Preparation Time: 5 minutes
Cooking Time: 10 to 15 minutes
Servings: 2
Ingredients:

- 1 small ginger knob, sliced into four 1-inch chunks
- 4 cups water
- Juice of 1 large lemon
- Maple syrup, to taste

Directions:

Add the ginger knob and water in a saucepan, then simmer over medium heat for 10 to 15 minutes.

Turn off the heat and then mix in the lemon juice. Strain the liquid to remove the ginger, then fold in the maple syrup and serve.

Nutrition: Calories: 32; Fat: 0.1 g; Carbs: 8.6 g; Fiber: 0.1 g; Proteins: 0.1 g.

337 CLASSIC SWITCHEL

Preparation Time: 5 minutes
Cooking Time: 0 minutes
Servings: 4
Ingredients:

- 1-inch piece ginger, minced
- 2 tbsp. apple cider vinegar
- 2 tbsp. maple syrup
- 4 cups water
- ¼ tsp. sea salt, optional

Directions:

Combine all the ingredients in a glass. Stir to mix well.

Serve immediately or chill in the refrigerator for an hour before serving.

Nutrition: Calories: 110; Fat: 0 g; Carbs: 28.0 g; Proteins: 0 g.

338 LIME AND CUCUMBER ELECTROLYTE DRINK

Preparation Time: 5 minutes
Cooking Time: 0 minutes
Servings: 4
Ingredients:

- ¼ cup chopped cucumber
- 1 tbsp. fresh lime juice
- 1 tbsp. apple cider vinegar
- 2 tbsp. maple syrup
- ¼ tsp. sea salt, optional
- 4 cups water

Directions:

Combine all the ingredients in a glass. Stir to mix well.

Refrigerate overnight before serving.

Nutrition: Calories: 114; Fat: 0.1 g; Carbs: 28.9 g; Fiber: 0.3 g; Proteins: 0.3 g.

339 EASY AND FRESH MANGO MADNESS

Preparation Time: 5 minutes
Cooking Time: 0 minutes
Servings: 4
Ingredients:

- 1 cup chopped mango
- 1 cup chopped peach
- 1 banana
- 1 cup strawberries
- 1 carrot, peeled and chopped
- 1 cup water

Directions:

Put all the ingredients in a food processor, then blitz until glossy and smooth.

Serve immediately or chill in the refrigerator for an hour before serving.

Nutrition: Calories: 376; Fat: 22.0 g; Carbs: 19.0 g; Fiber: 14.0 g; Proteins: 5.0 g.

340 SIMPLE DATE SHAKE

Preparation Time: 10 minutes
Cooking Time: 0 minutes
Servings: 2
Ingredients:

- 5 Medjool dates, pitted, soaked in boiling water for 5 minutes
- ¾ cup unsweetened coconut milk
- 1 tsp. vanilla extract
- ½ tsp. fresh lemon juice
- ¼ tsp. sea salt, optional
- 1 ½ cups ice

Directions:

Put all the ingredients in a food processor, then blitz until it has a milkshake and smooth texture.

Serve immediately.

Nutrition: Calories: 380; Fat: 21.6 g; Carbs: 50.3 g; Fiber: 6.0 g; Proteins: 3.2 g.

341 BEET AND CLEMENTINE PROTEIN SMOOTHIE

Preparation Time: 10 minutes
Cooking Time: 0 minutes
Servings: 3
Ingredients:

- 1 small beet, peeled and chopped
- 1 clementine, peeled and broken into segments
- ½ ripe banana
- ½ cup raspberries
- 1 tbsp. chia seeds
- 2 tbsp. almond butter
- ¼ tsp. vanilla extract
- 1 cup unsweetened almond milk
- ⅛ tsp. fine sea salt, optional

Directions:

Combine all the ingredients in a food processor, then pulse on high for 2 minutes or until glossy and creamy.

Refrigerate for an hour and serve chilled.

Nutrition: Calories: 526; Fat: 25.4 g; Carbs: 61.9 g; Fiber: 17.3 g; Proteins: 20.6 g.

342 MATCHA LIMEADE

Preparation Time: 10 minutes
Cooking Time: 0 minutes
Servings: 4
Ingredients:

2 tbsp. matcha powder
¼ cup raw agave syrup
3 cups water, divided
1 cup fresh lime juice
3 tbsp. chia seeds

Directions:

Lightly simmer the matcha, agave syrup, and 1 cup of water in a saucepan over medium heat. Keep stirring until no matcha lumps.

Pour the matcha mixture into a large glass, then add the remaining ingredients and stir to mix well.

Refrigerate for at least an hour before serving.

Nutrition: Calories: 152; Fat: 4.5 g; Carbs: 26.8 g; Fiber: 5.3 g; Proteins: 3.7 g.

343 GREEN & MEAN

Preparation Time: 10 minutes
Cooking Time: 0 minutes
Servings: 1
Ingredients:

3 stalks of celery
3 bunches of kale
½ cup of sliced pineapple
½ apple, chopped
A handful of spinach
1 tbsp. of coconut oil
1 scoop of vanilla protein powder

Directions:

Place all the ingredients together in the blender and process until the desired consistency is achieved.

Pour the contents of the blender into a tall glass.

Serve immediately and enjoy!

Nutrition: Calories: 497; Proteins: 28 g; Carbs: 62 g; Fat: 17 g.

344 CHOCOLATE PEANUT DELIGHT

Preparation Time: 10 minutes
Cooking Time: 0 minutes
Servings: 1
Ingredients:

1 scoop of chocolate whey protein powder

1 cup of low-Fat Greek yogurt
1 whole banana
2 tbsp. of peanut butter
1 cup of ice

Directions:

Add all the ingredients to a blender and blend until smooth.

Enjoy!

Nutrition: Calories: 656; Proteins: 63 g; Carbs: 55 g; Fat: 21 g.

345 AMY'S HOMEMADE MASS GAINER

Preparation Time: 10 minutes
Cooking Time: 0 minutes
Servings: 1
Ingredients:

2 scoops of chocolate whey protein powder
2 cups of whole milk
½ cup of dry rolled oats
1 whole banana
2 tbsp. of organic almond butter
1 cup of crushed ice

Directions:

Add all the ingredients to a blender and mix until smooth

Enjoy

Nutrition: Calories: 970; Proteins: 75 g; Carbs: 90 g; Fat: 30 g.

346 THE NUTTY SMOOTHIE

Preparation Time: 10 minutes
Cooking Time: 0 minutes
Servings: 1
Ingredients:

1-oz. Hazelnut
1 oz. Macadamia Nuts
1 tbsp. chia seeds
1-2 packets Stevia, optional
2 cups water

Directions:

Add all the listed ingredients to a blender.

Blend on high until smooth and creamy.

Enjoy your smoothie!

Nutrition: Calories: 452; Fat: 43 g; Carbohydrates: 15 g; Proteins: 9 g.

347 THE FEISTY NUT SHAKE

Preparation Time: 10 minutes
Cooking Time: 0 minutes
Servings: 1
Ingredients:

¼ cup almonds, sliced
¼ cup macadamia nuts, whole
1 tbsp. flaxseed
¼ cup heavy cream, liquid
½ tbsp. cocoa powder
1 cup of water
1 tbsp. hemp seed
1 pack stevia

Directions:

Add listed ingredients to a blender.

Blend until you have a smooth and creamy texture.

Serve chilled and enjoy!

Nutrition: Calories: 590; Fat: 57 g; Carbohydrates: 17 g; Proteins: 12 g.

348 THE DASHING COCONUT AND MELON

Preparation Time: 10 minutes
Cooking Time: 0 minutes
Servings: 1
Ingredients:

½ cup melon, sliced
1 tbsp. coconut flakes, unsweetened
¼ cup whole milk yogurt
1 tbsp. coconut oil
1 tbsp. chia seeds
1 pack stevia
1 ½ cups water

Directions:

Add listed ingredients to a blender.

Blend until you have a smooth and creamy texture.

Serve chilled and enjoy!

Nutrition: Calories: 278; Fat: 21 g; Carbohydrates: 15 g; Proteins: 6 g.

349 CAYENNE SPICES CHOCOLATE SHAKE

Preparation Time: 10 minutes
Cooking Time: 0 minutes
Servings: 1
Ingredients:

½ pinch cayenne powder
2 tbsp. coconut oil, unrefined
¼ cup coconut cream
1 tbsp. chia seeds, whole
2 tbsp. cacao
Dash of vanilla extract
1 ½ cups water
Ice cubes

Directions:

Add listed ingredients to a blender.

Blend until you have a smooth and creamy texture.

Serve chilled and enjoy!

Nutrition: Calories: 258; Fat: 26 g; Carbohydrates: 3 g; Proteins: 3 g.

350 APPLE CELERY DETOX SMOOTHIE

Preparation Time: 10 minutes
Cooking Time: 0 minutes
Servings: 2
Ingredients:

3 tbsp. collard greens
2 ribs celery
3 springs mint
1 apple, chopped
2 tbsp. hazelnuts, raw
½ tsp. moringa
1 cup of water
1 cup ice

Directions:

Add all the listed ingredients to a blender.

Blend until you have a smooth and creamy texture.

Serve chilled and enjoy!

Nutrition: Calories: 115; Fat: 5 g; Carbohydrates: 14 g; Proteins: 3 g.

351 ZUCCHINI DETOX SMOOTHIE

Preparation Time: 10 minutes
Cooking Time: 0 minutes
Servings: 1
Ingredients:

1 zucchini
1 tbsp. sea beans
½ lemon, juiced
1 tsp. maqui berry powder
8 tbsp. grape tomatoes
6 tbsp. celery stocks
½ jalapeno pepper, seeded
1 cup of water
1 cup ice

Directions:

Add all the listed ingredients to the blender, except zucchini.

Add zucchini and blend the mixture.

Blend until smooth.

Serve chilled and enjoy!

Nutrition: Calories: 50; Fat: 0.5 g; Carbohydrates: 10 g; Proteins: 2.4 g.

352 CARROT DETOX SMOOTHIE

Preparation Time: 10 minutes
Cooking Time: 0 minutes
Servings: 2
Ingredients:

10 tbsp. carrot, chopped
1-inch ginger, peeled and chopped
1 tsp. cinnamon
1 banana, peeled
1-inch turmeric peeled, chopped
1 cup of coconut milk
1 cup ice

Directions:

Add all the listed ingredients to a blender.

Blend until smooth.

Serve chilled and enjoy!

Nutrition: Calories: 134; Fat: 3 g; Carbohydrates: 30 g; Proteins: 2 g.

353 PEAR JICAMA DETOX SMOOTHIE

Preparation Time: 10 minutes
Cooking Time: 0 minutes
Servings: 2
Ingredients:

3 tbsp. red kale
8 tbsp. jicama, peeled and chopped
1 lemon, juiced
1 pear, chopped
1 tsp. reishi mushroom
1 tbsp. flaxseed
1 cup of water
1 cup ice

Directions:

Add all the listed ingredients to a blender.

Blend until smooth.

Serve chilled and enjoy!

Nutrition: Calories: 102; Fat: 0 g; Carbohydrates: 24 g; Proteins: 2 g.

354 COCONUT PINEAPPLE DETOX SMOOTHIE

Preparation Time: 10 minutes
Cooking Time: 0 minutes
Servings: 2
Ingredients:

3 tbsp. Swiss Chard
2 tbsp. coconut flakes
1 tbsp. chia seeds
8 tbsp. pineapple, peeled and chopped
½ avocado pitted
1 orange, peeled
1 cup of water
1 cup ice

Directions:

Add all the listed ingredients to a blender.

Blend until smooth.

Serve chilled and enjoy!

Nutrition: Calories: 212; Fat: 0 g; Carbohydrates: 26 g; Proteins: 3 g.

355 PINEAPPLE COCONUT DETOX SMOOTHIE

Preparation Time: 10 minutes
Cooking Time: 0 minutes
Servings: 2
Ingredients:

4 cups kale, chopped
2 cups of coconut water
2 bananas
2 cups pineapple

Directions:

Add all the listed ingredients to a blender.

Blend until you have a smooth and creamy texture.

Serve chilled and enjoy!

Nutrition: Calories: 299; Fat: 1.1 g; Carbohydrates: 71.5 g; Proteins: 7.9 g.

356 AVOCADO DETOX SMOOTHIE

Preparation Time: 5 minutes
Cooking Time: 0 minutes
Servings: 3
Ingredients:

4 cups spinach, chopped
1 avocado, chopped
3 cups apple juice
2 apples, unpeeled, cored and chopped

Directions:

Add all the listed ingredients to a blender.

Blend until you have a smooth and creamy texture.

Serve chilled and enjoy!

Nutrition: Calories: 336; Fat: 13.8 g; Carbohydrates: 55.8 g; Proteins: 3 g.

357 LEMON LIME LAVENDER SMOOTHIE

Preparation Time: 10 minutes
Cooking Time: 0 minutes
Servings: 3
Ingredients:

1 ½ cups plant yogurt
3 tbsp. lemon juice
4 tbsp. lime juice
A drop lavender extract, culinary or ½ tsp. of culinary lavender buds
¼ cup of ice
½ tsp. turmeric (or even more to accomplish the desired color)
¼ cup shavings from fresh organic lemons and limes

Directions:

Combine all of the ingredients in a blender and serve chilled with citrus shavings and lavender buds at the top for a robust scent while you spoon!

Then add plant-based milk to a thin mixture.

Nutrition: Calories: 229; Fat: 1.1 g; Carbohydrates: 71.5 g; Proteins: 7.9 g.

358 JALAPENO LIME AND MANGO PROTEIN SMOOTHIE

Preparation Time: 10 minutes
Cooking Time: 0 minutes
Servings: 2
Ingredients:

A little banana
1 Cheribundi Tart Cherry Mango smoothie pack (or ¾ cup frozen mango)
A heaping tbsp. of chopped jalapeño (about ½ a little pepper)
1 cup unsweetened original almond milk (or coconut milk)
1 tbsp. flaxseed, ground
1 tbsp. chia seeds, ground
2 tbsp. hemp seed, ground
½ lime, newly squeezed
½ an avocado (optional)

Directions:

Combine all the ingredients within a blender and work for approximately 45 seconds until smooth.

Pour right into a glass and revel in!

Nutrition: Calories: 219; Fat: 1.1 g; Carbohydrates: 1.5 g; Proteins: 7.9 g.

359 CINNAMON APPLE SMOOTHIE

Preparation Time: 10 minutes
Cooking Time: 0 minutes
Servings: 2
Ingredients:

- 1 small apple, sliced
- ½ cup rolled oats
- ½ tsp. cinnamon
- ½ tsp. nutmeg
- 1 tbsp. almond butter
- ½ cup unsweetened coconut milk three to four cubes of ice
- ½ cup cool water

Directions:

Combine oats and water inside a blender and allow it to rest for two minutes; therefore, the oats can soften.

Bring all the remaining ingredients to the blender and blend for approximately 30 seconds until smooth.

Pour right into a glass and sprinkle with just a little spare cinnamon and nutmeg. Enjoy!

Nutrition: Calories: 232; Fat: 1.1 g; Carbohydrates: 14.5 g; Proteins: 7.9 g.

360 BANANA WEIGHT LOSS JUICE

Preparation Time: 10 minutes
Cooking Time: 0 minutes
Servings: 1
Ingredients:

- ⅓ cup of water
- 1 apple, sliced
- 1 orange, sliced
- 1 banana, sliced
- 1 tsp. lemon juice

Directions:

Looking to boost your weight loss? The key is taking in fewer calories; this recipe can get you there.

Simply place everything into your blender. Blend on high for twenty seconds, and then pour into your glass.

Nutrition: Calories: 289; Total Carbohydrate: 2 g; Cholesterol: 3 mg; Total Fat: 17 g; Fiber: 2 g; Proteins: 7 g; Sodium: 163 mg.

361 CITRUS DETOX JUICE

Preparation Time: 10 minutes
Cooking Time: 0 minutes
Servings: 4
Ingredients:

- 3 cups water
- 1 lemon, sliced
- 1 grapefruit, sliced
- 1 orange, sliced

Directions:

While starting your new diet, it is going to be vital to stay hydrated. This detox juice is the perfect solution and offers some extra flavor.

Begin by peeling and slicing up your fruit. Once this is done, place it in a pitcher of water and infuse the water overnight.

Nutrition: Calories: 269; Total Carbohydrate: 2 g; Total Fat: 14 g; Fiber: 2 g; Proteins: 7 g.

362 METABOLISM WATER

Preparation Time: 10 minutes
Cooking Time: 0 minutes
Servings: 1
Ingredients:

- 3 cups water
- 1 cucumber, sliced
- 1 lemon, sliced
- 2 mint leaves
- Ice

Directions:

At some point, we probably all wish for a quicker metabolism! With the lemon acting as an energizer, cucumber for a refreshing taste, and mint to help your stomach digest, this water is perfect!

All you will have to do is get out a pitcher. Place all the ingredients in, and allow the ingredients to soak overnight for maximum benefits!

Nutrition: Calories: 301; Total Carbohydrate: 2 g; Cholesterol: 13 mg; Total Fat: 17 g; Fiber: 4 g; Proteins: 8 g; Sodium: 201 mg.

363 STRESS RELIEF DETOX DRINK

Preparation Time: 5 minutes
Cooking Time: 0 minutes
Servings: 1
Ingredients:

- 1 pitcher of water
- Mint
- 1 lemon, sliced
- Basil
- 1 cup of strawberries, sliced
- Ice

Directions:

Life can be a stressful event. Luckily, there is water to help keep you cool, calm, and collected! The lemon works like an energizer, the basil is a natural antidepressant, and mint can help your stomach do its job better. As for the strawberries, those are just for some sweetness!

When you are ready, take all the ingredients and place them into a pitcher of water overnight and enjoy the next day.

Nutrition: Calories: 189; Total Carbohydrate: 2 g; Cholesterol: 73 mg; Total Fat: 17 g; Fiber: 0 g; Proteins: 7 g; Sodium: 163 mg.

364 STRAWBERRY PINK DRINK

Preparation Time: 10 minutes
Cooking Time: 5 minutes
Servings: 4
Ingredients:

- 1 cup of water., boiling
- 2 tbsp. sugar
- 1 Acai Tea Bag
- 1 cup coconut milk
- ½ cup frozen strawberries

Directions:

If you are looking for a little treat, this is going to be the recipe for you! You will begin by boiling your cup of water and seep the tea bag in for at least five minutes.

When the tea is set, add in the sugar and coconut milk. Be sure to stir well to spread the sweetness throughout the tea.

Finally, add in your strawberries, and you can enjoy your freshly made pink drink!

Nutrition: Calories: 321; Total Carbohydrate: 2 g; Cholesterol: 13 mg; Total Fat: 17 g; Fiber: 2 g; Proteins: 9 g; Sodium: 312 mg.

365 AVOCADO PUDDING

Preparation Time: 10 minutes
Cooking Time: 0 minutes
Servings: 8
Ingredients:

- 2 ripe avocados, peeled, pitted, and cut into pieces
- 1 tbsp fresh lime juice
- 14 oz. can coconut milk
- 80 drops of liquid stevia
- 2 tsp vanilla extract

Directions:

Add all ingredients into the blender and blend until smooth.

Serve and enjoy.

Nutrition: Calories: 209; Total Carbohydrate: 6 g; Total Fat: 7 g; Fiber: 2 g; Proteins: 17 g.

366 RASPBERRY CHIA PUDDING

Preparation Time: 3 hours & 10 minutes
Cooking Time: 0 minutes
Servings: 2
Ingredients:

- 4 tbsp. chia seeds
- 1 cup coconut milk
- ½ cup raspberries

Directions:

Add raspberry and coconut milk in a blender and blend until smooth.

Pour the mixture into the Mason jar.

Add chia seeds in a jar and stir well.

Close the jar tightly with the lid and shake well.

Place in refrigerator for 3 hours.

Serve chilled and enjoy.

Nutrition: Calories: 189; Total Carbohydrate: 6 g; Cholesterol: 3 mg; Total Fat: 7 g; Fiber: 4 g; Proteins: 12 g; Sodium: 293 mg.

367 MANDARIN SMOOTHIE

Preparation Time: 10 minutes
Cooking Time: 0 minutes
Servings: 2
Ingredients:

4 mandarins
½ cup ice cubes
¼ cup unsweetened oat or nut milk
a pinch of sea salt
1 frozen banana
1 tsp. freshly grated turmeric or ½ tsp. ground turmeric
2 drops of vanilla extract

Directions:

Add all ingredients into a blender and blend for approximately 1-2 minutes or until smooth.

Then pour into a glass and enjoy.

Nutrition: Calories: 420; Fat: 12 g; Proteins: 23 g; Sugar: 13 g.

368 KIWI, GRAPEFRUIT, AND LIME SMOOTHIE

Preparation Time: 10 minutes
Cooking Time: 0 minutes
Servings: 2
Ingredients:

1 grapefruit, chopped
1 kiwi fruit
2 mandarins
1 pear, chopped
1 ½ tbsp. honey
2 cups ice cubes

Directions:

Add all ingredients into a blender, and blend for approximately 1-2 minutes or until smooth. Then pour into a glass and enjoy.

Nutrition: Calories: 400; Fat: 10 g; Proteins: 20 g; Sugar: 10 g.

369 BERRY RED SMOOTHIE

Preparation Time: 10 minutes
Cooking Time: 0 minutes
Servings: 2
Ingredients:

½ cup raspberries
½ cup strawberries
1 banana
2 cups pomegranate juice
½ cup plain yogurt

Directions:

Peel the banana, cut it into chunks and then put it into the blender.

Add the raspberries, the strawberries, and the pomegranate juice to the banana in the blender.

Pulse the ingredients a couple of times.

Finally, add the yogurt to the mixture and blend until smooth.

Transfer the smoothie into glasses and serve immediately.

Nutrition: Calories: 220; Fat: 2 g; Proteins: 3 g; Sugar: 11 g.

370 BLUEBERRY KIWI SMOOTHIE

Preparation Time: 10 minutes
Cooking Time: 0 minutes
Servings: 2

Ingredients:

1 cup blueberries
2 kiwis
½ cup plain yogurt

Directions:

Peel the kiwis and put them in the blender.

Put the blueberries and the yogurt in the blender as well.

Blend ingredients until smooth.

Transfer the smoothie to a glass and top it with blueberries.

Nutrition: Calories: 200; Fat: 10 g; Proteins: 9 g; Sugar: 6 g.

371 REFRESHING CUCUMBER SMOOTHIE

Preparation Time: 10 minutes
Cooking Time: 0 minutes
Servings: 2
Ingredients:

1 small cucumber
1 stalk celery
½ of avocado
½ of apple
1 kiwi
1 sprig of fresh mint
2 tbsp. fresh lemon juice
1 cup iced water

Directions:

Cut the cucumber into chunks.

Peel the avocado and remove the stone. Cut half of the avocado into chunks.

Peel the kiwi and cut it into chunks.

Cut the apple in half and remove the core. Cut half of the apple into chunks.

Put all the fruits and the rest of the ingredients in the blender and mix until smooth.

Nutrition: Calories: 340; Fat: 15 g; Proteins: 12 g; Sugar: 19 g.

372 LEMON MOUSSE

Preparation Time: 10 minutes
Cooking Time: 0 minutes
Servings: 2

Ingredients:

14 oz. coconut milk
12 drops liquid stevia
½ tsp. lemon extract
¼ tsp. turmeric

Directions:

Place coconut milk can in the refrigerator overnight. Scoop out thick cream into a mixing bowl.

Add remaining ingredients to the bowl and whip using a hand mixer until smooth.

Transfer mousse mixture to a zip-lock bag and pipe into small serving glasses. Place in refrigerator.

Serve chilled and enjoy.

Nutrition: Calories: 189; Total Carbohydrate: 2 g; Cholesterol: 13 mg; Total Fat: 7 g; Fiber: 2 g; Proteins: 15 g; Sodium: 321 mg.

373 CHOCÓ CHIA PUDDING

Preparation Time: 10 minutes
Cooking Time: 0 minutes
Servings: 6
Ingredients:

2 ½ cups coconut milk
2 scoops stevia extract powder
6 tbsp. cocoa powder
½ cup chia seeds
½ tsp. vanilla extract
⅛ cup xylitol
⅛ tsp. salt

Directions:

Add all ingredients into the blender and mix until smooth.

Pour mixture into the glass container and place in refrigerator.

Serve chilled and enjoy.

Nutrition: Calories: 178; Total Carbohydrate: 3 g; Cholesterol: 3 mg; Total Fat: 17 g; Proteins: 9 g.

374 SPICED BUTTERMILK

Preparation Time: 5 minutes
Cooking Time: 0 minutes
Servings: 2
Ingredients:

¾ tsp. ground cumin
¼ tsp. sea salt
⅛ tsp. ground black pepper
2 mint leaves
⅛ tsp. lemon juice
¼ cup cilantro leaves
1 cup chilled water
1 cup vegan yogurt, unsweetened
Ice as needed

Directions:

Place all the ingredients in the order in a food processor or blender, except for cilantro and ¼ tsp. cumin, and then pulse for 2 to 3 minutes at high speed until smooth.

Pour the milk into glasses, top with cilantro and cumin, and then serve.

Nutrition: Calories: 211; Total Carbohydrate: 7 g; Cholesterol: 13 mg; Total Fat: 18 g; Fiber: 3 g; Proteins: 17 g; Sodium: 289 mg.

375 TURMERIC LASSI

Preparation Time: 5 minutes
Cooking Time: 0 minutes
Servings: 2
Ingredients:

1 tsp. grated ginger
1/8 tsp. ground black pepper
1 tsp. turmeric powder
1/8 tsp. cayenne
1 tbsp. coconut sugar
1/8 tsp. salt
1 cup vegan yogurt
1 cup almond milk

Directions:

Place all the ingredients in the order in a food processor or blender and then pulse for 2 to 3 minutes at high speed until smooth.

Pour the lassi into two glasses and then serve.

Nutrition: Calories: 392; Fat: 10 g; Proteins: 18 g; Sugar: 8 g.

376 BROWNIE BATTER ORANGE CHIA SHAKE

Preparation Time: 5 minutes
Cooking Time: 0 minutes
Servings: 2
Ingredients:

2 tbsp. cocoa powder
3 tbsp. chia seeds
1/4 tsp. salt
4 tbsp. chocolate chips
4 tsp. coconut sugar
1/2 tsp. orange zest
1/2 tsp. vanilla extract, unsweetened
2 cup almond milk

Directions:

Place all the ingredients in the order in a food processor or blender and then pulse for 2 to 3 minutes at high speed until smooth.

Pour the smoothie into two glasses and then serve.

Nutrition: Calories: 290; Fat: 11 g; Proteins: 20 g; Sugar: 9 g.

377 SAFFRON PISTACHIO BEVERAGE

Preparation Time: 5 minutes
Cooking Time: 0 minutes
Servings: 2
Ingredients:

8 strands of saffron
1 tbsp. cashews
1/4 tsp. ground ginger
2 tbsp. pistachio

1/8 tsp. cloves
1/4 tsp. ground black pepper
1/4 tsp. cardamom powder
3 tbsp. coconut sugar
1/4 tsp. cinnamon
1/8 tsp. fennel seeds
1/4 tsp. poppy seeds

Directions:

Place all the ingredients in the order in a food processor or blender and then pulse for 2 to 3 minutes at high speed until smooth.

Pour the smoothie into two glasses and then serve.

Nutrition: Calories: 394; Fat: 5 g; Proteins: 12 g; Sugar: 4 g.

378 MEXICAN HOT CHOCOLATE MIX

Preparation Time: 5 minutes
Cooking Time: 0 minutes
Servings: 2
Ingredients:

For the Hot Chocolate Mix:

1/3 cup chopped dark chocolate
1/8 tsp. cayenne
1/8 tsp. salt
1/2 tsp. cinnamon
1/4 cup coconut sugar
1 tsp. cornstarch
3 tbsp. cocoa powder
1/2 tsp. vanilla extract, unsweetened

For Servings:

2 cups milk, warmed

Directions:

Place all the ingredients of hot chocolate mix in the order in a food processor or blender and then pulse for 2 to 3 minutes at high speed until ground.

Stir 2 tablespoons of the chocolate mix into a glass of milk until combined and then serve.

Nutrition: Calories: 160; Fat: 6 g; Proteins: 26 g; Sugar: 7 g.

379 PUMPKIN SPICE FRAPPUCCINO

Preparation Time: 5 minutes
Cooking Time: 0 minutes
Servings: 2
Ingredients:

1/2 tsp. ground ginger
1/8 tsp. allspice
1/2 tsp. ground cinnamon
2 tbsp. coconut sugar
1/8 tsp. nutmeg
1/4 tsp. ground cloves
1 tsp. vanilla extract, unsweetened
2 tsp. instant coffee
2 cups almond milk, unsweetened
1 cup of ice cubes

Directions:

Place all the ingredients in the order in a food processor or blender and

then pulse for 2 to 3 minutes at high speed until smooth.

Pour the Frappuccino into two glasses and then serve.

Nutrition: Calories: 490; Fat: 9 g; Proteins: 12 g; Sugar: 11 g.

380 COOKIE DOUGH MILKSHAKE

Preparation Time: 5 minutes
Cooking Time: 0 minutes
Servings: 2
Ingredients:

2 tbsp. cookie dough
5 dates, pitted
2 tsp. chocolate chips
1/2 tsp. vanilla extract, unsweetened
1/2 cup almond milk, unsweetened
1 1/2 cup almond milk ice cubes

Directions:

Place all the ingredients in the order in a food processor or blender and then pulse for 2 to 3 minutes at high speed until smooth.

Pour the milkshake into two glasses and then serve with some cookie dough balls.

Nutrition: Calories: 240; Fat: 13 g; Proteins: 21 g; Sugar: 9 g.

381 STRAWBERRY AND HEMP SMOOTHIE

Preparation Time: 5 minutes
Servings: 2
Ingredients:

3 cups fresh strawberries
2 tbsp. hemp seeds
1/2 tsp. vanilla extract, unsweetened
1/8 tsp. sea salt
2 tbsp. maple syrup
1 cup vegan yogurt
1 cup almond milk, unsweetened
1 cup of ice cubes
2 tbsp. hemp Protein

Directions:

Place all the ingredients in the order in a food processor or blender, except for Protein powder, and then pulse for 2 to 3 minutes at high speed until smooth.

Pour the smoothie into two glasses and then serve.

Nutrition: Calories: 510; Fat: 18 g; Proteins: 26 g; Sugar: 12 g.

382 BLUEBERRY, HAZELNUT, AND HEMP SMOOTHIE

Preparation Time: 5 minutes
Cooking Time: 0 minutes
Servings: 2
Ingredients:

2 tbsp. hemp seeds
1 1/2 cups frozen blueberries
2 tbsp. chocolate protein powder
1/2 tsp. vanilla extract, unsweetened

2 tbsp. chocolate hazelnut butter

1 small frozen banana

¼ cup almond milk

Directions:

Place all the ingredients in the order in a food processor or blender and then pulse for 2 to 3 minutes at high speed until smooth.

Pour the smoothie into two glasses and then serve.

Nutrition: Calories: 195; Fat: 14 g; Proteins: 36 g; Sugar: 10 g.

383 MANGO LASSI

Preparation Time: 5 minutes

Cooking Time: 0 minutes

Servings: 2

Ingredients:

1 ¼ cup mango pulp

1 tbsp. coconut sugar

⅛ tsp. salt

½ tsp. lemon juice

¼ cup almond milk, unsweetened

¼ cup chilled water

1 cup cashew yogurt

Directions:

Place all the ingredients in the order in a food processor or blender and then pulse for 2 to 3 minutes at high speed until smooth.

Pour the lassi into two glasses and then serve.

Nutrition: Calories: 420; Fat: 12 g; Proteins: 23 g; Sugar: 13 g.

384 MOCHA CHOCOLATE SHAKE

Preparation Time: 5 minutes

Cooking Time: 0 minutes

Servings: 2

Ingredients:

¼ cup hemp seeds

2 tsp. cocoa powder, unsweetened

½ cup dates, pitted

1 tbsp. instant coffee powder

2 tbsp. flax seeds

2 ½ cups almond milk, unsweetened

½ cup crushed ice

Directions:

Place all the ingredients in the order in a food processor or blender and then pulse for 2 to 3 minutes at high speed until smooth.

Pour the smoothie into two glasses and then serve.

Nutrition: Calories: 432; Fat: 18 g; Proteins: 14 g; Sugar: 12 g.

385 CHARD, LETTUCE AND GINGER SMOOTHIE

Preparation Time: 5 minutes

Servings: 2

Ingredients:

10 Chard leaves, chopped

1-inch piece of ginger, chopped

10 lettuce leaves, chopped

½ tsp. black salt

2 pears, chopped

2 tsp. coconut sugar

¼ tsp. ground black pepper

¼ tsp. salt

2 tbsp. lemon juice

2 cups water

Directions:

Place all the ingredients in the order in a food processor or blender and then pulse for 2 to 3 minutes at high speed until smooth.

Pour the smoothie into two glasses and then serve.

Nutrition: Calories: 240; Fat: 4 g; Proteins: 16 g; Sugar: 3 g.

386 RED BEET, PEAR AND APPLE SMOOTHIE

Preparation Time: 5 minutes

Cooking Time: 0 minutes

Servings: 2

Ingredients:

½ of medium beet, peeled, chopped

1 tbsp. chopped cilantro

1 orange, juiced

1 medium pear, chopped

1 medium apple, cored, chopped

¼ tsp. ground black pepper

⅛ tsp. rock salt

1 tsp. coconut sugar

¼ tsp. salt

1 cup of water

Directions:

Place all the ingredients in the order in a food processor or blender and then pulse for 2 to 3 minutes at high speed until smooth.

Pour the smoothie into two glasses and then serve.

Nutrition: Calories: 240; Fat: 4 g; Proteins: 16 g; Sugar: 3 g.

387 BERRY AND YOGURT SMOOTHIE

Preparation Time: 5 minutes

Cooking Time: 0 minutes

Servings: 2

Ingredients:

2 small bananas

3 cups frozen mixed berries

1 ½ cup cashew yogurt

½ tsp. vanilla extract, unsweetened

½ cup almond milk, unsweetened

Directions:

Place all the ingredients in the order in a food processor or blender and then pulse for 2 to 3 minutes at high speed until smooth.

Pour the smoothie into two glasses and then serve.

Nutrition: Calories: 291; Fat: 9 g; Proteins: 17 g; Sugar: 5 g.

388 CHOCOLATE AND CHERRY SMOOTHIE

Preparation Time: 5 minutes

Cooking Time: 0 minutes

Servings: 2

Ingredients:

4 cups frozen cherries

2 tbsp. cocoa powder

1 scoop of protein powder

1 tsp. maple syrup

2 cups almond milk, unsweetened

Directions:

Place all the ingredients in the order in a food processor or blender and then pulse for 2 to 3 minutes at high speed until smooth.

Pour the smoothie into two glasses and then serve.

Nutrition: Calories: 247; Fat: 3 g; Proteins: 18 g; Sugar: 3 g.

389 STRAWBERRY AND BANANA SHAKE

Preparation Time: 10 minutes

Cooking Time: 10 minutes

Servings: 2

Ingredients:

1 ½ cups fresh strawberries, hulled

1 large frozen banana, peeled

2 scoops of unsweetened vegan vanilla Protein powder

2 tbsp. hemp seeds

2 cups unsweetened hemp milk

Directions:

In a high-speed blender, place all the ingredients and pulse until creamy.

Pour into two glasses and serve immediately.

Nutrition: Calories: 259; Fat: 3 g; Proteins: 10 g; Sugar: 2 g.

390 CHOCOLATEY BANANA SHAKE

Preparation Time: 10 minutes

Cooking Time: 10 minutes

Servings: 2

Ingredients:

2 medium frozen bananas, peeled

4 dates, pitted

4 tbsp. peanut butter

4 tbsp. rolled oats

2 tbsp. cacao powder

2 tbsp. chia seeds

2 cups unsweetened soymilk

Directions:

Place all the ingredients in a high-speed blender and pulse until creamy.

Pour into two glasses and serve immediately.

Nutrition: Calories: 502; Fat: 4 g; Proteins: 11 g; Sugar: 9 g.

391 FRUITY TOFU SMOOTHIE

Preparation Time: 10 minutes
Cooking Time: 10 minutes
Servings: 2
Ingredients:

12 oz. silken tofu, pressed and drained
2 medium bananas, peeled
1 ½ cups fresh blueberries
1 tbsp. maple syrup
1 ½ cups unsweetened soymilk
¼ cup ice cubes

Directions:

Place all the ingredients in a high-speed
blender and pulse until creamy.
Pour into two glasses and serve
immediately.

Nutrition: Calories 235; Carbohydrates: 1.9
g; Proteins: 14.3 g; Fat: 18.9 g.

392 GREEN FRUITY SMOOTHIE

Preparation Time: 10 minutes
Cooking Time: 10 minutes
Servings: 2
Ingredients:

1 cup frozen mango, peeled, pitted, and
chopped
1 large frozen banana, peeled
2 cups fresh baby spinach
1 scoop unsweetened vegan vanilla
Protein powder
¼ cup pumpkin seeds
2 tbsp. hemp hearts
1 ½ cups unsweetened almond milk

Directions:

In a high-speed blender, place all the
ingredients and pulse until
creamy.
Pour into two glasses and serve
immediately.

Nutrition: Calories 206; Carbohydrates: 1.3
g; Proteins: 23.5 g; Fat: 11.9 g.

393 PROTEIN LATTE

Preparation Time: 10 minutes
Cooking Time: 10 minutes
Servings: 2
Ingredients:

2 cups hot brewed coffee
1 ¼ cups coconut milk
2 tsp. coconut oil
2 scoops unsweetened vegan vanilla
Protein powder

Directions:

Place all the ingredients in a high-speed
blender and pulse until creamy.
Pour into two serving mugs and serve
immediately.

Nutrition: Calories 483; Carbs: 5.2 g;
Proteins: 45.2 g; Fat: 31.2 g.

394 HEALTH BOOSTING JUICES

Preparation Time: 10 minutes
Cooking Time: 15 minutes

Servings: 2
Ingredients for a Red Juice:

4 beetroots, quartered
2 cups of strawberries
2 cups of blueberries

Ingredients for an orange juice:

4 green or red apples, halved
10 carrots
½ lemon, peeled
1" of ginger

Ingredients for a Yellow Juice:

2 green or red apples, quartered
4 oranges, peeled and halved
½ lemon, peeled
1" of ginger

Ingredients for Lime Juice:

6 stalks of celery
1 cucumber
2 green apples, quartered
2 pears, quartered

Ingredients for a Green Juice:

½ a pineapple, peeled and sliced
8 leaves of kale
2 fresh bananas, peeled

Directions:

Juice all ingredients in a juicer, chill,
and serve.

Nutrition: Calories 316; Carbs: 13.5 g;
Proteins: 37.8 g; Fat: 12.2 g.

395 THAI ICED TEA

Preparation Time: 5 minutes
Cooking Time: 10 minutes
Servings: 4
Ingredients:

4 cups water
1 can of light coconut milk (14 oz.)
¼ cup maple syrup
¼ cup muscovado sugar
1 tsp. vanilla extract
2 tbsp. loose-leaf black tea

Directions:

In a large saucepan, over medium heat
brings the water to a boil.
Turn off the heat and add in the tea,
cover and let steep for five
minutes.
Strain the tea into a bowl or jug. Add
the maple syrup, muscovado
sugar, and vanilla extract. Give it
a good whisk to blend all the
ingredients.
Set in the refrigerator to chill. Upon
serving, pour ¾ of the tea into
each glass, top with coconut milk,
and stir.

Tips:

Add a shot of dark rum to turn this
iced tea into a cocktail.
You could substitute the coconut milk
for almond or rice milk too.

Nutrition: Calories 844; Carbohydrates: 2.3
g; Proteins: 21.6 g; Fat: 83.1 g.

396 BERRY PROTEIN SHAKE

Preparation Time: 10 minutes
Cooking Time: 0 minutes
Servings: 1
Ingredients:

2 scoops whey protein powder
1 cup blueberries
1 cup blackberries
1 cup raspberries
1 cup of water
1 cup ice

Directions:

Add all the ingredients to a blender and
blend until smooth.
Enjoy!

Nutrition: Calories: 342; Proteins: 38 g;
Carbs: 42 g; Fat: 3 g.

397 FRESH STRAWBERRY SHAKE

Preparation Time: 10 minutes
Cooking Time: 0 minutes
Servings: 1
Ingredients:

2 scoops Vanilla Protein powder
1 cup strawberries
2 cups water
1 tbsp. flaxseed oil

Directions:

Add all the ingredients to a blender and
blend until smooth.
Enjoy!

Nutrition: Calories: 303; Proteins: 35 g;
Carbs: 15 g; Fat: 11 g.

398 CHOCO COFFEE ENERGY SHAKE

Preparation Time: 10 minutes
Cooking Time: 0 minutes
Servings: 1
Ingredients:

2 scoops chocolate protein powder
½ cup low-fat milk
1 cup of water
1 tbsp. instant coffee

Directions:

Add all the ingredients to a blender and
blend until smooth
Enjoy

Nutrition: Calories: 299; Proteins: 42 g;
Carbs: 14 g; Fat: 6 g.

399 LEAN AND MEAN PINEAPPLE SHAKE

Preparation Time: 10 minutes
Cooking Time: 0 minutes
Servings: 1
Ingredients:

1 cup chopped fresh pineapple
4 strawberries
1 banana
1 tbsp. low-fat Greek yogurt
1 scoop Vanilla Protein powder
1 cup of water

Directions:

Add all the ingredients to a blender and blend until smooth.
Enjoy!

Nutrition: Calories: 355; Proteins: 23 g; Carbs: 65 g; Fat: 3 g.

400 RASPBERRIES AND YOGURT SMOOTHIE

Preparation Time: 5 minutes
Cooking Time: 0 minutes
Servings: 2
Ingredients:

2 cups raspberries
½ cup Greek yogurt
½ cup almond milk
½ tsp. vanilla extract

Directions:

In your blender, combine the raspberries with the milk, vanilla, and the yogurt. Pulse well, divide into 2 glasses and serve for breakfast.

Nutrition: Calories: 245; Fat: 9.5 g; Carbs: 5.6 g; Protein: 1.6 g

SALADS AND SIDE DISHES

401 TUNA SALAD

Preparation Time: 10 minutes
Cooking Time: 0 minutes
Servings: 2
Ingredients:

12 oz. canned tuna in water, drained and flaked
¼ cup roasted red peppers, chopped
2 tbsp. capers, drained
8 kalamata olives, pitted and sliced
2 tbsp. olive oil
1 tbsp. parsley, chopped
1 tbsp. lemon juice
A pinch of salt and black pepper

Directions:

In a bowl, combine the tuna with roasted peppers and the rest of the ingredients. Toss, divide between plates and serve for breakfast.

Nutrition: Calories: 250; Fat: 17.3; Fiber: 0.8; Carbs: 2.7; Protein: 10.1

402 VEGGIE SALAD

Preparation Time: 5 minutes
Cooking Time: 0 minutes
Servings: 4
Ingredients:

2 tomatoes, cut into wedges
2 red bell peppers, chopped
1 cucumber, chopped
1 red onion, sliced
½ cup kalamata olives, pitted and sliced
2 oz. feta cheese, crumbled

¼ cup lime juice
½ cup olive oil
2 garlic cloves, minced
1 tbsp. oregano, chopped
Salt and black pepper to the taste

Directions:

In a large salad bowl, combine the tomatoes with the peppers and the rest of the ingredients except the cheese and toss.
Divide the salad into smaller bowls, sprinkle the cheese on top and serve for breakfast.

Nutrition: Calories: 327; Fat: 11.2; Fiber: 4.4; Carbs: 16.7; Protein: 6.4

403 SALMON AND BULGUR SALAD

Preparation Time: 25 minutes
Cooking Time: 10 minutes
Servings: 4
Ingredients:

1-pound salmon fillet, skinless and boneless
1 tbsp. olive oil
1 cup bulgur
1 cup parsley, chopped
¼ cup mint, chopped
3 tbsp. lemon juice
1 red onion, sliced
Salt and black pepper to the taste
2 cup hot water

Directions:

Heat up a pan with half of the oil over medium fire. Add the salmon, some salt and pepper. Cook for 5 minutes on each side, cool down, flake and put in a salad bowl.
In another bowl, mix the bulgur with hot water. Cover, leave aside for 25 minutes, drain and transfer to the bowl with the salmon.
Add the rest of the ingredients, toss and serve for breakfast.

Nutrition: Calories: 321; Fat: 11.3; Fiber: 7.9; Carbs: 30.8; Protein: 27.6

404 HERBED QUINOA AND ASPARAGUS

Preparation Time: 10 minutes
Cooking Time: 0 minutes
Servings: 4
Ingredients:

3 cups asparagus, steamed and roughly chopped
1 tbsp. olive oil
3 tbsp. balsamic vinegar
1 ¾ cups quinoa, cooked
2 tsp. mustard
Salt and black pepper to the taste
5 oz. baby spinach
½ cup parsley, chopped
1 tbsp. thyme, chopped

1 tbsp. tarragon, chopped

Directions:

In a salad bowl, combine the asparagus with the quinoa, spinach and the rest of the ingredients. Toss and keep in the fridge for 10 minutes before serving for breakfast.

Nutrition: Calories: 323; Fat: 11.3; Fiber: 3.4; Carbs: 16.4; Protein: 10

405 POTATO AND PANCETTA BOWLS

Preparation Time: 10 minutes
Cooking Time: 1 hour & 5 minutes
Servings: 4
Ingredients:

1-pound sweet potatoes, peeled and cut into small wedges
1 red onion, chopped
3 oz. pancetta, chopped
2 garlic cloves, minced
2 tbsp. olive oil
2 eggs, whisked
2 oz. goat cheese, crumbled
1 tbsp. parsley, chopped
A pinch of salt and black pepper

Directions:

Put potatoes in a pot, add water to cover; add salt and pepper and bring to a boil over medium heat. Simmer for 15 minutes, drain and put them in a bowl.
Heat up a pan with half of the oil over medium heat. Add the onion, the potatoes, the eggs and the rest of the ingredients. Toss and cook for 15 minutes.
Divide between plates and serve for breakfast.

Nutrition: Calories 230 g Protein: 12 g; Carbohydrates: 44 g; Fat: 14 g.

406 QUINOA SALAD

Preparation Time: 5 minutes
Cooking Time: 0 minutes
Servings: 4
Ingredients:

4 eggs, soft boiled, peeled and cut into wedges
2 cups baby arugula
2 cups cherry tomatoes, halved
1 cucumber, sliced
1 cup quinoa, cooked
1 cup almonds, chopped
1 avocado, peeled, pitted and sliced
1 tbsp. olive oil
½ cup mixed dill and mint, chopped
A pinch of salt and black pepper
Juice of 1 lemon

Directions:

In a large salad bowl, combine the eggs with the arugula and the rest of the ingredients. Toss, divide between plates and serve for breakfast.

Nutrition: Calories: 519; Fat: 32.4; Fiber: 11; Carbs: 43.3; Protein: 19.1

407 CORN SALAD

Preparation Time: 10 minutes
Cooking Time: 10 minutes
Servings: 4
Ingredients:

4 ears of sweet corn, husked
1 avocado, peeled, pitted and chopped
½ cup basil, chopped
A pinch of salt and black pepper
1-pound shrimp, peeled and deveined
1 and ½ cups cherry tomatoes, halved
¼ cup olive oil

Directions:

Put the corn in a pot and add water to cover. Bring to a boil over medium heat, cook for 6 minutes, drain, cool down. Cut corn from the cob and put it in a bowl.
Thread the shrimp onto skewers and brush with some of the oil.
Place the skewers on the preheated grill. Cook over medium heat for 2 minutes on each side, remove from skewers and add over the corn.
Add the rest of the ingredients to the bowl. Toss, divide between plates and serve for breakfast.

Nutrition: calories 371 Protein: 18 g; Carbohydrates: 50 g; Fat: 22 g.

408 BROWN LENTILS SALAD

Preparation Time: 10 minutes
Cooking Time: 35 minutes
Servings: 4
Ingredients:

2 yellow onions, chopped
4 garlic cloves, minced
2 cups brown lentils
1 tbsp. olive oil
A pinch of salt and black pepper
½ tsp. sweet paprika
½ tsp. ginger, grated
3 cups water
¼ cup lemon juice
¾ cup Greek yogurt
3 tbsp. tomato paste

Directions:

Heat up a pot with the oil over medium-high heat. Add the onions and sauté for 2 minutes.
Add the garlic and the lentils, stir and cook for 1 minute more.
Add the water, bring to a simmer and cook covered for 30 minutes.
Add the lemon juice and the remaining ingredients except for the yogurt. Toss, divide the mix into bowls, top with the yogurt and serve.

Nutrition: Calories: 294; Fat: 3; Fiber: 8; Carbs: 49; Protein: 21

409 QUICK ZUCCHINI BOWL

Preparation Time: 10 minutes
Cooking Time: 10 minutes
Servings: 4
Ingredients:

½ pound pasta
2 tbsp. olive oil
6 crushed garlic cloves
1 tsp. red chili
2 finely sliced spring onions
3 tsp. chopped rosemary
1 large zucchini cut up in half, lengthways and sliced
5 large portabella mushrooms
1 can of tomatoes
4 tbsp. Parmesan cheese
Fresh ground black pepper

Directions:

Cook the pasta.
Take a large-sized frying pan and place over medium heat.
Add oil and allow the oil to heat up.
Add garlic, onion and chili and sauté for a few minutes until golden.
Add zucchini, rosemary and mushroom, and sauté for a few minutes.
Increase the heat to medium-high and add tinned tomatoes to the sauce until thick.
Drain your boiled pasta and transfer to a serving platter.
Pour the tomato mix on top and mix using tongs.
Garnish with Parmesan cheese and freshly ground black pepper.
Enjoy!

Nutrition: Calories: 361; Fat: 12 g; Carbohydrates: 47 g; Protein: 14 g.

410 HEALTHY BASIL PLATTER

Preparation Time: 25 minutes
Cooking Time: 15 minutes
Servings: 4
Ingredients:

2 pieces of red pepper seeded and cut up into chunks
2 pieces of red onion cut up into wedges
2 mild red chilies, diced and seeded
3 coarsely chopped garlic cloves
1 tsp. golden caster sugar
2 tbsp. olive oil (plus additional for serving)
2 pounds small ripe tomatoes quartered up
12 oz. dried pasta
Just a handful of basil leaves
2 tbsp. grated Parmesan

Directions:

Preheat the oven to 392°F.
Take a large-sized roasting tin and scatter pepper, red onion, garlic and chilies.
Sprinkle sugar on top.
Drizzle olive oil then season with pepper and salt.
Roast the veggies in your oven for 15 minutes.
Take a large-sized pan and cook the pasta in boiling, salted water until al dente.
Drain them.
Remove the veggies from the oven and tip the pasta into the veggies.
Toss well and tear basil leaves on top.
Sprinkle Parmesan and enjoy!

Nutrition: Calories: 452; Fat: 8 g; Carbohydrates: 88 g; Protein: 14 g.

411 SPICED CHICKPEAS BOWLS

Preparation Time: 10 minutes
Cooking Time: 30 minutes
Servings: 4
Ingredients:

15 oz. canned chickpeas, drained and rinsed
¼ tsp. cardamom, ground
½ tsp. cinnamon powder
1 ½ tsp. turmeric powder
1 tsp. coriander, ground
1 tbsp. olive oil
A pinch of salt and black pepper
¾ cup Greek yogurt
½ cup green olives, pitted and halved
½ cup cherry tomatoes, halved
1 cucumber, sliced

Directions:

Spread the chickpeas on a lined baking sheet. Add the cardamom, cinnamon, turmeric, coriander, oil, salt and pepper. Toss and bake at 375°F for 30 minutes.
In a bowl, combine the roasted chickpeas with the rest of the ingredients. Toss and serve for breakfast.

Nutrition: Calories 519; Fat: 34.5; Fiber: 13.3; Carbs: 49.8; Protein: 12

412 EGGPLANT SALAD

Preparation Time: 20 minutes
Cooking Time: 15 minutes
Servings: 8
Ingredients:

1 large eggplant, washed and cubed
1 tomato, seeded and chopped
1 small onion, diced
2 tbsp. parsley, chopped
2 tbsp. extra virgin olive oil
2 tbsp. distilled white vinegar
½ cup feta cheese, crumbled
Salt as needed

Directions:

Preheat your outdoor grill to medium-high. Pierce the eggplant a few times using a knife/fork. Cook the eggplants on your grill for about 15 minutes until they are charred.)

Keep it on the side and allow them to cool. Remove the skin from the eggplant and dice the pulp. Transfer the pulp to a mixing bowl and add parsley, onion, tomato, olive oil, feta cheese and vinegar.

Mix well and chill for 1 hour. Season with salt and enjoy!

Nutrition: Calories: 99; Fat: 7 g; Carbohydrates: 7 g; Protein: 3.4 g.

413 GARBANZO BEAN SALAD

Preparation Time: 10 minutes
Cooking Time: 0 minutes
Servings: 4
Ingredients:

1 ½ cups cucumber, cubed
15 oz. canned garbanzo beans, drained and rinsed
3 oz. black olives, pitted and sliced
1 tomato, chopped
¼ cup red onion, chopped
5 cups salad greens
A pinch of salt and black pepper
½ cup feta cheese, crumbled
3 tbsp. olive oil
1 tbsp. lemon juice
¼ cup parsley, chopped

Directions:

In a salad bowl, combine the garbanzo beans with the cucumber, tomato, and the rest of the ingredients, except the cheese, and toss.

Divide the mix into small bowls. Sprinkle the cheese on top, and serve for breakfast.

Nutrition: Calories: 268; Fat: 16 g; Carbs: 24 g; Protein: 9 g.

414 PEARL COUSCOUS SALAD

Preparation Time: 15 minutes
Cooking Time: 0 minutes
Servings: 6

Ingredients:
For Lemon Dill Vinaigrette:

Juice of 1 large-sized lemon
⅓ cup of extra virgin olive oil
1 tsp. of dill weed
1 tsp. of garlic powder
Salt as needed
Pepper

For Israeli Couscous:

2 cups of Pearl Couscous
Extra virgin olive oil
2 cups of halved grape tomatoes
Water as needed

⅓ cup of finely chopped red onions
½ of a finely chopped English cucumber
15 oz. of chickpeas
14 oz. can of artichoke hearts (roughly chopped up)
½ cup of pitted Kalamata olives
15-20 pieces of fresh basil leaves, roughly torn and chopped up
3 oz. of fresh baby mozzarella

Directions:

Prepare the vinaigrette by taking a bowl and add the ingredients listed under vinaigrette. Mix them well and keep aside. Take a medium-sized heavy pot and place it over medium heat.

Add 2 tablespoons of olive oil and allow it to heat up. Add couscous and keep cooking until golden brown. Add 3 cups of boiling water and cook the couscous according to the package instructions.

Once done, drain in a colander and keep aside. Take another large-sized mixing bowl and add the remaining ingredients, except for the cheese and basil.

Add the cooked couscous and basil to the mix and mix everything well. Give the vinaigrette a nice stir and whisk it into the couscous salad. Mix well.

Adjust the seasoning as required. Add mozzarella cheese. Garnish with some basil. Enjoy!

Nutrition: Calories: 393; Fat: 13 g; Carbohydrates: 57 g; Protein: 13 g.

415 MEDITERRANEAN BREAKFAST SALAD

Preparation Time: 15 minutes
Cooking Time: 10 minutes
Servings: 2
Ingredients:

4 eggs (optional)
10 cups arugula
½ seedless cucumber, chopped
1 cup cooked quinoa, cooled
1 large avocado
1 cup natural almonds, chopped
½ cup mixed herbs like mint and dill, chopped
2 cups halved cherry tomatoes and/or heirloom tomatoes cut into wedges
Extra virgin olive oil
1 lemon
Sea salt, to taste
Freshly ground black pepper, to taste

Directions:

Cook the eggs by soft-boiling them. Bring a pot of water to a boil,

then reduce heat to a simmer. Gently lower all the eggs into the water and allow them to simmer for 6 minutes.

Remove the eggs from water and run cold water on top to stop the cooking. Process set aside and peel when ready to use.

In a large bowl, combine the arugula, tomatoes, cucumber, and quinoa. Divide the salad into 2 containers. Store in the fridge for 2 days.

Nutrition: Calories: 252; Carbs: 18 g; Fat: 16 g; Protein: 10 g.

416 BROWN RICE SALAD

Preparation Time: 10 minutes
Cooking Time: 0 minutes
Servings: 4

Ingredients:

9 oz. brown rice, cooked
7 cups baby arugula
15 oz. canned garbanzo beans, drained and rinsed
4 oz. feta cheese, crumbled
¾ cup basil, chopped
A pinch of salt and black pepper
2 tbsp. lemon juice
¼ tsp. lemon zest, grated
¼ cup olive oil

Directions:

In a salad bowl, combine the brown rice with the arugula, the beans, and the rest of the ingredients. Toss and serve cold for breakfast.

Nutrition: Calories: 473; Fat: 22 g; Carbs: 53 g; Protein: 13 g.

417 SHRIMP VEGGIE PASTA SALAD

Preparation Time: 50 minutes
Cooking Time: 10 minutes
Servings: 6
Ingredients:

1 lb. shrimp, peeled and deveined
8 oz. asparagus, sliced
Salt and pepper to taste
12 oz. farfalle, penne or macaroni pasta, cooked
2 tbsp. parsley, chopped
½ cup shallots, sliced thinly
¼ cup Parmesan cheese, grated
2 tbsp. freshly squeezed lemon juice
½ cup mayonnaise
2 tsp. garlic, minced
1 tsp. Worcestershire sauce
1 tsp. Dijon mustard
1 lemon, sliced into wedges

Directions:

Preheat your oven to 400°F.

Arrange the shrimp and asparagus in a baking pan.

Season with salt and pepper.

Roast in the oven for 10 minutes.

Let cool. Transfer to a bowl.

Stir in the cooked pasta, parsley and shallots.

Sprinkle the Parmesan cheese on top.

In another bowl, combine the lemon juice, mayonnaise, garlic, Worcestershire sauce and Dijon mustard.

Add this mixture to the pasta salad.

Toss to coat evenly.

Refrigerate for at least 30 minutes before serving.

Garnish with lemon wedges.

Nutrition: Calories: 429; Fat: 17.1 g; Saturated Fat: 2.8 g; Carbohydrates 45.6 g; Fiber: 7.2 g; Protein: 25 g.

418 PEA SALAD

Preparation Time: 40 minutes
Cooking Time: 0 minutes
Servings: 6
Ingredients:

1 cup chickpeas, rinsed and drained
1 ½ cups peas, divided
Salt to taste
3 tbsp. olive oil
½ cup buttermilk
Pepper to taste
8 cups pea greens
3 carrots, shaved
1 cup snow peas, trimmed

Directions:

Add the chickpeas and half of the peas to your food processor.

Season with salt.

Pulse until smooth. Set aside.

In a bowl, toss the remaining peas in oil, milk, salt and pepper.

Transfer the mixture to your food processor.

Process until pureed.

Transfer this mixture to a bowl.

Arrange the pea greens on a serving plate.

Top with the shaved carrots and snow peas.

Stir in the pea and milk dressing.

Serve with the reserved chickpea hummus.

Nutrition: Calories: 214; Fat: 8.6 g; Saturated Fat: 1.5 g; Carbohydrates 27.3 g; Fiber: 8.4 g; Protein: 8 g.

419 SNAP PEA SALAD

Preparation Time: 1 hour
Cooking Time: 0 minutes
Servings: 6
Ingredients:

2 tbsp. mayonnaise
¾ tsp. celery seed
¼ cup cider vinegar
1 tsp. yellow mustard
1 tbsp. sugar

Salt and pepper to taste
4 oz. radishes, sliced thinly
12 oz. sugar snap peas, sliced thinly

Directions:

In a bowl, combine the mayonnaise, celery seeds, vinegar, mustard, sugar, salt and pepper.

Stir in the radishes and snap peas.

Refrigerate for 30 minutes.

Nutrition: Calories: 69; Fat: 3.7 g; Saturated Fat: 0.6 g; Carbohydrates 7.1 g; Fiber: 1.8 g; Protein: 2 g.

420 PINTO AND GREEN BEAN FRY WITH COUSCOUS

Preparation Time: 5 minutes
Cooking Time: 15 minutes
Servings: 4
Ingredients:

½ cup water
⅓ cup couscous (semolina or whole-wheat)
2 tbsp. extra-virgin olive oil
1 small onion, chopped
½ tbsp. minced garlic
1 cup green beans, cut into 1-inch pieces
1 cup fresh or frozen corn
1½ tsp. chili powder
½ tsp. ground cumin
1 large tomato, finely chopped
1 (14-oz.) can pinto beans, drained and rinsed
1 tsp. salt

Directions:

Bring the water to a boil in a small saucepan. Remove from the heat and stir in the couscous. Cover the pan and let sit for 10 minutes. Gently fluff the couscous with a fork.

While the couscous is cooking, heat the olive oil in a large skillet over medium heat. Add the onion and garlic and stir for 1 minute.

Add the green beans and stir for 4 minutes, until they begin to soften.

Add the corn, stir for another 2 minutes, then add the chili powder and cumin, and stir to coat the vegetables.

Add the tomato and simmer for 3 or 4 minutes. Stir in the pinto beans and couscous and cook for 3 to 4 minutes, until everything is heated throughout. Stir often.

Stir in the salt and serve hot or warm.

Nutrition: Calories: 267; Total Fat: 8 g; Total Carbs: 41 g; Fiber: 10 g; Sugar: 4 g; Protein: 10 g; Sodium: 601 mg.

421 INDONESIAN-STYLE SPICY FRIED TEMPEH STRIPS

Preparation Time: 5 minutes

Cooking Time: 20 minutes
Servings: 4
Ingredients:

1 cup sesame oil, or as needed
1 (12-oz.) package tempeh, cut into narrow 2-inch strips
2 medium onions, sliced
1½ tbsp. tomato paste
3 tsp. tamari or soy sauce
1 tsp. dried red chili flakes
½ tsp. brown sugar
2 tbsp. lime juice

Directions:

Heat the sesame oil in a large wok or saucepan over medium-high heat. Add more sesame oil as needed to raise the level to at least 1 inch.

As soon as the oil is hot but not smoking, add the tempeh slices and cook, stirring frequently, for 10 minutes, until a light golden color on all sides.

Add the onions and stir for another 10 minutes, until the tempeh and onions are brown and crispy.

Remove with a slotted spoon and add to a large bowl lined with several sheets of paper towel.

While the tempeh and onions are cooking, whisk together the tomato paste, tamari or soy sauce, red chili flakes, brown sugar, and lime juice in a small bowl.

Remove the paper towel from the large bowl and pour the sauce over the tempeh strips. Mix well to coat.

Nutrition: Calories: 317; Total Fat: 23 g; Total Carbs: 15 g; Sugar: 4 g; Protein: 17 g; Sodium: 266 mg.

422 CUCUMBER TOMATO CHOPPED SALAD

Preparation Time: 15 minutes
Cooking Time: 0 minutes
Servings: 6
Ingredients:

½ cup light mayonnaise
1 tbsp. lemon juice
1 tbsp. fresh dill, chopped
1 tbsp. chives, chopped
½ cup feta cheese, crumbled
Salt and pepper to taste
1 red onion, chopped
1 cucumber, diced
1 radish, diced
3 tomatoes, diced
Chives, chopped

Directions:

Combine the mayo, lemon juice, fresh dill, chives, feta cheese, salt and pepper in a bowl.

Mix well.

Stir in the onion, cucumber, radish and tomatoes.

Coat evenly.

Garnish with the chopped chives.

Nutrition: Calories: 187; Fat: 16.7 g; Saturated Fat: 4.1 g; Carbohydrates 6.7 g; Fiber: 2 g; Protein: 3.3 g.

423 ZUCCHINI PASTA SALAD

Preparation Time: 4 minutes
Cooking Time: 0 minutes
Servings: 15
Ingredients:

- 5 tbsp. olive oil
- 2 tsp. Dijon mustard
- 3 tbsp. red-wine vinegar
- 1 clove garlic, grated
- 2 tbsp. fresh oregano, chopped
- 1 shallot, chopped
- ¼ tsp. red pepper flakes
- 16 oz. zucchini noodles
- ¼ cup Kalamata olives, pitted
- 3 cups cherry tomatoes, sliced in half
- ¾ cup Parmesan cheese, shaved

Directions:

Mix the olive oil, Dijon mustard, red-wine vinegar, garlic, oregano, shallot and red pepper flakes in a bowl.

Stir in the zucchini noodles.

Sprinkle on top the olives, tomatoes and Parmesan cheese.

Nutrition: Calories: 299; Fat: 24.7 g; Saturated Fat: 5.1 g; Carbohydrates 11.6 g; Fiber: 2.8 g; Protein: 7 g.

424 FRIED RICE AND VEGETABLES

Preparation Time: 5 minutes
Cooking Time: 25 minutes
Servings: 4
Ingredients:

- ¾ cup uncooked short- or long-grain white rice
- 1 ½ cups water
- 2 tbsp. sesame oil, divided
- 2 large eggs, lightly beaten
- 2 carrots, diced
- 4 oz. (1¼ cups) sliced white mushrooms
- 1 tbsp. minced garlic
- 6 green onions, white and green parts, sliced and divided
- 2 tbsp. tamari or soy sauce
- ½ cup frozen green peas, defrosted

Directions:

Rinse the rice and add to a small saucepan. Add the water and bring to a boil.

Reduce the heat to low, cover, and simmer for 15 minutes, until the water is absorbed. Fluff with a fork and set aside.

While the rice is cooking, heat ½ tablespoon of the sesame oil in a large saucepan or wok over medium heat.

Add the eggs and cook without stirring for 5 minutes, until the egg is dry. Remove to a plate and cut into small strips. Set aside.

Return the saucepan or wok to the heat. Heat the remaining 2 ½ tablespoons of sesame oil. Add the carrots and stir for 2 minutes.

Add the mushrooms, garlic, and white parts of the green onions. Stir for 3 more minutes.

Add the cooked rice and tamari or soy sauce. Cook, stirring frequently, for 10 minutes, until the rice is sticky.

Toss in the green parts of the green onions, peas, and egg and stir to mix. Remove from the heat and serve hot with extra tamari or soy sauce, if desired.

Nutrition: Calories: 271; Total Fat: 10 g; Total Carbs: 37 g; Fiber:3 g; Sugar: 4 g; Protein: 9 g; Sodium: 567 mg.

425 SPANISH-STYLE SAFFRON RICE WITH BLACK BEANS

Preparation Time: 5 minutes
Cooking Time: 25 minutes
Servings: 4
Ingredients:

- 2 cups vegetable stock
- ¼ tsp. saffron threads (optional)
- 1 ½ tbsp. extra-virgin olive oil
- 1 small red or yellow onion, halved and thinly sliced
- 1 tbsp. minced garlic
- 1 tsp. turmeric
- 2 tsp. paprika
- 1 cup long-grain white rice, well-rinsed
- 1 (14-oz.) can black beans, drained and rinsed
- ½ cup green beans, halved or quartered
- 1 small red bell pepper, chopped
- 1 tsp. salt

Directions:

In a small pot, heat the vegetable stock until boiling. Add the saffron, if using, and remove from the heat.

Meanwhile, heat the olive oil in a large nonstick skillet over medium heat.

Add the onion, garlic, turmeric, paprika, and rice and stir to coat.

Pour in the stock, and mix in the black beans, green beans, and red bell pepper.

Bring to a boil. Reduce the heat to medium-low, cover, and simmer until the rice is tender and most of the liquid has been absorbed, about 20 minutes.

Stir in the salt and serve hot.

Nutrition: Calories: 332; Total Fat: 5 g; Total Carbs: 63 g; Fiber: 9 g; Sugar: 2 g; Protein: 11 g; Sodium: 658 mg.

426 EGG AVOCADO SALAD

Preparation Time: 10 minutes
Cooking Time: 0 minutes
Servings: 4
Ingredients:

- 1 avocado
- 6 hard-boiled eggs, peeled and chopped
- 1 tbsp. mayonnaise
- 2 tbsp. freshly squeezed lemon juice
- ¼ cup celery, chopped
- 2 tbsp. chives, chopped
- Salt and pepper to taste

Directions:

Add the avocado to a large bowl.

Mash the avocado using a fork.

Stir in the egg and mash the eggs.

Add the mayo, lemon juice, celery, chives, salt and pepper.

Chill in the refrigerator for at least 30 minutes before serving.

Nutrition: Calories: 224; Fat: 18 g; Saturated Fat: 3.9 g; Carbohydrates 6.1 g; Fiber: 3.6 g; Protein: 10.6 g.

427 PEPPER TOMATO SALAD

Preparation Time: 1 hour, 25 minutes
Cooking Time: 0 minutes
Servings: 8
Ingredients:

- 2 tbsp. balsamic vinegar
- 2 tbsp. olive oil
- ½ tsp. Dijon mustard
- 2 tsp. fresh basil leaves, chopped
- 1 tbsp. fresh chives, chopped
- 1 tsp. sugar
- Pepper to taste
- 2 cups yellow bell peppers, sliced into rings
- 1 cups orange bell pepper, sliced into rings
- 4 tomatoes, sliced into rounds
- ¼ cup blue cheese, crumbled

Directions:

Mix the vinegar, olive oil, mustard, basil, chives, sugar and pepper in a bowl.

Arrange the tomatoes and pepper rings on a serving plate.

Sprinkle the crumbled blue cheese on top.

Drizzle with the dressing.

Chill in the refrigerator for 1 hour before serving.

Nutrition: Calories: 116; Fat: 7 g; Saturated Fat: 2 g; Carbohydrates 11 g; Fiber: 2 g; Protein: 3 g.

428 SIMPLE LEMON DAL

Preparation Time: 5 minutes
Cooking Time: 25 minutes
Servings: 4
Ingredients:
For the lentils:
- 1 cup dried red lentils, well-rinsed
- 2 ½ cups water
- ½ tsp. turmeric
- ½ tsp. ground cumin
- 2 tbsp. lemon juice
- ⅓ cup fresh parsley, chopped
- 1 tsp. salt

For finishing:
- 1 tbsp. extra-virgin olive oil
- 2 tsp. minced garlic
- ½ tsp. dried red chili flakes or ¼ tsp. cayenne pepper

Directions:
- Add the lentils to a medium saucepan and pour in the water. Stir in the turmeric and cumin and bring to a boil.
- Reduce the heat to medium-low, cover, and simmer, stirring occasionally, for 20 minutes, until the lentils are soft and the mixture has thickened.
- Stir in the lemon juice, parsley, and salt, and remove the pan from the heat.
- In a small saucepan, heat the oil over medium-high heat. When hot, add the garlic and red chili flakes or cayenne and stir for 1 minute.
- Quickly pour the oil into the cooked lentils, cover, and let sit for 5 minutes.
- Stir the lentils and serve immediately.

Nutrition: Calories: 207; Total Fat: 4 g; Total Carbs: 30 g; Fiber: 15 g; Sugar: 1 g; Protein: 13 g; Sodium: 589 mg.

429 CAULIFLOWER LATKE

Preparation Time: 15 minutes
Cooking Time: 30 minutes
Servings: 4
Ingredients:
- 12 oz. cauliflower rice, cooked
- 1 egg, beaten
- ⅓ cup cornstarch
- Salt and pepper to taste
- ¼ cup vegetable oil, divided
- Chopped onion chives

Direction:
- Squeeze excess water from the cauliflower rice using paper towels.
- Place the cauliflower rice in a bowl.
- Stir in the egg and cornstarch.
- Season with salt and pepper.
- Fill 2 tablespoons of oil into a pan over medium heat.

Add 2 to 3 tablespoons of the cauliflower mixture into the pan.
Cook for 3 minutes on each side.
Repeat until you've used up the rest of the batter.
Garnish with chopped chives.

Nutrition: Calories: 209; Fiber: 1.9 g; Protein: 3.4 g.

430 PENNE WITH VEGGIES

Preparation Time: 5 minutes
Cooking Time: 25 minutes
Servings: 6
Ingredients:
- 2 tsp. olive oil
- 2 cloves garlic, crushed and minced
- ½ cup shallots, chopped
- 2 tbsp. dry white wine
- 1 cup Brussels sprouts, trimmed and chopped
- 6 cups bok choy, chopped
- 6 cups cooked penne pasta
- 1 tbsp. vegetable oil spread
- Salt and pepper to taste
- 2 tsp. dried Italian seasoning
- 3 tbsp. Parmesan cheese, grated

Directions:
- Pour the oil into a pan over medium heat.
- Cook the garlic and shallots for 3 minutes.
- Pour in the wine.
- Scrape the browned bits using a wooden spoon.
- Stir in the Brussels sprouts. Cook for 3 minutes.
- Stir in the bok choy and cook for 2 to 3 minutes.
- Toss the pasta in the veggies.
- Add the vegetable oil to the mix.
- Season with salt, pepper and Italian seasoning.
- Sprinkle the Parmesan cheese on top.

Nutrition: Calories: 127; Fat: 4 g; Saturated Fat: 1 g; Carbohydrates 17 g; Fiber: 3 g; Protein: 6 g.

431 MARINATED VEGGIE SALAD

Preparation Time: 4 hours, 30 minutes
Cooking Time:
Servings: 6
Ingredients:
- 1 zucchini, sliced
- 4 tomatoes, sliced into wedges
- ¼ cup red onion, sliced thinly
- 1 green bell pepper, sliced
- 2 tbsp. fresh parsley, chopped
- 2 tbsp. red-wine vinegar
- 2 tbsp. olive oil
- 1 clove garlic, minced
- 1 tsp. dried basil
- 2 tbsp. water
- Pine nuts, toasted and chopped

Directions:

In a bowl, combine the zucchini, tomatoes, red onion, green bell pepper and parsley.
Pour the vinegar and oil into a glass jar with a lid.
Add the garlic, basil and water.
Seal the jar and shake well to combine.
Pour the dressing into the vegetable mixture.
Cover the bowl.
Marinate in the refrigerator for 4 hours.
Garnish with the pine nuts before serving.

Nutrition: Calories: 65; Fat: 4.7 g; Saturated Fat: 0.7 g; Carbohydrates 5.3 g; Fiber: 1.2 g; Protein: 0.9 g.

432 ROASTED BRUSSELS SPROUTS

Preparation Time: 30 minutes
Cooking Time: 20 minutes
Servings: 4
Ingredients:
- 1 lb. Brussels sprouts, sliced in half
- 1 shallot, chopped
- 1 tbsp. olive oil
- Salt and pepper to taste
- 2 tsp. balsamic vinegar
- ¼ cup pomegranate seeds
- ¼ cup goat cheese, crumbled

Directions:
Preheat your oven to 400°F.
Coat the Brussels sprouts with oil.
Sprinkle with salt and pepper.
Transfer to a baking pan.
Roast in the oven for 20 minutes.
Drizzle with vinegar.
Sprinkle with the seeds and cheese before serving.

Nutrition: Calories: 117; Fiber: 4.8 g; Protein: 5.8 g.

433 BRUSSELS SPROUTS & CRANBERRIES

Preparation Time: 10 minutes
Cooking Time: 0 minutes
Servings: 6
Ingredients:
- 3 tbsp. lemon juice
- ¼ cup olive oil
- Salt and pepper to taste
- 1 lb. Brussels sprouts, sliced thinly
- ¼ cup dried cranberries, chopped
- ½ cup pecans, toasted and chopped
- ½ cup Parmesan cheese, shaved

Directions:
Mix the lemon juice, olive oil, salt and pepper in a bowl.
Toss the Brussels sprouts, cranberries and pecans in this mixture.
Sprinkle the Parmesan cheese on top.

Nutrition: Calories: 245; Protein: 6.4 g; Fiber: 5 g.

434 ARUGULA SALAD

Preparation Time: 15 minutes
Cooking Time: 0 minutes
Servings: 4
Ingredients:
- 6 cups fresh arugula leaves
- 2 cups radicchio, chopped
- ¼ cup low-fat balsamic vinaigrette
- ¼ cup pine nuts, toasted and chopped

Directions:
- Arrange the arugula leaves in a serving bowl.
- Sprinkle the radicchio on top.
- Drizzle with the vinaigrette.
- Sprinkle the pine nuts on top.

Nutrition: Calories: 85; Fat: 6.6 g; Saturated Fat: 0.5 g; Carbohydrates 5.1 g; Fiber: 1 g; Protein: 2.2 g.

435 MEDITERRANEAN SALAD

Preparation Time: 20 minutes
Cooking Time: 5 minutes
Servings: 2
Ingredients:
- 2 tsp. balsamic vinegar
- 1 tbsp. basil pesto
- 1 cup lettuce
- ¼ cup broccoli florets, chopped
- ½ cup zucchini, chopped
- ¼ cup tomato, chopped
- ¼ cup yellow bell pepper, chopped
- 2 tbsp. feta cheese, crumbled

Directions:
- Arrange the lettuce on a serving platter.
- Top with broccoli, zucchini, tomato and bell pepper.
- In a bowl, mix the vinegar and pesto.
- Drizzle the dressing on top.
- Sprinkle the feta cheese and serve.

Nutrition: Calories: 100; Fat: 6 g; Saturated Fat: 1 g; Carbohydrates 7 g; Protein: 4 g.

436 RAINBOW MANGO SALAD

Preparation Time: 10 minutes
Cooking Time: 0 minutes
Servings: 2
Ingredients:
- 1 mango, peeled, destoned, cubed
- ¼ of onion, chopped
- ½ cup cherry tomatoes halved
- ½ of cucumber, deseeded, sliced
- ½ of green bell pepper, deseeded, sliced

Extra:
- ⅓ tsp. salt
- ¼ tsp. cayenne pepper
- ¼ of key lime, juiced

Directions:
- Take a medium bowl and place the mango pieces in it. Add onion, tomatoes, cucumber, and bell pepper; then drizzle with lime juice.

Season with salt and cayenne pepper. Toss until combined, and let the salad rest in the refrigerator for a minimum of 20 minutes.

Nutrition: Calories: 108; Fats: 0.5 g; Protein: 1 g; Carbohydrates: 28.1 g; Fiber: 3.3 g.

437 SATISFYING SPRING SALAD

Preparation Time: 5 minutes
Cooking Time: 10 minutes
Servings: 2
Ingredients:
- 4 oz. arugula
- ½ cup cherry tomatoes halved
- ¼ cup basil leaves
- ½ key lime, juiced
- 2 tbsp. walnuts

Extra:
- ¼ tsp. salt
- ⅛ tsp. cayenne pepper
- ½ tbsp. tahini butter

Directions:
- Prepare the dressing: take a small bowl, place key lime juice in it. Add tahini butter, salt, and cayenne pepper; then whisk until combined.
- Take a medium bowl. Place arugula, tomatoes, and basil leaves in it. Pour in the dressing and then massage using your hands.
- Let the salad rest for 20 minutes. Then taste to adjust seasoning and then serve.

Nutrition: Calories: 87.3; Fats: 7 g; Protein: 1.4 g; Carbohydrates: 6 g; Fiber: 1.3 g.

438 THE RAW GREEN DETOX SALAD

Preparation Time: 5 minutes
Cooking Time: 0 minutes
Servings: 2
Ingredients:
- ½ of cucumber, deseeded
- 4 oz. arugula
- ⅛ tsp. salt
- 1 tbsp. key lime juice
- 1 tbsp. olive oil

Extra:
- ⅛ tsp. cayenne pepper

Directions:
- Cut the cucumber into slices. Add to a salad bowl, and then add arugula in it.
- Mix lime juice and oil until combined. Pour over the salad, and then season with salt and cayenne pepper.
- Toss until mixed and then serve.

Nutrition: Calories: 142; Fats: 12.5 g; Protein: 1.6 g; Carbohydrates: 7.8 g; Fiber: 1 g.

439 DANDELION SALAD

Preparation Time: 10 minutes
Cooking Time: 7 minutes
Servings: 2
Ingredients:
- ½ of onion, peeled, sliced
- 5 strawberries, sliced
- 2 cups dandelion greens, rinsed
- 1 tbsp. key lime juice
- 1 tbsp. grapeseed oil

Extra:
- ¼ tsp. salt

Directions:
- Take a medium skillet pan, place it over medium heat, add oil and let it heat until warm.
- Add onion, season with ⅛ teaspoon of salt, stir until mixed and then cook for 3 to 5 minutes until tender and golden brown.
- Meanwhile, take a small bowl. Place slices of strawberries in it. Drizzle with ½ tablespoon of lime juice and then toss until coated.
- When onions have turned golden brown, stir in remaining lime juice. Stir until mixed, and then cook for 1 minute.
- Remove pan from heat and transfer onions into a large salad bowl. Add strawberries and juices and dandelion greens, then sprinkle with the remaining salt. Toss until mixed and then serve.

Nutrition: Calories: 204; Fats: 16.1 g; Protein: 7 g; Carbohydrates: 10.6 g; Fiber: 2.8 g.

440 SPICY WAKAME SALAD

Preparation Time: 15 minutes
Cooking Time: 0 minutes
Servings: 2
Ingredients:
- 1 cup wakame stems
- ½ tbsp. chopped red bell pepper
- ½ tsp. onion powder
- ½ tbsp. key lime juice

Extra:
- ½ tbsp. agave syrup
- ½ tbsp. sesame seeds
- ½ tbsp. sesame oil

Directions:
- Place wakame stems in a bowl and cover with water. Let them soak for 10 minutes, and then drain.
- Meanwhile, prepare the dressing. Take a small bowl, add lime juice, onion, agave syrup, and sesame oil in it; then whisk until blended.
- Place drained wakame stems in a large dish. Add bell pepper, pour in the dressing, and then toss until coated.

Sprinkle sesame seeds over the salad and then serve.

Nutrition: Calories: 106; Fats: 7.3 g; Protein: 3 g; Carbohydrates: 8 g; Fiber: 1.7 g.

441 AVO-ORANGE SALAD DISH

Preparation Time: 5 minutes
Cooking Time: 0 minutes
Servings: 2
Ingredients:

1 orange, peeled, sliced
4 cups greens
½ of avocado, peeled, pitted, diced
2 tbsp. slivered red onion
½ cup cilantro

Extra:

¼ tsp. salt
¼ cup olive oil
2 tbsp. lime juice
2 tbsp. orange juice

Directions:

Prepare the dressing. Place cilantro in a food processor. Pour in orange juice, lime juice, and oil. Add salt and then pulse until blended.

Tip the dressing into a mason jar. Add remaining ingredients and toss until coated. Add to a salad bowl, or serve in the jar.

Nutrition: Calories: 228; Fats: 18.9 g; Protein: 3.3 g; Carbohydrates: 14.7 g; Fiber: 7 g.

442 NOURISHING ELECTRIC SALAD

Preparation Time: 5 minutes
Cooking Time: 0 minutes
Servings: 2
Ingredients:

½ of a medium cucumber, deseeded, chopped
6 leaves of lettuce, broke into pieces
4 mushrooms, chopped
6 cherry tomatoes, chopped
10 olives

Extra:

½ of lime, juiced
1 tsp. olive oil
¼ tsp. salt

Directions:

Take a medium salad bowl. Place all the ingredients to it and then toss until mixed.

Nutrition: Calories: 129; Fats: 7 g; Protein: 2 g; Carbohydrates: 14 g; Fiber: 4 g.

443 SUPERFOOD FONIO SALAD

Preparation Time: 10 minutes
Cooking Time: 5 minutes
Servings: 2
Ingredients:

½ cup cooked chickpeas
¼ cup chopped cucumber
½ cup chopped red pepper
½ cup cherry tomatoes halved

½ cup fonio

Extra:

⅓ tsp. salt
1 tbsp. grapeseed oil
⅛ tsp. cayenne pepper
1 key lime, juiced
1 cup spring water

Directions:

Take a medium saucepan, place it over high heat, pour in water, and bring it to boil.

Add fonio, switch heat to the low level, cook for 1 minute, and then remove the pan from heat.

Cover the pan with its lid, let fonio rest for 5 minutes, fluff by using a fork, and then let it cool for 15 minutes.

Take a salad bowl, place lime juice and oil in it and then stir in salt and cayenne pepper until combined.

Add remaining ingredients including fonio, toss until mixed, and then serve.

Nutrition: Calories: 145; Fats: 3 g; Protein: 6 g; Carbohydrates: 24.5 g; Fiber: 5.5 g.

444 HEALTHY CHICKPEA ROAST SALAD

Preparation Time: 10 minutes
Cooking Time: 20 minutes
Servings: 2
Ingredients:

½ of cucumber, deseeded, sliced
2 avocados, peeled, pitted, cubed
1 medium white onion, peeled, diced
2 cups cooked chickpeas
¼ cup chopped coriander

Extra:

1 tsp. onion powder
½ tsp. cayenne pepper
1 tsp. of sea salt
2 tbsp. hemp seeds, shelled
1 key lime, juiced
1 tbsp. olive oil

Directions:

Switch on the oven, then set it to 425°F and let it preheat.

Meanwhile, take a baking sheet, place chickpeas on it, season with salt, onion powder, and pepper, drizzle with oil and then toss until combined.

Bake the chickpeas for 20 minutes or until golden brown and crisp, then let them cool for 10 minutes.

Transfer chickpeas to a bowl, add remaining ingredients and stir until combined.

Nutrition: Calories: 208.3; Fats: 8 g; Protein: 6.4 g; Carbohydrates: 30 g; Fiber: 8 g.

445 AMARANTH TABBOULEH SALAD

Preparation Time: 5 minutes
Cooking Time: 10 minutes
Servings: 2
Ingredients:

1 small white onion, peeled, chopped
1 cup cooked amaranth
½ of cucumber, deseeded, chopped
1 cup cooked chickpeas
½ of medium red bell pepper, chopped

Extra:

⅓ tsp. sea salt
⅛ tsp. cayenne pepper
2 tbsp. key lime juice

Directions:

Take a small bowl, place lime juice in it, add salt and stir until combined.

Place remaining ingredients in a salad bowl and drizzle with lime juice mixture. Toss until mixed, and then serve.

Nutrition: Calories: 214; Fats: 4.5 g; Protein: 6.5 g; Carbohydrates: 37 g; Fiber: 9 g.

446 ZUCCHINI AND MUSHROOM BOWL

Preparation Time: 5 minutes
Cooking Time: 8 minutes
Servings: 2
Ingredients:

2 zucchinis, spiralized
½ of medium red bell pepper, sliced
½ cup sliced mushrooms
½ of medium green bell pepper, sliced
½ of medium white onion, peeled, sliced

Extra:

⅓ tsp. salt
⅛ tsp. cayenne pepper
1 tbsp. grapeseed oil

Directions:

Take a large skillet pan. Place it over medium-high heat, add oil, and when hot, add onion, mushrooms, and bell peppers; then cook for 3 to 5 minutes until tender-crisp.

Add zucchini noodles. Toss until mixed, and then cook for 2 minutes until warm.

Nutrition: Calories: 168; Fats: 2 g; Protein: 0.9 g; Carbohydrates: 36 g; Fiber: 6 g.

447 PEAR & STRAWBERRY SALAD

Preparation Time: 15 minutes
Cooking Time: 0 minutes
Servings: 4
Ingredients:

4 cups romaine lettuce, torn
2 pears, cored and sliced
1 cup fresh strawberries, hulled and sliced
¼ cup walnuts, chopped
3 tbsp. olive oil
2 tbsp. fresh key lime juice

1 tbsp. agave nectar

Directions:

In a salad bowl, place all ingredients and toss to coat well.

Serve immediately.

Nutrition: Calories: 8 g; Fats: 1.8 g; Cholesterol: 0 mg; Carbohydrates: 25.2 g; Fiber: 5.1 g; Protein: 2.8 g.

448 RASPBERRY & ARUGULA SALAD

Preparation Time: 15 minutes
Cooking Time: 0 minutes
Servings: 2
Ingredients:
Salad:

3 cups fresh baby arugula
1 cup fresh raspberries
¼ cup walnuts, chopped

Dressing:

1 tbsp. olive oil
1 tbsp. fresh key lime juice
½ tsp. agave nectar
Sea salt, as needed

Directions:

For the salad:

Place all ingredients in a salad bowl and mix.

For the dressing:

Place all ingredients in another bowl and beat until well combined.

Pour the dressing over the salad and toss to coat well.

Serve immediately.

Nutrition: Calories: 202; Fats: 1.6 g; Cholesterol: 0 mg; Carbohydrates: 11.4 g; Fiber: 5.6 g; Protein: 5.3 g.

449 MIXED BERRIES SALAD

Preparation Time: 15 minutes
Cooking Time: 15 minutes
Servings: 4
Ingredients:

1 cup fresh strawberries, hulled and sliced
½ cup fresh blackberries
½ cup fresh blueberries
½ cup fresh raspberries
6 cups fresh arugula
2 tbsp. olive oil
Sea salt, as needed

Directions:

In a salad bowl, place all ingredients and toss to coat well.

Serve immediately.

Nutrition: Calories: 105; Fats: 1 g; Cholesterol: 0 mg; Carbohydrates: 10.1 g; Fiber: 3.6 g; Protein: 1.6 g.

450 APPLE & KALE SALAD

Preparation Time: 15 minutes
Cooking Time: 15 minutes
Servings: 4
Ingredients:

3 large apples, cored and sliced

6 cups fresh baby kale
¼ cup walnuts, chopped
2 tbsp. olive oil
1 tbsp. agave nectar
Sea salt, as needed

Directions:

In a salad bowl, place all ingredients and toss to coat well.

Serve immediately.

Nutrition: Calories: 260; Fats: 1.3 g; Cholesterol: 0 mg; Carbohydrates: 38.4 g; Fiber: 6.3 g; Protein: 5.3 g.

451 MANGO & ARUGULA SALAD

Preparation Time: 15 minutes
Cooking Time: 15 minutes
Servings: 6
Ingredients:

2 ½ cups mangoes; peeled, pitted and sliced
2 ½ cups avocados; peeled, pitted and sliced
1 red onion, sliced
6 cups fresh baby arugula
¼ cup fresh mint leaves, chopped
2 tbsp. fresh orange juice
Sea salt, as needed

Directions:

Place all ingredients in a salad bowl and gently toss to combine.

Cover and refrigerate to chill before serving.

Nutrition: Calories: 182; Fats: 2.6 g; Cholesterol: 0 mg; Carbohydrates: 18.8 g; Fiber: 6.2 g; Protein: 2.6 g.

452 ORANGE & KALE SALAD

Preparation Time: 10 minutes
Cooking Time: 10 minutes
Servings: 2
Ingredients:
Salad:

3 cups fresh kale, tough ribs removed and torn
2 oranges, peeled and segmented
2 tbsp. fresh cranberries

Dressing:

2 tbsp. olive oil
2 tbsp. fresh orange juice
½ tsp. agave nectar
Sea salt, as needed

Directions:

For the salad:

Place all ingredients in a salad bowl and mix.

For the dressing:

Place all ingredients in another bowl and beat until well combined.

Pour the dressing over the salad and toss to coat well.

Serve immediately.

Nutrition: Calories: 272; Fats: 2 g; Cholesterol: 0 mg; Carbohydrates: 35.7 g; Fiber: 6.3 g; Protein: 4.8 g.

453 ZUCCHINI & TOMATO SALAD

Preparation Time: 15 minutes
Cooking Time: 15 minutes
Servings: 4
Ingredients:

2 medium zucchinis, sliced thinly
2 cups plum tomatoes, sliced
2 tbsp. olive oil
2 tbsp. fresh key lime juice
Pinch of sea salt

Directions:

In a salad bowl, place all ingredients and gently toss to combine.

Serve immediately.

Nutrition: Calories: 93; Fats: 1.1 g; Cholesterol: 0 mg; Carbohydrates: 6.9 g; Fiber: 2.2 g; Protein: 2 g.

454 TOMATO & ARUGULA SALAD

Preparation Time: 15 minutes
Cooking Time: 15 minutes
Servings: 4
Ingredients:

6 cups fresh baby arugula
2 cups cherry tomatoes
2 scallions, chopped
2 tbsp. olive oil
2 tbsp. fresh orange juice
Sea salt, as needed

Directions:

In a salad bowl, place all ingredients and toss to combine.

Cover the bowl and refrigerate for about 6–8 hours.

Remove from the refrigerator and toss well before serving.

Nutrition: Calories: 90; Fats: 1.1 g; Cholesterol: 0 mg; Carbohydrates: 6 g; Fiber: 1.8 g; Protein: 1.8 g.

455 WARM AVO AND QUINOA SALAD

Preparation Time: 5 minutes
Cooking Time: 12 minutes
Servings: 4
Ingredients:

4 ripe avocados, quartered
1 cup quinoa
0.9 lb. Chickpeas, drained
1 oz. flat-leaf parsley

Directions:

Add quinoa to a pot with 2 cups of water. Bring to boil then simmer for 12 minutes or until all the water has evaporated. The grains should be glassy and swollen.

Toss the quinoa with all other ingredients and season with salt and pepper to taste.

Serve with olive oil and lemon wedges. Enjoy!

Nutrition: Calories: 354; Fat: 16 g; Carbohydrates: 31 g; Protein: 15 g; Fiber: 15 g.

456 CHICKPEAS & QUINOA SALAD

Preparation Time: 20 minutes
Cooking Time: 20 minutes
Servings: 8
Ingredients:

  1 ¼ cups spring water
  1 cup quinoa, rinsed
  Sea salt, as needed
  2 cups cooked chickpeas
  1 medium red bell pepper, seeded and chopped
  1 medium green bell pepper, seeded and chopped
  2 large cucumbers, chopped
  ½ cup onion, chopped
  3 tbsp. olive oil
  4 tbsp. fresh basil leaves, chopped

Directions:

  In a pan, add the water over high heat and bring to a boil.
  Add the quinoa and salt and cook until boiling.
  Now, adjust the heat to low and simmer, covered for about 15–20 minutes or until all the liquid is absorbed.
  Remove from the heat and set aside, covered for about 5–10 minutes.
  Uncover and with a fork, fluff the quinoa.
  In a salad bowl, place quinoa with the remaining ingredients and gently toss to coat.
  Serve immediately.

Nutrition: Calories: 215; Fats: 1 g; Cholesterol: 0 mg; Carbohydrates: 30.5 g; Fiber: 5.6 g; Protein: 7.5 g.

457 QUINOA, TOMATO & MANGO SALAD

Preparation Time: 15 minutes
Cooking Time: 0 minutes
Servings: 4
Ingredients:

  2 cups mango; peeled, pitted and chopped
  1 cup cooked quinoa
  1 green bell pepper, seeded and chopped
  1 cup cherry tomato, halved
  ½ cup fresh parsley, chopped
  ¼ cup onion, sliced
  2 garlic cloves, minced
  2 tbsp. fresh key lime juice
  1 ½ tbsp. olive oil
  Pinch of sea salt

Directions:

  In a salad bowl, place all ingredients and gently stir to combine.

Refrigerate for about 1–2 hours before serving.

Nutrition: Calories: 270; Fats: 1.2 g; Cholesterol: 0 mg; Carbohydrates: 45.3 g; Fiber: 5.7 g; Protein: 7.8 g.

458 ZESTY CITRUS SALAD

Preparation Time: 5 minutes
Cooking Time: 0 minutes
Servings: 2
Ingredients:

  4 slices of onion
  ½ of avocado, peeled, pitted, sliced
  4 oz. arugula
  1 orange, zested, peeled, sliced
  1 tsp. agave syrup

Extra:

  ⅛ tsp. salt
  ⅛ tsp. cayenne pepper
  2 tbsp. key lime juice
  2 tbsp. olive oil

Directions:

  Distribute avocado, oranges, onion, and arugula between two plates.
  Mix together oil, salt, cayenne pepper, agave syrup and lime juice in a small bowl and then stir until mixed.
  Drizzle the dressing over the salad and then serve.

Nutrition: Calories: 265; Fats: 24 g; Protein: 3.8 g; Carbohydrates: 11.6 g; Fiber: 6.4 g.

459 ZUCCHINI HUMMUS WRAP

Preparation Time: 10 minutes
Cooking Time: 8 minutes
Servings: 2
Ingredients:

  ½ cup iceberg lettuce
  1 zucchini, sliced
  2 cherry tomatoes, sliced
  2 spelled flour tortillas
  4 tbsp. homemade hummus

Extra:

  ¼ tsp. salt
  ⅛ tsp. cayenne pepper
  1 tbsp. grapeseed oil

Directions:

  Take a grill pan, grease its oil and let it preheat over medium-high fire.
  Meanwhile, place zucchini slices in a large bowl, sprinkle with salt and cayenne pepper. Drizzle with oil and then toss until coated.
  Arrange zucchini slices on the grill pan and then cook for 2 to 3 minutes per side until developed grill marks.
  Assemble tortillas and for this, heat the tortilla on the grill pan until warm and develop grill marks and spread 2 tbsp. of hummus over each tortilla.

Distribute grilled zucchini slices over the tortillas, top with lettuce and tomato slices, and then wrap tightly.

Nutrition: Calories: 264.5; Fats: 5.1 g; Protein: 8.5 g; Carbohydrates: 34.5 g; Fiber: 5 g.

460 BASIL AND AVOCADO SALAD

Preparation Time: 10 minutes
Cooking Time: 0 minutes
Servings: 2
Ingredients:

  ½ cup avocado, peeled, pitted, chopped
  ½ cup basil leaves
  ½ cup cherry tomatoes
  2 cups cooked spelled noodles

Extra:

  1 tsp. agave syrup
  1 tbsp. key lime juice
  2 tbsp. olive oil

Directions:

  Take a large bowl, place pasta in it, add tomato, avocado, and basil in it and then stir until mixed.
  Take a small bowl, add agave syrup and salt in it. Pour in lime juice and olive oil, and then whisk until combined.
  Pour lime juice mixture over pasta, toss until combined, and then serve.

Nutrition: Calories: 387; Fats: 16.6 g; Protein: 9.4 g; Carbohydrates: 54.3 g; Fiber: 8.6 g.

461 GRILLED ROMAINE LETTUCE SALAD

Preparation Time: 10 minutes
Cooking Time: 10 minutes
Servings: 2
Ingredients:

  2 small heads of romaine lettuce, cut in half
  1 tbsp. chopped basil
  1 tbsp. chopped red onion
  ¼ tsp. onion powder
  ½ tbsp. agave syrup

Extra:

  ½ tsp. salt
  ¼ tsp. cayenne pepper
  2 tbsp. olive oil
  1 tbsp. key lime juice

Directions:

  Take a large skillet pan, place it over medium heat and when warmed, arrange lettuce heads in it. Cut-side down, and then cook for 4 to 5 minutes per side until golden brown on both sides.
  When done, transfer lettuce heads to a plate and then let them cool for 5 minutes.

Meanwhile, prepare the dressing. Place remaining ingredients in a small bowl and then stir until combined.

Drizzle the dressing over lettuce heads and then serve.

Nutrition: Calories: 130; Fats: 2 g; Protein: 2 g; Carbohydrates: 24 g; Fiber: 4 g.

462 KALE AND SPROUTS SALAD

Preparation Time: 5 minutes
Cooking Time: 0 minutes
Servings: 2
Ingredients:

2 cups kale leaves
1 cup sprouts
1 cup cherry tomato
½ of avocado, peeled, pitted, diced
1 key lime, juiced

Extra:

1 tsp. agave syrup
½ tbsp. olive oil
⅛ tsp. cayenne pepper

Directions:

Take a small bowl and place lime juice in it. Add oil and agave syrup and then stir until mixed.

Take a salad bowl and place remaining ingredients in it. Drizzle with the lime juice mixture and then toss until mixed.

Nutrition: Calories: 179.2; Fats: 14.1 g; Protein: 3.7 g; Carbohydrates: 13.5 g; Fiber: 6.1 g.

463 DANDELION AND STRAWBERRY SALAD

Preparation Time: 10 minutes
Cooking Time: 7 minutes
Servings: 2
Ingredients:

½ of onion, peeled, sliced
5 strawberries, sliced
2 cups dandelion greens, rinsed
1 tbsp. key lime juice
1 tbsp. grapeseed oil

Extra:

¼ tsp. salt

Directions:

Take a medium skillet pan and place it over medium heat. Add oil and let it heat until warm.

Add onion, season with ⅛ teaspoon of salt, stir until mixed and then cook for 3 to 5 minutes until tender and golden brown.

Meanwhile, take a small bowl and place slices of strawberries in it. Drizzle with ½ tablespoon of lime juice and then toss until coated.

When onions have turned golden brown, stir in remaining lime juice. Stir until mixed, and then cook for 1 minute.

Remove pan from heat. Transfer onions into a large salad bowl and add strawberries along with their juices and dandelion greens. Sprinkle with remaining salt.

Toss until mixed and then serve.

Storage instructions:

Divide the salad evenly between two meal prep containers. Cover with a lid, and then store the containers in the refrigerator for up to 5 days.

Nutrition: Calories: 204; Fats: 16.1 g; Protein: 7 g; Carbohydrates: 10.6 g; Fiber: 2.8 g.

464 BASIL SALAD

Preparation Time: 10 minutes
Cooking Time: 0 minutes
Servings: 2
Ingredients:

½ cup avocado, peeled, pitted, chopped
½ cup basil leaves
½ cup cherry tomatoes
2 cups cooked spelled noodles

Extra:

1 tsp. agave syrup
1 tbsp. key lime juice
2 tbsp. olive oil

Directions:

Take a large bowl, place pasta in it, add tomato, avocado, and basil and then stir until mixed.

Take a small bowl, add agave syrup and salt in it. Pour in lime juice and olive oil, and then whisk until combined.

Pour lime juice mixture over pasta. Toss until combined, and then serve.

Storage instructions:

Divide the salad evenly between two meal prep containers. Cover with a lid, and then store the containers in the refrigerator for up to 5 days.

Nutrition: Calories: 387; Fats: 16.6 g; Protein: 9.4 g; Carbohydrates: 54.3 g; Fiber: 8.6 g.

465 CITRUS SALAD

Preparation Time: 5 minutes
Cooking Time: 0 minutes
Servings: 2
Ingredients:

4 slices of onion
½ of avocado, peeled, pitted, sliced
4 oz. arugula
1 orange, zested, peeled, sliced
1 tsp. agave syrup

Extra:

⅛ tsp. salt
⅛ tsp. cayenne pepper

2 tbsp. key lime juice
2 tbsp. olive oil

Directions:

Distribute avocado, oranges, onion, and arugula between two plates.

Mix together oil, salt, cayenne pepper, agave syrup and lime juice in a small bowl. Stir until mixed.

Drizzle the dressing over the salad and then serve.

Storage instructions:

Divide the salad evenly between two meal containers, cover with a lid, and then store the containers in the refrigerator for up to 5 days.

Nutrition: Calories: 265; Fats: 24 g; Protein: 3.8 g; Carbohydrates: 611.6 g; Fiber: 4 g.

466 MANGO SALAD

Preparation Time: 10 minutes
Cooking Time: 0 minutes
Servings: 2
Ingredients:

1 mango, peeled, destoned, cubed
¼ of onion, chopped
½ cup cherry tomatoes, halved
½ of cucumber, deseeded, sliced
½ of green bell pepper, deseeded, sliced

Extra:

⅓ tsp. salt
¼ tsp. cayenne pepper
¼ of key lime, juiced

Directions:

Take a medium bowl. Place the mango pieces in it. Add onion, tomatoes, cucumber, and bell pepper. Drizzle with lime juice.

Season with salt and cayenne pepper. Toss until combined, and let the salad rest in the refrigerator for a minimum of 20 minutes.

Storage instructions:

Divide salad between two meal prep containers. Cover with a lid and then store the containers in the refrigerator for up to 3 days.

Nutrition: Calories: 108; Fats: 0.5 g; Protein: 1 g; Carbohydrates: 28.1 g; Fiber: 3.3 g.

467 CUCUMBER AND ARUGULA SALAD

Preparation Time: 5 minutes
Cooking Time: 0 minutes
Servings: 2
Ingredients:

½ of cucumber, deseeded
4 oz. arugula
⅛ tsp. salt
1 tbsp. key lime juice
1 tbsp. olive oil

Extra:

⅛ tsp. cayenne pepper

Directions:

Cut the cucumber into slices. Add to a salad bowl and then add arugula in it.

Mix together lime juice and oil until combined. Pour over the salad, and then season with salt and cayenne pepper.

Toss until mixed and then serve.

Storage instructions:

Divide the salad evenly between two containers, cover with a lid, and then store the containers in the refrigerator for up to 5 days.

Nutrition: Calories: 142; Fats: 12.5 g; Protein: 1.6 g; Carbohydrates: 7.8 g; Fiber: 1 g.

468 GREEK SALAD WRAPS

Preparation Time: 15 minutes

Cooking Time: 10 minutes

Servings: 2

Ingredients:

- 1 ½ cups seedless cucumber, peeled and chopped (about 1 large cucumber)
- 1 cup chopped tomato (about 1 large tomato)
- ½ cup finely chopped fresh mint
- 1 (2.25-oz.) can sliced black olives (about ½ cup), drained
- ¼ cup diced red onion (about ¼ onion)
- 2 tbsp. extra-virgin olive oil
- 1 tbsp. red wine vinegar
- ¼ tsp. freshly ground black pepper
- ¼ tsp. kosher or sea salt
- ½ cup crumbled goat cheese (about 2 oz.)
- 4 whole-wheat flatbread wraps or soft whole-wheat tortillas

Directions:

In a large bowl, mix together the cucumber, tomato, mint, olives, and onion until well combined.

In a small bowl, whisk together the oil, vinegar, pepper, and salt. Drizzle the dressing over the salad, and mix gently.

With a knife, spread the goat cheese evenly over the four wraps. Spoon a quarter of the salad filling down the middle of each wrap.

Fold up each wrap: Start by folding up the bottom, then fold one side over and fold the other side over the top. Repeat with the remaining wraps and serve.

Nutrition: Calories: 262; Total Fat: 15 g; Saturated Fat: 5 g; Cholesterol: 15 mg; Sodium: 529 mg; Total Carbohydrates: 23 g; Fiber: 4 g; Protein: 7 g.

469 GOLDEN SPRING ROLLS

Preparation Time: 10 minutes

Cooking Time: 18 minutes

Servings: 4

Ingredients:

- 4 spring roll wrappers
- ½ cup cooked vermicelli noodles
- 1 tsp. sesame oil
- 1 tbsp. freshly minced ginger
- 1 tbsp. soy sauce
- 1 clove garlic, minced
- ½ red bell pepper, deseeded and chopped
- ½ cup chopped carrot
- ½ cup chopped mushrooms
- ¼ cup chopped scallions
- Cooking spray

Directions:

Spritz the air fry basket with cooking spray and set aside.

Heat the sesame oil in a saucepan on medium fire. Sauté the garlic and ginger in the sesame oil for 1 minute, or until fragrant. Add soy sauce, carrot, red bell pepper, mushrooms and scallions. Sauté for 5 minutes or until the vegetables become tender. Mix in vermicelli noodles. Turn off the heat and remove them from the saucepan. Allow to cool for 10 minutes.

Lay out one spring roll wrapper with a corner pointed toward you. Scoop the noodle mixture on the spring roll wrapper and fold the corner up over the mixture. Fold left and right corners toward the center and continue to roll to make firmly sealed rolls.

Arrange the spring rolls in the basket and spritz with cooking spray.

Place the basket on the air fry position.

Select Air Fry, set temperature to 340°F (171°C) and set Time to 12 minutes. Flip the spring rolls halfway through the cooking time.

When done, the spring rolls will be golden brown and crispy.

Serve warm.

Nutrition: Calories: 137; Fat: 15 g; Protein 10 g.

470 GOLDEN CABBAGE AND MUSHROOM SPRING ROLLS

Preparation Time: 20 minutes

Cooking Time: 14 minutes

Servings: 14

Ingredients:

- 2 tbsp. vegetable oil
- 4 cups sliced Napa cabbage
- 5 oz. (142 g;) shiitake mushrooms, diced
- 3 carrots, cut into thin matchsticks
- 1 tbsp. minced fresh ginger
- 1 tbsp. minced garlic
- 1 bunch scallions, white and light green parts only, sliced
- 2 tbsp. soy sauce
- 1 (4-oz. / 113-g;) package cellophane noodles
- ¼ tsp. cornstarch
- 1 (12-oz. / 340-g;) package frozen spring roll wrappers, thawed
- Cooking spray

Directions:

Heat the olive oil in a nonstick skillet over medium-high fire until shimmering.

Add the cabbage, carrots, and mushrooms and sauté for 3 minutes or until tender.

Add the garlic, scallions, and ginger and sauté for 1 minute or until fragrant.

Mix in the soy sauce and turn off the heat. Discard any liquid that remains in the skillet and allow to cool for a few minutes.

Bring a pot of water to a boil, then turn off the heat and pour in the noodles. Let sit for 10 minutes or until the noodles are al dente. Transfer 1 cup of the noodles to the skillet and toss with the cooked vegetables. Reserve the remaining noodles for other use.

Dissolve the cornstarch in a small water dish; then place the wrappers on a clean work surface. Dab the edges of the wrappers with cornstarch.

Scoop up 3 tablespoons of filling in the center of each wrapper; then fold the corner in front of you over the filling. Tuck the wrapper under the filling; then fold the corners on both sides into the center. Keep rolling to seal the wrapper. Repeat with remaining wrappers. Spritz the air fry basket with cooking spray. Arrange the wrappers in the basket and spritz with cooking spray.

Place the basket on the air fry position.

Select Air Fry, set temperature to 400°F (205°C) and set Time to 10 minutes. Flip the wrappers halfway through the cooking time.

When cooking is complete, the wrappers will be golden brown.

Serve immediately.

Nutrition: Calories: 161; proteins: 8 g; Fat: 88 g; Carbs: 32 g.

471 VEGGIE SALSA WRAPS

Preparation Time: 5 minutes
Cooking Time: 7 minutes
Servings: 4
Ingredients:

    1 cup red onion, sliced
    1 zucchini, chopped
    1 poblano pepper, deseeded and finely chopped
    1 head lettuce
    ½ cup salsa
    8 oz. (227 g.) Mozzarella cheese

Directions:

    Place the red onion, zucchini, and poblano pepper in the air fryer basket. Select the Air Fry function and cook at 390°F (199°C) for 7 minutes, or until they are tender and fragrant.

    Divide the veggie mixture among the lettuce leaves and spoon the salsa over the top. Finish off with Mozzarella cheese. Wrap the lettuce leaves around the filling.

    Serve immediately.

Nutrition: Calories 140; Fat: 4 g; Fiber: 3 g; Carbohydrates: 5 g; Protein:7 g.

472 NUGGET AND VEGGIE TACO WRAPS

Preparation Time: 5 minutes
Cooking Time: 15 minutes
Servings: 4
Ingredients:

    1 tbsp. water
    4 pieces commercial vegan nuggets, chopped
    1 small yellow onion, diced
    1 small red bell pepper, chopped
    2 cobs grilled corn kernels
    4 large corn tortillas
    Mixed greens, for garnish

Directions:

    Over a medium heat, sauté the nuggets in the water with the onion, corn kernels and bell pepper in a skillet, then remove from the heat.

    Fill the tortillas with the nuggets and vegetables and fold them up. Transfer to the air fryer basket. Select the Air Fry function and cook at 400°F (204°C) for 15 minutes.

    Once crispy, serve immediately, garnished with the mixed greens.

Nutrition: Calories 140 Fat: 4g Fiber: 3g Carbohydrates: 5g; Protein: 7 g.

473 AVOCADO AND TOMATO WRAPS

Preparation Time: 10 minutes
Cooking Time: 5 minutes

Servings: 5
Ingredients:

    10 egg roll wrappers
    3 avocados, peeled and pitted
    1 tomato, diced
    Salt and ground black pepper, to taste
    Cooking spray

Directions:

    Spritz a pan with cooking spray.

    Put the tomato and avocados in a food processor. Sprinkle with salt and ground black pepper. Pulse to mix and coarsely mash until smooth.

    Unfold the wrappers on a clean work surface, then divide the mixture in the center of each wrapper. Roll the wrapper up and press to seal.

    Transfer the rolls to the pan and spritz with cooking spray.

    Select Air Fry. Set temperature to 350°Fahrenheit (180°Celsius) and set Time to 5 minutes. Press Start to begin preheating.

    Once the oven has preheated, place the pan into the oven. Flip the rolls halfway through the cooking time.

    When cooked, the rolls should be golden brown.

    Serve immediately.

Nutrition: Calories: 419; Total Fat: 14 g; Total Carbohydrates: 39 g; Protein: 33 g.

474 SWEET POTATO AND SPINACH BURRITOS

Preparation Time: 15 minutes
Cooking Time: 30 minutes
Servings: 6 burritos
Ingredients:

    2 sweet potatoes, peeled and cut into a small dice
    1 tbsp. vegetable oil
    Kosher salt and ground black pepper, to taste
    6 large flour tortillas
    1 (16-oz.) can refried black beans, divided
    1 ½ cups baby spinach, divided
    6 eggs, scrambled
    ¾ cup grated Cheddar cheese, divided
    ¼ cup salsa
    ¼ cup sour cream
    Cooking spray

Directions:

    Put the sweet potatoes in a large bowl, then drizzle with vegetable oil and sprinkle with salt and black pepper. Toss to coat well.

    Place the potatoes in the perforated pan.

    Select Air Fry. Set temperature to 400°Fahrenheit (205°Celsius) and

set Time to 10 minutes. Press Start to begin preheating.

    Once preheated, place the pan into the oven. Flip the potatoes halfway through the cooking time.

    When done, the potatoes should be lightly browned. Remove the potatoes from the oven.

    Unfold the tortillas on a clean work surface. Divide the black beans, spinach, air-fried sweet potatoes, scrambled eggs, and cheese on top of the tortillas.

    Fold the long side of the tortillas over the filling, then fold in the shorter side to wrap the filling to make the burritos.

    Wrap the burritos in aluminum foil and put in the pan.

    Select Air Fry. Set temperature to 350°Fahrenheit (180°Celsius) and set Time to 20 minutes. Place the pan into the oven. Flip the burritos halfway through the cooking time.

    Remove the burritos from the oven and spread with sour cream and salsa. Serve immediately.

Nutrition: Calories: 385; Total Fat: 9 g; Total Carbohydrates: 32 g; Protein: 13 g.

475 CHERRY TOMATO GRATIN

Preparation Time: 15 minutes
Cooking Time: 20 minutes
Servings: 4
Ingredients:

    2 tbsp. olive oil
    ½ cup cherry tomatoes halved
    ½ cup mayonnaise, Keto-friendly
    ½ cup vegan Mozzarella cheese, cut into pieces
    1 oz. (28 g;) vegan Parmesan cheese, shredded
    1 tbsp. basil pesto
    Pepper and salt
    1 cup watercress

Directions:

    Let the oven heat up to 400°F. Grease a baking pan with olive oil.

    Combine the cherry tomatoes, mayo, vegan Mozzarella cheese, ½ oz. (14 g;) of Parmesan cheese, basil pesto, salt, and black pepper baking pan.

    Scatter with the remaining Parmesan.

    Baking time: 20 minutes

    Remove them from the oven and divide among four plates. Top with watercress and olive oil, and slice to serve.

Nutrition: Calories: 254; Fat: 12.1 g; Fiber: 9.3 g; Carbohydrates: 11.1 g; Protein: 9.5 g.

476 FENNEL-PARMESAN FARRO

Preparation Time: 15 minutes

Cooking Time: 50 minutes
Servings: 4-6
Ingredients:

¼ cup minced fresh parsley
1 onion, chopped fine
1 oz. Parmesan cheese, grated (½ cup)
1 small fennel bulb, stalks discarded, bulb halved, cored, and chopped fine
1 tsp. minced fresh thyme or ¼ tsp. dried
1 ½ cups whole farro
2 tsp. sherry vinegar
3 garlic cloves, minced
3 tbsp. extra-virgin olive oil
Salt and pepper

Directions:

Bring 4 quarts of water to boil in a Dutch oven. Put in farro and 1 tablespoon of salt. Return to boil and cook until grains are soft with a slight chew, 15 to 30 minutes.

Drain farro. Return to now-empty pot and cover to keep warm. Heat 2 tbsp. oil in a 12-inch frying pan on moderate heat until it starts to shimmer.

Put in onion, fennel, and ¼ teaspoon of salt and cook, stirring intermittently, till they become tender, 8 to 10 minutes. Add in garlic and thyme and cook until aromatic, approximately half a minute.

Put in remaining 1 tablespoon of oil and farro and cook, stirring often, until heated through, approximately 2 minutes.

Remove from the heat. Mix in Parmesan, parsley, and vinegar. Sprinkle with salt and pepper to taste. Serve.

Nutrition: Calories: 338; Carbs: 56 g; Fat: 10 g; Protein: 11 g.

477 CREAMY ZOODLES

Preparation Time: 15 minutes
Cooking Time: 10 minutes
Servings: 4
Ingredients:

1 ¼ cups heavy whipping cream
¼ cup mayonnaise
Salt and ground black pepper, as required
30 oz. zucchini, spiralized
3 oz. Parmesan cheese, grated
2 tbsp. fresh mint leaves
2 tbsp. butter, melted

Directions:

The heavy cream must be added to a pan then bring to a boil.

Lower the heat to low and cook until reduced in half.

Put in the pepper, mayo, and salt; cook until mixture is warm enough.

Add the zucchini noodles and gently stir to combine.

Stir in the Parmesan cheese.

Divide the zucchini noodles onto four serving plates and immediately drizzle with the melted butter.

Serve immediately.

Nutrition: Calories: 241; Fat: 11.4 g; Fiber: 7.5 g; Carbohydrates: 3.1 g; Protein: 5.1 g.

478 BLACK BEAN VEGGIE BURGER

Preparation Time: 15 minutes
Cooking Time: 20 minutes
Servings: 2
Ingredients:

½ onion (chopped small)
1 (14-oz.) can of black beans (well-drained)
slices of bread (crumbled)
½ tsp. of seasoned salt
1 tsp. of garlic powder
1 tsp. of onion powder
½ cup of almond flour
Dash salt (to taste)
Dash pepper (to taste)
Oil for frying (divide)

Directions:

Combine onions and sauté and pour it into the small frying pan. Fry them until they are soft. This process usually takes between 3 and 5 minutes.

Get a large bowl. Mash the black beans inside it. Ensure that the beans are almost smooth.

Sauté your onions and crumble the bread.

In the bowl, add the sautéed onions, mashed black beans, crumbled bread, seasoned salt, garlic powder, and onion powder. Ensure you mix to combine well.

Add some flour to the ingredients by adding 1teaspoon of per time. Stir everything together until it is well combined.

While mixing, make sure that it is very thick.

To achieve this, you should use your hand to work your flour well.

Make the mixed black beans into patties.

Ensure that each of the patties is approximately ½ inch thick.

The best way to do this is to make a ball with black beans.

After doing this, flatten the ball gently. Place your frying pan on medium-low heat. Add some oil.

Fry your black bean patties in the frying pan until it is slightly firm and lightly browned on each side.

This usually takes about 3 minutes.

Ensure you adjust the head well because if the pan is too hot, the bean burgers will be brown in the middle and will not be well cooked in the middle.

To serve, assemble your veggie burgers and enjoy it with all the fixings.

Serve them with a little ketchup or hot sauce.

To increase the nutrition of the meal, you can add a nice green salad.

Nutrition: Calories: 376; Fat: 15.1 g; Fiber: 12.9 g; Carbohydrates: 9.4 g; Protein: 11.6 g.

479 RED CURRY

Preparation Time: 20 minutes
Cooking Time: 15-20 minutes
Servings: 6
Ingredients:

1 cup broccoli florets
1 large handful of fresh spinach
4 tbsp. coconut oil
¼ medium onion
1 tsp. garlic, minced
1 tsp. fresh ginger, peeled and minced
2 tsp. soy sauce
1 tbsp. red curry paste
½ cup coconut cream

Directions:

Add half the coconut oil to a saucepan and heat over medium-high heat.

When the oil is hot, put the onion in the pan and sauté for 3-4 minutes, until it is semi-translucent.

Sauté garlic, stirring, just until fragrant, about 30 seconds.

Lower the heat to medium-low and add broccoli florets. Sauté, stirring, for about 1-2 minutes.

Now, add the red curry paste. Sauté until the paste is fragrant, then mix everything.

Add the spinach on top of the vegetable mixture. When the spinach begins to wilt, add the coconut cream and stir.

Add the rest of the coconut oil, the soy sauce, and the minced ginger. Bring to a simmer for 5-10 minutes.

Serve hot.

Nutrition: Calories: 265; Fat: 7.1 g; Fiber: 6.9 g; Carbohydrates: 2.1 g; Protein: 4.4 g.

480 SWEET-AND-SOUR TEMPEH

Preparation Time: 10 minutes
Cooking Time: 25 minutes
Servings: 4
Ingredients:
Tempeh:

1 package tempeh

¾ cup vegetable broth
2 tbsp. soy sauce
2 tbsp. olive oil

Sauce:

1 can pineapple juice
2 tbsp. brown sugar
¼ cup white vinegar
1 tbsp. cornstarch
1 red bell pepper
1 chopped white onion

Directions:

Place a skillet on high heat. Pour in the vegetable broth and tempeh in it.

Add the soy sauce to the tempeh. Let it cook until it softens. This usually takes 10 minutes.

When it is well cooked, remove the tempeh and keep the liquid. We will use it for the sauce.

Put the tempeh in another skillet placed on medium heat.

Sauté it with olive oil and cook until the tempeh is browned. This should take 3 minutes.

Place a pot of the reserved liquid from the cooked tempeh on medium heat.

Add the pineapple juice, vinegar, brown sugar, and cornstarch. Stir everything together until it's well combined.

Let it simmer for 5 minutes.

Add the onion and pepper to the sauce.

Stir in until the sauce is thick.

Reduce the heat, add the cooked tempeh and pineapple chunks to the sauce. Leave it to simmer together.

Remove from heat and serve with any grain food of your choice.

Nutrition: Calories: 312; Fat: 10 g; Fiber: 4.1 g; Carbohydrates: 2.1 g; Protein: 5.2 g.

481 MEXICAN CASSEROLE WITH BLACK BEANS

Preparation Time: 20 minutes
Cooking Time: 20 minutes
Servings: 6
Ingredients:

2 cups of minced garlic cloves
2 cups of Monterey Jack and cheddar
¾ cup of salsa
2 ½ cups chopped red pepper
2 tsp. ground cumin
2 cans black beans
12 corn tortillas
2 chopped tomatoes
½ cup of sliced black olives
2 cups of chopped onion

Directions:

Let the oven heat to 350°F.

Place a large pot over medium heat.

Pour the onion, garlic, pepper, cumin, salsa, and black beans in the pot

— Cook the ingredients for 3 minutes, stirring frequently.

Arrange the tortillas in the baking dish.

Ensure they are well spaced and even overlapping the dish if necessary.

Spread half of the bean's mixture on the tortillas. Sprinkle with the cheddar.

Repeat the process across the tortillas until everything is well stuffed.

Cover the baking dish with foil paper and place in the oven.

Bake it for 15 minutes. Remove from the oven to cool down a bit.

Garnish the casserole with olives and tomatoes.

Nutrition: Calories: 325; Fat: 9.4 g; Fiber: 11.2 g; Carbohydrates: 3.1 g; Protein: 12.6 g.

482 BAKED ZUCCHINI GRATIN

Preparation Time: 25 minutes
Cooking Time: 30 minutes
Servings: 2
Ingredients:

1 large zucchini, cut into ¼-inch-thick slices
Pink Himalayan salt
1-oz. Brie cheese, rind trimmed off
1 tbsp. butter
Freshly ground black pepper
⅓ cup shredded Gruyere cheese
¼ cup crushed pork rinds

Directions:

Preheat the oven to 400°F.

When the zucchini has been "weeping" for about 30 minutes, in a small saucepan over medium-low flame, heat the Brie and butter, occasionally stirring, until the cheese has melted.

The mixture is thoroughly combined in about 2 minutes.

Arrange the zucchini in an 8-inch baking dish, so the zucchini slices are overlapping a bit.

Season with pepper.

Pour the Brie mixture over the zucchini, and top with the shredded Gruyere cheese.

Sprinkle the crushed pork rinds over the top.

Bake for about 25 minutes, until the dish is bubbling and the top is nicely browned, and serve.

Nutrition: Calories: 324; Fat: 11.5 g; Fiber: 5.1 g; Carbohydrates: 2.2 g; Protein: 5.1 g.

483 VEGGIE GREEK MOUSSAKA

Preparation Time: 20 minutes
Cooking Time: 30 minutes
Servings: 6
Ingredients:

2 large eggplants, cut into strips
1 cup diced celery

1 cup diced carrots
1 small white onion, chopped
3 eggs
2 tsp. olive oil
2 cups grated Parmesan
1 cup ricotta cheese
2 cloves garlic, minced
1 tsp. Italian seasoning blend
Salt to taste

Sauce:

½ cups heavy cream
¼ cup butter, melted
1 cup grated mozzarella cheese
2 tsp. Italian seasoning
¾ cup almond flour

Directions:

Preheat the oven to 350°F.

Lay the eggplant strips, sprinkle with salt, and let it sit there to exude liquid. Heat olive oil heat and sauté the onion, celery, garlic, and carrots for 5 minutes.

Mix the eggs, 1 cup of Parmesan cheese, ricotta cheese, and salt in a bowl; set aside.

Pour the heavy cream into a pot and bring to heat over a medium fire while continually stirring.

Stir in the remaining Parmesan cheese and one teaspoon of Italian seasoning. Turn the heat off and set aside.

To lay the moussaka, spread a small amount of the sauce at the bottom of the baking dish.

Pat dry the eggplant strips and makes a single layer on the sauce.

A layer of ricotta cheese must be spread on the eggplants. Sprinkle some veggies on it, and repeat everything

In a small bowl, evenly mix the melted butter, almond flour, and one teaspoon of dries Italian seasoning.

Spread the top of the moussaka layers with it and sprinkle the top with mozzarella cheese.

Bake for 25 minutes until the cheese is slightly burned. Slice the moussaka and serve warm.

Nutrition: Calories: 398; Fat: 15.1 g; Fiber: 11.3 g; Carbohydrates: 3.1 g; Protein: 5.9 g.

484 GOUDA CAULIFLOWER CASSEROLE

Preparation Time: 15 minutes
Cooking Time: 15 minutes
Servings: 4
Ingredients:

2 heads cauliflower, cut into florets
⅓ cup butter, cubed
2 tbsp. melted butter
1 white onion, chopped

Salt and black pepper to taste
¼ almond milk
½ cup almond flour
1 ½ cups grated gouda cheese

Directions:

Preheat oven to 350°F and put the cauliflower florets in a large microwave-safe bowl.

Sprinkle with a bit of water, and steam in the microwave for 4 to 5 minutes.

Melt the ⅓ cup of butter in a saucepan over medium heat and sauté the onion for 3 minutes.

Add the cauliflower, season with salt and black pepper, and mix in almond milk. Simmer for 3 minutes.

Mix the remaining melted butter with almond flour.

Stir into the cauliflower as well as half of the cheese. Sprinkle the top with the remaining cheese and bake for 10 minutes until the cheese has melted and golden brown.

Plate the bake and serve with salad.

Nutrition: Calories: 349; Fat: 9.4 g; Fiber: 12.1 g; Carbohydrates: 4.1 g; Protein: 10 g.

485 SPINACH AND ZUCCHINI LASAGNA

Preparation Time: 15 minutes
Cooking Time: 30 minutes
Servings: 4
Ingredients:

2 zucchinis, sliced
Salt and black pepper to taste
2 cups ricotta cheese
2 cups shredded mozzarella cheese
3 cups tomato sauce
1 cup baby spinach

Directions:

Let the oven heat to 375°F and grease a baking dish with cooking spray.

Put the zucchini slices in a colander and sprinkle with salt.

Let sit and drain liquid for 5 minutes and pat dry with paper towels.

Mix the ricotta, mozzarella cheese, salt, and black pepper to evenly combine and spread ¼ cup of the mixture in the bottom of the baking dish.

Layer ⅓ of the zucchini slices. Spread 1 cup of tomato sauce over, and scatter a ⅓ cup of spinach on top. Repeat process.

Grease one end of foil with cooking spray and cover the baking dish with the foil.

Let it bake for about 35 minutes. Bake further for 5 to 10 minutes or

until the cheese has a nice golden-brown color.

Remove the dish. Let it cool for 5 minutes; make slices of the lasagna, and serve warm.

Nutrition: Calories: 376; Fat: 14.1 g; Fiber: 11.3 g; Carbohydrates: 2.1 g; Protein: 9.5 g.

486 LEMON CAULIFLOWER "COUSCOUS" WITH HALLOUMI

Preparation Time: 5 minutes
Cooking Time: 5 minutes
Servings: 2
Ingredients:

4 oz. halloumi, sliced
cauliflower head, cut into small florets
¼ cup chopped cilantro
¼ cup chopped parsley
¼ cup chopped mint
½ lemon juiced
Salt and black pepper to taste
Sliced avocado to garnish

Directions:

Heat the pan and add oil

Add the halloumi and fry on both sides until golden brown, set aside. Turn the heat off.

Next, pour the cauliflower florets in a food processor and pulse until it crumbles and resembles couscous.

Transfer to a bowl and steam in the microwave for 2 minutes. They should be slightly cooked but crunchy.

Stir in the cilantro, parsley, mint, lemon juice, salt, and black pepper.

Garnish the couscous with avocado slices and serve with grilled halloumi and vegetable sauce.

Nutrition: Calories: 312; Fat: 9.4 g; Fiber: 11.9 g; Carbohydrates: 1.2 g; Protein: 8.5 g.

487 SPICY CAULIFLOWER STEAKS WITH STEAMED GREEN BEANS

Preparation Time: 15 minutes
Cooking Time: 20 minutes
Servings: 4
Ingredients:

2 heads cauliflower, sliced lengthwise into 'steaks.'
¼ cup olive oil
¼ cup chili sauce
2 tsp. erythritol
Salt and black pepper to taste
2 shallots, diced
1 bunch green beans, trimmed
2 tbsp. fresh lemon juice
1 cup of water
Dried parsley to garnish

Directions:

In a bowl or container, mix the olive oil, chili sauce, and erythritol.

Brush the cauliflower with the mixture. Grill for 6 minutes. Flip the cauliflower and cook further for 6 minutes.

Let the water boil. Place the green beans in a sieve, and set over the steam from the boiling water.

Cover with a clean napkin to keep the steam trapped in the sieve.

Cook for 6 minutes.

Next, remove to a bowl and toss with lemon juice.

Remove the grilled caulis to a plate; sprinkle with salt, pepper, shallots, and parsley. Serve with the steamed green beans.

Nutrition: Calories: 329; Fat: 10.4 g; Fiber: 3.1 g; Carbohydrates: 4.2 g; Protein: 8.4 g.

488 CHEESY CAULIFLOWER FALAFEL

Preparation Time: 20 minutes
Cooking Time: 15 minutes
Servings: 4
Ingredients:

1 head cauliflower, cut into florets
⅓ cup silvered ground almonds
3 tbsp. cheddar cheese, shredded
½ tsp. mixed spice
Salt and chili pepper to taste
2tbsp. coconut flour
2 fresh eggs
2 tbsp. ghee

Directions:

Blend the florets in a blender until a grain meal consistency is formed.

Pour the rice in a bowl. Add the ground almonds, mixed spice, salt, cheddar cheese, chili pepper, coconut flour, and mix until evenly combined.

Beat the eggs in a bowl until creamy in color and mix with the cauliflower mixture.

Shape ¼ cup each into patties.

Melt ghee and fry the patties for 5 minutes on each side to be firm and browned.

Remove onto a wire rack to cool; share into serving plates, and top with tahini sauce.

Nutrition: Calories: 287; Fat: 9.2 g; Fiber: 4.1 g; Carbohydrates: 3.2 g; Protein: 13.2 g.

489 TOFU SESAME SKEWERS WITH WARM KALE SALAD

Preparation Time: 2 hours
Cooking Time: 25 minutes
Servings: 4
Ingredients:

14 oz. firm tofu
4 tsp. sesame oil
2 lemon, juiced
1 tbsp. sugar-free soy sauce
1 tsp. garlic powder

1 tbsp. coconut flour
½ cup sesame seeds

Warm Kale Salad:

2 cups chopped kale
2 tsp. + 2 tsp. olive oil
1 white onion, thinly sliced
2 cloves garlic, minced
1 cup sliced white mushrooms
1 tsp. chopped rosemary
Salt and black pepper to season
1 tbsp. balsamic vinegar

Directions:

In a bowl, mix sesame oil, lemon juice, soy sauce, garlic powder, and coconut flour.

Wrap the tofu in a paper towel, squeeze out as much liquid from it, and cut it into strips.

Stick on the skewers, height-wise.

Place onto a plate, pour the soy sauce mixture over, and turn in the sauce to be adequately coated.

Heat the griddle pan over high heat.

Pour the sesame seeds into a plate and roll the tofu skewers in the seeds for a generous coat.

Grill the tofu in the griddle pan to be golden brown on both sides, about 12 minutes.

Heat 2 tablespoons of olive oil in a skillet over medium heat and sauté onion to begin browning for 10 minutes with continuous stirring.

Add the remaining olive oil and mushrooms.

Continue cooking for 10 minutes. Add garlic, rosemary, salt, pepper, and balsamic vinegar.

Cook for 1 minute.

Put the kale in a salad bowl; when the onion mixture is ready, pour it on the kale and toss well.

Serve the tofu skewers with the warm kale salad and a peanut butter dipping sauce.

Nutrition: Calories: 276; Fat: 11.9 g; Fiber: 9.4 g; Carbohydrates: 21 g; Protein: 10.3 g.

490 BRUSSEL SPROUTS WITH SPICED HALLOUMI

Preparation Time: 20 minutes
Cooking Time: 30 minutes
Servings: 2
Ingredients:

10 oz. halloumi cheese, sliced
1 tbsp. coconut oil
½ cup unsweetened coconut, shredded
1 tsp. chili powder
½ tsp. onion powder
½-pound Brussels sprouts, shredded
4 oz. butter
Salt and black pepper to taste
Lemon wedges for serving

Directions:

In a bowl, mix the shredded coconut, chili powder, salt, coconut oil, and onion powder.

Then, toss the halloumi slices in the spice mixture.

The grill pan must be heated then cook the coated halloumi cheese for 2-3 minutes.

Transfer to a plate to keep warm.

The half butter must be melted in a pan, add, and sauté the Brussels sprouts until slightly caramelized.

Then, season with salt and black pepper.

Dish the Brussels sprouts into serving plates with the halloumi cheese and lemon wedges.

Melt left butter and drizzle over the Brussels sprouts and halloumi cheese. Serve.

Nutrition: Calories: 276; Fat: 9.5 g; Fiber: 9.1 g; Carbohydrates: 4.1 g; Protein: 5.4 g.

491 VEGETABLE PATTIES

Preparation Time: 15 minutes
Cooking Time: 20 minutes
Servings: 4
Ingredients:

1 tbsp. olive oil
1 onion, chopped
1 garlic clove, minced
½ head cauliflower, grated
1 carrot, shredded
1 tbsp. coconut flour
½ cup Gruyere cheese, shredded
½ cup Parmesan cheese, grated
3 eggs, beaten
½ tsp. dried rosemary
Salt and black pepper, to taste

Directions:

Cook onion and garlic in warm olive oil over medium heat, until soft, for about 3 minutes.

Stir in grated cauliflower and carrot and cook for a minute; allow cooling and set aside.

To the cooled vegetables, add the rest of the ingredients. Form balls from the mixture, then press each ball to form a burger patty.

Set oven to 400°F and bake the burgers for 20 minutes.

Flip and bake for another 10 minutes or until the top becomes golden brown.

Nutrition: Calories: 315; Fat: 12.1; Fiber: 8.6 g; Carbohydrates: 3.3 g; Protein: 5.8 g.

492 VEGAN SANDWICH WITH TOFU & LETTUCE SLAW

Preparation Time: 15 minutes
Cooking Time: 15 minutes
Servings: 2

Ingredients:

¼-pound firm tofu, sliced
2 low carb buns
1 tbsp. olive oil

Marinade:

2 tbsp. olive oil
Salt and black pepper to taste
1 tsp. allspice
½ tbsp. xylitol
1 tsp. thyme, chopped
1 habanero pepper, seeded and minced
2 green onions, thinly sliced
1 garlic clove

Lettuce slaw:

½ small iceberg lettuce, shredded
½ carrot, grated
½ red onion, grated
2 tsp. liquid stevia
1 tbsp. lemon juice
2 tbsp. olive oil
½ tsp. Dijon mustard
Salt and black pepper to taste

Directions:

Put the tofu slices in a bowl.

Blend the marinade ingredients for a minute.

Cover the tofu with this mixture and place in the fridge to marinate for 1 hour.

In a container, combine the lemon juice, stevia, olive oil, Dijon mustard, salt, and pepper.

Stir in the lettuce, carrot, and onion; set aside.

Heat oil, cook the tofu on both sides for 6 minutes in total.

Remove to a plate.

To the buns, add the tofu and top with the slaw. Close the buns and serve.

Nutrition: Calories: 315; Fat: 10.4 g; Fiber: 15.1 g; Carbohydrates: 9.4 g; Protein: 8.4 g.

493 PUMPKIN AND CAULIFLOWER CURRY

Preparation Time: 15 minutes
Cooking Time: 7 to 8 hours
Servings: 6
Ingredients:

1 tbsp. extra-virgin olive oil
4 cups coconut milk
1 cup diced pumpkin
1 cup cauliflower florets
1 red bell pepper, diced
1 zucchini, diced
1 sweet onion, chopped
1 tsp. grated fresh ginger
1 tsp. minced garlic
1 tbsp. curry powder
2 cups shredded spinach
1 avocado, diced, for garnish

Directions:

Lightly grease the slow cooker with olive oil.

Add the coconut milk, pumpkin, cauliflower, bell pepper, zucchini, onion, ginger, garlic, and curry powder.

Cover and cook on low for 7 to 8 hours.

Stir in the spinach.

Garnish each bowl with a spoonful of avocado and serve.

Nutrition: Calories: 501; Fat: 44.0 g; Protein: 7.0 g; Carbs: 19.0 g; Net carbs: 9.0 g; Fiber: 10.0 g.

494 CAULIFLOWER EGG BAKE

Preparation Time: 10 minutes
Cooking Time: 25 minutes
Servings: 6
Ingredients:

1 ½ pounds (680 g;) cauliflower, broken into small florets
½ cup Greek yogurt
4 eggs, beaten
6 oz. (170 g;) ham, diced
1 cup Swiss cheese, preferably freshly grated

Directions:

Place the cauliflower into a deep saucepan; cover with water and bring to a boil over high heat; immediately reduce the heat to medium-low.

Let it simmer, covered, for approximately 6 minutes. Drain and mash with a potato masher.

Add in the yogurt, eggs and ham; stir until everything is well combined and incorporated.

Scrape the mixture into a lightly greased casserole dish. Top with the grated Swiss cheese and transfer to a preheated at 390°F (199°C) oven.

Bake for 15 to 20 minutes or until cheese bubbles and browns. Bon appétit!

Nutrition: Calories: 237; Fat: 13.6 g; Protein: 20.2 g; Carbs: 7.1 g; Net carbs: 4.8 g; Fiber: 2.3 g.

495 ZUCCHINI CASSEROLE

Preparation Time: 15 minutes
Cooking Time: 45 minutes
Servings: 4
Ingredients:

Nonstick cooking spray
2 cups zucchini, thinly sliced
2 tbsp. leeks, sliced
½ tsp. salt
Freshly ground black pepper, to taste
½ tsp. dried basil
½ tsp. dried oregano
½ cup Cheddar cheese, grated
¼ cup heavy cream
4 tbsp. Parmesan cheese, freshly grated

1 tbsp. butter, room temperature
1 tsp. fresh garlic, minced

Directions:

Start by preheating your oven to 370°F (188°C). Lightly grease a casserole dish with a nonstick cooking spray.

Place 1 cup of the zucchini slices in the dish; add 1 tablespoon of leeks; sprinkle with salt, pepper, basil, and oregano. Top with ¼ cup of Cheddar cheese. Repeat the layers one more time.

In a mixing dish, thoroughly whisk the heavy cream with Parmesan, butter, and garlic. Spread this mixture over the zucchini layer and cheese layers.

Place in the preheated oven and bake for about 40 to 45 minutes until the edges are nicely browned. Sprinkle with chopped chives, if desired. Bon appétit!

Nutrition: Calories: 156; Fat: 12.8 g; Protein: 7.5 g; Carbs: 3.6 g; Net carbs: 2.8 g; Fiber: 0.8 g.

496 CHINESE CAULIFLOWER RICE WITH EGGS

Preparation Time: 7 minutes
Cooking Time: 8 minutes
Servings: 3
Ingredients:

½ pound (227 g;) fresh cauliflower
1 tbsp. sesame oil
½ cup leeks, chopped
1 garlic, pressed
Sea salt and freshly ground black pepper, to taste
½ tsp. Chinese five-spice powder
1 tsp. oyster sauce
½ tsp. light soy sauce
1 tbsp. Shaoxing wine
3 eggs

Directions:

Pulse the cauliflower in a food processor until it resembles rice.

Heat the sesame oil in a pan over medium-high heat; sauté the leeks and garlic for 2 to 3 minutes. Add the prepared cauliflower rice to the pan, along with salt, black pepper, and Chinese five-spice powder.

Next, add oyster sauce, soy sauce, and wine. Let it cook, stirring occasionally, until the cauliflower is crisp-tender, about 5 minutes.

Then, add the eggs to the pan; stir until everything is well combined. Serve warm and enjoy!

Nutrition: Calories: 132; Fats: 8.8 g; Protein: 7.2 g; Carbs: 6.2 g; Net Carbs: 4.4 g; Fiber: 1.8 g.

497 MUSHROOM STROGANOFF

Preparation Time: 5 minutes
Cooking Time: 10 minutes
Servings: 3
Ingredients:

2 tbsp. olive oil
½ shallot, diced
3 cloves garlic, chopped
12 oz. (340 g;) brown mushrooms, thinly sliced
2 cups tomato sauce

Directions:

Heat the olive oil in a stockpot over medium-high heat. Then, sauté the shallot for about 3 minutes until tender and fragrant.

Now, stir in the garlic and mushrooms and cook them for 1 minute more until aromatic.

Fold in the tomato sauce and bring to a boil; turn the heat to medium-low, cover, and continue to simmer for 5 to 6 minutes.

Salt to taste and serve over cauliflower rice if desired. Enjoy!

Nutrition: Calories: 137; Fats: 9.3 g; Protein: 3.4 g; Carbs: 7.1 g; Net Carbs: 5.3 g; Fiber: 1.8 g.

498 ZUCCHINI FRITTERS

Preparation Time: 10 minutes
Cooking Time: 5 minutes
Servings: 6
Ingredients:

1 pound (454 g.) zucchini, grated and drained
1 egg
1 tsp. fresh Italian parsley
½ cup almond meal
½ cup goat cheese, crumbled
Sea salt and ground black pepper, to taste
½ tsp. red pepper flakes, crushed
2 tbsp. olive oil

Directions:

Mix all ingredients, except for the olive oil, in a large bowl. Let it sit in your refrigerator for 30 minutes.

Heat the oil in a non-stick frying pan over medium heat; scoop the heaped tablespoon of the zucchini mixture into the hot oil.

Cook for 3 to 4 minutes; then, gently flip the fritters over and cook on the other side. Cook in a couple of batches.

Transfer to a paper towel to soak up any excess grease. Serve and enjoy!

Nutrition: Calories: 110; Fats: 8.8 g; Protein: 5.8 g; Carbs: 3.2 g; Net Carbs: 2.2 g; Fiber: 1.0 g.

499 CHEESE STUFFED SPAGHETTI SQUASH

Preparation Time: 15 minutes
Cooking Time: 50 to 60 minutes
Servings: 4
Ingredients:

½-pound (227 g.) spaghetti squash, halved, scoop out seeds
1 tsp. olive oil
½ cup Mozzarella cheese, shredded
½ cup cream cheese
½ cup full-fat Greek yogurt
2 eggs
1 garlic clove, minced
½ tsp. cumin
½ tsp. basil ½ tsp. mint
Sea salt and ground black pepper, to taste

Directions:

Place the squash halves in a baking pan; drizzle the insides of each squash half with olive oil.

Bake in the preheated oven at 370°F (188°C) for 45 to 50 minutes or until the interiors are easily pierced through with a fork.

Now, scrape out the spaghetti squash "noodles" from the skin in a mixing bowl. Add the remaining ingredients and mix to combine well.

Carefully fill each of the squash halves with the cheese mixture. Bake at 350°F (180°C) for 5 to 10 minutes, until the cheese is bubbling and golden brown. Bon appétit!

Nutrition: Calories: 220; Fats: 17.6 g; Protein: 9.0 g; Carbs: 6.8 g; Net Carbs: 5.9 g; Fiber: 0.9 g.

500 COTTAGE KALE STIR-FRY

Preparation Time: 10 minutes
Cooking Time: 10 minutes
Servings: 3
Ingredients:

½ tbsp. olive oil
1 tsp. fresh garlic, chopped
9 oz. (255 g.) kale, torn into pieces
½ cup Cottage cheese, creamed
½ tsp. sea salt

Directions:

Heat the olive oil in a saucepan over a moderate flame. Now, cook the garlic until just tender and aromatic.

Then, stir in the kale and continue cooking for about 10 minutes until all liquid evaporates.

Fold in the Cottage cheese and salt; stir until everything is heated through. Enjoy!

Nutrition: Calories: 94; Fats: 4.5 g; Protein: 7.0 g; Carbs: 6.2 g; Net Carbs: 3.5 g; Fiber: 2.7 g.

501 HERBED EGGPLANT AND KALE BAKE

Preparation Time: 20 minutes
Cooking Time: 40 minutes
Servings: 6
Ingredients:

1 (¾-pound / 340 g.) eggplant, cut into ½-inch slices
1 tbsp. olive oil
1 tbsp. butter, melted
8 oz. (227 g.) kale leaves, torn into pieces
14 oz. (397 g.) garlic-and-tomato pasta sauce, without sugar
⅓ cup cream cheese
1 cup Asiago cheese, shredded
½ cup Gorgonzola cheese, grated
2 tbsp. ketchup, without sugar
1 tsp. hot pepper
1 tsp. basil
1 tsp. oregano
½ tsp. rosemary

Directions:

Place the eggplant slices in a colander and sprinkle them with salt. Allow it to sit for 2 hours. Wipe the eggplant slices with paper towels.

Brush the eggplant slices with olive oil; cook in a cast-iron grill pan until nicely browned on both sides, about 5 minutes.

Melt the butter in a pan over medium flame. Now, cook the kale leaves until wilted. In a mixing bowl, combine the three types of cheese.

Transfer the grilled eggplant slices to a lightly greased baking dish. Top with the kale. Then, add a layer of ½ of the cheese blend.

Pour the tomato sauce over the cheese layer. Top with the remaining cheese mixture. Sprinkle with seasoning.

Bake in the preheated oven at 350°F (180°C) until cheese is bubbling and golden brown, about 35 minutes. Bon appétit!

Nutrition: Calories: 231; Fats: 18.6 g; Protein: 10.5 g; Carbs: 6.7 g; Net Carbs: 4.3 g; Fiber: 2.4 g.

502 BROCCOLI AND CAULIFLOWER MASH

Preparation Time: 2 minutes
Cooking Time: 13 minutes
Servings: 3
Ingredients:

½-pound (227 g.) broccoli florets
½-pound (227 g.) cauliflower florets
Kosher salt and ground black pepper, to season
½ tsp. garlic powder
1 tsp. shallot powder
4 tbsp. whipped cream cheese
1½ tbsp. butter

Directions:

Microwave the broccoli and cauliflower for about 13 minutes until they have softened completely. Transfer to a food processor and add in the remaining ingredients.

Process the ingredients until everything is well combined.

Taste and adjust the seasoning. Bon appétit!

Nutrition: Calories: 163; Fats: 12.8 g; Protein: 4.7 g; Carbs: 7.2 g; Net Carbs: 3.7 g; Fiber: 3.5 g.

503 CHEESY STUFFED PEPPERS

Preparation Time: 15 minutes
Cooking Time: 40 minutes
Servings: 4
Ingredients:

2 tbsp. olive oil
4 red bell peppers, halved and seeded
1 cup ricotta cheese
½ cup gorgonzola cheese, crumbled
2 cloves garlic, minced
1 ½ cups tomatoes, chopped
1 tsp. dried basil
Salt and black pepper, to taste
½ tsp. oregano

Directions:

Let the oven heat up to 350°F.

In a bowl, mix garlic, tomatoes, gorgonzola, and ricotta cheeses.

Stuff the pepper halves and remove them to the baking dish. Season with oregano, salt, cayenne pepper, black pepper, and basil.

Bake during 40 minutes.

Nutrition: Calories: 295; Fat: 12.4 g; Fiber: 10.1 g; Carbohydrates: 5.4 g; Protein: 13.2 g.

504 CREAMY SPINACH

Preparation Time: 5 minutes
Cooking Time: 5 minutes
Servings: 4
Ingredients:

1 tbsp. butter, room temperature
1 clove garlic, minced
10 oz. (283 g.) spinach
½ tsp. garlic salt
¼ tsp. ground black pepper, or more to taste
½ tsp. cayenne pepper
3 oz. (85 g.) cream cheese
½ cup double cream

Directions:

Melt the butter in a saucepan preheated over medium flame. Once hot. Cook garlic for 30 seconds.

Now, add the spinach; cover the pan for 2 minutes to let the spinach wilt. Season with salt, black pepper, and cayenne pepper.

Stir in cheese and cream; stir until the cheese melts. Serve immediately.

Nutrition: Calories: 167; Fats: 15.1 g; Protein: 4.4 g; Carbs: 5.0 g; Net Carbs: 3.3 g; Fiber: 1.7 g.

505 FRIED CABBAGE

Preparation Time: 10 minutes
Cooking Time: 15 minutes
Servings: 3
Ingredients:

4 oz. (113 g.) bacon, diced
1 medium-sized onion, chopped
2 cloves garlic, minced
½ tsp. caraway seeds
1 bay laurel
½ tsp. cayenne pepper
1 pound (454 g.) red cabbage, shredded
¼ tsp. ground black pepper, to season
1 cup beef bone broth

Directions:

Heat up a nonstick skillet over a moderate flame. Cook the bacon for 3 to 4 minutes, stirring continuously; set aside.

In the same skillet, sauté the onion for 2 to 3 minutes or until it has softened. Now, sauté the garlic and caraway seeds for 30 seconds more or until aromatic.

Then, add in the remaining ingredients and stir to combine. Reduce the temperature to medium-low, cover, and cook for 10 minutes longer; stirring periodically to ensure even cooking.

Serve in individual bowls, garnished with the reserved bacon. Enjoy!

Nutrition: Calories: 242; Fats: 22.2 g; Protein: 6.5 g; Carbs: 6.8 g; Net Carbs: 4.9 g; Fiber: 1.9 g.

506 CUMIN GREEN CABBAGE STIR-FRY

Preparation Time: 10 minutes
Cooking Time: 20 minutes
Servings: 2
Ingredients:

2 tbsp. olive oil
1 (1-inch) piece fresh ginger, grated
½ tsp. cumin seeds
1 shallot, chopped
½ cup chicken stock
¾ pound (340 g.) green cabbage, sliced
¼ tsp. turmeric powder
½ tsp. coriander powder

Kosher salt and cayenne pepper, to taste

Directions:

Heat the olive oil in a saucepan over medium fire; then, sauté the ginger and cumin seeds until fragrant.

Add in the shallot and continue sautéing an additional 2 to 3 minutes or until just tender and aromatic. Pour in the chicken stock to deglaze the pan.

Add the cabbage wedges, turmeric, coriander, salt, and cayenne pepper. Cover and cook for 15 to 18 minutes or until your cabbage has softened. Make sure to stir occasionally.

Serve in individual bowls and enjoy!

Nutrition: Calories: 169; Fats: 13.0 g; Protein: 2.6 g; Carbs: 7.0 g; Net Carbs: 2.9 g; Fiber: 4.1 g.

507 GREEK VEGGIE BRIAM

Preparation Time: 10 minutes
Cooking Time: 30 minutes
Servings: 4
Ingredients:

⅓ cup good-quality olive oil, divided
1 onion, thinly sliced
1 tbsp. minced garlic
¾ small eggplant, diced
2 zucchinis, diced
2 cups chopped cauliflower
1 red bell pepper, diced
2 cups diced tomatoes
2 tbsp. chopped fresh parsley
2 tbsp. chopped fresh oregano
Sea salt, for seasoning
Freshly ground black pepper, for seasoning
1 ½ cups crumbled feta cheese
¼ cup pumpkin seeds

Directions:

Preheat the oven. Set the oven to broil and lightly grease a 9-by-13-inch casserole dish with olive oil.

Sauté the aromatics in a medium stockpot over medium heat, warm 3 tablespoons of the olive oil. Add the onion and garlic and sauté until they've softened for about 3 minutes.

Sauté the vegetables. Stir in the eggplant, cook, stirring occasionally.

Add the zucchini, cauliflower, and red bell pepper and cook for 5 minutes.

Stir in the tomatoes, parsley, and oregano and cook, stirring it from time to time, until the vegetables are tender, about 10 minutes. Season it with salt and pepper.

Broil. Put vegetable mix in the casserole dish and top with the crumbled feta. Broil until the cheese is melted.

Serve. Divide the casserole between four plates and top it with the pumpkin seeds. Drizzle with the remaining olive oil.

Nutrition: Calories: 341; Fat: 5.1 g; Fiber: 11 g; Carbohydrates: 1.2 g.

508 BRAISED CREAM KALE

Preparation Time: 4 minutes
Cooking Time: 11 minutes
Servings: 5
Ingredients:

2 tbsp. olive oil
1 shallot, chopped
6 cups kale, torn into pieces
½ tsp. fresh garlic, minced
2 tbsp. dry white wine
¼ tsp. red pepper flakes, crushed
Sea salt and ground black pepper, to taste
½ cup double cream

Directions:

Heat the olive oil in a large, heavy-bottomed sauté pan over moderate heat. Now, sauté the shallot until it is tender or about 4 minutes.

Stir in the kale and continue cooking for 2 minutes more. Remove any excess liquid and stir in the garlic; continue cooking for one minute or so.

Add a splash of wine to deglaze the pan. Then, add the red pepper, salt, black pepper, and double cream to the pan.

Turn the heat to simmer. Continue to simmer, covered, for a further 4 minutes. Serve warm and enjoy!

Nutrition: Calories: 130; Fats: 10.5 g; Protein: 3.7 g; Carbs: 6.1 g; Net Carbs: 3.1 g; Fiber: 3.0 g.

509 WHITE WINE-DIJON BRUSSELS SPROUTS

Preparation Time: 10 minutes
Cooking Time: 10 minutes
Servings: 3
Ingredients:

6 oz. (170 g.) smoked bacon, diced
12 Brussels sprouts, trimmed and halved
¼ tsp. ground bay leaf
¼ tsp. dried oregano
¼ tsp. dried sage
¼ tsp. freshly cracked black pepper, or more to taste
Sea salt, to taste
½ cup dry white wine
1 tsp. Dijon mustard

Directions:

Heat up a nonstick skillet over medium-high heat. Once hot, cook the bacon for 1 minute.

Add the Brussels sprouts and seasoning and continue sautéing, adding white wine and stirring until the bacon is crisp and the Brussels sprouts are tender. It will take about 9 minutes.

Then, stir in the mustard, remove from the heat, and serve immediately. Enjoy!

Nutrition: Calories: 298; Fats: 22.4 g; Protein: 9.6 g; Carbs: 6.4 g; Net Carbs: 3.4 g; Fiber: 3.0 g.

510 PAPRIKA RICED CAULIFLOWER

Preparation Time: 4 minutes
Cooking Time: 6 minutes
Servings: 4
Ingredients:

1 tbsp. butter
1 pound (454 g.) cauliflower florets
2 cloves garlic, minced
1 tbsp. smoked paprika
Flaky salt, to taste

Directions:

Melt the butter in a frying pan over a moderate flame.

Pulse the cauliflower in your food processor until your cauliflower has broken down into rice-sized chunks for approximately 6 seconds.

Add the cauliflower rice to the frying pan and cook, covered, for 5 minutes. Stir in the garlic and smoked paprika. Continue to sauté an additional minute or so.

Season with salt to taste and serve immediately. Bon appétit!

Nutrition: Calories: 57; Fats: 3.2 g; Protein: 2.3 g; Carbs: 6.1 g; Net Carbs: 3.8 g; Fiber: 2.3 g.

511 WAX BEANS WITH TOMATO-MUSTARD SAUCE

Preparation Time: 9 minutes
Cooking Time: 6 minutes
Servings: 4
Ingredients:

1 tbsp. butter
2 garlic cloves, thinly sliced
½-pound (227 g.) wax beans, trimmed
½ cup tomato sauce
2 tbsp. dry white wine
½ tsp. mustard seeds
Sea salt and ground black pepper, to taste

Directions:

Melt the butter in a saucepan over a medium-high flame. Now, sauté

the garlic until aromatic but not browned.

Stir in the wax beans, tomato sauce, wine, and mustard seeds. Season with salt and black pepper to taste.

Turn the heat to medium-low, partially cover and continue cooking for 6 minutes longer or until everything is heated through. Bon appétit!

Nutrition: Calories: 56; Fats: 3.5 g; Protein: 1.5 g; Carbs: 6.0 g; Net Carbs: 3.8 g; Fiber: 2.2 g.

512 LEEK, MUSHROOM, AND ZUCCHINI STEW

Preparation Time: 5 minutes
Cooking Time: 15 minutes
Servings: 4
Ingredients:

½ cup leeks, chopped
1 pound (454 g.) brown mushrooms, chopped
1 tsp. garlic, minced
1 medium-sized zucchini, diced
2 ripe tomatoes, puréed

Directions:

Heat up a lightly greased soup pot over medium-high heat. Now, sauté the leeks until just tender about 3 minutes.

Stir in the mushrooms, garlic, and zucchini. Continue sautéing for an additional 2 minutes or until tender and aromatic.

Add in the tomatoes and 2 cups of water. Season with Sazón spice, if desired. Reduce the temperature to simmer and continue cooking, covered, for 10 to 12minutes more. Bon appétit!

Nutrition: Calories: 108; Fat: 7.5 g; Protein: 3.1 g; Carbs: 7.0 g; Net Carbs: 4.5 g; Fiber: 2.5 g.

513 ALMOND AND RIND CRUSTED ZUCCHINI FRITTERS

Preparation Time: 13 minutes
Cooking Time: 2 minutes
Servings: 2
Ingredients:

2 tbsp. olive oil
3 eggs, whisked
1 tsp. garlic, pressed
½-pound (227 g.) zucchini, grated
⅓ cup almond meal
2 tbsp. pork rinds
¼ tsp. paprika
Sea salt and ground black pepper, to taste
½ cup Swiss cheese, shredded

Directions:

Add the grated zucchini to a colander. Add ½ teaspoon of salt, toss and let it sit for 10 minutes. After that, drain the zucchini completely using a cheese cloth.

Heat the olive oil in a skillet over medium-high flame. In a mixing bowl, combine the zucchini with the remaining ingredients until everything is well incorporated.

Make the fritters, flattening them with a spatula; cook for 2 minutes on both sides. Bon appétit!

Nutrition: Calories: 462; Fat: 36.0 g; Protein: 27.5 g; Carbs: 7.6 g; Net Carbs: 4.8 g; Fiber: 2.8 g.

514 SPICED CAULIFLOWER CHEESE BAKE

Preparation Time: 20 minutes
Cooking Time: 20 minutes
Servings: 4
Ingredients:

½ tsp. butter, melted
1 (½-pound / 227 g.) head cauliflower, broken into florets
½ cup Swiss cheese, shredded
½ cup Mexican blend cheese, room temperature
½ cup Greek yogurt
1 cup cooked ham, chopped
1 roasted chili pepper, chopped
½ tsp. porcini powder
1 tsp. garlic powder
1 tsp. shallot powder
½ tsp. cayenne pepper
¼ tsp. dried sage
½ tsp. dried oregano
Sea salt and ground black pepper, to taste

Directions:

Start by preheating your oven to 340°F (171°C). Then, coat the bottom and sides of a casserole dish with ½ teaspoon of melted butter.

Empty the cauliflower into a pot and cover it with water. Let it cook for 6 minutes until it is nice and tender (mashable). Mash the prepared cauliflower with a potato ricer press or potato masher.

Now, stir in the cheese; stir until the cheese has melted. Add Greek yogurt, chopped ham, roasted pepper, and spices.

Place the mixture in the prepared casserole dish; bake in the preheated oven for 20 minutes. Let it sit for about 10 minutes before cutting. Serve and enjoy!

Nutrition: Calories: 189; Fat: 11.3 g; Protein: 14.9 g; Carbs: 5.7 g; Net Carbs: 4.6 g; Fiber: 1.1 g.

515 ROASTED ASPARAGUS

Preparation Time: 10 minutes
Cooking Time: 15 minutes
Servings: 5
Ingredients:

4 tbsp. butter, melted
4 tbsp. Pecorino Romano cheese, grated
1 ½ pounds (680 g.) asparagus, trimmed
½ tsp. cayenne pepper
Sea salt and cracked black pepper, to taste
1 tbsp. Sriracha sauce
1 tbsp. fresh cilantro, roughly chopped

Directions:

Toss your asparagus with the melted butter, cheese, cayenne pepper, salt, black pepper, and Sriracha sauce; toss until well coated.
Place the asparagus on a roasting pan. Roast in the preheated oven at 420°F (216°C) for 10 minutes.
Rotate the pan and continue cooking for an additional 4 to 5 minutes. Serve immediately garnished with fresh cilantro. Bon appétit!

Nutrition: Calories: 141; Fat: 11.5 g; Protein: 5.6 g; Carbs: 5.5 g; Net Carbs: 2.6 g; Fiber: 2.9 g.

516 MOZZARELLA ITALIAN PEPPERS

Preparation Time: 7 minutes
Cooking Time: 13 minutes
Servings: 5
Ingredients:

4 tbsp. canola oil
1 yellow onion, sliced
1 ⅓ pounds (605 g.) Italian peppers, deveined and sliced
1 tsp. Italian seasoning mix
Sea salt and cayenne pepper, to season
2 balls buffalo Mozzarella, drained and halved

Directions:

Heat the canola oil in a saucepan over a medium-low flame. Now, sauté the onion until just tender and translucent.
Add in the peppers and spices. Cook for about 13 minutes, adding a splash of water to deglaze the pan.
Divide between serving plates; top with cheese and serve immediately. Enjoy!

Nutrition: Calories: 175; Fat: 11.0 g; Protein: 10.4 g; Carbs: 7.0 g; Net Carbs: 5.1 g; Fiber: 1.9 g.

517 QUESO FRESCO AVOCADO SALSA

Preparation Time: 5 minutes
Cooking Time: 0 minutes
Servings: 4
Ingredients:

2 tomatoes, diced
3 scallions, chopped
1 poblano pepper, chopped
1 garlic clove, minced
2 ripe avocados, peeled, pitted and diced
1 tbsp. extra-virgin olive oil
2 tbsp. fresh lime juice
Sea salt and ground black pepper, to season
¼ cup queso fresco, crumbled

Directions:

Place the tomatoes, scallions, poblano pepper, garlic and avocado in a serving bowl. Drizzle olive oil and lime juice over everything.
Season with salt and black pepper.
To serve, top with crumbled queso fresco and enjoy!

Nutrition: Calories: 189; Fat: 16.0 g; Protein: 3.6 g; Carbs: 6.9 g; Net Carbs: 2.7 g; Fiber: 4.2 g.

518 INDIAN WHITE CABBAGE STEW

Preparation Time: 8 minutes
Cooking Time: 22 minutes
Servings: 3
Ingredients:

6 oz. (170 g.) Goan chorizo sausage, sliced
2 cloves garlic, finely chopped
1 tsp. Indian spice blend
1 pound (454 g.) white cabbage, outer leaves removed and finely shredded
¾ cup cream of celery soup

Directions:

Heat a large-sized wok over a moderate flame. Now, sear the Goan chorizo sausage until no longer pink; reserve.
Cook the garlic and Indian spice blend in the pan drippings until they are aromatic. Now, stir in the cabbage and cream of celery soup.
Turn the temperature to medium-low. Cover, and continue simmering for an additional 22 minutes or until tender and heated through.
Add the reserved Goan chorizo sausage; ladle into individual bowls and serve. Enjoy!

Nutrition: Calories: 236; Fat: 17.7 g; Protein: 9.8 g; Carbs: 6.1 g; Net Carbs: 3.7 g; Fiber: 2.4 g.

519 BAKED EGGPLANT ROUNDS

Preparation Time: 10 minutes
Cooking Time: 35 minutes
Servings: 6
Ingredients:

1 pound (454 g.) eggplant, peeled and sliced
2 tsp. Italian seasoning blend
½ tsp. cayenne pepper
½ tsp. salt
1½ cups marinara sauce
1 cup Mozzarella cheese
2 tbsp. fresh basil leaves, snipped

Directions:

Begin by preheating your oven to 380°F (193°C). Line a baking pan with parchment paper.
Now, arrange the eggplant rounds on the baking pan. Season with the Italian blend, cayenne pepper, and salt.
Bake for 25 to 28 minutes, flipping the rounds halfway through baking time.
Next, remove from the oven and top with the marinara sauce and Mozzarella cheese.
Bake for 6 to 8 minutes more until Mozzarella is bubbling. Garnish with fresh basil leaves just before serving.

Nutrition: Calories: 92; Fat: 4.8 g; Protein: 5.2 g; Carbs: 5.2 g; Net Carbs: 2.3 g; Fiber: 2.9 g.

520 FENNEL AVGOLEMONO

Preparation Time: 10 minutes
Cooking Time: 20 minutes
Servings: 6
Ingredients:

2 tbsp. olive oil
1 celery stalk, chopped
1 pound (454 g.) fennel bulbs, sliced
1 garlic clove, minced
1 bay laurel
1 thyme sprig
cups chicken stock
Sea salt and ground black pepper, to season
2 eggs
1 tbsp. freshly squeezed lemon juice

Directions:

Heat the olive oil in a heavy-bottomed pot over a medium-high flame. Now, sauté the celery and fennel until they have softened but not browned, about 8 minutes.
Add in the garlic, bay laurel, and thyme sprig; continue sautéing until aromatic an additional minute or so.
Add the chicken stock, salt, and black pepper to the pot. Bring to a boil. Reduce the heat to medium-low and let it simmer, partially covered, for approximately 13 minutes.

Discard the bay laurel and then, blend your soup with an immersion blender.

Whisk the eggs and lemon juice; gradually pour 2cups of the hot soup into the egg mixture, whisking constantly.

Return the soup to the pot and continue stirring for a few minutes or just until thickened. Serve warm.

Nutrition: Calories: 85; Fat: 6.2 g; Protein: 2.8 g; Carbs: 6.0 g; Net Carbs: 3.5 g; Fiber: 2.5 g.

521 SPINACH AND BUTTERNUT SQUASH STEW

Preparation Time: 10 minutes
Cooking Time: 30 minutes
Servings: 4
Ingredients:

2 tbsp. olive oil
1 Spanish onion, peeled and diced
1 garlic clove, minced
½-pound (227 g.) butternut squash, diced
1 celery stalk, chopped
3 cups vegetable broth
Kosher salt and freshly cracked black pepper, to taste
4 cups baby spinach
4 tbsp. sour cream

Directions:

Heat the olive oil in a soup pot over a moderate flame. Now, sauté the Spanish onion until tender and translucent.

Then, cook the garlic until just tender and aromatic.

Stir in the butternut squash, celery, broth, salt, and black pepper. Turn the heat to simmer and let it cook, covered, for 30 minutes.

Fold in the baby spinach leaves and cover with the lid; let it sit in the residual heat until the baby spinach wilts completely.

Serve dolloped with cold sour cream. Enjoy!

Nutrition: Calories: 150; Fat: 11.6 g; Protein: 2.5 g; Carbs: 6.8 g; Net Carbs: 4.5 g; Fiber: 2.3 g.

522 BROCCOLI CHEESE

Preparation Time: 10 minutes
Cooking Time: 15 minutes
Servings: 5
Ingredients:

3 tbsp. olive oil
1 tsp. garlic, minced
1 ½ pounds (680 g.) broccoli florets
½ tsp. flaky salt
½ tsp. ground black pepper
½ tsp. paprika
½ cup cream of mushrooms soup
6 oz. (170 g.) Swiss cheese, shredded

Directions:

Heat 1 tablespoon of the olive oil in a nonstick frying pan over a moderate flame. Then, sauté the garlic until just tender and fragrant.

Preheat your oven to 390°F (199°C). Now, brush the sides and bottom of a casserole dish with 1 tablespoon of olive oil.

Parboil the broccoli in salted water until it is crisp-tender; discard any excess water and transfer the boiled broccoli florets to the prepared casserole dish. Scatter the sautéed garlic around the broccoli florets.

Drizzle the remaining tablespoon of olive oil; sprinkle the salt, black pepper, and paprika over your broccoli. Pour in the cream of mushroom soup.

Top with the Swiss cheese and bake for approximately 18 minutes until the cheese bubbled all over. Bon appétit!

Nutrition: Calories: 180; Fat: 10.3 g; Protein: 13.5 g; Carbs: 7.6 g; Net Carbs: 4.0 g; Fiber: 3.6 g.

523 ZA'ATAR CHANTERELLE STEW

Preparation Time: 15 minutes
Cooking Time: 50 minutes
Servings: 4
Ingredients:

½ tsp. Za'atar spice
4 tbsp. olive oil
½ cup shallots, chopped
2 bell peppers, chopped
1 poblano pepper, finely chopped
8 oz. (227 g.) Chanterelle mushroom, sliced
½ tsp. garlic, minced
Sea salt and freshly cracked black pepper, to taste
1 cup tomato purée
3 cups vegetable broth
1 bay laurel

Directions:

Combine the Za'atar with 3 tablespoons of olive oil in a small saucepan. Cook over a moderate flame until hot; make sure not to burn the zaatar. Set aside for 1hour to cool and infuse.

In a heavy-bottomed pot, heat the remaining tablespoon of olive oil. Now, sauté the shallots and bell peppers until just tender and fragrant.

Stir in the poblano pepper, mushrooms, and garlic; continue to sauté until the mushrooms have softened.

Next, add in the salt, black pepper, tomato purée, broth, and bay laurel. Once your stew begins to boil, turn the heat down to a simmer.

Let it simmer for about 40 minutes until everything is thoroughly cooked. Ladle into individual bowls and drizzle each serving with Za'atar oil. Bon appétit!

Nutrition: Calories: 156; Fat: 13.8 g; Protein: 1.4 g; Carbs: 6.0 g; Net Carbs: 3.1 g; Fiber: 2.9 g.

524 DUO-CHEESE BROCCOLI CROQUETTES

Preparation Time: 10 minutes
Cooking Time: 10 minutes
Servings: 5
Ingredients:

1 pound (454 g.) broccoli florets
1 tbsp. fresh parsley, minced
½ tsp. paprika
Sea salt and ground black pepper, to taste
3 eggs
1 cup Romano cheese, preferably freshly grated
oz. (142 g.) Swiss cheese, sliced
2 tbsp. olive oil

Directions:

Pulse the broccoli florets in your food processor until small rice-sized pieces are formed.

Mix the chopped broccoli florets with parsley, paprika, salt, pepper, eggs, and Romano cheese. Shape the mixture into bite-sized balls; flatten the balls with your hands or fork.

Heat the olive oil in a frying pan over a moderate flame.

Cook for 4 to 5 minutes; turn over, top with the Swiss cheese, and continue cooking on the other side for a further 4 minutes or until thoroughly cooked. Bon appétit!

Nutrition: Calories: 324; Fat: 24.1 g; Protein: 19.9 g; Carbs: 5.8 g; Net Carbs: 3.5 g; Fiber: 2.3 g.

525 BELL PEPPER AND TOMATO SATARAŠ

Preparation Time: 5 minutes
Cooking Time: 15 minutes
Servings: 3
Ingredients:

3 tsp. olive oil
1 onion, chopped
2 garlic cloves, minced
3 bell peppers, deveined and sliced

1 tomato, puréed

Directions:

Heat the olive oil in a saucepan over moderate flame. Then, sweat the onion until translucent.

Stir in the garlic and bell peppers and sauté for 2 minutes more or until aromatic. Stir in the puréed tomato.

Cover, reduce the temperature to medium-low, and continue cooking for 12 minutes or until the peppers have softened and the cooking liquid has evaporated.

Salt to taste and serve in individual bowls. Bon appétit!

Nutrition: Calories: 84; Fat: 4.6 g; Protein: 1.6 g; Carbs: 6.5 g; Net Carbs: 4.7 g; Fiber: 1.8 g.

526 PROVENÇAL RATATOUILLE

Preparation Time: 15 minutes
Cooking Time: 35 minutes
Servings: 6
Ingredients:

2 tbsp. olive oil
2 garlic cloves, finely minced
1 red pepper, sliced
1 yellow pepper, sliced
1 green pepper, sliced
1 shallot, sliced
1 large-sized zucchini, sliced
3 tomatoes, sliced
1 cup vegetable broth
Sea salt, to taste
½ tsp. dried oregano
½ tsp. dried parsley flakes
½ tsp. paprika
½ tsp. ground black pepper - eggs

Directions:

Start by preheating your oven to 400°F (205°C). Brush the sides and bottom of a baking pan with olive oil.

Layer all vegetables into the prepared pan and cover tightly with foil. Pour in the vegetable broth. Season with salt, oregano, parsley, paprika, and ground black pepper.

Bake for about 25 minutes.

Create six indentations in the hot ratatouille. Break an egg into each indentation. Bake until the eggs are set or about 9 minutes. Enjoy!

Nutrition: Calories: 440; Fat: 45.0 g; Protein: 6.4 g; Carbs: 5.6 g; Net Carbs: 4.6 g; Fiber: 1.0 g.

527 MOZZARELLA ROASTED PEPPERS

Preparation Time: 5 minutes
Cooking Time: 15 minutes

Servings: 4
Ingredients:

2 tsp. olive oil
4 Italian sweet peppers, deveined and halved
Salt and black pepper, to taste
¼ tsp. red pepper flakes
8 oz. (227 g.) Mozzarella cheese

Directions:

Put your oven on broil. Drizzle the pepper halves with olive oil. Season the peppers with salt, black pepper, and red pepper flakes.

Top the pepper halves with Mozzarella cheese. Arrange the stuffed peppers on a parchment-lined baking tray.

Roast for 12 to 15 minutes until the cheese is browned on top and the peppers are tender and blistered. Bon appétit!

Nutrition: Calories: 215; Fat: 15.1 g; Protein: 13.5 g; Carbs: 6.7 g; Net Carbs: 4.7 g; Fiber: 2.0 g.

528 ITALIAN TOMATO AND CHEESE STUFFED PEPPERS

Preparation Time: 15 minutes
Cooking Time: 10 minutes
Servings: 2
Ingredients:

1 tbsp. canola oil
1 garlic clove, pressed
½ cup celery, finely chopped
½ Spanish onion, finely chopped
4 oz. (113 g.) pork, ground
Sea salt, to taste
1 tsp. Italian seasoning mix
2 sweet Italian peppers, deveined and halved
1 large-sized Roma tomato, puréed
½ cup Cheddar cheese, grated

Directions:

Heat the canola oil in a sauté pan over medium-high flame. Now, sauté the garlic, celery, and onion until they have softened.

Stir in the ground pork and cook for a further 3 minutes or until no longer pink. Sprinkle with salt and Italian seasoning mix. Divide the filling mixture between the pepper halves.

Add the puréed tomato to a lightly greased baking dish; place the stuffed peppers in the baking dish.

Bake in the preheated oven at 390°F (199°C) for 20 minutes. Top with the Cheddar cheese and bake an additional 4 to 6 minutes or until

the cheese is bubbling. Serve warm and enjoy!

Nutrition: Calories: 312; Fat: 21.4 g; Protein: 20.2 g; Carbs: 5.7 g; Net Carbs: 3.8 g; Fiber: 1.9 g.

529 MUSHROOM MÉLANGE

Preparation Time: 10 minutes
Cooking Time: 15 minutes
Servings: 6
Ingredients:

4 tbsp. olive oil
1 bell pepper, sliced
½ cup leeks, finely diced
2 cloves garlic, smashed
2 pounds (907 g.) brown mushrooms, sliced
2 cups chicken broth
1 cup tomato sauce
½ tsp. dried oregano
½ tsp. chili powder
½ tsp. paprika
½ tsp. ground black pepper
Sea salt, to taste

Directions:

Heat the oil in a heavy-bottomed pot over medium-high flame. Now, sauté bell pepper along with the leeks for about 5 minutes.

Stir in the garlic and mushrooms, and continue sautéing an additional minute or so. Add in a splash of chicken broth to deglaze the bottom of the pan.

After that, add in the tomato sauce and seasonings. Bring to a boil and immediately reduce the heat to simmer.

Partially cover and cook for 8 to 10 minutes more or until the mushrooms are cooked through.

Ladle into individual bowls and serve with cauli rice if desired. Bon appétit!

Nutrition: Calories: 124; Fat: 9.2 g; Protein: 4.6 g; Carbs: 5.8 g; Net Carbs: 4.3 g; Fiber: 1.5 g.

530 GREEN CABBAGE WITH TOFU

Preparation Time: 5 minutes
Cooking Time: 15 minutes
Servings: 3
Ingredients:

6 oz. (170 g.) tofu, diced
½ shallot, chopped
2 garlic cloves, finely chopped
1 (1 ½-pound / 680-g.) head green cabbage, cut into strips
½ cup vegetable broth

Directions:

Heat up a lightly oiled sauté pan over moderate heat. Now, cook the tofu until brown and crisp; set aside.

Then, sauté the shallot and garlic until just tender and fragrant. Add in the green cabbage and beef bone broth; stir to combine.

Reduce the heat to medium-low and continue cooking for an additional 13 minutes. Season with salt to taste, top with reserved tofu and serve warm. Bon appétit!

Nutrition: Calories: 168; Fat: 11.7 g; Protein: 10.5 g; Carbs: 5.2 g; Net Carbs: 2.9 g; Fiber: 2.3 g.

531 MUSHROOM AND BELL PEPPER OMELET

Preparation Time: 5 minutes
Cooking Time: 5 minutes
Servings: 4
Ingredients:

2 tbsp. olive oil
1 cup Chanterelle mushrooms, chopped
2 bell peppers, chopped
1 white onion, chopped
eggs

Directions:

Heat the olive oil in a nonstick skillet over moderate heat. Now, cook the mushrooms, peppers, and onion until they have softened.

In a mixing bowl, whisk the eggs until frothy. Add the eggs to the skillet, reduce the heat to medium-low, and cook approximately 5 minutes until the center starts to look dry. Do not overcook.

Taste and season with salt to taste. Bon appétit!

Nutrition: Calories: 240; Fat: 17.5 g; Protein: 12.3 g; Carbs: 6.1 g; Net Carbs: 4.3 g; Fiber: 1.8 g.

532 PARMIGIANO-REGGIANO CHEESE BROILED AVOCADOS

Preparation Time: 10 minutes
Cooking Time: 5 minutes
Servings: 6
Ingredients:

3 avocados, pitted and halved
½ tsp. red pepper flakes, crushed
½ tsp. Himalayan salt
3 tbsp. extra-virgin olive oil
1 tbsp. Parmigiano-Reggiano cheese, grated

Directions:

Begin by preheating your oven for broil.

Then, cut a crisscross pattern about ¾ of the way through on each avocado half with a sharp knife.

Sprinkle red pepper and salt over the avocado halves. Drizzle olive oil over them and top with the grated Parmigiano-Reggiano cheese.

Transfer the avocado halves to a roasting pan and cook under the broiler for approximately 5 minutes. Enjoy!

Nutrition: Calories: 196; Fat: 18.8 g; Protein: 2.6 g; Carbs: 6.4 g; Net Carbs: 1.9 g; Fiber: 4.5 g.

533 ROMAINE LETTUCE BOATS

Preparation Time: 10 minutes
Cooking Time: 3 minutes
Servings: 4
Ingredients:

½-pound (227 g.) pork sausage, sliced
1 green bell pepper, deveined and chopped
1 garlic clove, minced
½ cup tomato purée
¼ tsp. ground black pepper
½ tsp. fennel seeds
Himalayan salt, to taste
1 head Romaine lettuce, separated into leaves
2 scallions, chopped

Directions:

Preheat a nonstick frying pan over a moderate flame. Then, sear the pork sausage until no longer pink, crumbling with a fork.

Stir in the bell pepper and garlic, and continue sautéing an additional minute or so or until fragrant.

Fold in the tomato purée. Season with black pepper, fennel seeds, and salt. Stir well and continue cooking for 2 minutes more; remove from the heat.

Arrange the lettuce boats on a serving platter. Then, top each boat with the sausage mixture. Garnish with scallions and serve immediately. Bon appétit!

Nutrition: Calories: 231; Fat: 18.1 g; Protein: 10.2 g; Carbs: 5.6 g; Net Carbs: 3.5 g; Fiber: 2.1 g.

534 GRUYERE CELERY BOATS

Preparation Time: 10 minutes
Cooking Time: 35 minutes
Servings: 2
Ingredients:

1 jalapeño pepper, deveined and minced
¼ tsp. sea salt
¼ tsp. ground black pepper
1 tsp. granulated garlic
3 tbsp. scallions, minced
½ tsp. caraway seeds
2 oz. (57 g.) Gruyere cheese
3 celery stalks, halved

Directions:

In a mixing bowl, thoroughly combine the minced jalapeño with sea salt, black pepper, garlic, scallions, caraway seeds, and Gruyere cheese.

Spread this mixture over the celery stalks. Then, arrange them on a parchment-lined baking tray.

Roast in the preheated oven at 360°F (182°C) for 35 minutes or until cooked through.

Nutrition: Calories: 195; Fat: 17.1 g; Protein: 2.5 g; Carbs: 7.0 g; Net Carbs: 2.0 g; Fiber: 5.0 g.

535 PEASANT STIR-FRY

Preparation Time: 10 minutes
Cooking Time: 20 minutes
Servings: 5
Ingredients:

2 tbsp. olive oil
1 yellow onion, sliced
3 garlic cloves, halved
8 bell peppers, deveined and cut into strips
1 tomato, chopped
½ tsp. ground black pepper
½ tsp. paprika
½ tsp. kosher salt
2 eggs

Directions:

Heat the olive oil in a frying pan over medium-low flame. Now, sweat the onion for 3 to 4 minutes or until tender.

Next, stir in the garlic and peppers; continue sautéing for 5 minutes. Then, add in the tomato, black pepper, paprika, and kosher salt.

Partially cover and continue cooking for a further 6 to 8 minutes.

Fold in the eggs and stir fry for another 5 minutes. Serve warm and enjoy!

Nutrition: Calories: 115; Fat: 7.5 g; Protein: 3.4 g; Carbs: 6.0 g; Net Carbs: 4.5 g; Fiber: 1.5 g.

536 CAULIFLOWER SOUP

Preparation Time: 4 minutes
Cooking Time: 15 minutes
Servings: 4
Ingredients:

2 green onions, chopped
½ tsp. ginger-garlic paste
1 celery stalk, chopped
1 pound (454 g.) cauliflower florets
3 cups vegetable broth

Directions:

Heat up a lightly oiled soup pot over a medium-high flame. Now, sauté the green onions until they have softened.

Stir in the ginger-garlic paste, celery, cauliflower, and vegetable broth;

bring to a rapid boil. Turn the heat to medium-low.

Continue to simmer for 13 minutes more or until heated through; heat off.

Puree the soup in your blender until creamy and uniform. Enjoy!

Nutrition: Calories: 70; Fat: 1.6 g; Protein: 6.2 g; Carbs: 7.0 g; Net Carbs: 4.0 g; Fiber: 3.0 g.

537 AVOCADO SAUCED CUCUMBER NOODLES

Preparation Time: 15 minutes
Cooking Time: 0 minutes
Servings: 2
Ingredients:

½ tsp. sea salt
1 cucumber, spiralized
1 California avocado, pitted, peeled and mashed
1 tbsp. olive oil
½ tsp. garlic powder
½ tsp. paprika
1 tbsp. fresh lime juice

Directions:

Toss your cucumber with salt and let it sit for 30 minutes; discard the excess water and pat dry.

In a mixing bowl, thoroughly combine the avocado with olive oil, garlic powder, paprika, and lime juice.

Add the sauce to the cucumber noodles and serve immediately. Bon appétit!

Nutrition: Calories: 195; Fat: 17.2 g; Protein: 2.6 g; Carbs: 7.6 g; Net Carbs: 3.0 g; Fiber: 4.6 g.

538 ZUCCHINI NOODLES WITH MUSHROOM SAUCE

Preparation Time: 10 minutes
Cooking Time: 10 minutes
Servings: 3
Ingredients:

1 ½ tbsp. olive oil
3 cups button mushrooms, chopped
2 cloves garlic, smashed
1 cup tomato purée
1 pound (454 g.) zucchini, spiralized
Salt and ground black pepper, to taste
⅓ cup Pecorino Romano cheese, preferably freshly grated

Directions:

Heat the olive oil in a saucepan over a moderate flame. Then, cook the mushrooms until tender and fragrant or about 4 minutes.

Stir in the garlic and continue to sauté for an additional 30 seconds or until just tender and aromatic. Fold in the tomato purée and zucchini.

Reduce the heat to medium-low, partially cover and let it cook for about 6 minutes or until heated through. Season with salt and black pepper to taste.

Divide your zoodles and sauce between serving plates. Top with Pecorino Romano cheese and serve warm. Bon appétit!

Nutrition: Calories: 161; Fat: 10.5 g; Protein: 10.0 g; Carbs: 7.4 g; Net Carbs: 4.0 g; Fiber: 3.4 g.

539 GOAT CHEESE EGGPLANT CASSEROLE

Preparation Time: 10 minutes
Cooking Time: 25 minutes
Servings: 3
Ingredients:

1 (1-pound / 454-g.) eggplant, cut into rounds
2 bell peppers, deveined and quartered
2 vine-ripe tomatoes, sliced
3 tbsp. olive oil
Sea salt and freshly ground black pepper, to taste
½ tsp. red pepper flakes, crushed
½ tsp. sumac
½ cup sour cream
1 ½ cups goat cheese
2 tbsp. green onions, chopped

Directions:

Place your eggplant and peppers in a baking pan. Top with the sliced tomatoes. Drizzle olive oil over the vegetables.

Season with salt, black pepper, crushed red pepper, and sumac. Bake in the preheated oven at 420°F (216°C) for 15 minutes. Rotate the pan and bake for an additional 10 minutes.

Top with sour cream and goat cheese. Garnish with green onions and serve. Enjoy!

Nutrition: Calories: 476; Fat: 41.4 g; Protein: 18.4 g; Carbs: 7.2 g; Net Carbs: 3.6 g; Fiber: 3.6 g.

540 MUSHROOM RED WINE CHILI

Preparation Time: 10 minutes
Cooking Time: 15 minutes
Servings: 3
Ingredients:

3 oz. (85 g.) bacon, diced
1 brown onion, chopped
2 cloves garlic, minced
¾ pound (340 g.) brown mushrooms, sliced
3 tbsp. dry red wine
½ tsp. freshly ground black pepper
1 tsp. chili powder
2 bay laurels
Sea salt, to taste

Directions:

Heat a soup pot over a medium-high flame and fry the bacon; once the bacon is crisp, remove from the pot and reserve.

Now, cook the brown onion and garlic until they have softened or about 6 minutes. Stir in the mushrooms and sauté them for 3 to 4 minutes longer.

Turn the heat to simmer; add the other ingredients and continue cooking for 10 minutes more, until most of the cooking liquid has evaporated.

Ladle into bowls and top with the reserved bacon. Bon appétit!

Nutrition: Calories: 160; Fats: 11.3 g; Protein: 6.9 g; Carbs: 6.0 g; Net Carbs: 4.7 g; Fiber: 1.3 g.

541 MINUTES VEGETARIAN PASTA

Preparation Time: 5 minutes
Cooking Time: 16 minutes
Servings: 4
Ingredients:

3 shallots, chopped
¼ tsp. red pepper flakes
¼ cup vegan parmesan cheese
2 tbsp. olive oil
2 garlic cloves, minced
8-oz. spinach leaves
8-oz. linguine pasta
1 pinch salt
1 pinch black pepper

Directions:

Boil salted water in a large pot and add pasta.

Cook for about 6 minutes and drain the pasta in a colander.

Heat olive oil over medium heat in a large skillet and add the shallots.

Cook for about 5 minutes until soft and caramelized and stir in the spinach, garlic, red pepper flakes, salt and black pepper.

Cook for about 5 minutes and add pasta and 2 ladles of pasta water.

Stir in the parmesan cheese and dish out in a bowl to serve.

Nutrition: Calories: 25; Fat: 2.0 g; Protein: 5.2 g; Carbohydrates: 5.3 g; Fiber: 4g; Sodium: 18 mg.

542 CHIPOTLE, PINTO, AND GREEN BEAN AND CORN SUCCOTASH

Preparation Time: 5 minutes
Cooking Time: 10 minutes
Servings: 2
Ingredients:

2 tbsp. extra-virgin olive oil
1 ½ cups fresh or frozen corn
1 cup green beans, chopped

2 green onions, white and green parts, sliced
½ tbsp. minced garlic
1 medium tomato, chopped
1 tsp. chili powder
½ tsp. chipotle powder
½ tsp. ground cumin
1 (14-oz.) can pinto beans, drained and rinsed
1 tsp. sea salt, or to taste

Directions:

Heat the olive oil in a large skillet over medium heat. Add the corn, green beans, green onions, and garlic and stir for 5 minutes.

Add the tomato, chili powder, chipotle powder, and cumin and stir for 3 minutes, until the tomato starts to soften.

In a bowl, mash some of the pinto beans with a fork. Add all of the beans to the skillet and stir for 2 minutes, until the beans are heated through.

Remove from the heat and stir in the salt. Serve hot or warm.

Nutrition: Calories: 391; Total Fat: 16 g; Total Carbs: 53 g; Fiber: 15 g; Sugar: 4 g; Protein: 15 g; Sodium: 253 mg.

543 BROCCOLI SALAD

Preparation Time: 5 minutes
Cooking Time: 25 minutes
Servings: 6
Ingredients:

2 tbsp. sherry vinegar
¼ cup olive oil
2 tsp. fresh thyme, chopped
1 tsp. Dijon mustard
1 tsp. honey
Salt to taste
8 cups broccoli florets, steamed or roasted
2 red onions, sliced thinly
½ cup Parmesan cheese, shaved
¼ cup pecans, toasted and chopped

Directions:

Mix the sherry vinegar, olive oil, thyme, mustard, honey and salt in a bowl.

In a serving bowl, combine the broccoli florets and onions.

Drizzle the dressing on top.

Sprinkle with the pecans and Parmesan cheese before serving.

Nutrition: Calories: 199; Fat: 17.4 g; Saturated fat: 2.9; Carbohydrates: 7.5 g; Fiber: 2.8 g; Protein: 5.2 g.

544 POTATO CARROT SALAD

Preparation Time: 15 minutes
Cooking Time: 10 minutes
Servings: 6
Ingredients:

Water
6 potatoes, sliced into cubes
3 carrots, sliced into cubes
1 tbsp. milk
1 tbsp. Dijon mustard
¼ cup mayonnaise
Pepper to taste
2 tsp. fresh thyme, chopped
1 stalk celery, chopped
2 scallions, chopped
1 slice turkey bacon, cooked crispy and crumbled

Directions:

Fill your pot with water.
Place it over medium-high heat.
Boil the potatoes and carrots for 10 minutes or until tender.
Drain and let cool.
In a bowl, mix the milk mustard, mayo, pepper and thyme.
Stir in the potatoes, carrots and celery.
Coat evenly with the sauce.
Cover and refrigerate for 4 hours.
Top with the scallions and turkey bacon bits before serving.

Nutrition: Calories: 106 Fat: 5.3 g; Saturated Fat: 1 g; Carbohydrates: 12.6 g; Fiber: 1.8 g; Protein: 2 g.

545 MIXED VEGETABLE MEDLEY

Preparation Time: 5 minutes
Cooking Time: 20 minutes
Servings: 2
Ingredients:

1 stick (½ cup) unsalted butter, divided
1 large potato, cut into ½-inch dice
1 onion, chopped
½ tbsp. minced garlic
1 cup green beans, chopped
2 ears fresh sweet corn, kernels removed
1 red bell pepper, seeded and cut into strips
2 cups sliced white mushrooms
Salt
Freshly ground black pepper

Directions:

Heat half of the butter in a large nonstick skillet over medium-high flame. When the butter is frothy, add the potato and cook, stirring frequently, for 15 minutes, until golden.

Turn the heat down slightly if the butter begins to burn.

Add the remaining butter, turn down the heat to medium, and add the onion, garlic, green beans, and corn. Cook, stirring frequently, for 5 minutes.

Add the red bell pepper and mushrooms. Stir for another 5 minutes, until the vegetables are tender and the mushrooms have

browned but are still plump. Add more butter, if necessary.

Remove from heat and season with salt and pepper. Serve hot.

Nutrition: Calories: 688; Total Fat: 48 g; Total Carbs: 63 g; Fiber: 11 g; Sugar: 11 g; Protein: 11 g; Sodium: 360 mg.

546 SPICY LENTILS WITH SPINACH

Preparation Time: 5 minutes
Cooking Time: 25 minutes
Servings: 4
Ingredients:

1 cup dried red lentils, well-rinsed
2 ½ cups water
1 tbsp. extra-virgin olive oil
1 tbsp. minced garlic
1 tsp. ground cumin
½ tsp. ground coriander
½ tsp. turmeric
¼ tsp. cayenne pepper
1 medium tomato, chopped
1 (16-oz.) package spinach
1 tsp. salt
Freshly ground black pepper

Directions:

In a medium saucepan, bring the lentils and water to a boil.

Partially cover the pot, reduce the heat to medium, and simmer, stirring occasionally, until the lentils are tender, about 15 minutes.

Drain the lentils and set aside.

In a large nonstick skillet, heat the olive oil over medium heat. When hot, add garlic, cumin, coriander, turmeric, and cayenne. Sauté for 2 minutes.

Stir in the tomato and cook for another 3 to 5 minutes, until the tomato begins to break apart and the mixture thickens somewhat.

Add handfuls of the spinach at a time, stirring until wilted.

Stir in the drained lentils and cook for another few minutes.

Season with salt and freshly ground black pepper and serve hot.

Nutrition: Calories: 237; Total Fat: 5 g; Total Carbs: 35 g; Fiber: 18 g; Sugar: 2 g; Protein: 16 g; Sodium: 677 mg.

547 PARMESAN ASPARAGUS

Preparation Time: 10 minutes
Cooking Time: 5 minutes
Servings: 2
Ingredients:

1 egg, lightly beaten
10 asparagus spears, trimmed and cut woody ends
1 tbsp. heavy cream
⅓ cup parmesan cheese, grated
⅓ cup almond flour
½ tsp. paprika

Directions:

Spray air fryer basket with cooking spray.

In a shallow dish, whisk together egg and cream until well mix.

In a separate dish, mix together almond flour, parmesan cheese, paprika, and salt.

Dip asparagus spear into the egg mixture then coat with almond flour mixture.

Place coated asparagus into the air fryer basket and cook at 350°F for 5 minutes.

Nutrition: Calories: 166; Fat: 11.3 g; Carbohydrates: 7 g; Sugar 2.7 g; Protein: 12.3 g; Cholesterol: 105 mg.

548 GREEK VEGETABLES

Preparation Time: 10 minutes
Cooking Time: 20 minutes
Servings: 4
Ingredients:

1 carrot, sliced
1 parsnip, sliced
1 green bell pepper, chopped
1 courgetti, chopped
¼ cup cherry tomatoes, cut in half
6 tbsp. olive oil
2 tsp. garlic puree
1 tsp. mustard
1 tsp. mixed herbs
Pepper
Salt

Directions:

Add cherry tomatoes, carrot, parsnip, bell pepper, and courgetti into the air fryer basket.

Drizzle olive oil over vegetables and cook at 350°F for 15 minutes.

In a mixing bowl, mix together the remaining ingredients. Add vegetables into the mixing bowl and toss well.

Return vegetables to the air fryer basket and cook at 400°F for 5 minutes more.

Serve and enjoy.

Nutrition: Calories: 66; Fat: 1.5 g; Carbohydrates: 12.7 g; Sugar 5.3 g; Protein: 1.8 g; Cholesterol: 1 mg.

549 LEMON GARLIC CAULIFLOWER

Preparation Time: 10 minutes
Cooking Time: 10 minutes
Servings: 2
Ingredients:

3 cups cauliflower
1 tbsp. fresh parsley, chopped
½ tsp. lemon juice
1 tbsp. pine nuts
½ tsp. dried oregano
1 ½ tsp. olive oil
Pepper

Salt

Directions:

Add cauliflower, oregano, oil, pepper, and salt into the mixing bowl and toss well.

Add cauliflower into the air fryer basket and cook at 375°F for 10 minutes.

Transfer cauliflower into the serving bowl. Add pine nuts, parsley, and lemon juice and toss well.

Serve and enjoy.

Nutrition: Calories: 99 Fat: 6.7 g; Carbohydrates: 8.9 g; Sugar 3.8 g; Protein: 3.7 g; Cholesterol: 0 mg.

550 BALSAMIC BRUSSELS SPROUTS

Preparation Time: 10 minutes
Cooking Time: 20 minutes
Servings: 4
Ingredients:

1 lb. brussels sprouts, remove ends and cut in half
1 tbsp balsamic vinegar
2 tbsp. olive oil
Pepper
Salt

Directions:

Add brussels sprouts, vinegar, oil, pepper, and salt into the mixing bowl and toss well.

Add brussels sprouts into the air fryer basket and cook at 360 F for 15-20 minutes. Toss halfway through.

Serve and enjoy.

Nutrition: Calories: 110; Fat: 7.4 g; Carbohydrates: 10.4 g; Sugar 2.5 g; Protein: 3.9 g; Cholesterol: 0 mg.

551 FLAVORFUL BUTTERNUT SQUASH

Preparation Time: 10 minutes
Cooking Time: 15 minutes
Servings: 4
Ingredients:

4 cups butternut squash, cut into 1-inch pieces
1 tsp Chinese five-spice powder
1 tbsp. Truvia
2 tbsp. olive oil

Directions:

Add butternut squash and remaining ingredients into the mixing bowl and mix well.

Add butternut squash into the air fryer basket and cook at 400°F for 15 minutes. Shake basket halfway through.

Serve and enjoy.

Nutrition: Calories: 83; Fat: 7.1 g; Carbohydrates: 6.7 g; Sugar 2.2 g; Protein: 0.6 g; Cholesterol: 0 mg.

552 CRISPY GREEN BEANS

Preparation Time: 10 minutes
Cooking Time: 10 minutes
Servings: 4
Ingredients:

2 cups green beans, ends trimmed
2 tbsp. parmesan cheese, shredded
1 tbsp. fresh lemon juice
1 tsp. Italian seasoning
2 tsp. olive oil
¼ tsp. salt

Directions:

Preheat the Cosori Air Fryer to 400°F.

Brush green beans with olive oil and season with Italian seasoning and salt.

Place green beans into the air fryer basket and cook for 8-10 minutes. Shake basket 2-3 times.

Transfer green beans to a serving plate.

Pour lemon juice over beans and sprinkle shredded cheese on top of beans.

Serve and enjoy.

Nutrition: Calories: 64; Fat: 4.3 g; Carbohydrates: 4.4 g; Sugar 1 g; Protein: 3.3 g; Cholesterol: 6 mg.

553 ROASTED ZUCCHINI

Preparation Time: 10 minutes
Cooking Time: 10 minutes
Servings: 4

Ingredients:

2 medium zucchinis, cut into 1-inch slices
1 tsp. lemon zest
1 tbsp. olive oil
Pepper
Salt

Directions:

Toss zucchini with lemon zest, oil, pepper, and salt.

Arrange zucchini slices into the air fryer basket and cook at 350 F for 10 minutes. Turn halfway through.

Serve and enjoy.

Nutrition:

Calories: 46; Fat: 3.7 g; Carbohydrates: 3.4 g; Sugar 1.7 g; Protein: 1.2 g; Cholesterol: 0 mg.

554 AIR FRIED CARROTS, ZUCCHINI & SQUASH

Preparation Time: 10 minutes
Cooking Time: 35 minutes
Servings: 2
Ingredients:

1 lb. yellow squash, cut into ¾-inch half-moons
1 lb. zucchini, cut into ¾-inch half-moons
½ lb. carrots, peeled and cut into 1-inch pieces

6 tsp. olive oil

1 tbsp. tarragon, chopped

Pepper

Salt

Directions:

In a bowl, toss carrots with 2 teaspoons of oil. Add carrots into the air fryer basket and cook at 400 F for 5 minutes.

In a mixing bowl, toss squash, zucchini, remaining oil, pepper, and salt.

Add squash and zucchini mixture into the air fryer basket with carrots and cook for 30 minutes. Shake basket 2-3 times.

Sprinkle with tarragon and serve.

Nutrition: Calories: 176; Fat: 17.3 g; Carbohydrates: 6.2 g; Sugar 3.2 g; Protein: 2.5 g; Cholesterol: 0 mg.

555 CRISPY & SPICY EGGPLANT

Preparation Time: 10 minutes

Cooking Time: 20 minutes

Servings: 4

Ingredients:

1 eggplant, cut into 1-inch pieces

½ tsp. Italian seasoning

1 tsp. paprika

½ tsp. red pepper

1 tsp. garlic powder

2 tbsp. olive oil

Directions:

Add eggplant and remaining ingredients into the bowl and toss well.

Spray air fryer basket with cooking spray.

Add eggplant into the air fryer basket and cook at 375 F for 20 minutes. Shake basket halfway through.

Serve and enjoy.

Nutrition: Calories: 99; Fat: 7.5 g; Carbohydrates: 8.7 g; Sugar 4.5 g; Protein: 1.5 g; Cholesterol: 0 mg.

556 CURRIED EGGPLANT SLICES

Preparation Time: 10 minutes

Cooking Time: 10 minutes

Servings: 4

Ingredients:

1 large eggplant, cut into ½-inch slices

1 garlic clove, minced

1 tbsp. olive oil

½ tsp. curry powder

⅛ tsp. turmeric

Salt

Directions:

Preheat the Cosori Air Fryer to 300°F.

In a small bowl, mix together oil, garlic, curry powder, turmeric, and salt and rub all over eggplant slices.

Add eggplant slices into the air fryer basket and cook for 10 minutes or until lightly browned.

Serve and enjoy.

Nutrition: Calories: 61; Fat: 3.8 g; Carbohydrates: 7.2 g; Sugar 3.5 g; Protein: 1.2 g; Cholesterol: 0 mg.

557 SPICED GREEN BEANS

Preparation Time: 10 minutes

Cooking Time: 10 minutes

Servings: 2

Ingredients:

2 cups green beans

⅛ tsp. ground allspice

¼ tsp. ground cinnamon

½ tsp. dried oregano

2 tbsp. olive oil

¼ tsp. ground coriander

¼ tsp. ground cumin

⅛ tsp. cayenne pepper

½ tsp. salt

Directions:

Add all ingredients into the medium bowl and toss well.

Grease air fryer basket with cooking spray.

Add green beans into the air fryer basket and cook at 370°F for 10 minutes. Shake basket halfway through.

Serve and enjoy.

Nutrition: Calories: 158; Fat: 14.3 g; Carbohydrates: 8.6 g; Sugar 1.6 g; Protein: 2.1 g; Cholesterol: 0 mg.

558 AIR FRYER BASIL TOMATOES

Preparation Time: 10 minutes

Cooking Time: 25 minutes

Servings: 4

Ingredients:

4 large tomatoes, halved

1 garlic clove, minced

1 tbsp. vinegar

1 tbsp. olive oil

2 tbsp. parmesan cheese, grated

½ tsp. fresh parsley, chopped

1 tsp. fresh basil, minced

Pepper

Salt

Directions:

Preheat the Cosori Air Fryer to 320°F.

In a bowl, mix together oil, basil, garlic, vinegar, pepper, and salt. Add tomatoes and stir to coat.

Place tomato halves into the air fryer basket and cook for 20 minutes.

Sprinkle parmesan cheese over tomatoes and cook for 5 minutes more.

Serve and enjoy.

Nutrition: Calories: 87; Fat: 5.4 g; Carbohydrates: 7.7 g; Sugar 4.8 g; Protein: 3.9 g; Cholesterol: 5 mg.

559 AIR FRYER RATATOUILLE

Preparation Time: 10 minutes

Cooking Time: 15 minutes

Servings: 6

Ingredients:

1 eggplant, diced

1 onion, diced

3 tomatoes, diced

1 red bell pepper, diced

1 green bell pepper, diced

1 tbsp. vinegar

2 tbsp. olive oil

2 tbsp. herb de Provence

2 garlic cloves, chopped

Pepper

Salt

Directions:

Preheat the Cosori Air Fryer to 400°F.

Add all ingredients into the bowl and toss well and transfer into the air fryer safe dish.

Place dish into the air fryer basket and cook for 15 minutes. Stir halfway through.

Serve and enjoy.

Nutrition: Calories: 91; Fat: 5 g; Carbohydrates: 11.6 g; Sugar 6.4 g; Protein: 1.9 g; Cholesterol: 0 mg.

560 GARLICKY CAULIFLOWER FLORETS

Preparation Time: 10 minutes

Cooking Time: 20 minutes

Servings: 4

Ingredients:

5 cups cauliflower florets

½ tsp. cumin powder

½ tsp. ground coriander

6 garlic cloves, chopped

4 tbsp. olive oil

½ tsp. salt

Directions:

Add cauliflower florets and remaining ingredients into the large mixing bowl and toss well.

Add cauliflower florets into the air fryer basket and cook at 400 F for 20 minutes. Shake basket halfway through.

Serve and enjoy.

Nutrition: Calories: 159; Fat: 14.2 g; Carbohydrates: 8.2 g; Sugar 3.1 g; Protein: 2.8 g; Cholesterol: 0 mg.

561 PARMESAN BRUSSELS SPROUTS

Preparation Time: 10 minutes

Cooking Time: 12 minutes

Servings: 4

Ingredients:

1 lb. Brussels sprouts, remove stems and halved

¼ cup parmesan cheese, grated

2 tbsp. olive oil

Pepper

Salt

Directions:

116

Preheat the Cosori Air Fryer to 350°F.

In a mixing bowl, toss Brussels sprouts with oil, pepper, and salt.

Transfer Brussels sprouts into the air fryer basket and cook for 12 minutes. Shake basket halfway through.

Sprinkle with parmesan cheese and serve.

Nutrition: Calories: 129; Fat: 8.7 g; Carbohydrates: 10.6 g; Sugar 2.5 g; Protein: 5.9 g; Cholesterol: 4 mg.

562 FLAVORFUL TOMATOES

Preparation Time: 10 minutes
Cooking Time: 15 minutes
Servings: 4
Ingredients:

4 Roma tomatoes, sliced, remove seeds pithy portion
1 tbsp. olive oil
½ tsp. dried thyme
2 garlic cloves, minced
Pepper
Salt

Directions:

Preheat the Cosori Air Fryer to 390°F.

Toss sliced tomatoes with oil, thyme, garlic, pepper, and salt.

Arrange sliced tomatoes into the air fryer basket and cook for 15 minutes.

Serve and enjoy.

Nutrition: Calories: 55; Fat: 3.8 g; Carbohydrates: 5.4 g; Sugar 3.3 g; Protein: 1.2 g; Cholesterol: 0 mg.

563 HEALTHY ROASTED CARROTS

Preparation Time: 10 minutes
Cooking Time: 12 minutes
Servings: 4
Ingredients:

2 cups carrots, peeled and chopped
1 tsp. cumin
1 tbsp. olive oil
¼ fresh coriander, chopped

Directions:

Toss carrots with cumin and oil and place them into the air fryer basket.

Cook at 390°F for 12 minutes.

Garnish with fresh coriander and serve.

Nutrition: Calories: 55; Fat: 3.6 g; Carbohydrates: 5.7 g; Sugar 2.7 g; Protein: 0.6 g; Cholesterol: 0 mg.

564 CURRIED CAULIFLOWER WITH PINE NUTS

Preparation Time: 10 minutes
Cooking Time: 10 minutes
Servings: 4
Ingredients:

1 small cauliflower head, cut into florets
2 tbsp. olive oil
¼ cup pine nuts, toasted
1 tbsp. curry powder
¼ tsp. salt

Directions:

Preheat the Cosori Air Fryer to 350°F.

In a mixing bowl, toss cauliflower florets with oil, curry powder, and salt.

Add cauliflower florets into the air fryer basket and cook for 10 minutes. Shake basket halfway through.

Transfer cauliflower into the serving bowl. Add pine nuts and toss well.

Serve and enjoy.

Nutrition: Calories: 139; Fat: 13.1 g; Carbohydrates: 5.5 g; Sugar 1.9 g; Protein: 2.7 g; Cholesterol: 0 mg.

565 THYME SAGE BUTTERNUT SQUASH

Preparation Time: 10 minutes
Cooking Time: 12 minutes
Servings: 4
Ingredients:

2 lbs. butternut squash, cut into chunks
1 tsp. fresh thyme, chopped
1 tbsp. fresh sage, chopped
1 tbsp. olive oil
Pepper
Salt

Directions:

Preheat the Cosori Air Fryer to 390°F.

In a mixing bowl, toss butternut squash with thyme, sage, oil, pepper, and salt.

Add butternut squash into the air fryer basket and cook for 10 minutes. Shake basket well and cook for 2 minutes more.

Serve and enjoy.

Nutrition: Calories: 50; Fat: 3.8 g; Carbohydrates: 4.2 g; Sugar 2.5 g; Protein: 1.4 g; Cholesterol: 0 mg.

566 GRILLED CAULIFLOWER

Preparation Time: 15 minutes
Cooking Time: 40 minutes
Servings: 4
Ingredients:

1 large head of cauliflower, leaves removed and stem trimmed
Salt, as required
4 tbsp. unsalted butter
¼ cup hot sauce
1 tbsp. ketchup
1 tbsp. soy sauce
½ cup mayonnaise
2 tbsp. white miso
1 tbsp. fresh lemon juice
½ tsp. ground black pepper

2 scallions, thinly sliced

Directions:

Sprinkle the cauliflower with salt evenly.

Arrange the cauliflower head in a large microwave-safe bowl.

With a plastic wrap, cover the bowl.

With a knife, pierce the plastic a few times to vent.

Microwave on high for about 5 minutes.

Remove from the microwave and set aside to cool slightly.

In a small saucepan, add butter, hot sauce, ketchup and soy sauce over medium heat and cook for about 2-3 minutes, stirring occasionally.

Brush the cauliflower head with warm sauce evenly.

Place the water tray in the bottom of the Power XL Smokeless Electric Grill.

Place about 2 cups of lukewarm water into the water tray.

Place the drip pan over the water tray and then arrange the heating element.

Now, place the grilling pan over the heating element.

Set the temperature settings according to the manufacturer's directions.

Cover the grill with a lid and let it preheat.

After preheating, remove the lid and grease the grilling pan.

Place the cauliflower head over the grilling pan.

Cover with the lid and cook for about 10 minutes.

Turn the cauliflower over and brush with warm sauce.

Cover with the lid and cook for about 25 minutes, flipping and brushing with warm sauce after every 10 minutes.

In a bowl, place the mayonnaise, miso, lemon juice, and pepper and beat until smooth.

Spread the mayonnaise mixture onto a plate and arrange the cauliflower on top.

Nutrition: Calories: 261; Total Fat: 22 g; Saturated Fat: 8.9 g; Cholesterol: 38 mg; Sodium: 300 mg; Total Carbs:15.1 g; Fiber: 2.5 g; Sugar: 5.4 g; Protein: 3.3 g.

567 STUFFED ZUCCHINI

Preparation Time: 20 minutes
Cooking Time: 24 minutes
Servings: 6
Ingredients:

3 medium zucchinis, sliced in half lengthwise
1 tsp. vegetable oil

3 cup corn, cut off the cob
1 cup Parmesan cheese, shredded
⅔ cup sour cream
¼ tsp. hot sauce
Olive oil cooking spray

Directions:

Cut the ends off the zucchini and slice in half lengthwise.

Scoop out the pulp from each half of zucchini, leaving the shell.

For the filling: in a large pan of boiling water, add the corn over medium heat and cook for about 5-7 minutes.

Drain the corn and set aside to cool.

In a large bowl, add corn, half of the parmesan cheese, sour cream and hot sauce and mix well.

Spray the zucchini shells with cooking spray evenly.

Place the water tray in the bottom of the Power XL Smokeless Electric Grill.

Place about 2 cups of lukewarm water into the water tray.

Place the drip pan over the water tray and then arrange the heating element.

Now, place the grilling pan over the heating element.

Set the temperature settings according to the manufacturer's directions.

Cover the grill with a lid and let it preheat.

After preheating, remove the lid and grease the grilling pan.

Place the zucchini halves over the grilling pan, flesh side down.

Cover with the lid and cook for about 8-10 minutes.

Remove the zucchini halves from the grill.

Spoon filling into each zucchini half evenly and sprinkle with remaining parmesan cheese.

Place the zucchini halves over the grilling pan.

Cover with the lid and cook for about 8 minutes.

Serve hot.

Nutrition: Calories: 198; Total Fat: 10.8 g; Saturated Fat: 6 g; Cholesterol: 21 mg; Sodium: 293 mg; Total Carbs: 19.3 g; Fiber: 3.2 g; Sugar: 4.2 g; Protein: 9.6 g.

568 VINEGAR VEGGIES

Preparation Time: 15 minutes
Cooking Time: 10 minutes
Servings: 4
Ingredients:

3 golden beets, trimmed, peeled and sliced thinly
3 carrots, peeled and sliced lengthwise
1 cup zucchini, sliced
1 onion, sliced
½ cup yam, sliced thinly
2 tbsp. fresh rosemary
1 garlic clove, minced
Salt and ground black pepper, as required
3 tbsp. vegetable oil
2 tsp. balsamic vinegar

Directions:

Place all ingredients in a bowl and toss to coat well.

Refrigerate to marinate for at least 30 minutes.

Place the water tray in the bottom of the Power XL Smokeless Electric Grill.

Place about 2 cups of lukewarm water into the water tray.

Place the drip pan over the water tray and then arrange the heating element.

Now, place the grilling pan over the heating element.

Plugin the Power XL Smokeless Electric Grill and press the 'Power' button to turn it on.

Then press the 'Fan" button.

Set the temperature settings according to the manufacturer's directions.

Cover the grill with a lid and let it preheat.

After preheating, remove the lid and grease the grilling pan.

Place the vegetables over the grilling pan.

Cover with the lid and cook for about 5 minutes per side.

Serve hot.

Nutrition: Calories: 184; Total Fat: 10.7 g; Saturated Fat: 2.2 g; Cholesterol: 0 mg; Sodium: 134 mg; Total Carbs: 21.5 g; Fiber: 4.9 g; Sugar: 10 g; Protein: 2.7 g.

569 GARLICKY MIXED VEGGIES

Preparation Time: 15 minutes
Cooking Time: 8 minutes
Servings: 4
Ingredients:

1 bunch fresh asparagus, trimmed
6 oz. fresh mushrooms, halved
6 Campari tomatoes, halved
1 red onion, cut into 1-inch chunks
3 garlic cloves, minced
2 tbsp. olive oil
Salt and ground black pepper, as required

Directions:

In a large bowl, add all ingredients and toss to coat well.

Place the water tray in the bottom of the Power XL Smokeless Electric Grill.

Place about 2 cups of lukewarm water into the water tray.

Place the drip pan over the water tray and then arrange the heating element.

Now, place the grilling pan over the heating element.

Plugin the Power XL Smokeless Electric Grill and press the 'Power' button to turn it on.

Then press the 'Fan" button.

Set the temperature settings according to the manufacturer's directions.

Cover the grill with a lid and let it preheat.

After preheating, remove the lid and grease the grilling pan.

Place the vegetables over the grilling pan.

Cover with the lid and cook for about 8 minutes, flipping occasionally.

Nutrition: Calories: 137; Total Fat: 7.7 g; Saturated Fat: 1.1 g; Cholesterol: 0 mg; Sodium: 54 mg; Total Carbs: 15.6 g; Fiber: 5.6 g; Sugar: 8.9 g; Protein: 5.8 g.

570 MEDITERRANEAN VEGGIES

Preparation Time: 5 minutes
Cooking Time: 10 minutes
Servings: 4
Ingredients:

1 cup mixed bell peppers, chopped
1 cup eggplant, chopped
1 cup zucchini, chopped
1 cup mushrooms, chopped
½ cup onion, chopped
½ cup sun-dried tomato vinaigrette dressing

Directions:

In a large bowl, add all ingredients and toss to coat well.

Refrigerate to marinate for about 1 hour.

Place the water tray in the bottom of the Power XL Smokeless Electric Grill.

Place about 2 cups of lukewarm water into the water tray.

Place the drip pan over the water tray and then arrange the heating element.

Now, place the grilling pan over the heating element.

Plugin the Power XL Smokeless Electric Grill and press the 'Power' button to turn it on.

Then press the 'Fan" button.

Set the temperature settings according to the manufacturer's directions.

Cover the grill with a lid and let it preheat.

After preheating, remove the lid and grease the grilling pan.

Place the vegetables over the grilling pan.

Cover with the lid and cook for about 8-10 minutes, flipping occasionally.

Nutrition: Calories: 159; Total Fat: 11.2 g; Saturated Fat: 2 g; Cholesterol: 0 mg; Sodium: 336 mg; Total Carbs: 12.3 g; Fiber: 1.9 g; Sugar: 9.5 g; Protein: 1.6 g.

571 MARINATED VEGGIE SKEWERS

Preparation Time: 20 minutes
Cooking Time: 10 minutes
Servings: 4
Ingredients:
For Marinade:

- 2 garlic cloves, minced
- 2 tsp. fresh basil, minced
- 2 tsp. fresh oregano, minced
- ½ tsp. cayenne pepper
- Sea Salt and ground black pepper, as required
- 2 tbsp. fresh lemon juice
- 2 tbsp. olive oil

For Veggies:

- 2 large zucchinis, cut into thick slices
- 8 large button mushrooms, quartered
- 1 yellow bell pepper, seeded and cubed
- 1 red bell pepper, seeded and cubed

Directions:

For the marinade: in a large bowl, add all the ingredients and mix until well combined.

Add the vegetables and toss to coat well.

Cover and refrigerate to marinate for at least 6-8 hours.

Remove the vegetables from the bowl and thread onto pre-soaked wooden skewers.

Place the water tray in the bottom of the Power XL Smokeless Electric Grill.

Place about 2 cups of lukewarm water into the water tray.

Place the drip pan over the water tray and then arrange the heating element.

Now, place the grilling pan over the heating element.

Plugin the Power XL Smokeless Electric Grill and press the 'Power' button to turn it on.

Then press the 'Fan' button.

Set the temperature settings according to the manufacturer's directions.

Cover the grill with a lid and let it preheat.

After preheating, remove the lid and grease the grilling pan.

Place the skewers over the grilling pan. Cover with the lid and cook for about 8-10 minutes, flipping occasionally. Serve hot.

Nutrition: Calories: 122; Total Fat: 7.8 g; Saturated Fat: 1.2 g; Cholesterol: 0 mg;

Sodium: 81 mg; Total Carbs: 12.7 g; Fiber: 3.5 g; Sugar: 6.8g Protein: 4.3 g.

572 PINEAPPLE & VEGGIE SKEWERS

Preparation Time: 20 minutes
Cooking Time: 15 minutes
Servings: 6
Ingredients:

- ⅓ cup olive oil
- 1 ½ tsp. dried basil
- ¾ tsp. dried oregano
- Salt and ground black pepper, as required
- 2 zucchinis, cut into 1-inch slices
- 2 yellow squash, cut into 1-inch slices
- ½ pound whole fresh mushrooms
- 1 red bell pepper, cut into chunks
- 1 red onion, cut into chunks
- 12 cherry tomatoes
- 1 fresh pineapple, cut into chunks

Directions:

In a bowl, add oil, herbs, salt and black pepper and mix well.

Thread the veggies and pineapple onto pre-soaked wooden skewers.

Brush the veggies and pineapple with the oil mixture evenly.

Place the water tray in the bottom of the Power XL Smokeless Electric Grill.

Place about 2 cups of lukewarm water into the water tray.

Place the drip pan over the water tray and then arrange the heating element.

Now, place the grilling pan over the heating element.

Plugin the Power XL Smokeless Electric Grill and press the 'Power' button to turn it on.

Then press the 'Fan' button.

Set the temperature settings according to the manufacturer's directions.

Cover the grill with a lid and let it preheat.

After preheating, remove the lid and grease the grilling pan.

Place the skewers over the grilling pan.

Cover with the lid and cook for about 10-15 minutes, flipping occasionally.

Serve hot.

Nutrition: Calories: 220; Total Fat: 11.9 g; Saturated Fat: 1.7 g; Cholesterol: 0 mg; Sodium: 47 mg; Total Carbs: 30 g; Fiber: 5 g; Sugar: 20.4 g; Protein: 4.3 g.

573 BUTTERED CORN

Preparation Time: 10 minutes
Cooking Time: 20 minutes
Servings: 6
Ingredients:

- 6 fresh whole corn on the cob
- ½ cup butter, melted
- Salt, as required

Directions:

Husk the corn and remove all the silk.

Brush each corn with melted butter and sprinkle with salt.

Place the water tray in the bottom of the Power XL Smokeless Electric Grill.

Place about 2 cups of lukewarm water into the water tray.

Place the drip pan over the water tray and then arrange the heating element.

Now, place the grilling pan over the heating element.

Plugin the Power XL Smokeless Electric Grill and press the 'Power' button to turn it on.

Then press the 'Fan' button.

Set the temperature settings according to the manufacturer's directions.

Cover the grill with a lid and let it preheat.

After preheating, remove the lid and grease the grilling pan.

Place the corn over the grilling pan.

Cover with the lid and cook for about 20 minutes, rotating after every 5 minutes and brushing with butter once halfway through.

Serve warm.

Nutrition: Calories: 268; Total Fat: 17.2 g; Saturated Fat: 10 g; Cholesterol: 41 mg; Sodium: 159 mg; Total Carbs: 29 g; Fiber: 4.2 g; Sugar: 5 g; Protein: 5.2 g.

574 GUACAMOLE

Preparation Time: 15 minutes
Cooking Time: 4 minutes
Servings: 4
Ingredients:

- 2 ripe avocados, halved and pitted
- 2 tsp. vegetable oil
- 3 tbsp. fresh lime juice
- 1 garlic clove, crushed
- ¼ tsp. ground chipotle chile
- Salt, as required
- ¼ cup red onion, chopped finely
- ¼ cup fresh cilantro, chopped finely

Directions:

Brush the cut sides of each avocado half with oil.

Place the water tray in the bottom of the Power XL Smokeless Electric Grill.

Place about 2 cups of lukewarm water into the water tray.

Place the drip pan over the water tray and then arrange the heating element.

Now, place the grilling pan over the heating element.

Plugin the Power XL Smokeless Electric Grill and press the 'Power' button to turn it on.

Then press the 'Fan" button.

Set the temperature settings according to the manufacturer's directions.

Cover the grill with a lid and let it preheat.

After preheating, remove the lid and grease the grilling pan.

Place the avocado halves over the grilling pan, cut side down.

Cook, uncovered for about 2-4 minutes.

Transfer the avocados onto the cutting board and let them cool slightly.

Remove the peel and transfer the flesh into a bowl.

Add the lime juice, garlic, chipotle and salt, and with a fork, mash until almost smooth.

Stir in onion and cilantro and refrigerate, covered for about 1 hour before serving.

Nutrition: Calories: 230; Total Fat: 21.9 g; Saturated Fat: 4.6g Cholesterol: 0 mg; Sodium: 46 mg; Total Carbs: 9.7 g; Fiber: 6.9 g; Sugar: 0.8 g; Protein: 2.1 g.

575 POTATO LATKE

Preparation Time: 15 minutes
Cooking Time: 10 minutes
Servings: 6
Ingredients:

3 eggs, beaten
1 onion, grated
1 ½ tsp. baking powder
Salt and pepper to taste
2 lb. potatoes, peeled and grated
¼ cup all-purpose flour
4 tbsp. vegetable oil
Chopped onion chives

Directions:

Prep your oven to 400°F.

Scourge eggs, onion, baking powder, salt and pepper.

Squeeze moisture from the shredded potatoes using a paper towel.

Add potatoes to the egg mixture.

Stir in the flour.

Fill the oil into a pan over medium heat.

Cook a small amount of the batter for 3 to 4 minutes per side.

Repeat. Garnish with the chives.

Nutrition: Calories: 266; Carbohydrates: 34.6 g; Protein: 7.6 g.

576 BROCCOLI RABE

Preparation Time: 15 minutes
Cooking Time: 15 minutes
Servings: 8
Ingredients:

2 oranges, sliced in half

1 lb. broccoli rabe
2 tbsp. sesame oil, toasted
Salt and pepper to taste
1 tbsp. sesame seeds, toasted

Directions:

Fill the oil into a pan over medium heat.

Add the oranges and cook until caramelized.

Transfer to a plate.

Put the broccoli in the pan and cook for 8 minutes.

Squeeze the oranges to release juice in a bowl.

Stir in the oil, salt and pepper.

Coat the broccoli rabe with the mixture.

Sprinkle seeds on top.

Nutrition: Calories: 59; Carbohydrates: 4.1 g; Protein: 2.2 g.

577 HONEY ALMOND RICOTTA SPREAD WITH PEACHES

Preparation Time: 5 minutes
Cooking Time: 8 minutes
Servings: 4
Ingredients:

½ cup Fisher Sliced Almonds
1 cup whole milk ricotta
¼ tsp. almond extract
zest from an orange, optional
1 tsp. honey
hearty whole-grain toast
English muffin or bagel
extra Fisher sliced almonds
sliced peaches
extra honey for drizzling

Directions:

Cut peaches into a proper shape and then brush them with olive oil. After that, set it aside. Take a bowl; combine the ingredients for the filling. Set aside.

Then just preheat the grill to medium. Place peaches cut side down onto the greased grill. Close lid cover and then just grill until the peaches have softened, approximately 6-10 minutes, depending on the size of the peaches.

Then you will have to place peach halves onto a serving plate. Put a spoon of about 1 tablespoon of ricotta mixture into the cavity (you are also allowed to use a small scooper).

Sprinkle it with slivered almonds, crushed amaretti cookies, and honey. Decorate with the mint leaves.

Nutrition: Calories: 187; Protein: 7 g; Fat: 9 g; Carbs: 18 g.

578 GREEK YOGURT PANCAKES

Preparation Time: 10 minutes
Cooking Time: 5 minutes
Servings: 2
Ingredients:

1 cup all-purpose flour
1 cup whole-wheat flour
¼ tsp. salt
4 tsp. baking powder
1 tbsp. sugar
1 ½ cups unsweetened almond milk
2 tsp. vanilla extract
2 large eggs
½ cup plain 2% Greek yogurt
Fruit, for serving
Maple syrup, for serving

Directions:

First, you will have to pour the curds into the bowl and mix them well until creamy. After that, you will have to add egg whites and mix them well until combined.

Then take a separate bowl, pour the wet mixture into the dry mixture. Stir to combine. The batter will be extremely thick.

Then, simply spoon the batter onto the sprayed pan heated too medium-high. The batter must make 4 large pancakes.

Then, you will have to flip the pancakes once when they start to bubble a bit on the surface. Cook until golden brown on both sides.

Nutrition: Calories: 166; Protein: 14 g; Fat: 5 g; Carbs: 52 g.

579 5-MINUTE HEIRLOOM TOMATO & CUCUMBER TOAST

Preparation Time: 10 minutes
Cooking Time: 6-10 minutes
Servings: 1
Ingredients:

1 small Heirloom tomato
1 Persian cucumber
1 tsp. olive oil
1 pinch oregano
Kosher salt and pepper as desired
2 tsp. Low-fat whipped cream cheese
2 pieces Trader Joe's Whole Grain Crispbread or your choice
1 tsp. balsamic glaze

Directions:

Dice the cucumber and tomato. Combine all the fixings, except for the cream cheese. Smear the cheese on the bread and add the mixture. Top it off with the balsamic glaze and serve.

Nutrition: Calories: 239; Carbs: 32 g; Fat: 11 g; Protein: 7 g.

580 GREEK YOGURT WITH WALNUTS AND HONEY

Preparation Time: 5 minutes
Cooking Time: 0 minutes
Servings: 4
Ingredients:

- 4 cups Greek yogurt, fat-free, plain or vanilla
- ½ cup California walnuts, toasted, chopped
- 3 tbsp. honey or agave nectar
- Fresh fruit, chopped or granola, low-fat (both optional)

Directions:

Spoon yogurt into 4 individual cups. Sprinkle 2 tablespoons of walnuts over each and drizzle 2 tablespoons of honey over each. Top with fruit or granola, whichever is preferred.

Nutrition: Calories 300; Fat: 10 g; Carbs: 25 g; Protein: 29 g.

581 TAHINI PINE NUTS TOAST

Preparation Time: 5 minutes
Cooking Time: 0 minutes
Servings: 2
Ingredients:

- 2 whole-wheat bread slices, toasted
- 1 tsp. water
- 1 tbsp. tahini paste
- 2 tsp. feta cheese, crumbled
- Juice of ½ lemon
- 2 tsp. pine nuts
- A pinch of black pepper

Directions:

In a bowl, mix the tahini with the water and the lemon juice, whisk well, and spread over the toasted bread slices. Top each serving with the remaining ingredients and serve for breakfast.

Nutrition: Calories: 142; Fat: 7.6 g; Carbs: 13.7 g; Protein: 5.8 g.

582 FETA - AVOCADO & MASHED CHICKPEA TOAST

Preparation Time: 10 minutes
Cooking Time: 15 minutes
Servings: 4
Ingredients:

- 15 oz. can Chickpeas
- 2 oz. - ½ cup Diced feta cheese
- 1 Pitted avocado

Fresh juice:

- 2 tsp. Lemon (or 1 tbsp. orange)
- ½ tsp. Black pepper
- 2 tsp. Honey
- 4 slices Multigrain toast

Directions:

Toast the bread. Drain the chickpeas in a colander. Scoop the avocado flesh into the bowl. Use a large fork/potato masher to mash them until the mix is spreadable.

Pour in the lemon juice, pepper, and feta. Combine and divide onto the four slices of toast. Drizzle using the honey and serve.

Nutrition: Calories: 337; Carbs: 43 g; Fat: 13 g; Protein: 13 g.

583 BLUEBERRY, HAZELNUT, AND LEMON BREAKFAST GRAIN SALAD

Preparation Time: 5 minutes
Cooking Time: 10 minutes
Servings: 8
Ingredients:

- 1 cup steel-cut oats
- 1 cup dry golden quinoa
- ½ cup dry millet
- 3 tbsp. olive oil, divided
- ¾ tsp. salt
- 1 x 1" piece fresh ginger, peeled and cut into coins
- 2 large lemons, zest and juice
- ½ cup maple syrup
- 1 cup Greek yogurt
- ¼ tsp. nutmeg
- 2 cups hazelnuts, roughly chopped and toasted
- 2 cups blueberries or mixed berries
- 4 ½ cups water

Directions:

Grab a mesh strainer and add the oats, quinoa, and millet. Wash well then pop to one side. Find a 3-quart saucepan; add 1 tablespoon of the oil, and pop over medium heat.

Add the grains and cook for 2-3 minutes to toast. Pour in the water, salt, ginger coins, and lemon zest. Bring to the boil then cover and turn down the heat. Leave to simmer for 20 minutes.

Turn off the heat and leave to sit for five minutes. Fluff with a fork, remove the ginger then leave to cool for at least an hour. Grab a large bowl and add the grains.

Take a medium bowl and add the remaining olive oil, lemon juice, maple syrup, yogurt, and nutmeg. Whisk well to combine. Pour this over the grains and stir well.

Add the hazelnuts and blueberries, stir again then pop into the fridge overnight. Serve and enjoy.

Nutrition: Calories 363; Fat: 11 g; Carbs: 60 g; Protein: 7 g.

584 BLUEBERRY GREEK YOGURT PANCAKES

Preparation Time: 15 minutes
Cooking Time: 15 minutes
Servings: 6
Ingredients:

- 1 ¼ cup all-purpose flour
- 2 tsp. baking powder
- 1 tsp. baking soda
- ¼ tsp. salt
- ¼ cup sugar
- 3 eggs
- 3 tbsp. vegan butter unsalted, melted
- ½ cup milk
- 1 ½ cups Greek yogurt plain, non-fat
- ½ cup blueberries optional

Toppings:

- Greek yogurt
- Mixed berries – blueberries, raspberries and blackberries

Directions:

In a large bowl, whisk together the flour, salt, baking powder and baking soda. In a separate bowl, whisk together butter, sugar, eggs, Greek yogurt, and milk until the mixture is smooth.

Then add in the Greek yogurt mixture from step to the dry mixture in step 1, mix to combine, allow the patter to sit for 20 minutes to get a smooth texture – if using blueberries fold them into the pancake batter.

Heat the pancake griddle, spray with non-stick butter spray or just brush with butter. Pour the batter, in ¼ cupfuls, onto the griddle.

Cook until the bubbles on top burst and create small holes, lift up the corners of the pancake to see if they're golden browned on the bottom.

With a wide spatula, flip the pancake and cook on the other side until lightly browned. Serve.

Nutrition: Calories: 258; Carbohydrates: 33 g; Fat: 8 g; Protein: 11 g.

585 CHEESY GARDEN VEGGIE CRUSTLESS QUICHE

Preparation Time: 5 minutes
Cooking Time: 25 minutes
Servings: 4
Ingredients:

- ½ tbsp. grass-fed butter, divided
- 6 eggs
- ¾ cup heavy (whipping) cream
- 1 oz. goat cheese, divided
- ½ cup sliced mushrooms, chopped
- ¼ cup scallion, white and green parts, chopped
- 1 cup shredded fresh spinach
- 10 cherry tomatoes, cut in half

Directions:

Preheat the oven. Set the oven temperature to 350°F. Grease a 9-inch pie plate with ½ teaspoon of butter and set it aside.

Mix the quiche base. In a medium bowl, whisk the eggs, cream, and 2 ounces of the cheese until it's all well blended. Set it aside.

Sauté the vegetables. In a small skillet over medium-high heat, melt the remaining butter. Add the mushrooms and scallion and sauté them until they've softened, about 2 minutes. Add the spinach and sauté until it's wilted, about 2 minutes.

Assemble and bake. Spread the vegetable mixture in the bottom of the pie plate and pour the egg-and-cream mixture over the vegetables. Scatter the cherry tomatoes and the remaining 1 ounce of goat cheese on top. Bake for 20 to 25 minutes until the quiche is cooked through, puffed, and lightly browned.

Serve. Cut the quiche into wedges and divide it between four plates. Serve it warm or cold.

Nutrition: Macronutrients: Fat: 75%; Protein: 20%; Carbs: 5% Calories: 355; Total fat: 30 g; Total carbs: 5 g; Fiber: 1 g; Net carbs: 4 g; Sodium: 228 mg; Protein: 18 g.

586 MEDITERRANEAN FILLING STUFFED PORTOBELLO MUSHROOMS

Preparation Time: 10 minutes
Cooking Time: 35 minutes
Servings: 4
Ingredients:

4 large portobello mushroom caps
3 tbsp. good-quality olive oil, divided
1 cup chopped fresh spinach
1 red bell pepper, chopped
1 celery stalk, chopped
½ cup chopped sun-dried tomato
¼ onion, chopped
1 tsp. minced garlic
1 tsp. chopped fresh oregano
2 cups chopped pecans
¼ cup balsamic vinaigrette
Sea salt, for seasoning
Freshly ground black pepper, for seasoning

Directions:

Preheat the oven. Set the oven temperature to 350°F. Line a baking sheet with parchment paper.

Prepare the mushrooms. Use a spoon to scoop the black gills out of the mushrooms. Massage 2 tablespoons of olive oil all over

the mushroom caps and place the mushrooms on the prepared baking sheet. Set them aside.

Prepare the filling. In a large skillet over medium-high heat, warm the remaining 1 tablespoon of olive oil. Add the spinach, red bell pepper, celery, sun-dried tomato, onion, garlic, and oregano and sauté until the vegetables are tender, about 10 minutes. Stir in the pecans and balsamic vinaigrette and season the mixture with salt and pepper.

Assemble and bake. Stuff the mushroom caps with the filling and bake for 20 to 25 minutes until they're tender and golden.

Serve. Place one stuffed mushroom on each of four plates and serve them hot.

Nutrition: Macronutrients: Fat: 80%; Protein: 7%; Carbs: 13% Calories: 595; Total fat: 56 g; Total carbs: 18 g; Fiber: 9 g; Net carbs: 9 g; Sodium: 51m g; Protein: 10 g.

587 ZUCCHINI ROLL MANICOTTI

Preparation Time: 15 minutes
Cooking Time: 30 minutes
Servings: 4
Ingredients:

Olive oil cooking spray
4 zucchinis
2 tbsp. good-quality olive oil
1 red bell pepper, diced
½ onion, minced
1 tsp. minced garlic
1 cup goat cheese
1 cup shredded mozzarella cheese
1 tbsp. chopped fresh oregano
Sea salt, for seasoning
Freshly ground black pepper, for seasoning
2 cups low-carb marinara sauce, divided
½ cup grated Parmesan cheese

Directions:

Preheat the oven. Set the temperature to 375°F. Lightly grease a 9-by-13-inch baking dish with olive oil cooking spray.

Prepare the zucchini. Cut the zucchini lengthwise into ⅛-inch-thick slices and set them aside.

Make the filling. In a medium skillet over medium-high heat, warm the olive oil. Add the red bell pepper, onion, and garlic and sauté until they've softened, about 4 minutes. Remove the skillet from the heat and transfer the vegetables to a medium bowl. Stir the goat cheese, mozzarella, and oregano into the vegetables. Season it all with salt and pepper.

Assemble the manicotti. Spread 1 cup of the marinara sauce in the bottom of the baking dish. Lay a zucchini slice on a clean cutting board and place a couple of tablespoons of filling at one end. Roll the slice up and place it in the baking dish, seam-side down. Repeat with the remaining zucchini slices. Spoon the remaining sauce over the rolls and top with the Parmesan.

Bake. Bake the rolls for 30 to 35 minutes until the zucchini is tender and the cheese is golden.

Serve. Spoon the rolls onto four plates and serve them hot.

Nutrition: Macronutrients: Fat: 63%; Protein: 14%; Carbs: 23% Calories: 342; Total fat: 24 g; Total carbs: 14 g; Fiber: 3 g; Net carbs: 11 g; Sodium: 331 mg; Protein: 20 g.

588 SPINACH ARTICHOKE STUFFED PEPPERS

Preparation Time: 10 minutes
Cooking Time: 20 minutes
Servings: 4
Ingredients:

4 red bell peppers, halved and seeded
2 tbsp. good-quality olive oil, for drizzling
Sea salt, for seasoning
Freshly ground black pepper, for seasoning
2 cups finely chopped cauliflower
10 oz. chopped fresh spinach
2 cups chopped marinated artichoke hearts
1 cup cream cheese, softened
1 ½ cups shredded mozzarella cheese, divided
½ cup sour cream - tbsp. mayonnaise - tsp. minced garlic

Directions:

Preheat the oven. Set the temperature to 400°F. Line a baking sheet with parchment paper.

Prepare the peppers. Place the red bell peppers cut-side up on the baking sheet. Lightly grease them all over with olive oil and season them with salt and pepper.

Make the filling. In a large bowl, mix together the cauliflower, spinach, artichoke hearts, cream cheese, ¾ cup of the mozzarella, and the sour cream, mayonnaise, and garlic.

Stuff and bake. Stuff the peppers with the filling and sprinkle with the remaining ¾ cup of mozzarella. Bake them for 20 to 25 minutes until the filling is heated through, bubbly, and lightly browned.

Serve. Place one stuffed pepper on each of the four plates and serve them hot.

Nutrition: Macronutrients: Fat: 72%; Protein: 16%; Carbs: 12% Calories: 523; Total fat: 43 g; Total carbs: 19 g; Fiber: 7 g; Net carbs: 12 g; Sodium: 355 mg; Protein: 19 g.

589 PESTO-GLAZED CAULIFLOWER STEAKS WITH FRESH BASIL AND MOZZARELLA

Preparation Time: 10 minutes
Cooking Time: 20 minutes
Servings: 4
Ingredients:

Olive oil cooking spray
1 head cauliflower, cut into "steaks" about 1 inch thick
¼ cup Spinach Basil Pesto
1 cup shredded mozzarella cheese
¼ cup chopped marinated artichoke hearts
¼ cup chopped sun-dried tomatoes
¼ cup sliced olives
1 tbsp. pine nuts

Directions:

Preheat the oven. Set the temperature to 400°F. Lightly grease a baking sheet with olive oil cooking spray.

Assemble the cauliflower steaks and place them in a single layer on the baking sheet. Spread 1 tablespoon of pesto on each. Sprinkle with the mozzarella and top with the artichoke hearts, sun-dried tomatoes, olives, and pine nuts.

Bake the cauliflower for 20 minutes until the edges are crispy and the cheese is bubbly and melted.

Divide the cauliflower between four plates and serve it hot.

Nutrition: Macronutrients: Fat: 65%; Protein: 18%; Carbs: 17% Calories: 316; Total fat: 23 g; Total carbs: 14 g; Fiber: 6 g; Net carbs: 8 g; Sodium: 465 mg; Protein: 14 g.

590 ZUCCHINI PASTA WITH SPINACH, OLIVES, AND ASIAGO

Preparation Time: 10 minutes
Cooking Time: 10 minutes
Servings: 4
Ingredients:

3 tbsp. good-quality olive oil
2 tbsp. grass-fed butter
1 ½ tbsp. minced garlic
1 cup packed fresh spinach
½ cup sliced black olives
½ cup halved cherry tomatoes
1 tbsp. chopped fresh basil
3 zucchini, spiralized

Sea salt, for seasoning
Freshly ground black pepper, for seasoning
½ cup shredded Asiago cheese

Directions:

Sauté the vegetables. In a large skillet over medium-high heat, warm the olive oil and butter. Add the garlic and sauté until it's tender, about 2 minutes. Stir in the spinach, olives, tomatoes, and basil and sauté until the spinach is wilted, about 4 minutes. Stir in the zucchini noodles, toss to combine them with the sauce, and cook until the zucchini is tender, about 2 minutes.

Season with salt and pepper. Divide the mixture between four bowls and serve topped with the Asiago.

Nutrition: Macronutrients: Fat: 80%; Protein: 13%; Carbs: 7% Calories: 199; Total fat: 18 g; Total carbs: 4 g; Fiber: 1 g; Net carbs: 3 g; Sodium: 363 mg; Protein: 6 g.

591 VEGETARIAN CHILI WITH AVOCADO AND SOUR CREAM

Preparation Time: 10 minutes
Cooking Time: 25 minutes
Servings: 8
Ingredients:

2 tbsp. good-quality olive oil
½ onion, finely chopped
1 Red bell pepper, diced
1 Jalapeño peppers, chopped
1 tbsp. minced garlic
1 tbsp. chili powder
1 tsp. ground cumin
2 cups canned diced tomatoes
2 cups pecans, chopped
1 cup sour cream
2 avocado, diced
1 tbsp. chopped fresh cilantro

Directions:

Sauté the vegetables. In a large pot over medium-high heat, warm the olive oil. Add the onion, red bell pepper, jalapeño peppers, and garlic and sauté until they've softened, about 4 minutes. Stir in the chili powder and cumin, stirring to coat the vegetables with the spices.

Cook the chili. Stir in the tomatoes and pecans and bring the chili to a boil, then reduce the heat to low and simmer until the vegetables are soft and the flavors mellow, about 20 minutes.

Serve. Ladle the chili into bowls and serve it with sour cream, avocado, and cilantro.

Nutrition: Macronutrients: Fat: 80%; Protein: 7%; Carbs: 13% Calories: 332; Total

fat: 32 g; Total carbs: 11 g; Fiber: 6 g; Net carbs: 5 g; Sodium: 194 mg; Protein: 5 g.

592 VEGETABLE VODKA SAUCE BAKE

Preparation Time: 10 minutes
Cooking Time: 30 minutes
Servings: 4
Ingredients:

3 tbsp. melted grass-fed butter, divided
4 cups mushrooms, halved
4 cups cooked cauliflower florets
1 ½ cups purchased vodka sauce
¾ cup heavy (whipping) cream
½ cup grated Asiago cheese
Sea salt, for seasoning
Freshly ground black pepper, for seasoning
1 cup shredded provolone cheese
1 tbsp. chopped fresh oregano

Directions:

Preheat the oven. Set the oven temperature to 350°F and use 1 tablespoon of the melted butter to grease a 9-by-13-inch baking dish.

Mix the vegetables. In a large bowl, combine the mushrooms, cauliflower, vodka sauce, cream, Asiago, and the remaining 2 tablespoons of butter. Season the vegetables with salt and pepper.

Bake. Transfer the vegetable mixture to the baking dish and top it with the provolone cheese. Bake for 30 to 35 minutes until it's bubbly and heated through.

Serve. Divide the mixture between four plates and top with the oregano.

Nutrition: Macronutrients: Fat: 75%; Protein: 10%; Carbs: 15% Calories: 537; Total fat: 45 g; Total carbs: 14 g; Fiber: 6 g; Net carbs: 8 g; Sodium: 527 mg; Protein: 19 g.

593 EASY CHEESY ARTICHOKES

Preparation Time: 5 minutes
Cooking Time: 5 minutes
Servings: 3
Ingredients:

3 medium-sized artichokes, cleaned and trimmed
3 cloves garlic, smashed
3 tbsp. butter, melted
Sea salt, to taste
½ tsp. cayenne pepper
¼ tsp. ground black pepper, or more to taste
lemon, freshly squeezed
1 cup Monterey-Jack cheese, shredded
1 tbsp. fresh parsley, roughly chopped

Directions:

Start by adding 1 cup of water and a steamer basket to the Instant Pot.

Place the artichokes in the steamer basket; add garlic and butter.

Secure the lid. Choose "Manual" mode and High pressure; cook for 8 minutes. Once cooking is complete, use a quick pressure release; carefully remove the lid.

Season your artichokes with salt, cayenne pepper, and black pepper. Now, drizzle them with lemon juice.

Top with cheese and parsley and serve immediately. Bon appétit!

Nutrition: Calories: 173; Fat: 12.5g; Carbs: 9g; Protein: 8.1g; Sugars: 0.9 g.

594 CHINESE BOK CHOY

Preparation Time: 2 minutes
Cooking Time: 8 minutes
Servings: 4
Ingredients:

2 tbsp. butter, melted
2 cloves garlic, minced
(½-inch) slice fresh ginger root, grated
½ pounds Bok choy, trimmed
1 cup vegetable stock
Celery salt and ground black pepper to taste
1 tsp. Five-spice powder
1 tbsp. soy sauce

Directions:

Press the "Sauté" button to heat up the Instant Pot. Now, warm the butter and sauté the garlic until tender and fragrant.

Now, add grated ginger and cook for a further 40 seconds.

Add Bok choy, stock, salt, black pepper, and Five-spice powder.

Secure the lid. Choose "Manual" mode and High pressure; cook for 6 minutes. Once cooking is complete, use a quick pressure release; carefully remove the lid.

Drizzle soy sauce over your Bok choy and serve immediately. Bon appétit!

Nutrition: Calories: 83; Fat: 6.1 g; Carbs: 5.7 g; Protein: 3.2 g; Sugars: 2.4 g.

595 GREEN CABBAGE WITH BACON

Preparation Time: 2 minutes
Cooking Time: 8 minutes
Servings: 4
Ingredients:

2 tsp. olive oil
4 slices bacon, chopped
1 head green cabbage, cored and cut into wedges
2 cups vegetable stock
Sea salt, to taste
½ tsp. whole black peppercorns
1 tsp. cayenne pepper

2 bay leaf
Directions:

Press the "Sauté" button to heat up the Instant Pot. Then, heat olive oil and cook the bacon until it is nice and delicately browned.

Next, add the remaining ingredients; gently stir to combine.

Secure the lid. Choose "Manual" mode and High pressure; cook for 3 minutes. Once cooking is complete, use a quick pressure release; carefully remove the lid.

Serve warm and enjoy!

Nutrition: Calories: 166; Fat: 13 g; Carbs: 7.1 g; Protein: 6.8 g; Sugars: 2.7 g.

596 WARM BROCCOLI SALAD BOWL

Preparation Time: 2 minutes
Cooking Time: 8 minutes
Servings: 4
Ingredients:

1 pound broccoli, broken into florets
1 tbsp. balsamic vinegar
2 garlic cloves, minced
1 tsp. mustard seeds
1 tsp. cumin seeds
Salt and pepper, to taste
1 cup Cottage cheese, crumbled
1 cup of water

Directions:

Place 1 cup of water and a steamer basket in your Instant Pot.

Place the broccoli in the steamer basket.

Secure the lid. Choose "Manual" mode and High pressure; cook for 5 minutes. Once cooking is complete, use a quick pressure release; carefully remove the lid.

Then, toss your broccoli with the other ingredients. Serve and enjoy!

Nutrition: Calories: 95; Fat: 3.1 g; Carbs: 8.1 g; Protein: 9.9 g; Sugars: 3.8 g.

597 CREAMED SPINACH WITH CHEESE

Preparation Time: 2 minutes
Cooking Time: 8 minutes
Servings: 4
Ingredients:

2 tbsp. butter, melted
½ cup scallions, chopped
2 cloves garlic, smashed
½ pounds fresh spinach
1 cup vegetable broth, preferably homemade
1 cup cream cheese, cubed
Seasoned salt and ground black pepper, to taste
½ tsp. dried dill weed

Directions:

Press the "Sauté" button to heat up the Instant Pot. Then, melt the

butter; cook the scallions and garlic until tender and aromatic.

Add the remaining ingredients and stir to combine well.

Secure the lid. Choose "Manual" mode and High pressure; cook for 2 minutes. Once cooking is complete, use a quick pressure release; carefully remove the lid.

Ladle into individual bowls and serve warm. Bon appétit!

Nutrition: Calories: 283; Fat: 23.9 g; Carbs: 9 g; Protein: 10.7 g; Sugars: 3.2 g.

598 TURNIP GREENS WITH SAUSAGE

Preparation Time: 2 minutes
Cooking Time: 8 minutes
Servings: 4
Ingredients:

2 tsp. sesame oil
2 pork sausages, casing removed sliced
2 garlic cloves, minced
1 medium-sized leek, chopped
1 pound turnip greens
1 cup turkey bone stock
Sea salt, to taste
¼ tsp. ground black pepper, or more to taste
1 bay leaf
1 tbsp. black sesame seeds

Directions:

Press the "Sauté" button to heat up the Instant Pot. Then, heat the sesame oil; cook the sausage until nice and delicately browned; set aside.

Add the garlic and leeks; continue cooking in pan drippings for a minute or two.

Add the greens, stock, salt, black pepper, and bay leaf.

Secure the lid. Choose "Manual" mode and Low pressure; cook for 3 minutes. Once cooking is complete, use a quick pressure release; carefully remove the lid.

Serve garnished with black sesame seeds and enjoy!

Nutrition: Calories: 149; Fat: 7.2 g; Carbs: 9 g; Protein: 14.2 g; Sugars: 2.2 g.

599 ASPARAGUS WITH COLBY CHEESE

Preparation Time: 2 minutes
Cooking Time: 8 minutes
Servings: 4
Ingredients:

½ pounds fresh asparagus
2 tbsp. olive oil
2 garlic cloves, minced
Sea salt, to taste
¼ tsp. ground black pepper
½ cup Colby cheese, shredded

Directions:

Add 1 cup of water and a steamer basket to your Instant Pot.

Now, place the asparagus on the steamer basket; drizzle your asparagus with olive oil. Scatter garlic over the top of the asparagus.

Season with salt and black pepper.

Secure the lid. Choose "Manual" mode and High pressure; cook for 1 minute. Once cooking is complete, use a quick pressure release; carefully remove the lid.

Transfer the prepared asparagus to a nice serving platter and scatter shredded cheese over the top. Enjoy!

Nutrition: Calories: 164; Fat: 12.2 g; Carbs: 8.1 g; Protein: 7.8 g; Sugars: 3.3 g.

600 MEDITERRANEAN AROMATIC ZUCCHINI

Preparation Time: 2 minutes
Cooking Time: 8 minutes
Servings: 4
Ingredients:

2 tbsp. olive oil
2 garlic cloves, chopped
1 pound zucchini, sliced
½ cup tomato purée
1 ½ cup water
tsp. dried thyme
½ tsp. dried oregano
½ tsp. dried rosemary

Directions:

Press the "Sauté" button to heat up the Instant Pot. Then, heat the olive oil; sauté the garlic until aromatic.

Add the remaining ingredients.

Secure the lid. Choose "Manual" mode and Low pressure; cook for 3 minutes. Once cooking is complete, use a quick pressure release; carefully remove the lid. Bon appétit!

Nutrition: Calories: 85; Fat: 7.1 g; Carbs: 4.7 g; Protein: 1.6 g; Sugars: 3.3 g.

601 CHANTERELLES WITH CHEDDAR CHEESE

Preparation Time: 2 minutes
Cooking Time: 8 minutes
Servings: 4
Ingredients:

2 tbsp. olive oil
2 cloves garlic, minced
(1-inch) ginger root, grated
½ tsp. dried dill weed
1 tsp. dried basil
½ tsp. dried thyme
16 oz. Chanterelle mushrooms, brushed clean and sliced
½ cup water
½ cup tomato purée

tbsp. dry white wine
⅓ tsp. freshly ground black pepper
Kosher salt, to taste
1 cup Cheddar cheese

Directions:

Press the "Sauté" button to heat up the Instant Pot. Then, heat the olive oil; sauté the garlic and grated ginger for 1 minute or until aromatic.

Add dried dill, basil, thyme, Chanterelles, water, tomato purée, dry white wine, black pepper, and salt.

Secure the lid. Choose "Manual" mode and Low pressure; cook for 5 minutes. Once cooking is complete, use a quick pressure release; carefully remove the lid.

Top with shredded cheese and serve immediately. Bon appétit!

Nutrition: Calories: 218; Fat: 15.1 g; Carbs: 9.5 g; Protein: 9.9 g; Sugars: 2.3 g.

MEAT RECIPES

602 SEASONED PORK CHOPS

Preparation Time: 10 minutes
Cooking Time: 15 minutes
Servings: 8
Ingredients:

2 garlic cloves, minced
Freshly ground black pepper, to taste
1 lime, juiced
1 tbsp. fresh basil, chopped
1 tbsp. Old Bay seafood seasoning
½ cup apple cider vinegar
½ cup olive oil
8 boneless pork chops, cut into ½ inch thick

Directions:

Add the minced garlic, black pepper, lime juice, basil, seasoning, apple cider vinegar, and olive oil to a Ziploc bag.

Place the pork chops in this bag and seal it. Shake it well to coat the pork and place it in the refrigerator for 6 hours. Continue flipping and shaking the bag every 1 hour.

Meanwhile, preheat your outdoor grill over medium-high heat.

Remove the pork chops from the Ziploc bag and discard its marinade.

Grill all the marinated pork chops for 7 minutes per side until their internal temperature reaches 145°F (63°C). Serve warm on a plate.

Nutrition: Calories: 412; Fats: 26.4 g; Total Carbs: 1.0 g; Fiber: 0.1 g; Protein: 40.0 g.

603 GARLICKY PORK ROAST

Preparation Time: 20 minutes
Cooking Time: 2 hours
Servings: 6
Ingredients:

3 pounds (1.4 kg) pork tenderloin
2 garlic cloves, minced
1 tbsp. olive oil
1 tbsp. dried rosemary

Directions:

Preheat the oven to 375°F (190°C).

Mix the garlic, olive oil, and rosemary in a bowl, then rub this mixture all over the pork tenderloin.

Place the pork tenderloin in a roasting pan and roast in the preheated oven for about 2 hours, or until the internal temperature reaches 145°F (63°C).

Once roasted, remove the tenderloin from the oven. Slice and serve warm.

Nutrition: Calories: 274; Fats: 7.4 g; Total Carbs: 1.4 g; Fiber: 0.7 g; Protein: 47.7 g.

604 SPICED PORK TENDERLOIN

Preparation Time: 10 minutes
Cooking Time: 2 hours
Servings: 4
Ingredients:

2 tsp. minced garlic
1 tbsp. fresh cilantro
dash ground black pepper
2 ½ tsp. ground cumin
1 tsp. salt
1 tbsp. chili powder
2 pounds (907 g.) pork tenderloin, cubed

Directions:

In a bowl, add the garlic, cilantro, black pepper, cumin, salt, and chili powder. Mix these spices together.

Toss in the pork cubes and coat them well with the spice mixture.

Cover the pork cubes and refrigerate them for 45 minutes to marinate.

Meanwhile, preheat the oven to 225°F (107°C).

Arrange the spiced pork in a baking tray and roast for 2 hours, or until crispy.

Remove from the oven and serve on a plate.

Nutrition: Calories: 291; Fats: 8.9 g; Total Carbs: 3.1 g; Fiber: 1.6 g; Protein: 47.7 g.

605 CHICKEN PARMESAN WRAPS

Preparation Time: 10 minutes
Cooking Time: 20 minutes
Servings: 2
Ingredients:

Nonstick cooking spray

1-pound boneless, skinless chicken breasts

1 large egg

¼ cup buttermilk

⅔ cup whole-wheat panko or whole-wheat bread crumbs

½ cup grated Parmesan cheese (about 1 ½ oz.)

¾ tsp. garlic powder, divided

1 cup canned low-sodium or no-salt-added crushed tomatoes

1 tsp. dried oregano

6 (8-inch) whole-wheat tortillas, or whole-grain spinach wraps

1 cup fresh mozzarella cheese (about 4 oz.), sliced

1 ½ cups loosely packed fresh flat-leaf (Italian) parsley, chopped

Directions:

Preheat the oven to 425°F. Line a large, rimmed baking sheet with aluminum foil. Place a wire rack on the aluminum foil, and grease the rack with nonstick cooking spray. Set aside.

Put the chicken breasts in a large, zip-top plastic bag. With a rolling pin or meat mallet, pound the chicken so it is evenly flattened, about ¼ inch thick.

Slice the chicken into six portions. (It's fine if you have to place 2 smaller pieces together to form six equal portions.)

In a wide, shallow bowl, whisk together the egg and buttermilk. In another wide, shallow bowl, mix together the panko crumbs, Parmesan cheese, and ½ teaspoon of garlic powder.

Dip each chicken breast portion into the egg mixture and then into the Parmesan crumb mixture, pressing the crumbs into the chicken so they stick. Place the chicken on the prepared wire rack.

Bake the chicken for 15 to 18 minutes, or until the internal temperature of the chicken reads 165°F on a meat thermometer and any juices run clear.

Transfer the chicken to a cutting board, and slice each portion diagonally into ½-inch pieces.

In a small, microwave-safe bowl, mix together the tomatoes, oregano, and the remaining ¼ tsp. of garlic powder.

Cover the bowl with a paper towel and microwave for about 1 minute on high, until very hot. Set aside.

Wrap the tortillas in a damp paper towel or dishcloth and microwave for 30 to 45 seconds on high, until warmed.

To assemble the wraps, divide the chicken slices evenly among the six tortillas and top with the cheese.

Spread 1 tbsp. of the warm tomato sauce over the cheese on each tortilla, and top each with about ¼ cup of parsley.

To wrap each tortilla, fold up the bottom of the tortilla, then fold one side over and fold the other side over the top. Serve the wraps immediately, with the remaining sauce for dipping.

Nutrition: Calories: 373; Total Fat: 10 g; Saturated Fat: 4 g; Cholesterol: 95 mg; Sodium: 591 mg; Total Carbohydrates: 33 g; Fiber: 8 g; Protein: 30 g.

606 FAST CHEESY BACON AND EGG WRAPS

Preparation Time: 15 minutes
Cooking Time: 10 minutes
Servings: 3
Ingredients:

3 corn tortillas

3 slices bacon, cut into strips

2 scrambled eggs

3 tbsp. salsa

1 cup grated Pepper Jack cheese

3 tbsp. cream cheese, divided

Cooking spray

Directions:

Spritz the air fry basket with cooking spray.

Unfold the tortillas on a clean work surface, divide the bacon and eggs in the middle of the tortillas, and then spread with scatter and salsa with cheeses. Fold the tortillas over.

Arrange the tortillas in the basket.

Place the basket on the air fry position.

Select Air Fry, set temperature to 390°F (199°C) and set Time to 10 minutes. Flip the tortillas halfway through the cooking time.

When cooking is complete, the cheeses will be melted and the tortillas will be lightly browned.

Serve immediately.

Nutrition: Calories: 133; Fat: 19 g; Protein: 8 g.

607 CHICKEN WRAPS WITH RICOTTA CHEESE

Preparation Time: 30 minutes
Cooking Time: 5 minutes
Servings: 12
Ingredients:

2 large-sized chicken breasts, cooked and shredded

2 spring onions, chopped

10 oz. (284 g.) Ricotta cheese

1 tbsp. rice vinegar

1 tbsp. molasses

1 tsp. grated fresh ginger

¼ cup soy sauce

⅓ tsp. sea salt

¼ tsp. ground black pepper, or more to taste

48 wonton wrappers

Cooking spray

Directions:

Spritz the perforated pan with cooking spray.

Combine all the ingredients, except for the wrappers in a large bowl. Toss to mix well.

Unfold the wrappers on a clean work surface, then divide and spoon the mixture in the middle of the wrappers.

Dab a little water on the edges of the wrappers, then fold the edge close to you over the filling. Tuck the edge under the filling and roll up to seal.

Arrange the wraps in the pan.

Select Air Fry. Set temperature to 375°Fahrenheit (190°Celsius) and Time to 5 minutes. Press Start to begin preheating.

Once preheated, place the pan into the oven. Flip the wraps halfway through the cooking time.

When cooking is complete, the wraps should be lightly browned.

Serve immediately.

Nutrition: Calories: 250; Total Fat: 10.1 g; Total Carbohydrates: 4.9 g; Protein: 34.2 g.

608 BACON AND EGG WRAPS WITH SALSA

Preparation Time: 15 minutes
Cooking Time: 10 minutes
Servings: 3
Ingredients:

3 corn tortillas

3 slices bacon, cut into strips

2 scrambled eggs

3 tbsp. salsa

1 cup grated Pepper Jack cheese

2 tbsp. cream cheese, divided

Cooking spray

Directions:

Spritz the perforated pan with cooking spray.

Unfold the tortillas on a clean work surface, divide the bacon and eggs in the middle of the tortillas, then spread with salsa and scatter with cheeses. Fold the tortillas over.

Arrange the tortillas in the pan.

Select Air Fry. Set temperature to 390°Fahrenheit (199°Celsius) and Time to 10 minutes. Press Start to begin preheating.

Once the oven has preheated, place the pan into the oven. Flip the tortillas halfway through the cooking time.

When cooking is complete, the cheeses will be melted and the tortillas will be lightly browned.

Serve immediately.

Nutrition: Calories: 290; Total Fat: 10.5 g; Total Carbohydrates: 23.2 g; Protein: 27.3 g.

609 CHICKEN-LETTUCE WRAPS

Preparation Time: 15 minutes
Cooking Time: 12 to 16 minutes
Servings: 2 to 4
Ingredients:

1 pound (454 g.) boneless, skinless chicken thighs, trimmed
1 tsp. vegetable oil
1 tbsp. lime juice
1 shallot, minced
1 tbsp. fish sauce, plus extra for serving
1 tsp. packed brown sugar
1 garlic clove, minced
⅛ tsp. red pepper flakes
1 mango, peeled, pitted, and cut into ¼inch pieces
⅓ cup chopped fresh mint
⅓ cup chopped fresh cilantro
⅓ cup chopped fresh Thai basil
1 head Bibb lettuce, leaves separated (8 oz. / 227 g.)
¼ cup chopped dry-roasted peanuts
Thai chiles, stemmed and sliced thin

Directions:

Pat the chicken dry with paper towels and rub with oil. Place the chicken in the air fryer basket. Select the Air Fry function and cook at 400°Fahrenheit (204°Celsius) for 12 to 16 minutes, or until the chicken registers 175°Fahrenheit (79°Celsius), flipping and rotating chicken halfway through cooking.

Meanwhile, whisk lime juice, shallot, fish sauce, sugar, garlic, and pepper flakes together in a large bowl; set aside.

Transfer chicken to cutting board, let cool slightly, then shred into bite-size pieces using 2 forks. Add the shredded chicken, mango, mint, cilantro, and basil to bowl with dressing and toss to coat.

Serve the chicken in the lettuce leaves, passing peanuts, Thai chiles, and extra fish sauce separately.

Nutrition: Calories: 311; Fat: 11 g; Carbohydrate: 22 g; Protein: 31 g.

610 CHICKEN PITA

Preparation Time: 10 minutes
Cooking Time: 9 to 11 minutes
Servings: 4
Ingredients:

2 boneless, skinless chicken breasts, cut into 1-inch cubes
1 small red onion, sliced
1 red bell pepper, sliced
⅓ cup Italian salad dressing, divided
½ tsp. dried thyme
4 pita pockets, split
2 cups torn butter lettuce
1 cup chopped cherry tomatoes

Directions:

Select the Bake function and preheat Maxx to 380°Fahrenheit (193°Celsius).

Place the chicken, onion, and bell pepper in the air fryer basket. Drizzle with 1 tablespoon of the Italian salad dressing, add the thyme and toss.

Bake for 9 to 11 minutes, or until the chicken is 165°Fahrenheit (74°Celsius) on a food thermometer, stirring once during cooking time.

Transfer the chicken and vegetables to a bowl and toss with the remaining salad dressing.

Assemble sandwiches with pita pockets, butter lettuce, and cherry tomatoes. Serve immediately.

Nutrition: Calories: 311; Fat: 11 g; Carbohydrates: 22 g; Protein: 31 g.

611 DELICIOUS QUINOA & DRIED FIGS

Preparation Time: 10 minutes
Cooking Time: 17 minutes
Servings: 2
Ingredients:

3 cups water
¼ cup cashew nut
8 dried apricots
4 dried figs
1 tsp. cinnamon

Directions:

In a pot, mix water and quinoa.
Let simmer for 15 minutes, until the water evaporates.
Chop dried fruit.
When quinoa is cooked, stir in all other ingredients.
Serve cold. Add milk, if desired.

Nutrition: Carbs: 44; Fat: 7 g; Protein: 13g; Calories: 285.

612 LETTUCE FAJITA MEATBALL WRAPS

Preparation Time: 10 minutes
Cooking Time: 10 minutes

Servings: 4
Ingredients:

1 pound (454 g.) 85% lean ground beef
½ cup salsa, plus more for serving
¼ cup chopped onions
¼ cup diced green or red bell peppers
1 large egg, beaten
1 tsp. fine sea salt - ½ tsp. chili powder
½ tsp. ground cumin
1 clove garlic, minced
Cooking spray

For Servings:

8 leaves Boston lettuce
Pico de Gallo or salsa
Lime slices

Directions:

Grease the air fryer basket with cooking spray.

In a large bowl, mix together all the ingredients until well combined.

Shape the meat mixture into eight 1-inch balls. Place the meatballs in the air fryer basket, leaving a little space between them.

Select the Air Fry function and cook at 350°F (177°C) for 10 minutes, or until cooked through and no longer pink inside and the internal temperature reaches 145°F (63°C).

Serve each meatball on a lettuce leaf, topped with Pico de Gallo or salsa. Serve with lime slices.

Nutrition: Calories: 576; Fat: 49 g; Total Carbohydrates: 8 g; Fiber: 2 g; Protein: 25 g.

613 KOREAN BEEF AND ONION TACOS

Preparation Time: 1 hour 15 minutes
Cooking Time: 12 minutes
Servings: 6
Ingredients:

2 tbsp. gochujang
1 tbsp. soy sauce
2 tbsp. sesame seeds
2 tsp. minced fresh ginger
2 cloves garlic, minced
2 tbsp. toasted sesame oil
2 tsp. sugar
½ tsp. kosher salt
1 ½ pounds (680 g.) thinly sliced beef chuck
1 medium red onion, sliced
6 corn tortillas, warmed
¼ cup chopped fresh cilantro
½ cup kimchi
½ cup chopped green onions

Directions:

Combine the ginger, garlic, gochujang, sesame seeds, soy sauce, sesame oil, salt, and sugar in a large bowl. Stir to mix well.

Dunk the beef chunk in the large bowl. Press to submerge, then wrap the bowl in plastic and refrigerate to marinate for at least 1 hour.

Remove the beef chunk from the marinade and transfer to the air fry basket. Add the onion to the basket.

Place the basket on the air fry position.

Select Air Fry, set temperature to 400°F (205°C) and Time to 12 minutes. Stir the mixture halfway through the cooking time.

When cooked, the beef will be well browned.

Unfold the tortillas on a clean work surface, divide the fried beef and onion on the tortillas. Spread the green onions, kimchi, and cilantro on top.

Serve immediately.

Nutrition: Calories: 181; Proteins: 3 g; Fat: 98 g; Carbs: 42 g.

614 CRUNCHY CHICKEN EGG ROLLS

Preparation Time: 10 minutes
Cooking Time: 24 minutes
Servings: 4
Ingredients:

1 pound (454 g.) ground chicken
2 tsp. olive oil
2 garlic cloves, minced
1 tsp. grated fresh ginger
2 cups white cabbage, shredded
1 onion, chopped
¼ cup soy sauce
8 egg roll wrappers
1 egg, beaten
Cooking spray

Directions:

Spritz the air fry basket with cooking spray.

Heat olive oil in a saucepan over medium heat. Sauté the garlic and ginger in the olive oil for 1 minute, or until fragrant. Add the ground chicken to the saucepan. Sauté for 5 minutes, or until the chicken is cooked through. Add the cabbage, onion and soy sauce and sauté for 5 to 6 minutes, or until the vegetables become soft. Remove the saucepan from the heat.

Unfold the egg roll wrappers on a clean work surface. Divide the chicken mixture among the wrappers and brush the edges of the wrappers with the beaten egg. Tightly roll up the egg rolls, enclosing the filling. Arrange the rolls in the basket.

Place the basket on the air fry position.

Select Air Fry, set temperature to 370°F (188°C) and Time to 12 minutes.

Flip the rolls halfway through the cooking time.

When cooked, the rolls will be crispy and golden brown.

Transfer to a platter and let cool for 5 minutes before serving.

Nutrition: Calories: 181; Proteins: 3 g; Fat: 98 g; Carbs: 42 g.

615 GOLDEN CHICKEN AND YOGURT TAQUITOS

Preparation Time: 15 minutes
Cooking Time: 12 minutes
Servings: 4
Ingredients:

1 cup cooked chicken, shredded
¼ cup Greek yogurt
¼ cup salsa
1 cup shredded Mozzarella cheese
Salt and ground black pepper, to taste
4 flour tortillas
Cooking spray

Directions:

Spritz the air fry basket with cooking spray.

Combine all the ingredients except for the tortillas, in a large bowl. Stir to mix well.

Make the taquitos: Unfold the tortillas on a clean work surface, then scoop up 2 tablespoons of the chicken mixture in the middle of each tortilla. Roll the tortillas up to wrap the filling.

Arrange the taquitos in the basket and spritz with cooking spray.

Place the basket on the air fry position.

Select Air Fry, set temperature to 380°F (193°C) and Time to 12 minutes. Flip the taquitos halfway through the cooking time.

When cooked, the taquitos should be golden brown and the cheese should be melted.

Serve immediately.

Nutrition: Calories: 153; Fat: 15 g; Protein: 9 g.

616 BASIL-RUBBED PORK CHOPS

Preparation Time: 15 minutes
Cooking Time: 25 minutes
Servings: 4
Ingredients:

4 (8-oz. / 227-g.) pork chops
lime, juiced
¼ cup fresh basil, chopped
4 garlic cloves, minced
Salt and freshly ground black pepper, to taste
1 tbsp. olive oil

Directions:

Place the pork chops in a baking tray and drizzle lime juice over them

to coat. Rub the basil, garlic, salt and black pepper over the chops.

Cover the chops and let stand for about 30 minutes.

Meanwhile, preheat an outdoor grill on medium heat, and lightly grease its grate with olive oil.

Transfer the marinated pork chops to the grill and cook for 10 minutes per side until the internal temperature reaches 145°F (63°C).

Let cool for about 5 minutes before serving.

Nutrition: Calories: 512; Fats: 28.5 g; Total Carbs: 2.1 g; Fiber: 0.2 g; Protein: 58.4 g.

617 KALAMATA PARSLEY TAPENADE AND SALTED LAMB CHOPS

Preparation Time: 15 minutes
Cooking Time: 25 minutes
Servings: 4
Ingredients:
Tapenade:

1 cup pitted Kalamata olive
1 tsp. minced garlic
2 tbsp. extra-virgin olive oil
2 tbsp. chopped fresh parsley
2 tsp. freshly squeezed lemon juice

Lamb chops:

2 (1-pound / 454-g.) racks French-cut lamb chops (8 bones each)
Sea salt and ground black pepper, to taste
tbsp. olive oil

Directions:
Make the tapenade:

In a food processor, add the olives, garlic, olive oil, parsley, and lemon juice and blend well until it becomes slightly chunky purée.

Add the purée to a container. Cover with a plastic wrap and reserve in the refrigerator until ready to use.

Prepare the lamb chops:

Preheat the oven to 450°F (235°C).

Sprinkle the lamb racks with salt and pepper.

Heat olive oil in a skillet over medium-high heat. Sear for about 5 minutes until the lamb racks are browned. Flip the lamb racks halfway through the cooking time.

Turn the racks and interlace the bones. Roast in the preheated oven for about 20 minutes to get medium-rare results.

Allow the lamb to rest for about 10 minutes, then slice into chops.

Serve the chops equally to 4 plates, then top with the tapenade before serving.

Nutrition: Calories: 347; Fats: 27.0 g; Total Carbs: 2.0 g; Fiber: 1.0 g; Protein: 20.0 g.

618 BEEF TENDERLOIN STEAKS WRAPPED WITH BACON

Preparation Time: 10 minutes
Cooking Time: 15 minutes
Servings: 4
Ingredients:

- 4 (4-oz. / 113-g.) beef tenderloin steaks
- Sea salt and ground black pepper to taste
- 8 bacon slices
- 1 tbsp. extra-virgin olive oil

Directions:

Preheat the oven to 450°F (235°C) and line the baking sheet with parchment paper.

Arrange the steaks on a flat surface. Sprinkle with salt and pepper.

Wrap each steak tightly at the edges with 2 bacon slices and use toothpicks to secure.

Heat the olive oil in a skillet over medium-high heat.

Pan sear each side of the steaks for about 4 minutes and transfer to the baking sheet.

Roast the steaks in the preheated oven for 6 minutes until they are well browned on both sides.

Transfer the steaks to a flat surface to cool for about 10 minutes.

Remove the toothpicks before serving.

Nutrition: Calories: 564; Fats: 48.0 g; Total Carbs: 0 g; Fiber: 0 g; Protein: 27.0 g.

619 SAUSAGE, BEEF AND CHILI RECIPE

Preparation Time: 20 minutes
Cooking Time: 8 hours
Servings: 6
Ingredients:

- pound (454 g.) mild bulk sausage
- pound (454 g.) ground beef
- 4 minced cloves garlic
- ½ chopped medium yellow onion
- diced green bell pepper
- (14 ½-oz. / 411-g.) can diced tomatoes with juices
- 1 ½ tsp. ground cumin
- 1 tbsp. chili powder
- 1 (6-oz. / 170-g.) can low-carb tomato paste
- ⅓ cup water

Toppings:

- 1 cup sour cream
- ½ cup sliced green onions
- tbsp. sliced jalapeños
- ½ cup shredded Cheddar cheese

Directions:

In a pot, add sausage and beef. Cook until browned. Break the clumps with a wooden spoon. Pat dry with paper towels. Reserve half of the meat for drippings.

Transfer the meat to a slow cooker. Add the reserved drippings, garlic, onion, bell pepper, tomatoes with juices, cumin, chili powder, tomato paste, and water. Mix well to combine.

Put the slow cooker lid on, then cook for about 8 hours until the vegetables become soft.

Transfer them to serving plates. Top with sour cream, green onions, sliced jalapeños, and shredded cheese before serving.

Nutrition: Calories: 388; Fats: 24.7 g; Total Carbs: 10.6 g; Fiber: 2.9 g; Protein: 33.4 g.

620 EGG WHITE SCRAMBLE WITH CHERRY TOMATOES & SPINACH

Preparation Time: 5 minutes
Cooking Time: 8-10 minutes
Servings: 4
Ingredients:

- 1 tbsp. olive oil
- 1 whole egg
- 10 egg whites
- ¼ tsp. black pepper
- ½ tsp. salt
- 1 garlic clove, minced
- 2 cups cherry tomatoes, halved
- 2 cups packed fresh baby spinach
- ½ cup light cream or Half & Half
- ¼ cup finely grated parmesan cheese

Directions:

Whisk the eggs, pepper, salt, and milk. Prepare a skillet using the med-high temperature setting. Toss in the garlic when the pan is hot to sauté for approximately 30 seconds.

Pour in the tomatoes and spinach and continue to sauté it for one additional minute. The tomatoes should be softened, and the spinach wilted.

Add the egg mixture into the pan using the medium heat setting. Fold the egg gently as it cooks for about two to three minutes. Remove from the burner, and sprinkle with cheese.

Nutrition: Calories: 142; Protein: 15 g; Fat: 2 g; Carbs: 4 g.

621 MARINATED STEAK SIRLOIN KABOBS

Preparation Time: 15 minutes
Cooking Time: 10 minutes
Servings: 3
Ingredients:
Marinade:

- 1 ½ tsp. paprika
- 1 tsp. ground cumin
- 1 tbsp. chili powder
- ½ tsp. garlic powder
- ½ tsp. salt
- Juice of 1 lime
- 2 tbsp. avocado oil

Kabobs:

- 1 pound (454 g.) boneless sirloin steak, sliced into 1-inch cubes
- red bell pepper
- green bell pepper
- ½ red onion, peeled and sliced into 1-inch pieces
- Sliced jalapeños, for garnish
- Special equipment:
- 6 bamboo skewers (about 10 inches / 25 cm long), soaked for at least 30 minutes

Directions:

Put the steak in a Ziploc bag, then set aside.

Make the marinade: In a small bowl, mix the paprika, cumin, chili, garlic, and salt, then mix well with a fork. Add the lime juice and avocado oil, and mix well. Transfer the mixture into the steak bag and seal tightly. Swing slowly to allow the pieces to coat evenly in the marinade. Transfer the bag into the refrigerator and chill for 45 minutes.

Preheat the grill to medium-high fire.

Deseed and remove membranes from the red and green bell peppers, then chop into 1-inch chunks.

Thread the marinated steak, onions, and peppers alternately onto the skewers.

Allow the kabobs to grill for 10 minutes or until browned.

Transfer to serving plates and garnish with the jalapeños before serving.

Nutrition: Calories: 428; Fats: 28.9 g; Total Carbs: 8.4 g; Fiber: 3.0 g; Protein: 33.0 g.

622 BEEF MINI MEATLOAVES WITH BACON WRAPPINGS

Preparation Time: 10 minutes
Cooking Time: 30 minutes
Servings: 8
Ingredients:

- 1 pound (454 g.) ground beef
- ⅓ cup nutritional yeast
- ¾ tsp. ground gray sea salt
- ¼ cup low-carb tomato sauce
- 1 tbsp. prepared yellow mustard
- ¼ tsp. ground black pepper
- 8 (1-oz. / 28-g.) strips bacon

Directions:

Preheat the oven to 350°F (180°C).

In a bowl, add the beef, yeast, salt, tomato sauce, mustard, and pepper. Mix well with your hands.

Make the mini meatloaves: Scoop out 1 tablespoon portions and roll to form a cylinder. Repeat with the remaining mixture to make 8 cylinders. Wrap each of the cylinders with one strip of bacon. Transfer the wrapped cylinders to a cast-iron pan (loose ends of the bacon facing down) with a spacing of ½ inch (1.25 cm) between cylinders.

Bake in the preheated oven for about 30 minutes or until an instant-read thermometer inserted in the center registers 165°F (74°C).

Adjust the oven broiler to high. Allow the mini meatloaves to broil for 2 minutes until the bacon is crispy.

Transfer to a serving platter to cool before serving.

Nutrition: Calories: 295; Fats: 21.2 g; Total Carbs: 3.2 g; Fiber: 1.0 g; Protein: 21.9 g.

623 SLOPPY JOES

Preparation Time: 15 minutes
Cooking Time: 40 minutes
Servings: 8
Ingredients:

¼ cup plus 1 ½ tsp. refined avocado oil
1 tsp. cumin seeds
1 small minced cloves garlic
1 minced piece fresh ginger root
¼ cup red onions, finely diced
pound (454 g.) ground beef
1 ⅔ cups low-carb tomato sauce
1 crushed whole dried chilis
¾ cup water
1 tsp. curry powder
½ tsp. paprika
1 tsp. finely ground gray sea salt
⅓ cup raw macadamia nut halves
2 tbsp. apple cider vinegar
½ cup unsweetened coconut milk
¼ cup chopped fresh cilantro leaves, plus more for garnish
endives, leaves separated, plus more for garnish

Directions:

Make Sloppy Joes: Add ¼ cup of oil, cumin seeds, garlic, ginger, and onions in a saucepan. Cook over medium heat for about 3 minutes until the onions are fragrant.

Add the beef to cook for about 8 minutes until it loses the pink color. Stir occasionally to break the beef into small clumps.

Add the tomato sauce, crushed chilis, water, curry powder, paprika, and salt. Stir thoroughly to mix. Cover the lid partially to allow the steam to escape. Bring to a boil before adjusting the heat to medium-low to simmer for 25 minutes.

In a frying pan over medium-low heat, add the remaining oil and macadamia nuts. Roast for about 3 minutes until lightly golden. Toss constantly.

After 25 minutes of simmering, add the vinegar and coconut milk to the meat mixture. Adjust to medium-high heat and cook for about 5 minutes until thickened.

Add the cilantro and roasted nuts into the meat mixture. Stir well to mix.

Divide the endive leaves equally on 8 plates. Top with Sloppy Joes using a spoon.

Garnish the meal with extra cilantro and endives before serving.

Nutrition: Calories: 340; Fats: 26.8 g; Total Carbs: 8.1 g; Fiber: 2.7 g; Protein: 16.5 g.

624 FETA FRITTATA

Preparation Time: 15 minutes
Cooking Time: 25 minutes
Servings: 2
Ingredients:

1 small clove garlic
1 green onion
2 large eggs
½ cup egg substitute
4 tbsp. crumbled feta cheese - divided
⅓ cup plum tomato
4 thin avocado slices
2 tbsp. reduced-fat sour cream

Directions:

Thinly slice/mince the onion, garlic, and tomato. Peel the avocado before slicing. Heat the pan using the medium temperature setting and spritz it with cooking oil.

Whisk the egg substitute, eggs, and feta cheese. Add the egg mixture into the pan. Cover and simmer for four to six minutes.

Sprinkle it using the rest of the feta cheese and tomato. Cover and continue cooking until the eggs are set or about two to three more minutes.

Wait for about five minutes before cutting it into halves. Serve with avocado and sour cream.

Nutrition: Calories: 460; Carbs: 8 g; Fat: 37 g; Protein: 24 g.

625 MEDITERRANEAN EGGS WHITE BREAKFAST SANDWICH WITH ROASTED TOMATOES

Preparation Time: 15 minutes
Cooking Time: 10 minutes
Servings: 2
Ingredients:

Salt and pepper to taste
¼ cup egg whites

1 tsp. chopped fresh herbs like rosemary, basil, parsley,
1 whole-grain seeded ciabatta roll
1 tsp. butter
1-2 slices Muenster cheese
1 tbsp. pesto
About ½ cup roasted tomatoes
10 oz. grape tomatoes
1 tbsp. extra-virgin olive oil
Black pepper and salt to taste

Directions:

First, you will have to melt the butter over medium heat in the small nonstick skillet. Then, mix the egg whites with pepper and salt.

Next, sprinkle it with fresh herbs. After that cook it for almost 3-4 minutes or until the eggs are done, then flip it carefully.

Meanwhile, toast ciabatta bread in the toaster. Place the egg on the bottom half of the sandwich rolls, then top with cheese

Add roasted tomatoes and the top half of the roll. To make a roasted tomato, preheat the oven to 400°F. Then, slice the tomatoes in half lengthwise.

Place on the baking sheet and drizzle with olive oil. Season it with pepper and salt and then roast in the oven for about 20 minutes. Skins will appear wrinkled when done.

Nutrition: Calories: 458; Protein: 21 g; Fat: 24 g; Carbs: 51 g.

626 SMOKED SALMON AND POACHED EGGS ON TOAST

Preparation Time: 10 minutes
Cooking Time: 4 minutes
Servings: 4
Ingredients:

2 oz. avocado smashed
2 slices of bread toasted
Pinch of kosher salt and cracked black pepper
¼ tsp freshly squeezed lemon juice
2 eggs see notes, poached
3.5 oz. smoked salmon
1 tbsp. thinly sliced scallions
Splash of Kikkoman soy sauce optional
Microgreens are optional

Directions:

Take a small bowl and then smash the avocado into it. Then, add the lemon juice and also a pinch of salt into the mixture. Mix well and set aside.

After that, poach the eggs and toast the bread for some time. Once the bread is toasted, spread the avocado on both slices and after that, add the smoked salmon to each slice.

Thereafter, carefully transfer the poached eggs to the respective toasts. Add a splash of Kikkoman soy sauce and some cracked pepper; then, just garnish with scallions and microgreens.

Nutrition: Calories: 459; Protein: 31 g; Fat: 22 g; Carbs: 33 g.

627 LOW-CARB BAKED EGGS WITH AVOCADO AND FETA

Preparation Time: 10 minutes
Cooking Time: 15 minutes
Servings: 2
Ingredients:

1 avocado
4 eggs
2-3 tbsp. crumbled feta cheese
Nonstick cooking spray
Pepper and salt to taste

Directions:

First, preheat the oven to 400°F. After that, put the gratin dishes right on the baking sheet.

Then, leave the dishes to heat in the oven for almost 10 minutes.

Break the eggs into individual ramekins. Then, let the avocado and eggs come to room temperature for at least 10 minutes. Next, peel the avocado properly and cut it each half into 6-8 slices.

Remove the dishes from the oven and spray them with non-stick spray. Then, you will have to arrange all the sliced avocados in the dishes and tip two eggs into each dish. Sprinkle with feta, add pepper and salt to taste, serve.

Nutrition: Calories: 280; Protein: 11 g; Fat: 23 g; Carbs: 10 g.

628 MEDITERRANEAN BREAKFAST EGG WHITE SANDWICH

Preparation Time: 15 minutes
Cooking Time: 30 minutes
Servings: 1
Ingredients:

1 tsp. vegan butter
¼ cup egg whites
1 tsp. chopped fresh herbs such as parsley, basil, rosemary
1 whole-grain seeded ciabatta roll
1 tbsp. pesto
1-2 slices muenster cheese (or other cheese such as provolone, Monterey Jack, etc.)
About ½ cup roasted tomatoes
Salt, to taste
Pepper, to taste

Roasted Tomatoes:

10 oz. grape tomatoes

1 tbsp. extra virgin olive oil
Kosher salt, to taste
Coarse black pepper, to taste

Directions:

In a small nonstick skillet over medium heat, melt the vegan butter. Pour in egg whites and season with salt and pepper. Sprinkle with fresh herbs, cook for 3-4 minutes or until egg is done, flip once.

In the meantime, toast the ciabatta bread in the toaster. Once done, spread both halves with pesto.

Place the egg on the bottom half of the sandwich roll, folding, if necessary. Add cheese, the roasted tomatoes and top half of roll sandwich.

For the roasted tomatoes, preheat the oven to 400°F. Slice tomatoes in half lengthwise. Then place them onto a baking sheet and drizzle with the olive oil, toss to coat.

Season with salt and pepper and roast in the oven for about 20 minutes, until the skin appears wrinkled.

Nutrition: Calories: 458; Carbohydrates: 51 g; Fat: 0 g; Protein: 21 g.

629 MEDITERRANEAN EGGS CUPS

Preparation Time: 10 minutes
Cooking Time: 20 minutes
Servings: 8
Ingredients:

1 cup spinach, finely diced
½ yellow onion, finely diced
½ cup sliced sun-dried tomatoes
4 large basil leaves, finely diced
Pepper and salt to taste
⅓ cup feta cheese crumbles
8 large eggs
¼ cup milk (any kind)

Directions:

Warm the oven to 375°F. Then, roll the dough sheet into a 12x8-inch rectangle and cut in half lengthwise.

After that, cut each half crosswise into 4 pieces, forming 8 (4x3-inch) pieces of dough. Then, press each into the bottom and up sides of the ungreased muffin cup.

Trim dough to keep the dough from touching, if essential. Set aside. Then, you will have to combine the eggs, salt, pepper in the bowl and beat it with a whisk until well mixed. Set aside.

Melt the butter in a 12-inch skillet over medium heat until sizzling; add bell peppers. You will have to cook it, stirring occasionally, 2-3 minutes or until crisply tender.

After that, add spinach leaves; continue cooking until spinach is wilted. Then just add egg mixture and prosciutto.

Divide the mixture evenly among prepared muffin cups. Finally, bake it for 14-17 minutes or until the crust is golden brown.

Nutrition: Calories: 240; Protein: 9 g; Fat: 16 g; Carbs: 13 g.

630 CHEESE, OLIVES AND SAUSAGE CASSEROLE

Preparation Time: 10 minutes
Cooking Time: 15 minutes
Servings: 2
Ingredients:

3 oz. sausage
1 oz. green olives, sliced
2 eggs
4 oz. coconut milk, unsweetened
3 tbsp. grated cheddar cheese

Seasoning:

¼ tsp. ground black pepper
⅓ tsp. salt
⅓ tsp. mustard powder

Directions:

Take a medium skillet pan, place it over medium heat and when hot, add sausage, crumble it and cook for 5 minutes until cooked.

Meanwhile, crack eggs in a medium bowl. Add milk, salt, black pepper, and mustard and whisk until blended.

When sausage had cooked, add sausage mixture into the eggs, add onion and olives, 2 tablespoons of cheese, and then stir until mixed.

Then spoon the mixture into a casserole dish, cover with a lid and let it refrigerate for 1 hour until chilled.

When ready to bake, turn on the oven, then set it to 350°F and let it preheat.

Sprinkle cheese on the top casserole and then bake it for 10 minutes until cheese has melted.

Serve.

Nutrition: Calories: 351; Fats: 30.6 g; Protein: 15.7 g; Net Carb: 1.7 g; Fiber: 0.9 g.

631 CURRIED GROUND SAUSAGE

Preparation Time: 5 minutes
Cooking Time: 15 minutes
Servings: 4
Ingredients:

5 oz. sausage, crumbled
1 tbsp green onion, sliced
2 oz. spinach
1-oz. chicken bone broth
1-oz. whipping cream
1 tbsp. avocado oil

½ tsp. garlic powder

1 Tbsp. curry powder

¼ cup of water

Directions:

Take a medium saucepan, place it over medium heat, add ½ tablespoon of oil and when hot, add ground sausage and cook for 4 to 5 minutes until cooked.

When done, transfer sausage to a bowl and add remaining oil. When hot, add green onion, sprinkle with garlic powder and cook for 2 minutes until sauté.

Sprinkle with curry powder, continue cooking for 30 seconds until fragrant. Pour in chicken broth and water, add sausage and spinach, stir until mixed and simmer for 5 minutes until thickened slightly.

Taste to adjust seasoning, stir in cream and then remove the pan from heat.

Serve.

Nutrition: Calories: 435; Fats: 42 g; Protein: 12 g; Net Carb: 1.4 g; Fiber: 0.8 g.

632 PORTOBELLO MUSHROOMS WITH SAUSAGE AND CHEESE

Preparation Time: 10 minutes

Cooking Time: 20 minutes

Servings: 2

Ingredients:

2 Portobello mushroom caps

2 oz. sausage

1 tbsp. melted butter, unsalted

1 tbsp. grated parmesan cheese

⅛ tsp. garlic powder

⅛ tsp. red chili powder

¼ tsp. salt

2 tsp. avocado oil

Directions:

Turn on the oven, then set it to 425°F and let it preheat.

Meanwhile, remove the stems from mushroom caps, chop them and then brush the caps with butter inside-out.

Take a frying pan, place it over medium heat, add oil and when hot, add sausage, crumble it, sprinkle with garlic powder and then cook for 5 minutes until cooked.

Stir in mushroom stems, season with salt and black pepper, continue cooking for 3 minutes, or until ready, and then remove the pan from heat.

Distribute sausage-mushroom mixture into mushroom caps, sprinkle cheese, and red chili powder on top and then bake for 10 to 12 minutes, until mushroom caps

have turned tender and cooked. Serve.

Nutrition: Calories: 310; Fats: 26 g; Protein: 10.7 g; Net Carb: 6.6 g; Fiber: 1.1 g.

633 SAUSAGE AND CAULIFLOWER RICE

Preparation Time: 5 minutes

Cooking Time: 15 minutes

Servings: 2

Ingredients:

7 oz. grated cauliflower

3 oz. sausage

green onion, sliced

½ tsp. garlic powder

1 tbsp. avocado oil

⅓ tsp salt

¼ tsp ground black pepper

6 tbsp water

Directions:

Take a medium skillet pan and place it over medium heat. Add 1 tablespoon of oil and when hot, add sausage and cook for 4 to 5 minutes until nicely browned.

Switch heat to medium-low level, pour in 4 tablespoons of water and then simmer for 5 to 7 minutes until sausage has thoroughly cooked.

Transfer sausage to a bowl and wipe clean the pan. Then return it over medium heat, add oil and when hot, add cauliflower rice and green onion. Sprinkle with garlic powder, salt, and black pepper.

Stir until mixed, drizzle with 2 tablespoons of water, and cook for 5 minutes until softened.

Add sausage, stir until mixed, cook for 1 minute until hot and then serve.

Nutrition: Calories: 333; Fats: 31.3 g; Protein: 9.1 g; Net Carb: 0.8 g; Fiber: 2.5 g.

634 CHEESY SAUSAGE AND EGG BAKE

Preparation Time: 5 minutes

Cooking Time: 18 minutes

Servings: 2

Ingredients:

4 oz. sausage

1 egg

1 tbsp. grated cheddar cheese

½ tbsp. grated mozzarella cheese

½ tbsp. grated parmesan cheese

¼ tsp. salt

⅛ tsp. ground black pepper

1 tsp. avocado oil

Directions:

Turn on the oven, then set it to 375°F and let it preheat.

Meanwhile, take a medium skillet pan and place it over medium heat. Add oil, and when hot, add

sausage and cook for 5 minutes until cooked.

Meanwhile, crack the egg in a medium bowl, add salt, black pepper, and cheeses, reserving 1 tablespoon of cheddar cheese and whisk until mixed.

When the sausage has cooked, transfer it to the bowl containing egg batter and stir until combined.

Take a baking pan. Grease it with oil, pour in sausage mixture, sprinkle remaining cheddar cheese in the top. Then bake for 10 to 12 minutes until cooked.

When done, let sausage cool for 5 minutes. Cut it into squares and then serve.

Nutrition: Calories: 439; Fats: 38.9 g; Protein: 19.7 g; Net Carb: 2.2 g; Fiber: 0 g.

635 SAUSAGE AND MARINARA CASSEROLE

Preparation Time: 5 minutes

Cooking Time: 12 minutes

Servings: 2

Ingredients:

2 oz. chorizo

4 oz. sausage

2 tbsp. avocado oil

4 oz. marinara sauce

1 tbsp. grated cheddar cheese

¼ tsp. salt

⅛ tsp. ground black pepper

¼ tsp. dried thyme

Directions:

Take a medium skillet pan and place it over medium heat. Add oil and, when hot, add chorizo and sausage and cook for 4 to 5 minutes until meat is no longer pink.

Add the marinara sauce into the pan. Stir in salt, black pepper, and thyme. Cook for 1 minute until hot and then transfer the meat mixture into a casserole dish.

Sprinkle cheese over the top of the casserole and then bake for 7 minutes until thoroughly cooked.

Serve.

Nutrition: Calories: 485; Fats: 44.4 g; Protein: 15.6 g; Net Carb: 3.7 g; Fiber: 1.1 g.

636 DOUBLE CHEESE MEATLOAF

Preparation Time: 10 minutes

Cooking Time: 20 minutes

Servings: 2

Ingredients:

2 slices of bacon, chopped, cooked

6 oz. of sausage

2 tbsp. grated mozzarella cheese

2 tbsp. grated cheddar cheese

⅓ tsp. salt

¼ tsp. ground black pepper
1 tsp. dried parsley
2 tbsp. marinara sauce
1 egg

Directions:

Turn on the oven. Then set it to 375°F and let it preheat.

Meanwhile, take a medium bowl and place all the ingredients in it, except for marinara. Stir until well combined.

Spoon the mixture into a mini loaf pan. Top with marinara, and then bake for 20 to 25 minutes until cooked through and done.

When done, let meatloaf cool for 5 minutes. Cut it into slices and then serve.

Nutrition: Calories: 578; Fats: 50.6 g; Protein: 27.4 g; Net Carb: 2.6 g; Fiber: 0.3 g.

637 SPINACH SAUSAGE BALL PASTA

Preparation Time: 10 minutes
Cooking Time: 12 minutes
Servings: 2
Ingredients:

½ pound cabbage, shredded
4 oz. sausage
1 oz. spinach, chopped
2 tbsp grated parmesan cheese
2 tbsp. marinara sauce
⅓ tsp. salt
¼ tsp. ground black pepper
2 tbsp. avocado oil

Directions:

Take a medium bowl. Put the sausage, spinach and cheese in it. Season with ⅓ teaspoon of salt and black pepper. Stir until well combined, and then shape the mixture into balls.

Take a medium skillet pan and place it over medium heat. Add tablespoon of oil and, when hot, add meatballs and cook for 3 to 4 minutes per side until cooked and nicely golden brown.

Transfer meatballs to a plate. Add remaining oil into the pan and, when hot, add cabbage and then cook for 3 minutes, until tender-crisp.

Return meatballs into the pan. Add marinara sauce, toss until well mixed and cook for 1 minute until hot. Serve.

Nutrition: Calories: 505; Fats: 41.6 g; Protein: 18.7 g; Net Carb: 6.5 g; Fiber: 6 g.

638 BEEF WITH CABBAGE NOODLES

Preparation Time: 5 minutes
Cooking Time: 18 minutes
Servings: 2

Ingredients:

4 oz. ground beef
1 cup chopped cabbage
4 oz. tomato sauce
½ tsp. minced garlic
½ cup of water
½ tbsp. coconut oil
½ tsp. salt
¼ tsp. Italian seasoning
⅛ tsp. dried basil

Directions:

Take a skillet pan and place it over medium heat. Add oil and, when hot, add beef and cook for 5 minutes until nicely browned.

Meanwhile, slice the cabbage into thin shred.

When the beef has cooked, add garlic, season with salt, basil, and Italian seasoning. Stir well and continue cooking for 3 minutes until beef has thoroughly cooked.

Pour in tomato sauce and water, stir well and bring the mixture to boil.

Then reduce heat to medium-low level. Add cabbage, stir well until well mixed and simmer for 3 to 5 minutes until cabbage is softened, covering the pan.

Uncover the pan and continue simmering the beef until most of the cooking liquid has evaporated.

Serve.

Nutrition: Calories: 188.5; Fats: 12.5 g; Protein: 15.5 g; Net Carb: 2.5 g; Fiber: 1 g.

639 ROAST BEEF AND MOZZARELLA PLATE

Preparation Time: 5 minutes
Cooking Time: 0 minutes
Servings: 2

Ingredients:

4 slices of roast beef
½ oz. chopped lettuce
1 avocado, pitted
1 oz. mozzarella cheese, cubed
½ cup mayonnaise
¼ tsp salt
⅛ tsp ground black pepper
2 tbsp. avocado oil

Directions:

Scoop out flesh from avocado and divide it evenly between two plates.

Add slices of roast beef, lettuce, and cheese and then sprinkle with salt and black pepper.

Serve with avocado oil and mayonnaise.

Nutrition: Calories: 267.7; Fats: 24.5 g; Protein: 9.5 g; Net Carb: 1.5 g; Fiber: 2 g.

640 GARLIC HERB BEEF ROAST

Preparation Time: 5 minutes

Cooking Time: 10 minutes
Servings: 2
Ingredients:

6 slices of beef roast
½ tsp. garlic powder
⅓ tsp. dried thyme
¼ tsp. dried rosemary
2 tbsp. butter, unsalted
⅓ tsp. salt
¼ tsp. ground black pepper

Directions:

Prepare the spice mix. Take a small bowl, place garlic powder, thyme, rosemary, salt, and black pepper. Stir until mixed.

Sprinkle spice mix on the beef roast.

Take a medium skillet pan and place it over medium heat. Add butter and, when it melts, add beef roast and then cook for 5 to 8 minutes until golden brown and cooked.

Serve.

Nutrition: Calories: 140; Fats: 12.7 g; Protein: 5.5 g; Net Carb: 0.1 g; Fiber: 0.2 g.

641 SPROUTS STIR-FRY WITH KALE, BROCCOLI, AND BEEF

Preparation Time: 5 minutes
Cooking Time: 8 minutes
Servings: 2
Ingredients:

3 slices of beef roast, chopped
2 oz. Brussels sprouts, halved
4 oz. broccoli florets
3 oz. kale
½ tbsp. butter, unsalted
⅛ tsp. red pepper flakes

Seasoning:

¼ tsp. garlic powder
¼ tsp. salt
⅛ tsp. ground black pepper

Directions:

Take a medium skillet pan and place it over medium heat. Add ¼ tablespoon of butter and, when it melts, add broccoli florets and sprouts. Sprinkle with garlic powder, and cook for 2 minutes.

Season vegetables with salt and red pepper flakes. Add chopped beef, stir until mixed and continue cooking for 3 minutes until browned on one side.

Then add kale along with the remaining butter. Flip the vegetables and cook for 2 minutes until kale leaves wilts.

Serve.

Nutrition: Calories: 125; Fats: 9.4 g; Protein: 4.8 g; Net Carb: 1.7 g; Fiber: 2.6 g.

642 BEEF AND VEGETABLE SKILLET

Preparation Time: 5 minutes
Cooking Time: 15 minutes
Servings: 2
Ingredients:

- 3 oz. spinach, chopped
- ½-pound ground beef
- 2 slices of bacon, diced
- 2 oz. chopped asparagus
- 3 tbsp. coconut oil
- 2 tsp. dried thyme
- ⅔ tsp. salt
- ½ tsp. ground black pepper

Directions:

- Take a skillet pan and place it over medium heat. Add oil and, when hot, add beef and bacon. Cook for 5 to 7 minutes until slightly browned.
- Then add asparagus and spinach and sprinkle with thyme. Stir well and cook for 7 to 10 minutes until thoroughly cooked.
- Season skillet with salt and black pepper and serve.

Nutrition: Calories: 332.5; Fats: 26 g; Protein: 23.5 g; Net Carb: 1.5 g; Fiber: 1 g.

643 BEEF, PEPPER AND GREEN BEANS STIR-FRY

Preparation Time: 5 minutes
Cooking Time: 18 minutes
Servings: 2
Ingredients:

- 6 oz. ground beef
- 2 oz. chopped green bell pepper
- 4 oz. green beans
- 3 tbsp. grated cheddar cheese
- ½ tsp. salt
- ¼ tsp. ground black pepper
- ¼ tsp. paprika

Directions:

- Take a skillet pan and place it over medium heat. Add ground beef and cook for 4 minutes until slightly browned.
- Then add bell pepper and green beans. Season with salt, paprika, and black pepper. Stir well and continue cooking for 7 to 10 minutes until beef and vegetables have cooked through.
- Sprinkle cheddar cheese on top. Then transfer pan under the broiler and cook for 2 minutes until cheese has melted and the top is golden brown. Serve.

Nutrition: Calories: 282.5; Fats: 17.6 g; Protein: 26.1 g; Net Carb: 2.9 g; Fiber: 2.1 g.

644 CHEESY MEATLOAF

Preparation Time: 5 minutes
Cooking Time: 4 minutes

Servings: 2
Ingredients:

- 4 oz. ground turkey
- egg
- 1 tbsp. grated mozzarella cheese
- ¼ tsp. Italian seasoning
- ½ tbsp. soy sauce
- ¼ tsp. salt
- ⅛ tsp. ground black pepper

Directions:

- Take a bowl, place all the ingredients in it, and stir until mixed.
- Take a heatproof mug, spoon in prepared mixture and microwave for 3 minutes at high heat setting until cooked.
- When done, let the meatloaf rest in the mug for 1 minute, then take it out, cut it into two slices and serve.

Nutrition: Calories: 196.5; Fats: 13.5 g; Protein: 18.7 g; Net Carb: 18.7 g; Fiber: 0 g.

645 ROAST BEEF AND VEGETABLE PLATE

Preparation Time: 10 minutes
Cooking Time: 10 minutes
Servings: 2
Ingredients:

- 2 scallions, chopped into large pieces
- ½ tbsp. coconut oil
- 4 thin slices of roast beef
- 4 oz. cauliflower and broccoli mix
- 1 tbsp butter, unsalted
- ½ tsp. salt
- ⅓ tsp. ground black pepper
- 1 tsp. dried parsley

Directions:

- Turn on the oven, then set it to 400°F, and let it preheat.
- Take a baking sheet and grease it with oil. Place slices of roast beef on one side, and top with butter.
- Take a separate bowl, add cauliflower and broccoli mix. Add scallions, drizzle with oil, season with remaining salt and black pepper. Toss until coated and then spread vegetables on the empty side of the baking sheet.
- Bake for 5 to 7 minutes until beef is nicely browned and vegetables are tender-crisp, tossing halfway.
- Distribute beef and vegetables between two plates and then serve.

Nutrition: Calories: 313; Fats: 26 g; Protein: 15.6 g; Net Carb: 2.8 g; Fiber: 1.9 g.

646 GRILLED MOROCCAN-SPICED RACK OF LAMB

Preparation Time: 15 minutes
Cooking Time: 30-35 minutes
Servings: 4
Ingredients:

For the spice blend:

- ⅓ cup finely chopped fresh cilantro
- ⅓ cup finely chopped fresh parsley
- ¼ cup freshly squeezed lemon juice of about 2 lemons
- 2 tbsp. extra virgin olive oil
- 2 tbsp. freshly sliced garlic, about 3 medium-sized teeth

For the spice and lamb sauce:

- 2 tbsp. bell pepper
- 1 tbsp. kosher salt
- 1 tsp. ground cumin
- 1 tsp. ground coriander
- 1 tsp. freshly ground black pepper
- ½ tsp. cinnamon
- ¼ tsp. cayenne pepper
- lamb chops, 7-10 ribs, sliced everything but a thin layer of art, about 1 ½ lb. each
- 2 tbsp. Dijon mustard

Directions:

For the spice mix:

- Combine the coriander, parsley, lemon juice, olive oil, and garlic in a medium bowl. Set aside.

For the Rub Spice:

- Combine the pepper, salt, cumin, coriander, black pepper, cinnamon, and cayenne pepper in a small bowl. Season the lamb chops with the spice blend.
- Light a fireplace full of coals. When all the charcoal is lit and covered with gray ash, pour and place the charcoal on 1 side of the charcoal grate. Place the grill in its place, cover the grill, and let it preheat for 5 minutes. Clean and grease the grill. Bring the lamb chops on the hot side, fat side down, and cook until golden, 3 to 5 minutes. Place the lamb on a cutting board.
- Brush a thin layer of mustard on the thick side of each rack of lamb. Gently squeeze the mixture of herbs and lemon into the mustard in each box and spread evenly.
- Put the meat back in the grill, close, but not directly above, the coals. Continue cooking until an immediately readable thermometer registers 130°F when placed at the bottom of the rack for 15 to 25 minutes. Remove from grill, leave uncovered for 10 minutes. Cut between ribs in chops, and serve immediately.

Nutrition: Calories: 374; Protein: 47.89 g; Fat: 19.11 g; Carbohydrates: 3.36 g.

647 LAMB BURGERS WITH TZATZIKI

Preparation Time: 10 minutes
Cooking Time: 20 minutes
Servings: 4
Ingredients:

- 1 lb. of grass-fed lamb
- ¼ cup chives finely chopped green onion or red onion if desired
- 2tbsp. chopped fresh dill
- ½ tsp dried oregano or about 1 tbsp. freshly chopped
- tbsp. finely chopped fresh mint
- A pinch of chopped red pepper
- Fine-grained sea salt to taste
- 3 tbsp. water
- 2 tsp. olive oil to grease the pan

For the tzatziki:

- 1 can coconut milk with all the cooled fat and 1 tbsp. the discarded liquid portion **
- cloves of garlic
- peeled cucumber without seeds, roughly sliced
- tbsp. freshly squeezed lemon juice
- tbsp. chopped fresh dill
- ¾ tsp fine grain sea salt
- Black pepper to taste

Directions:
To make the tzatziki:

- Place the garlic, cucumber, and lemon juice in the food processor and press until finely chopped. Add the coconut cream, dill, salt, and pepper, and mix until well blended.
- Put it in a jar with a lid and keep it in the refrigerator until it is served. The flavors become more intense over time when they cool in the fridge.

For burgers:

- Thoroughly mix the ground lamb in a bowl with the chives or red onion, dill, oregano, mint, red pepper, and water.
- Sprinkle the mixture with fine-grained sea salt and form 4 patties of the same size.
- Heat a large cast-iron skillet over medium heat and brush with a small amount of olive oil. Lightly sprinkle the pan with fine-grain sea salt.
- Bring the patties into the pan and cook on each side for about 4 minutes, adjusting the heat to prevent the outside from becoming too brown. Alternatively, you can grill the burgers.
- Remove from the pan and cover with tzatziki sauce.

Nutrition: Calories: 363; Protein: 35.33 g; Fat: 22.14 g; Carbohydrates: 6.83 g.

648 LAMB SLIDERS

Preparation Time: 5 minutes
Cooking Time: 15 minutes
Servings: 6
Ingredients:

- 1 lb. minced lamb or half veal, half lamb
- ½ sliced onion
- 2 garlic cloves minced
- 1 tbsp. dried dill
- ½ tsp. salt
- ½ tsp black pepper

Directions:

- Blend the ingredients gently in a large bowl until well combined. Overworking the meat will cause it to be tough.
- Form the meat into burgers.
- Grill or fry in a pan on medium-high heat until cooked through, 4-5 minutes per side. If preparing in a pan, sear both sides quickly, then throw the burgers in a 350°F oven for 10 min to finish cooking through.
- Serve with Tzatziki for dipping!

Nutrition: Calories: 207; Protein: 22.68 g; Fat: 11.89 g; Carbohydrates: 1.17 g.

649 TANDOORI LAMB TAIL

Preparation Time: 10 minutes
Cooking Time: 1hour, 10 minutes
Servings: 2-4
Ingredients:
Roast meat:

- 2 lb. minced lamb
- 1 diced onion
- 5 finely chopped garlic cloves
- 1 serrano pepper, chopped
- 5 tbsp. organic tomato puree
- 1 tsp. bell pepper
- 1 tsp. coriander powder
- 1 tsp. turmeric
- 1 tsp. salt
- ¼ tsp. freshly ground black pepper
- ¼ tsp. cumin powder
- ¼ tsp. ground cloves
- ¼ tsp. cinnamon (ground)
- A pinch freshly grated nutmeg
- eggs
- A small hand of chopped mint

"Ketchup" filling:

- 5 tbsp. organic tomato puree
- ¼ cup water
- A pinch of salt and pepper
- A pinch of garlic powder

Directions:

- Bring all the ingredients in a bowl, then mix and divide the mixture into a bowl with greased bread.
- Bake the bread at 350°C for 1 hour.

While the bread is baking, prepare the tomato sauce by mixing the ingredients in a pan over low heat.

When the bread is ready, apply ketchup and put it in the oven for 10 minutes.

Take off from the oven, then let stand for a few minutes to cool the juice, remove the meatloaf from the pan, and serve.

Nutrition: Calories: 506; Protein: 45.93 g; Fat: 30.01 g; Carbohydrates: 11.82 g.

650 SMOKED LAMB

Preparation Time: 30 minutes + smoke time
Cooking Time: 100 minutes
Servings: 4
Ingredients:

- 2.5kg boneless 5 lb. lamb shoulder
- 3-4 sprigs fresh rosemary
- Himalayan salt to taste
- Freshly ground black pepper to taste
- About 6 cups of cherry wood chips

Directions:

- Place 4 cups of wood chips to soak in water for at least an hour before smoking your lamb.
- Remove the fillet around the shoulder of the lamb, rinse it in cold water and dry it. Place the lamb on a cutting board (cut the thicker parts if necessary) and make several deep incisions along with the meat with a kitchen knife. Insert pieces of fresh rosemary into these incisions. Sprinkle generously with salt and pepper.
- Preheat your outdoor grill to 225°F. Lighting a single burner in the lowest setting should be the trick.
- Make 8 bags of wood chips. Cut a piece of heavy-duty 12 "x 24" aluminum foil for each bag (double if you are using lighter weight paper) and place about half a cup of damp wood chips at 1 end of the paper. Add a handful of dried chips and fold the sheet over the wood chips. Fold the 4 edges in the center at least twice, then make holes in the top and bottom of the bag with a fork or other sharp object.
- Lift the grill on the ignition element and place 2 bags directly on the heat source. Close and wait for the smoke to come out of the bags.
- Place the roast lamb on the other side of the grill and close the lid.
- Smoke the meat for about 6 hours and replace the bags with 2 new ones

every 90 minutes. If necessary, increase the heat under the new bag until the smoke comes out.

Try to keep the temperature of your grill as stable as possible at around 225°F. *Please note that it is not necessary to get massive amounts of smoke to get a good taste. However, if you feel you don't have enough, add more dry chips to your foil pouches or place an aluminum container with a handful of baked chips next to your existing foil pouches. *

When the lamb has smoked for 6 hours, remove it from the grill and wrap it in aluminum foil. Use a double layer to make sure no cooking juices leak out. You must preserve moisture at this time.

Place it back on the grill and crank up the heat to 350°F. Cook the meat for another 90 minutes, or until the meat becomes very tender and can be easily removed with a fork.

Take off the roast from the grill. Then let it sit for 10. Cut and serve sprinkled with the cooking juices.

Nutrition: Calories: 797; Protein: 136.98 g; Fat: 27.1 g; Carbohydrates: 1.97 g.

651 LAMB SOUVLAKI

Preparation Time: 15 minutes + marinate time
Cooking Time: 45 minutes
Servings: 2
Ingredients:

2 lbs. of Fat-free lamb, cut into 1-inch pieces
2 lemon juice
3 tbsp. olive oil
½ tsp salt
½ tsp freshly ground pepper
1 tbsp. dried oregano
2 garlic cloves, finely chopped
1 medium onion, thinly sliced

Directions:

Combine olive oil, lemon juice, salt, pepper, oregano, garlic, and onion in a large bowl. Place the slices of meat in the pan and mix so that the meat is completely covered with marinade. Cover and let cool for a minimum of 2 hours and a maximum of 24 hours. Bring chicken on metal or bamboo skewers.

Roast the skewer on all sides until golden.

Serve with pita bread.

Nutrition: Calories: 1396; Protein: 114.74 g; Fat: 99.7 g; Carbohydrates: 4.23 g.

652 LAMB SAAGWALI

Preparation Time: 15 minutes
Cooking Time: 50 minutes
Servings: 4
Ingredients:

2 to 3 lb. of fat-free lamb, cut into 1-inch cubes
4 tbsp. ghee, divided
2 dried red peppers
3 teeth
1-inch cinnamon stick
4 green cardamom pods
1 tbsp. coriander seeds
1 tsp. cumin seeds
1 large onion, diced
1 tsp. ginger and garlic paste
½ tsp. turmeric
3 tomatoes, diced
6 cups of spinach or a mixture of vegetables (mustard, kale, etc.)
1 tsp. coriander powder
1 tsp. cumin powder
1 tbsp. ground kasoori methi
½ tsp. garam masala powder
¼ cup cream
salt and pepper to taste

Directions:

Heat 2 tablespoons of ghee in a heavy-bottomed pan. Brown the lamb cubes and place them in a pressure cooker *. Cook up to 6-8 whistles. Remove from heat and set aside for steam to escape.

In the same pan used to brown the meat, add the red peppers, cinnamon, cardamom, and cloves. Jump until you smell it.

Add the coriander seeds and cumin seeds. As soon as they start to crack, add the onions.

Fry the onions until it's almost golden.

Add ginger and garlic paste and turmeric. Cook until the rough odor disappears.

Cover and simmer until the tomatoes are tender. Add the vegetables. Thoroughly mix the vegetables and simmer for 5 minutes.

Transfer to a blender. Mix until smooth.

Heat the remaining ghee in the prior pan and add the mixed vegetable mixture. Add the coriander, cumin and methi Kasuri.

Cover and simmer for ten minutes. Adjust the salt if necessary.

Cover and simmer the lamb for another 20 minutes, stirring frequently. Add water if necessary.

Add the cream and garam masala. Serve hot

Nutrition: Calories: 926; Protein: 72.1 g; Fat: 58.74 g; Carbohydrates: 33 g.

653 ROGAN JOSH

Preparation Time: 20 minutes
Cooking Time: 1 hour, 20 minutes
Servings: 4
Ingredients:

2 lbs. lamb shoulder cut into 1 to 2-inch pieces
2 tbsp. avocado oil or macadamia nut oil

Garlic and onion pasta:

1 medium onion
8 garlic cloves
Spice blend:
2 Bay leaves
10 whole cardamom pods
1 cinnamon stick
½ tsp. ground cloves
1 tsp. coriander
1 tsp. cumin
1 tbsp. bell pepper
1 tsp. cayenne pepper (reduce to ½ tsp if it is sensitive to spicy dishes. This dish is not so tasty, but in my opinion, it is a way)
¼ tsp. salt
1 tsp. pepper

Basic sauce:

Relatively good medium-sized, russet, and chopped fresh tomatoes, but leave them a little thick. (Remember the tomatoes are breaking up there, so don't make them too small)
¼ cup coconut milk or yogurt

Directions:

Put all the ingredients under the spice mix in a small bowl and keep cardamom, cinnamon, and bay leaves whole.

Blanch your fresh Roma tomatoes by soaking them in boiling water for about a minute or until they burst. Let them cool, peel them, cut them, and reserve them.

Add garlic and onion to a mixer and mix until a relatively fine paste is obtained and place in a small bowl on the side.

Now everything is ready to heat the oil in an oven over medium heat (or in a large pan)

Add the meat in batches if necessary and brown well on all sides.

Once all the meat is brown, put it back in the Dutch oven. Lower the heat and add the onion and garlic paste with the spice mixture.

Mix thoroughly and make sure not to crush the bay leaves. Stir for 3 to 5 minutes or until very aromatic.

Add the chopped and blanched Roma tomatoes and coconut milk and stir until smooth.

Once it has been combined and boiled again on low heat, lower the temperature and place the lid on the Dutch oven and simmer for 1 hour and 15 minutes.

Once cooked, serve with chopped fresh cilantro sprinkled on top.

Nutrition: Calories: 865; Protein: 60.23 g; Fat: 64.07 g; Carbohydrates: 9.88 g.

654 INTERMITTENT SLOW COOKER ASIAN PIG MEAT

Preparation Time: 20 minutes
Cooking Time: 3 hours
Servings: 2
Ingredients:

Porkchop
garlic paste
ginger paste
onion
chicken broth
gluten-free tamari sauce or coconut amino acids
5-spice Chinese herbs
green onion

Directions:

Bring the pork ribs to a slow cooker. Add the onions, garlic paste, ginger paste, and chicken broth. If the ribs are not completely covered, add a little broth before including them.

Cover and cook for 3 hours over low heat.

Cut the ribs apart and cover with aluminum foil. Set aside.

Use a blender to bombard well, then add the 5-spice tamari and Chinese. Reduce the excessively thick mixture and jam over medium-high heat.

Move the onions and broth to a clean saucepan on the slow cooker.

Brush the marinade with sliced green onions over the hot ribs.

Nutrition: Calories: 482; Fat: 38 g; Net Carbs: 4 g; Protein: 25 g; Carbs: 5 g; Fiber: 1 g.

655 INTERMITTENT SLOW COOKER KALUA PORK LETTUCE WRAPS

Preparation Time: 5 minutes
Cooking Time: 8 hours
Servings: 10
Ingredients:

liquid smoke
sea salt
tomatoes
pork butt or pork shoulder
bell pepper
olive oil
apple cider vinegar
iceberg lettuce

Directions:

Mix the salt with the liquid smoke.

Use a knife to make some small holes in the pork to help get the flavor in.

Stroke the salt mixture of liquid smoke into the food.

Place in your slow cooker and cook at low for 8 hours.

Mix the tomatoes, bell pepper, olive oil, and vinegar to make the salsa.

Chop the pork finely and enjoy a sauce scoop in lettuce wraps.

Nutrition: Calories: 394; Fat: 28 g; Net Carbs: 1 g; Protein: 32 g; Carbs: 2 g; Fiber: 1 g.

656 INTERMITTENT CROCKPOT PORK SHANKS WITH GRAVY

Preparation Time: 10 minutes
Cooking Time: 2 hours
Servings:
Ingredients:

Olive oil
onions
garlic cloves
lemon juice
pork shanks (on the bone)
chicken broth
dried bay leaves
Dijon mustard
ghee

Directions:

Heat 1 teaspoon of olive oil in a frying pan and fry pork until the skin is browned. Remove and set aside.

Apply the second teaspoon of olive oil to the same pan and add the onions and garlic until the onions caramelize. Deglaze pan with the lemon juice and scrape off any stuck pieces.

Place the shanks in a crockpot and pour the cooked onion.

Take the shanks from the crockpot and place them on a roasting tray.

Place the tray on the bottom rack once the oven is heated and cook until the skin is crisping and puffing up. Remove before serving and allow to rest.

Make gravy in the meantime. Spoon all the crockpot cooking juices and onions into a large saucepan on the stovetop.

Nutrition: Calories: 355; Fat: 30 g; Net Carbs: 3 g; Protein: 13 g; Carbs: 7 g; Fiber: 1 g.

657 GRILLED PORK PATTIES

Preparation Time: 10 minutes
Cooking Time: 7-8 minutes
Servings: 6
Ingredients:

½ pounds ground pork
½-pound ground turkey

serrano pepper, deseeded and minced
garlic cloves, finely minced
½ cup onion, finely minced
1 cup Romano cheese, grated
½ cup Asiago cheese, shredded
½ tsp. mustard seeds
½ tsp. dried marjoram
½ tsp. dried basil
½ tsp. paprika
Sea salt, to taste
Ground black pepper, to taste

Directions:

Begin by preheating a gas grill to high.

Mix all of the above ingredients until everything is well incorporated. Form the mixture into 6 patties with oiled hands.

Place on the preheated grill and cook for 7 to 8 minutes on each side until slightly charred. Bon appétit!

Nutrition: Calories: 515;35. Fat: 4 g; Carbs: 2.6 g; Protein: 44.3 g; Protein: 0.2 g.

658 PORK FILLETS WITH MUSTARD SAUCE

Preparation Time: 10 minutes
Cooking Time: 20 minutes
Servings: 4
Ingredients:

4 tbsp. butter, melted
1 pound pork fillets
1 tsp scallions, chopped
2 cloves garlic, minced
½ cup dry white wine
Sea salt, to taste
Freshly cracked black pepper, to taste
1 tsp. cayenne pepper
1 tsp. dried basil
1 tbsp. whole-grain Dijon mustard
4 tbsp. chicken stock

Directions:

Melt the butter in a frying pan at a moderate flame. Now, brown the pork fillets for about 3 minutes per side; reserve.

Then, in the pan drippings, continue cooking the scallions and garlic for a minute or so. Add in a splash of wine to scrape up the browned bits that stick to the pan's bottom.

Return the pork to the frying pan. Add in the remaining ingredients, partially cover, and cook an additional 13 minutes.

Spoon the sauce over the pork fillets and serve warm. Bon appétit!

Nutrition: Calories: 343; Fat: 17.5 g; Carbs: 5.4 g; Protein: 40 g; Protein: 1 g.

659 SUNDAY GROUND PORK BAKE

Preparation Time: 9 minutes
Cooking Time: 21 minutes
Servings: 4
Ingredients:
- 2 tbsp. butter
- 2 pounds ground pork
- 1 bell pepper, deseeded and chopped
- 1 serrano pepper, deseeded and chopped
- 1 stalk leek, chopped
- 2 garlic cloves, minced
- ½ cup chicken broth
- 2 eggs, beaten
- 1 tsp. paprika
- Sea salt, to taste
- Ground black pepper, to taste
- ½ cup cream cheese
- 1 cup heavy whipped cream

Directions:
Melt the butter in a frying pan at moderate heat. Now, cook the ground pork until no longer pink.
Add in the peppers, leek, and garlic and continue cooking approximately 7 minutes, or until tender and aromatic.
Pour the chicken broth and continue cooking for a further 6 minutes. Scoop the mixture into a lightly greased baking pan.
In a mixing bowl, whisk the egg, paprika, salt, black pepper, cream cheese, and heavy whipped cream. Pour the mixture into the prepared baking pan.
Bake in the preheated oven at 330°F for about 8 minutes until golden brown on the top. Bon appétit!

Nutrition: Calories: 620; Fat: 50 g; Carbs: 5.7 g; Protein: 33.9 g; Protein: 0.7 g.

660 PORK CUTLETS IN CHILI TANGY SAUCE

Preparation Time: 10 minutes
Cooking Time: 5 minutes
Servings: 3
Ingredients:
- 1 pound pork cutlets
- Sea salt, to taste
- Ground black pepper, to taste
- ½ tsp. thyme
- ½ tsp. rosemary
- 1 tsp. basil
- 1 tbsp. lard, room temperature

The Sauce:
- 1 tbsp. sherry
- ¼ cup sour cream
- ¼ cup beef bone broth
- 1 tsp. mustard
- ½ tsp. turmeric powder - ½ tsp. chili powder

Directions:
Season the pork cutlets using salt, pepper, thyme, rosemary, and basil.
Melt the lard in a pan on medium-high heat; now, sear pork cutlets for 3 minutes; flip and cook for 3 minutes on the other side. Reserve.
Deglaze your pan with sherry. Add the remaining ingredients and cook on medium-low heat until the sauce has thickened slightly.
Put the reserved pork and let it simmer for a couple of minutes or until everything is heated through. Scoop the sauce over pork cutlets and serve.

Nutrition: Calories: 288; Fat: 17.3 g; Carbs: 1.1 g; Protein: 0 g; Protein: 29.9 g.

661 HOLIDAY PORK BELLY WITH VEGETABLES

Preparation Time: 10 minutes
Cooking Time: 20 minutes
Servings: 2
Ingredients:
- 1 pound skinless pork belly
- Himalayan salt, to taste
- Freshly ground black pepper, to taste
- 1 tsp. dried parsley
- 1 tsp. dried basil
- ½ tsp. dried oregano
- 2 cloves garlic, pressed
- ½ cup shallots, sliced
- 1 red bell pepper, seeded and sliced
- 1 green bell pepper, seeded and sliced

Directions:
Poke holes on the pork using a fork. Rub the seasonings all over the pork belly. Place the pork in a lightly greased baking pan.
Top with garlic, shallots, and peppers. Transfer the pork belly to the preheated oven.
Bake at 390°F for about 18 minutes. Serve warm.

Nutrition: Calories: 607; Fat: 60 g; Carbs: 4.4 g; Protein: 0.7 g; Protein: 11.4 g.

662 FILIPINO NILAGA SOUP

Preparation Time: 10 minutes
Cooking Time: 45 minutes
Servings: 4
Ingredients:
- 2 tsp. butter
- 2 pound pork ribs, boneless and cut into small pieces
- 1 shallot, chopped
- 2 garlic cloves, minced
- (½-inch) piece fresh ginger, chopped
- 1 cup water
- 2 cups chicken stock
- 1 tbsp. patis (fish sauce)
- 1 cup fresh tomatoes, pureed
- 1 cup cauliflower "rice"
- Sea salt and ground black pepper, to taste

Directions:
Melt the butter in a pot at medium-high heat. Then, cook the pork ribs on all sides for 5 to 6 minutes.
Add the shallot, garlic, and ginger; cook an additional 3 minutes. Add the remaining ingredients.
Let it cook, covered, for 30 to 35 minutes. Ladle into individual bowls and serve.

Nutrition: Calories: 203; Fat: 8.4 g; Carbs: 3.7 g; Protein: 1.1 g; Protein: 27.1 g.

663 PORK TENDERLOIN WITH SOUTHERN CABBAGE

Preparation Time: 5 minutes
Cooking Time: 20 minutes
Servings: 2
Ingredients:
The Pork tenderloin:
- ½-pound pork tenderloin
- Celtic sea salt, to taste
- Freshly cracked black pepper, to taste
- ½ tsp. granulated garlic
- ¼ tsp. ginger powder
- ½ tsp. dried sage
- 1 tbsp. lard, room temperature

The Cabbage:
- 4 oz. cabbage, sliced into strips
- ⅓ cup vegetable broth
- 1 tbsp. sherry wine
- ½ tsp. mustard seeds
- Celtic sea salt, to taste
- ½ tsp. black peppercorns

Directions:
Season the pork with salt, black pepper, granulated garlic, ginger powder, and sage.
Melt the lard in a pan over moderate heat. Sear the pork for 7 to 8 minutes, turning periodically.
In a pan that is preheated over medium heat, bring the cabbage, broth, sherry, and mustard seeds to a boil over high heat.
Season with salt and black peppercorns; cook, stirring periodically, until the cabbage is tender, about 12 minutes; do not overcook.
Serve the pork with sautéed cabbage on the side. Bon appétit!

Nutrition: Calories: 254; Fat: 10.8 g; Carbs: 5.7 g; Protein: 1.6 g; Protein: 31.8 g.

664 PAPRIKA CRUSTED PORK CUTLETS

Preparation Time: 15 minutes
Cooking Time: 10 minutes
Servings: 4
Ingredients:
- 2 tbsp. sesame oil

2 eggs

cup Romano cheese, preferably freshly grated

½ tbsp. paprika

6 pork cutlets

Sea salt, to taste

Ground black pepper, to taste

Directions:

Put the sesame oil in a large frying pan and heat it at a medium-high flame.

Whisk the egg in a shallow dish. In another dish, place the Romano cheese and paprika. Season the pork cutlets with salt and black pepper.

Working one at a time, dip the pork cutlets into the eggs. Then dredge in the Romano cheese mixture, pressing to coat.

Fry the pork chops for approximately 4 minutes on each side. Move to a paper towel-lined plate and serve warm. Bon appétit!

Nutrition: Calories: 454; Fat: 21.5 g; Carbs: 1.1 g; Protein: 60.7 g; Protein: 0.4 g.

665 BEER-BRAISED BOSTON BUTT

Preparation Time: 20 minutes

Cooking Time: 1 hour, 35 minutes

Servings: 6

Ingredients:

2 tbsp. olive oil

2 pounds Boston butt, cut into cubes

½ tsp. paprika

1 tsp. mustard powder

Sea salt, to taste

Freshly ground black pepper, to taste

1 cup beer

Directions:

Put olive oil in a huge frying pan and heat it over moderate heat. Now, sear the Boston butt for 5 to 6 minutes, stirring periodically.

Sprinkle the cooked pork with paprika, mustard powder, salt, and black pepper. Pour the beer into the pan and gently stir to combine.

When the cooking juices reach boiling, turn the heat to medium-low. Allow it to simmer and partially covered, for at least 1 hour and 30 minutes.

Afterward, broil the pork under a preheated broiler for about 4 minutes. Bon appétit!

Nutrition: Calories: 238; Fat: 10.9 g; Carbs: 1.5 g; Protein: 28.5 g; Protein: 0.1 g.

666 PORK AND SAUSAGE ENDIVE WRAPS

Preparation Time: 10 minutes

Cooking Time: 15 minutes

Servings: 4

Ingredients:

2 tbsp. olive oil

½ pounds ground pork

1 oz. pork sausage, crumbled

½ cup yellow onions, chopped

1 bell peppers, chopped

1 jalapeno pepper, chopped

2 cloves garlic, finely chopped

¼ tsp. ground bay leaf

Sea salt, to taste

Ground black pepper, to taste

18 endive spears, rinsed

Directions:

Put olive oil in a huge saucepan and heat it over medium-high heat. Now, cook the ground pork and sausage until no longer pink or about 3 minutes, breaking the meat apart with a wide spatula.

Add in the onions and peppers and stir until the vegetables begin to soften. Add in the jalapeno, garlic, ground bay leaf, salt, and black pepper.

Continue stirring for an additional 30 seconds or until fragrant.

Spoon the meat mixture on top of each endive spear and serve warm.

Nutrition: Calories: 432; Fat: 30.1 g; Carbs: 6 g; Protein: 3.2 g.

667 LAHANA SARMASI (TURKISH STUFFED CABBAGE ROLLS)

Preparation Time: 10 minutes

Cooking Time: 1 hour & 30 minutes

Servings: 8

Ingredients:

16 cabbage leaves

½-pound Italian sausage, crumbled

1 pound ground pork

2 medium-sized leek, chopped

4 cloves garlic, halved

1 serrano pepper, sliced

2 tbsp. tomato paste

1 tbsp. pepper paste

1 tsp. mint

Kosher salt, to taste

1 tsp. red pepper flakes

2 cups chicken bone broth

2 bay leaves

Directions:

Place the salted water to a boil in a large pot. Now, put the cabbage leaves into this boiling water. Cook until just tender and rinse them under cold water; reserve.

In a lightly greased frying pan, brown the ground meat until no longer pink or about 4 minutes. Stir in the leeks, garlic, and serrano pepper; continue cooking for a father for 2 minutes.

Add in the tomato paste, pepper paste, mint, salt, and red pepper.

Pour the chicken bone broth over the cabbage rolls, add the bay leaves, and cover with aluminum foil. Bake for about 80 minutes. Serve warm.

Nutrition: Calories: 278; Fat: 21.7 g; Carbs: 5.1 g; Protein: 1.3 g.

668 PORK MEDALLIONS WITH AROMATIC HERB BUTTER

Preparation Time: 10 minutes

Cooking Time: 10 minutes

Servings: 6

Ingredients:

2 tbsp. olive oil

6 pork medallions

1 tsp. mustard powder

1 tsp. paprika

Sea salt, to taste

Freshly ground black pepper, to taste

⅔ cup butter, at room temperature

2 cloves garlic, smashed

½ tsp. dried thyme, crushed

1 tsp. dried rosemary, crushed

1 tbsp. lemon juice

Directions:

In a frying pan, warm the oil to medium-high heat. Cook the pork medallions for 4 to 5 minutes per side or until they achieve the reddish-brown exterior.

Now, season the pork medallions with mustard powder, paprika, salt, and black pepper.

Mix the remaining ingredients in a bowl. Serve the pork medallions with well-chilled herb butter. Enjoy!

Nutrition: Calories: 451; Fat: 31.7 g; Carbs: 0.8 g; Protein: 39.5 g.

669 GRILLED BACK RIBS

Preparation Time: 10 minutes

Cooking Time: 20 minutes

Servings: 4

Ingredients:

2 pounds back ribs

2 tbsp. coconut aminos

1 tsp. garlic powder

2 tsp. shallot powder

2 tbsp. monk fruit powder

Sea salt, to taste

Ground black pepper, to taste

2 tbsp. dry red wine

½ cup beef bone broth

2 tbsp. olive oil

Directions:

Bring all of the above ingredients in a ceramic dish. Cover and let it marinate in your refrigerator overnight; reserve the marinade.

Grill the back ribs over medium-high heat for about 5 minutes per side, basting them with the reserved

marinade. An instant thermometer should read 145°F.
Serve with mashed cauliflower if desired. Enjoy!

Nutrition: Calories: 570; Fat: 42.4 g; Carbs: 2.1 g; Protein: 45 g.

670 TERIYAKI BEEF STIR-FRY

Preparation Time: 10 minutes
Cooking Time: 15 minutes
Servings: 6
Ingredients:

½ tbsp. toasted sesame seed oil
½-pound bottom round steak, cut into bite-sized pieces
1 zucchini, sliced
1 onion, sliced
1 tbsp. coconut aminos
½ lime, zested and juiced
2 garlic cloves, grated
1 tsp. fresh ginger, minced
½ tsp. red pepper flakes, crushed
1 tbsp. rice vinegar
1 package (0.07-oz.) stevia

Directions:

Warm 1 tablespoon of oil in a wok over medium-high heat. Sear the beef for 5 to 6 minutes until brown around the edges; reserve.
Heat the remaining ½ tablespoon of sesame oil and stir fry the zucchini and onion for about 5 minutes.
Meanwhile, mix the remaining ingredients to make the sauce.
Put the sauce into the wok; return the reserved beef to the wok. Cook approximately 3 minutes over medium-high heat until thoroughly heated. Serve immediately.

Nutrition: Calories: 207; Fat: 11 g; Carbs: 1.1 g; Protein: 24.2 g.

671 GRILLED BEEF SHORT LOIN

Preparation Time: 5 minutes
Cooking Time: 25 minutes
Servings: 2
Ingredients:

½-pound beef short loin
1 tsp thyme sprigs, chopped
1 tsp rosemary sprig, chopped
½ tsp. garlic powder
Sea salt, to taste
Ground black pepper, to taste

Directions:

Bring all of the above ingredients in a re-sealable zipper bag. Shake until the beef short loin is well coated on all sides.
Cook on a preheated grill for 15 to 20 minutes, flipping once or twice during the cooking time.

Let it stand for 5 minutes before slicing and serving. Bon appétit!

Nutrition: Calories: 313; Fat: 11.6 g; Carbs: 0.1 g; Protein: 52 g.

672 ROSEMARY LIVER BURGERS

Preparation Time: 15 minutes
Cooking Time: 15 minutes
Servings: 15
Ingredients:

2 lb. ground grass-fed beef
1 lb. ground liver
¼–½ cup rosemary
¼ tsp. chili pepper flakes and black pepper
¼ tbsp. oregano

Directions:

Mix all the ingredients until they are well mixed.
Structure slim burger patties with your hands.
Flame broils the burgers until completely cooked through.

Nutrition: Calories: 324; Fat: 21 g; Carbs: 2.6 g; Protein: 6 g.

673 PAN-SEARED BEEF TONGUE

Preparation Time: 35 minutes
Cooking Time: 65 minutes
Servings: 4
Ingredients:

Whole beef tongue
3 cups water
1 tbsp. olive oil
desired seasoning

Directions:

Wash tongue in the sink.
Spot tongue in a weight cooker alongside 3 cups of water.
Weight cooks on the "stew" setting for 35 minutes.
Let the tongue rest in the broth for 30 minutes.
Remove the skin tongue.
Cut tongue into emblems.
Season tongue with salt pepper.
Skillet burn with olive oil for 2-3 minutes for each side.

Nutrition: Calories: 463; Fat: 6 g; Carbs: 5 g; Protein: 34 g.

674 INTERMITTENT ROASTED BONE MARROW

Preparation Time: 5 minutes
Cooking Time: 20 minutes
Servings: 2
Ingredients:

4 bone marrow halves
sea salt
freshly ground black pepper

Directions:

Preheat the stove to 350°F.

Spot the bones marrow side-up onto a profound plate.
Spot in the broiler for 20-25 minutes until brilliant and firm, and the vast majority of the fat has rendered off.
Season the marrow with ocean salt chips and naturally ground dark pepper.
Serve without anyone else as a starter or scoop out the marrow and spread on flame-broiled steak.

Nutrition: Calories: 440; Fat: 48 g; Carbs: 1.4 g; Protein: 4 g.

675 INTERMITTENT SPICY BEEF AVOCADO CUPS

Preparation Time: 5 minutes
Cooking Time: 15 minutes
Servings: 2
Ingredients:

beefsteak, chopped into small cubes
chili peppers
½ medium onion
2 tbsp. avocado oil
2 tbsp. gluten-free tamari sauce or coconut amino
1 large ripe avocado

Directions:

Add the avocado oil to a skillet on excessive warmth and cook the steak three-D shapes till accomplished simply as you will prefer.
Add peppers and onions to the skillet and prepare dinner until mellowed.
Use regularly avocado oil if vital. Return the steak blocks to the skillet and season with tamari sauce.
Spoon the beef combination over the avocado components and serve.

Nutrition: Calories: 570; Fat: 50 g; Carbs: 6.3 g; Protein: 19 g.

676 INTERMITTENT ROSEMARY ROAST BEEF AND WHITE RADISHES

Preparation Time: 10 minutes
Cooking Time: 60 minutes
Servings: 8
Ingredients:

3 lb. boneless beef roast
2 white daikon radishes
3 tbsp. rosemary
2 tbsp. salt, to taste
2 tbsp. olive oil

Directions:

Preheat oven to 400°F.
Spread olive oil, rosemary, and salt over the cheeseburger.
Detect the stripped and severed radishes at the base of a warming dish.

Detect the burger over the radishes and warmth for an hour.

Wrap the burger by utilizing foil and permit unwinding for 20 minutes sooner than serving.

Nutrition: Calories: 492; Fat: 39 g; Carbs: 4.1 g; Protein: 29 g.

677 INTERMITTENT BEEF LIVER WITH ASIAN DIP

Preparation Time: 10 minutes
Cooking Time: 15 minutes
Servings: 10
Ingredients:

4 lb. beef liver, whole
¼ cup tamari sauce
2 cloves garlic
2 tsp. fresh ginger
2 tsp. sesame oil

Directions:

Put the meat liver into a pot secured with water and heat to the point of boiling. Bubble for 2-3 minutes and afterward pour the water with the filth out. Top off with new water and bubble for 10 minutes.

In the interim, make the plunge by combining all the plunge ingredients.

Let the hamburger liver cool. At that point, cut it daintily and serve with the plunge.

Nutrition: Calories: 66; Fat: 2 g; Carbs: 2 g; Protein: 9 g.

678 MEATLOAF MUFFINS

Preparation Time: 5 minutes
Cooking Time: 45 minutes
Servings: 6
Ingredients:

1 pound ground beef
½ cup chopped spinach
large egg, lightly beaten
½ cup shredded mozzarella cheese
½ cup shredded parmesan cheese
¼ cup chopped yellow onion
¼ tbsp. seeded and minced jalapeno pepper

Directions:

Set the oven to 350°F. Lightly grease every muffin tin.

Put and mix all ingredients in a bowl.

Scoop an equal portion of meat mixture into each muffin tin and press down lightly.

Bake for 45 minutes.

Serve.

Nutrition: Calories: 198; Fat: 13.8 g; Carbs: 1.8 g; Protein: 11.9 g.

679 COFFEE BARBECUE PORK BELLY

Preparation Time: 15 minutes
Cooking Time: 60 minutes

Servings: 4
Ingredients:

½ cups beef stock
2 pounds of pork belly
2 tbsp. olive oil
1 batch Low Carb Barbecue Dry Rub
1 tbsp. Instant Espresso Powder

Directions:

Preheat the broiler to 350°F.

Warmth the hamburger stock in a little pan over medium warmth until hot, yet not bubbling

In a little bowl, combine the grill dry rub and coffee powder until very much mixed.

Spot the pork midsection, skin side up in a shallow dish and sprinkle 2 tablespoons of the olive oil over the top, scouring it over the whole pork tummy.

Pour the hot stock around the pork midsection and spread the dish firmly with aluminum foil. Prepare for 45 minutes. Cut into 8 thick cuts.

Warmth the remaining olive oil in a skillet over medium-high warmth and singe each cut for 3 minutes on each side or until the ideal degree of freshness is reached.

Nutrition: Calories: 464; Fat: 68 g; Carbs: 3.4 g; Protein: 24 g.

680 CHICKEN-BASIL ALFREDO WITH SHIRATAKI NOODLES

Preparation Time: 10 minutes
Cooking Time: 15 minutes
Servings: 2
Ingredients:
For the noodles:

1 (7-oz.) package Miracle Noodle Fettuccini Shirataki Noodles

For the sauce:

2 tbsp. olive oil
4 oz. cooked shredded chicken (I usually use a store-bought rotisserie chicken)
Pink Himalayan salt to taste
Freshly ground black pepper to taste
1 cup Alfredo Sauce, or any brand you like
¼ cup grated Parmesan cheese
2 tbsp. chopped fresh basil leaves

Directions:

In a colander, rinse the noodles with cold water (shirataki noodles naturally have a smell, and rinsing with cold water will help remove this).

Fill a large saucepan with water and bring to a boil over high heat. Add the noodles and boil for 2 minutes. Drain.

Transfer the noodles to a large, dry skillet over medium-low heat to evaporate any moisture. Do not grease the skillet; it must be dry. Transfer the noodles to a plate and set aside.

To make the sauce:

In the saucepan over medium heat, heat the olive oil. Add the cooked chicken. Season with pink Himalayan salt and pepper.

Pour the Alfredo sauce over the chicken, and cook until warm. Season with more pink Himalayan salt and pepper.

Add the dried noodles to the sauce mixture, and toss until combined.

Divide the pasta between two plates, top each with the Parmesan cheese and chopped basil, and serve.

Nutrition: Calories: 673; Total Fat: 61 g; Carbs: 4 g; Net Carbs: 4 g; Fiber: 0 g; Protein: 29 g.

681 GARLIC-PARMESAN CHICKEN WINGS

Preparation Time: 10 minutes
Cooking Time: 3 hours
Servings: 2
Ingredients:

8 tbsp. (1 stick) butter
2 garlic cloves, minced
tbsp. dried Italian seasoning
¼ cup grated Parmesan cheese, plus ½ cup
Pink Himalayan salt
Freshly ground black pepper
1 pound chicken wings

Directions:

With the crock insert in place, preheat the slow cooker to high. Line a baking sheet with aluminum foil or a silicone baking mat.

Put the butter, garlic, Italian seasoning, and ¼ cup of Parmesan cheese in the slow cooker, and season with pink Himalayan salt and pepper. Allow the butter to melt. Stir the ingredients until well mixed.

Add the chicken wings and stir until coated with the butter mixture.

Cover the slow cooker and cook for 2 hours and 45 minutes.

Preheat the broiler.

Transfer the wings to the prepared baking sheet, sprinkle the remaining ½ cup of Parmesan cheese over the wings. Cook under the broiler until crispy, about 5 minutes.

Serve hot.

Nutrition: Calories: 738; Total Fat: 66 g; Carbs: 4 g; Net Carbs: 4 g; Fiber: 0 g; Protein: 39 g.

682 CHICKEN SKEWERS WITH PEANUT SAUCE

Preparation Time: 10 minutes, plus 1 hour to marinate
Cooking Time: 15 minutes
Servings: 2
Ingredients:

chicken breast, cut into chunks
3 tbsp. soy sauce (or coconut aminos), divided
½ tsp. Sriracha sauce, plus ¼ tsp.
3 tsp. toasted sesame oil, divided
Ghee, for oiling
2 tbsp. peanut butter
Pink Himalayan salt
Freshly ground black pepper

Directions:

In a large zip-top bag, combine the chicken chunks with 2 tablespoons of soy sauce, ½ teaspoon of Sriracha sauce, and 2 teaspoons of sesame oil. Seal the bag, and let the chicken marinate for an hour or so in the refrigerator or up to overnight.

If you are using wood 8-inch skewers, soak them in water for 30 minutes before using.

I like to use my grill pan for the skewers, because I don't have an outdoor grill. If you don't have a grill pan, you can use a large skillet. Preheat your grill pan or grill to low. Oil the grill pan with ghee.

Thread the chicken chunks onto the skewers.

Cook the skewers over low heat for 10 to 15 minutes, flipping halfway through.

Meanwhile, mix the peanut dipping sauce. Stir together the remaining 1 tablespoon of soy sauce, ¼ teaspoon of Sriracha sauce, 1 teaspoon of sesame oil, and the peanut butter. Season with pink Himalayan salt and pepper.

Serve the chicken skewers with a small dish of peanut sauce.

Nutrition: Calories: 586; Total Fat: 29 g; Carbs: 6 g; Net Carbs: 5 g; Fiber: 1 g; Protein: 75 g.

683 BRAISED CHICKEN THIGHS WITH KALAMATA OLIVES

Preparation Time: 10 minutes
Cooking Time: 40 minutes
Servings: 2

Ingredients:

4 chicken thighs, skin on
Pink Himalayan salt
Freshly ground black pepper
2 tbsp. ghee
½ cup chicken broth
lemon, ½ sliced and ½ juiced
½ cup pitted Kalamata olives
1 tbsp. butter

Directions:

Preheat the oven to 375°F.

Pat the chicken thighs dry with paper towels, and season with pink Himalayan salt and pepper.

In a medium oven-safe skillet or high-sided baking dish over medium-high heat, melt the ghee. When the ghee has melted and is hot, add the chicken thighs, skin-side down, and leave them for about 8 minutes, or until the skin is brown and crispy.

Flip the chicken and cook for 2 minutes on the second side. Around the chicken thighs, pour in the chicken broth, and add the lemon slices, lemon juice, and olives.

Bake in the oven for about 30 minutes, until the chicken is cooked through.

Add the butter to the broth mixture.

Divide the chicken and olives between two plates and serve.

Nutrition: Calories: 567; Total Fat: 47 g; Carbs: 4 g; Net Carbs: 2 g; Fiber: 2 g; Protein: 33 g.

684 BUTTERY GARLIC CHICKEN

Preparation Time: 5 minutes
Cooking Time: 40 minutes
Servings: 2

Ingredients:

2 tbsp. ghee, melted
2 boneless skinless chicken breasts
Pink Himalayan salt
Freshly ground black pepper
1 tbsp. dried Italian seasoning
4 tbsp. butter
2 garlic cloves, minced
¼ cup grated Parmesan cheese

Directions:

Preheat the oven to 375°F. Choose a baking dish large enough to hold both chicken breasts and coat it with the ghee.

Pat dry the chicken breasts and season with pink Himalayan salt, pepper, and Italian seasoning. Place the chicken in the baking dish.

In a medium skillet over medium heat, melt the butter. Add the minced garlic, and cook for about 5 minutes. You want the garlic very lightly browned but not burned.

Remove the butter-garlic mixture from the heat, and pour it over the chicken breasts.

Roast the chicken in the oven for 30 to 35 minutes, until cooked through. Sprinkle some of the Parmesan cheese on top of each chicken breast. Let the chicken rest in the baking dish for 5 minutes.

Divide the chicken between two plates, spoon the butter sauce over the chicken, and serve.

Nutrition: Calories: 642; Total Fat: 45 g; Carbs: 2 g; Net Carbs: 2 g; Fiber: 0 g; Protein: 57 g.

685 CHEESY BACON AND BROCCOLI CHICKEN

Preparation Time: 10 minutes
Cooking Time: 1 hour
Servings: 2

Ingredients:

2 tbsp. ghee
2 boneless skinless chicken breasts
Pink Himalayan salt
Freshly ground black pepper
4 bacon slices
6 oz. cream cheese, at room temperature
2 cups frozen broccoli florets, thawed
½ cup shredded Cheddar cheese

Directions:

Preheat the oven to 375°F.

Choose a baking dish that is large enough to hold both chicken breasts and coat it with the ghee.

Pat dries the chicken breasts with a paper towel, and season with pink Himalayan salt and pepper.

Place the chicken breasts and the bacon slices in the baking dish, and bake for 25 minutes.

Transfer the chicken to a cutting board and use two forks to shred it. Season it again with pink Himalayan salt and pepper.

Place the bacon on a paper towel-lined plate to crisp up, and then crumble it.

In a medium bowl, mix to combine the cream cheese, shredded chicken, broccoli, and half of the bacon crumbles. Transfer the chicken mixture to the baking dish, and top with the Cheddar and the remaining half of the bacon crumbles.

Bake until the cheese is bubbling and browned, about 35 minutes, and serve.

Nutrition: Calories: 935; Total Fat: 66 g; Carbs: 10 g; Net Carbs: 8 g; Fiber: 3 g; Protein: 75 g.

686 PARMESAN BAKED CHICKEN

Preparation Time: 5 minutes
Cooking Time: 20 minutes
Servings: 2
Ingredients:

2 tbsp. ghee
2 boneless skinless chicken breasts
Pink Himalayan salt
Freshly ground black pepper
½ cup mayonnaise
¼ cup grated Parmesan cheese
1 tbsp. dried Italian seasoning
¼ cup crushed pork rinds

Directions:

Preheat the oven to 425°F. Choose a baking dish large enough to hold both chicken breasts and coat it with the ghee.

Pat dry the chicken breasts with a paper towel, season with pink Himalayan salt and pepper, and place in the prepared baking dish.

In a small bowl, mix to combine the mayonnaise, Parmesan cheese, and Italian seasoning.

Slather the mayonnaise mixture evenly over the chicken breasts, and sprinkle the crushed pork rinds on top of the mayonnaise mixture.

Bake until the topping is browned, about 20 minutes, and serve.

Nutrition: Calories: 850; Total Fat: 67 g; Carbs: 2 g; Net Carbs: 2 g; Fiber: 0 g; Protein: 60 g.

687 CRUNCHY CHICKEN MILANESE

Preparation Time: 10 minutes
Cooking Time: 10 minutes
Servings: 2
Ingredients:

2 boneless skinless chicken breasts
½ cup coconut flour
¼ tsp. ground cayenne pepper
Pink Himalayan salt - Freshly ground black pepper
egg, lightly beaten
½ cup crushed pork rinds
2 tbsp. olive oil

Directions:

Pound the chicken breasts with a heavy mallet until they are about ½ inch thick. (If you don't have a kitchen mallet, you can use the thick rim of a heavy plate.)

Prepare two separate prep plates and one small, shallow bowl.

On plate 1, put the coconut flour, cayenne pepper, pink Himalayan salt, and pepper. Mix together.

Crack the egg into the small bowl, and lightly beat it with a fork or whisk.

On plate 2, put the crushed pork rinds.

In a large skillet over medium-high heat, heat the olive oil.

Dredge 1 chicken breast on both sides in the coconut-flour mixture. Dip the chicken into the egg, and coat both sides. Dredge the chicken in the pork-rind mixture, pressing the pork rinds into the chicken so they stick. Place the coated chicken in the hot skillet and repeat with the other chicken breast.

Cook the chicken for 3 to 5 minutes on each side, until brown, crispy, and cooked through, and serve.

Nutrition: Calories: 604; Total Fat: 29 g; Carbs: 17 g; Net Carbs: 7 g; Fiber: 10 g; Protein: 65 g.

688 EGG BUTTER

Preparation Time: 5 minutes
Cooking Time: 0 minutes
Servings: 2
Ingredients:

2 large eggs, hard-boiled
3-oz. unsalted butter
½ tsp. dried oregano
½ tsp. dried basil
2 leaves of iceberg lettuce

Seasoning:

½ tsp. sea salt
¼ tsp. ground black pepper

Directions:

Peel the eggs, then chop them finely and place in a medium bowl.

Add remaining ingredients and stir well.

Serve egg butter wrapped in a lettuce leaf.

Nutrition: Calories: 159; Fats: 16.5 g; Protein: 3 g; Net Carb: 0.2 g; Fiber: 0 g.

689 SHREDDED CHICKEN IN A LETTUCE WRAP

Preparation Time: 5 minutes
Cooking Time: 15 minutes
Servings: 2
Ingredients:

2 leaves of iceberg lettuce
2 large chicken thighs
2 tbsp. shredded cheddar cheese
3 cups hot water
4 tbsp. tomato sauce

Seasoning:

½ tbsp. soy sauce
½ tbsp. red chili powder
¾ tsp. salt
½ tsp cracked black pepper

Directions:

Turn on the instant pot, place chicken thighs in it, and add remaining ingredients except for lettuce.

Stir until just mixed, shut the instant pot with a lid and cook for 15 minutes at high pressure. When done, release the pressure naturally.

Then open the instant pot, transfer the chicken to a cutting board and shred with two forks.

Evenly divide the chicken between two lettuce leaves, and drizzle with some of the cooking liquid, reserving the remaining liquid for later use as chicken broth.

Serve.

Nutrition: Calories: 143.5; Fats: 1.4 g; Protein: 21.7 g; Net Carb: 3.4 g; Fiber: 0.7 g.

690 CIDER CHICKEN

Preparation Time: 10 minutes
Cooking Time: 18 minutes
Servings: 2
Ingredients:

2 chicken thighs
¼ cup apple cider vinegar
1 tsp. liquid stevia

Seasoning:

½ tbsp. coconut oil
⅓ tsp. salt
¼ tsp. ground black pepper

Directions:

Turn on the oven, then set it to 450°F and let it preheat.

Meanwhile, place chicken in a bowl, drizzle with oil and then season with salt and black pepper

Take a baking sheet, place prepared chicken thighs on it, and bake for 10 to 15 minutes or until its internal temperature reaches 165°F.

In the meantime, take a small saucepan, place it over medium heat, pour in vinegar, stir in stevia and bring the mixture to boil.

Then switch heat to the low level and simmer sauce for 3 to 5 minutes until reduced by half, set aside until required.

When the chicken has roasted, brush it generously with prepared cider sauce, then turn on the broiler and bake the chicken for 3 minutes until golden brown.

Serve.

Nutrition: Calories: 182.5; Fats: 107.5 g; Protein: 15.5 g; Net Carb: 2.5 g; Fiber: 0 g.

691 BACON-WRAPPED CHICKEN BITES

Preparation Time: 10 minutes
Cooking Time: 20 minutes
Servings: 2
Ingredients:
  chicken thigh, debone, cut into small pieces
  4 slices of bacon, cut into thirds
  ¼ tbsp. garlic powder
Seasoning:
  ¼ tsp. salt
  ⅛ tsp. ground black pepper
Directions:
  Turn on the oven, then set it to 400°F and let it preheat.
  Cut chicken into small pieces, then place them in a bowl, add salt, garlic powder, and black pepper and toss until well coated.
  Wrap each chicken piece with a bacon strip, place in a baking dish and bake for 15 to 20 minutes until crispy, turning carefully every 5 minutes.
  Serve.
Nutrition: Calories: 153; Fats: 8.7 g; Protein: 15 g; Net Carb: 2.7 g; Fiber: 0.7 g.

692 CHEESY BACON WRAPPED CHICKEN

Preparation Time: 5 minutes
Cooking Time: 25 minutes
Servings: 2
Ingredients:
  2 chicken thighs, boneless
  2 strips of bacon
  2 tbsp. shredded cheddar cheese
Seasoning:
  ⅓ tsp. salt
  ⅔ tsp. paprika
  ¼ tsp. garlic powder
Directions:
  Turn on the oven, then set it to 400°F and let it preheat.
  Meanwhile, season chicken thighs with salt, paprika, and garlic on both sides, and then place them onto a baking sheet greased with oil.
  Top each chicken thighs with a bacon strip and then bake for 15 to 20 minutes until the chicken has cooked through, and bacon has crispy.
  When done, sprinkle cheese over chicken, continue baking for 5 minutes until cheese has melted and golden, and then serve.
Nutrition: Calories: 172.5; Fats: 11.5 g; Protein: 14.5 g; Net Carb: 0.5 g; Fiber: 0 g.

693 BEANS AND SAUSAGE

Preparation Time: 5 minutes

Cooking Time: 6 minutes
Servings: 2
Ingredients:
  4 oz. green beans
  4 oz. chicken sausage, sliced
  ½ tsp dried basil
  ½ tsp dried oregano
  ⅓ cup chicken broth, from chicken sausage
Seasoning:
  2 tbsp. avocado oil
  ¼ tsp. salt
  ⅛ tsp. ground black pepper
Directions:
  Turn on the instant pot, place all the ingredients in its inner pot and shut with lid, in the sealed position.
  Press the "manual" button, cook for 6 minutes at high-pressure settings and, when done, do quick pressure release.
  Serve immediately.
Nutrition: Calories: 151; Fats: 9.4 g; Protein: 11.7 g; Net Carb: 3.4 g; Fiber: 1.6 g.

694 PAPRIKA RUBBED CHICKEN

Preparation Time: 5 minutes
Cooking Time: 25 minutes
Servings: 2
Ingredients:
  2 chicken thighs, boneless
  ¼ tbsp. fennel seeds, ground
  ½ tsp. hot paprika
  ¼ tsp. smoked paprika
  ½ tsp. minced garlic
Seasoning:
  ¼ tsp. salt
  2 tbsp. avocado oil
Directions:
  Turn on the oven, then set it to 325°F and let it preheat.
  Prepare the spice mix. Take a small bowl, add all the ingredients in it, except for chicken, and stir until well mixed.
  Brush the mixture on all sides of the chicken. Rub it well into the meat, then place chicken onto a baking sheet and roast for 15 to 25 minutes until thoroughly cooked, basting every 10 minutes with the drippings.
  Serve.
Nutrition: Calories: 102.3; Fats: 8 g; Protein: 7.2 g; Net Carb: 0.3 g; Fiber: 0.3 g.

695 TERIYAKI CHICKEN

Preparation Time: 5 minutes
Cooking Time: 18 minutes
Servings: 2
Ingredients:
  2 chicken thighs, boneless
  2 tbsp. soy sauce

  2 tbsp. swerve sweetener
  2 tbsp. avocado oil
Directions:
  Take a skillet pan, place it over medium heat, add oil and when hot, add chicken thighs and cook for 5 minutes per side until seared.
  Then sprinkle sugar over chicken thighs, drizzle with soy sauce and bring the sauce to boil.
  Switch heat to medium-low level, continue cooking for 3 minutes until chicken is evenly glazed, and then transfer to a plate.
  Serve chicken with cauliflower rice.
Nutrition: Calories: 150; Fats: 9 g; Protein: 17.3 g; Net Carb: 0 g; Fiber: 0 g.

696 CHILI LIME CHICKEN WITH COLESLAW

Preparation Time: 35 minutes
Cooking Time: 8 minutes
Servings: 2
Ingredients:
  chicken thigh, boneless
  ¼ oz. coleslaw
  ¼ tsp. minced garlic
  ¾ tbsp. apple cider vinegar
  ½ of a lime, juiced, zested
Seasoning:
  ¼ tsp. paprika
  ¼ tsp. salt
  2 tbsp. avocado oil
  1 ½ tbsp. unsalted butter
Directions:
  Prepare the marinade. Take a medium bowl, add vinegar, oil, garlic, paprika, salt, lime juice, and zest and stir until well mixed.
  Cut chicken thighs into bite-size pieces. Toss until well mixed, and marinate it in the refrigerator for 30 minutes.
  Then take a skillet pan. Place it over medium-high heat, add butter and marinated chicken pieces. Cook for 8 minutes until golden brown and thoroughly cooked.
  Serve chicken with coleslaw.
Nutrition: Calories: 157.3; Fats: 12.8 g; Protein: 9 g; Net Carb: 1 g; Fiber: 0.5 g.

697 LIME GARLIC CHICKEN THIGHS

Preparation Time: 35 minutes
Cooking Time: 15 minutes
Servings: 2
Ingredients:
  2 boneless chicken thighs, skinless
  ¾ tsp. garlic powder
  ½ tsp. all-purpose seasoning
  ½ of lime, juiced, zested
  ½ tbsp. avocado oil
Directions:

Take a medium bowl, place chicken in it, and sprinkle with garlic powder, all-purpose seasoning, and lime zest.

Drizzle with lime juice, toss until well coated and let chicken thighs marinate for 30 minutes.

Then take a medium skillet pan, place it over medium heat, add oil and when hot, place marinated chicken thighs in it and cook for 5 to 7 minutes per side until thoroughly cooked.

Serve.

Nutrition: Calories: 260; Fats: 15.6 g; Protein: 26.8 g; Net Carb: 1.3 g; Fiber: 0.6 g.

698 BACON RANCH DEVILED EGGS

Preparation Time: 5 minutes
Cooking Time: 0 minutes
Servings: 2
Ingredients:

slice of bacon, chopped, cooked
⅔ tsp. ranch dressing
½ tbsp. mayonnaise
⅓ tsp. mustard paste
eggs, boiled

Seasoning:

¼ tsp. paprika

Directions:

Peel the boiled eggs, then slice in half lengthwise and transfer the egg yolks to a medium bowl by using a spoon.

Mash the egg yolk, add remaining ingredients, except for bacon and paprika and stir until well combined.

Pipe the egg yolk mixture into egg whites, sprinkle with bacon and paprika and then serve.

Nutrition: Calories: 260; Fats: 24 g; Protein: 8.9 g; Net Carb: 0.6 g; Fiber: 0.1 g.

699 DEVILED EGGS WITH MUSHROOMS

Preparation Time: 5 minutes
Cooking Time: 0 minutes
Servings: 2
Ingredients:

tbsp. chopped mushroom
tsp. mayonnaise
½ tsp. apple cider vinegar
tsp. butter, unsalted
eggs, boiled
Seasoning:
¼ tsp. salt
⅛ tsp. ground black pepper
¼ tsp. dried parsley

Directions:

Peel the boiled eggs. Then slice in half lengthwise and transfer the egg yolks to a medium bowl by using a spoon.

Mash the egg yolk, add remaining ingredients and stir until well combined.

Pipe the egg yolk mixture into egg whites, sprinkle with black pepper and then serve.

Nutrition: Calories: 130.5; Fats: 10.9 g; Protein: 7.1 g; Net Carb: 0.6 g; Fiber: 0.1 g.

700 CHICKEN AND PEANUT STIR-FRY

Preparation Time: 5 minutes
Cooking Time: 15 minutes
Servings: 2
Ingredients:

2 chicken thighs, cubed
½ cup broccoli florets
¼ cup peanuts
1 tbsp. sesame oil
½ tbsp. soy sauce

Seasoning:

½ tsp. garlic powder

Directions:

Take a skillet pan and place it over medium heat. Add ½ tablespoon of oil and when hot, add chicken cubes and cook for 4 minutes until browned on all sides.

Then add broccoli florets and continue cooking for 2 minutes until tender-crisp.

Add remaining ingredients, stir well and cook for another 2 minutes.

Serve.

Nutrition: Calories: 266; Fats: 19 g; Protein: 18.5 g; Net Carb: 4 g; Fiber: 2.5 g.

701 CHICKEN SCARPARIELLO WITH SPICY SAUSAGE

Preparation Time: 10 minutes
Cooking Time: 45 minutes
Servings: 6
Ingredients:

2 pound boneless chicken thighs
Sea salt, for seasoning
Freshly ground black pepper, for seasoning
3 tbsp. good-quality olive oil, divided
½-pound Italian sausage (sweet or hot)
2 tbsp. minced garlic
2 pimiento, chopped
¼ cup dry white wine
2 cup chicken stock
2 tbsp. chopped fresh parsley

Directions:

Preheat the oven. Set the oven temperature to 425°F.

Brown the chicken and sausage. Pat the chicken thighs to dry using paper towels and season them lightly with salt and pepper. In a large oven-safe skillet over medium-high heat, warm 2 tablespoons of olive oil. Add the chicken thighs and sausage to the skillet and brown them on all sides, turning them carefully, about 10 minutes.

Bake the chicken and sausage. Bring the skillet into the oven and bake for 25 minutes or until the chicken is cooked through. Take the skillet out of the oven, transfer the chicken and sausage to a plate, and put the skillet over medium heat on the stovetop.

Make the sauce. Warm the remaining 1 tablespoon of olive oil. Add the garlic and pimiento and sauté for 3 minutes. Pour the white wine and deglaze the skillet by using a spoon to scrape up any browned bits from the bottom of the skillet. Pour in the chicken stock and bring it to a boil, then reduce the heat to low and simmer until the sauce reduces by about half, about 6 minutes.

Finish and serve. Put back the chicken and sausage to the skillet. Toss it to coat it with the sauce, and serve it topped with the parsley.

Nutrition: Calories: 370; Total fat: 30 g; Total carbs: 3 g; Fiber: 0 g; Net carbs: 3 g; Sodium: 314 mg; Protein: 19 g.

702 ALMOND CHICKEN CUTLETS

Preparation Time: 10 minutes
Cooking Time: 15 minutes
Servings: 4
Ingredients:

2 eggs
½ tsp. garlic powder
1 cup almond flour
1 tbsp. chopped fresh oregano
4 (4-oz.) boneless skinless chicken breasts, pounded to about ¼ inch thick
¼ cup good-quality olive oil
2 tbsp. grass-fed butter

Directions:

Bread the chicken. Whisk together the eggs, garlic powder in a medium bowl, and set it aside. Stir together the almond flour and oregano on a plate and set the plate next to the egg mixture. Pat the chicken breasts to dry using paper towels and dip them into the egg mixture. Remove excess egg; then roll the chicken in the almond flour until they are coated.

Fry the chicken. In a large skillet over medium-high heat, warm the olive oil and butter. Add the breaded chicken breasts and fry them, turning them once, until they are cooked through, very crispy, and golden brown, 14 to 16 minutes in total.

Serve. Place one cutlet on each of the four plates and serve them immediately.

Nutrition: Calories: 328; Total fat: 23 g; Total carbs: 0 g; Fiber: 0 g; Net carbs: 0 g; Sodium: 75 mg; Protein: 28 g.

703 SLOW COOKER CHICKEN CACCIATORE

Preparation Time: 15 minutes
Cooking Time: 10 minutes
Servings: 4
Ingredients:

¼ cup good-quality olive oil
4 (4-oz.) boneless chicken breasts, each cut into three pieces
1 onion, chopped
2 celery stalks, chopped
1 cup sliced mushrooms
1 tbsp. minced garlic
1 (28-oz.) can sodium-free diced tomatoes
½ cup red wine
½ cup tomato paste
1 tbsp. dried basil
1 tsp. dried oregano
⅛ tsp. red pepper flakes

Directions:

Brown the chicken. In a skillet at medium-high heat, warm the olive oil. Add the chicken breasts and brown them, turning them once, about 10 minutes in total.

Cook in the slow cooker. Place the chicken in the slow cooker and stir in the onion, celery, mushrooms, garlic, tomatoes, red wine, tomato paste, basil, oregano, and red pepper flakes. Cook it on high for approximately 3 to 4 hours or on low for 6 to 8 hours, until the chicken is fully cooked and tender.

Serve. Divide the chicken and sauce between four bowls and serve it immediately.

Nutrition: Calories: 383; Total fat: 26 g; Total carbs: 11 g; Fiber: 4 g; Net carbs: 7 g; Sodium: 116 mg; Protein: 26 g.

704 CHEESY CHICKEN SUN-DRIED TOMATO PACKETS

Preparation Time: 15 minutes
Cooking Time: 40 minutes
Servings: 4
Ingredients:

1 cup goat cheese
½ cup chopped oil-packed sun-dried tomatoes
1 tsp. minced garlic

½ tsp. dried basil - ½ tsp. dried oregano
4 (4-oz.) boneless chicken breasts
Sea salt, for seasoning
Freshly ground black pepper, for seasoning
1 tbsp. olive oil

Directions:

Preheat the oven. Set the oven temperature to 375°F.

Prepare the filling. In a medium bowl, put the goat cheese, sun-dried tomatoes, garlic, basil, and oregano; then mix until everything is well blended.

Stuff the chicken. Make a horizontal slice in the middle of each chicken breast to make a pocket, making sure not to cut through the sides or ends. Spoon one-quarter of the filling into each breast, folding the skin and chicken meat over the slit. Secure the pockets with a toothpick. Lightly season the breasts with salt and pepper.

Brown the chicken. In a large oven-safe skillet over medium heat, warm the olive oil. Add the breasts and sear them, turning them once, until they are golden, about 8 minutes in total.

Bake the chicken. Bring the skillet into the oven and bake the chicken for 30 minutes or until it's cooked through.

Serve. Remove the toothpicks. Divide the chicken into 4 plates and serve them immediately.

Nutrition: Calories: 388; Total fat: 29 g; Total carbs: 4 g; Fiber: 1 g; Net carbs: 3 g; Sodium: 210 mg; Protein: 28 g.

705 TUSCAN CHICKEN SAUTÉ

Preparation Time: 10 minutes
Cooking Time: 35 minutes
Servings: 4
Ingredients:

1 pound boneless chicken breasts, each cut into three pieces
Sea salt, for seasoning
Freshly ground black pepper, for seasoning
3 tbsp. olive oil
2 tbsp. minced garlic
¾ cup chicken stock
1 tsp. dried oregano
½ tsp. dried basil
½ cup heavy (whipping) cream
½ cup shredded Asiago cheese
1 cup fresh spinach
¼ cup sliced Kalamata olives

Directions:

Prepare the chicken. Pat, the chicken, breasts dry and lightly season them with salt and pepper.

Sauté the chicken. In a large skillet over medium-high heat, warm the olive oil. Add the chicken and sauté until it is golden brown and just cooked through, about 15 minutes in total. Transfer the chicken to a plate and set it aside.

Make the sauce. Put the garlic to the skillet, then sauté until it's softened for about 2 minutes. Stir in the chicken stock, oregano, and basil, scraping up any browned bits in the skillet. Bring to a boil, then reduce the heat to low and simmer until the sauce is reduced by about one-quarter, about 10 minutes.

Finish the dish. Stir in the cream, Asiago, and simmer, stirring the sauce frequently, until it has thickened about 5 minutes. Put back the chicken to the skillet along with any accumulated juices. Stir in the spinach and olives and simmer until the spinach is wilted for about 2 minutes.

Serve. Divide the chicken and sauce between four plates and serve it immediately.

Nutrition: Calories: 483; Total fat: 38 g; Total carbs: 5 g; Fiber: 1 g; Net carbs: 3 g; Sodium: 332 mg; Protein: 31 g.

706 EASY CHICKEN TACOS

Preparation Time: 5 minutes
Cooking Time: 27 minutes
Servings: 4
Ingredients:

1 pound ground chicken
½ cups Mexican cheese blend
1 tbsp. Mexican seasoning blend
1 tsp. butter, room temperature
2 small-sized shallots, peeled and finely chopped
2 clove garlic, minced
1 cup tomato puree
½ cup salsa
4 slices bacon, chopped

Directions:

In a saucepan, put butter then melt in over a moderately high flame. Now, cook the shallots until tender and fragrant.

Then, sauté the garlic, chicken, and bacon for about 5 minutes, stirring continuously and crumbling with a fork. Add the Mexican seasoning blend.

Fold in the tomato puree and salsa; continue to simmer for 5 to 7 minutes over medium-low heat; reserve.

- Line a baking pan with wax paper. Place 4 piles of the shredded cheese on the baking pan and gently press them down with a wide spatula to make "taco shells."
- Bake in the preheated oven at 365°F for 6 to 7 minutes or until melted. Allow these taco shells to cool for about 10 minutes.

Nutrition: Calories: 535; Fat: 33.3 g; Carbs: 4.8 g; Protein: 47.9 g; Fiber: 1.9 g.

707 CHEESY BACON-WRAPPED CHICKEN WITH ASPARAGUS SPEARS

Preparation Time: 20 minutes
Cooking Time: 30 minutes
Servings: 4
Ingredients:

- 4 chicken breasts
- 8 bacon slices
- 1 pound (454 g) asparagus spears
- 1 tbsp. fresh lemon juice
- ½ cup Manchego cheese, grated

From the cupboard:

- 1 tbsp. olive oil, divided
- Salt, to taste
- Freshly ground black pepper, to taste

Directions:

- Set the oven to 400°F. Line a baking sheet using parchment paper, then grease with 1 tablespoon of olive oil.
- Put the chicken breasts in a large bowl, and sprinkle with salt and black pepper. Toss to combine well.
- Wrap every chicken breast with 2 slices of bacon. Place the chicken on the baking sheet, then bake in the preheated oven for 25 minutes or until the bacon is crispy.
- Preheat the grill to high, then brush with the remaining olive oil.
- Place the asparagus spears on the grill grate, and sprinkle with salt. Grill for 5 minutes or until fork-tender. Flip the asparagus frequently during the grilling.
- Transfer the bacon-wrapped chicken breasts to four plates. Drizzle with lemon juice, and scatter with Manchego cheese. Spread the hot asparagus spears on top to serve.

Nutrition: Calories: 455; Total fat: 38.1 g; Net carbs: 2 g; Protein: 26.1 g.

708 BACON-WRAPPED CHICKEN WITH CHEDDAR CHEESE

Preparation Time: 10 minutes
Cooking Time: 4 hours
Servings: 6
Ingredients:

- 2 large chicken breasts, each cut into 6 pieces
- 6 slices of streaky bacon, each cut in half widthways
- 4 garlic cloves, crushed
- ½ cup Cheddar cheese, grated

From the cupboard:

- 1 tbsp. olive oil
- Salt, to taste
- Freshly ground black pepper, to taste

Directions:

- Grease the inside of the slow cooker with olive oil.
- Wrap each piece of chicken breast with each half of the bacon slice, and arrange them in the slow cooker. Sprinkle with garlic, salt, and black pepper.
- Put the lid and then cook on LOW for 4 hours.
- Set the oven to 350°F (180°C).
- Transfer the cooked bacon-wrapped chicken to a baking dish, then scatter with cheese.
- Cook in the preheated oven for 5 minutes or until the cheese melts.
- Take it off from the oven and serve warm.

Nutrition: Calories: 308; Total fat: 20.8 g; Total carbs: 2.9 g; Fiber: 0 g; Net carbs: 2.9 g; Protein: 26.1 g.

709 DELIGHTFUL TERIYAKI CHICKEN UNDER PRESSURE

Preparation Time: 5 minutes
Cooking Time: 20 minutes
Servings: 8
Ingredients:

- 3 cup chicken broth
- ¾ cup brown sugar
- 2 tbsp. ground ginger
- 2 tsp pepper
- 3 pounds boneless and skinless chicken thighs
- ¼ cup apple cider vinegar
- ¾ cup low-sodium soy sauce
- 20 oz. canned pineapple, crushed
- 2 tbsp. garlic powder

Directions:

- Mix all of the ingredients, excluding the chicken. Add the chicken meat and turn to coat. Seal the lid, press POULTRY, and cook for 20 minutes at High. Do a quick pressure release by turning the valve to an "open" position.

Nutrition: Calories: 352; Carbs: 31 g; Fat: 11 g; Protein: 31 g.

710 TURKEY AND POTATOES WITH BUFFALO SAUCE

Preparation Time: 10 minutes
Cooking Time: 20 minutes
Servings: 2

Ingredients:

- 3 tbsp. olive oil
- 4 tbsp. buffalo sauce
- 1-pound sweet potatoes, cut into cubes
- ½-pound turkey breast, cut into pieces
- ½ tsp. garlic powder
- onion, diced
- ½ cup water

Directions:

- Heat 1 tablespoon of olive oil on SAUTÉ mode at High. Stir-fry onion in hot oil for about 3 minutes. Stir in the remaining ingredients. Seal the lid, set to PRESSURE COOK/MANUAL mode for 20 minutes at high pressure.
- When cooking is over, do a quick pressure release by turning the valve to an "open" position.

Nutrition: Calories: 377; Carbs: 32 g; Fat: 9 g; Protein: 14 g.

711 EXQUISITE PEAR AND ONION GOOSE

Preparation Time: 15 minutes
Cooking Time: 20 minutes
Servings: 8
Ingredients:

- 2 cups chicken broth
- ½ tbsp. butter
- ½ cup slice onions
- ½ pounds goose, chopped into large pieces
- ½ tbsp. balsamic vinegar
- ¾ tsp. cayenne pepper
- pears, peeled and sliced
- ¼ tsp. garlic powder
- ½ tsp. pepper

Directions:

- Melt the butter on SAUTÉ. Add the goose and cook until it becomes golden on all sides. Transfer to a plate. Add the onions and cook for 2 minutes. Return the goose to the cooker.
- Add the rest of the ingredients. Stir well to combine and seal the lid. Select PRESSURE COOK/MANUAL mode, and set the timer to 18 minutes at High Pressure. Do a quick pressure release. Serve and enjoy!

Nutrition: Calories: 313; Carbs: 14 g; Fat: 8 g; Protein: 38 g.

712 TURKEY BREAST WITH FENNEL AND CELERY

Preparation Time: 10 minutes
Cooking Time: 15 minutes
Servings: 3
Ingredients:

- 2 pounds boneless and skinless turkey breast

½ cup fennel bulb, chopped

½ cup celery with leaves, chopped

¼ cups chicken stock

¼ tsp. pepper

¼ tsp. garlic powder

Directions:

Throw all ingredients in your pressure cooker. Give it a good stir and seal the lid. Press PRESSURE COOK/MANUAL, and cook for 15 minutes at High. Do a quick pressure release. Shred the turkey with two forks.

Nutrition: Calories: 272; Carbs: 7 g; Fat: 4 g; Protein: 48 g.

713 PANCETTA AND CHICKEN RISOTTO

Preparation Time: 15 minutes

Cooking Time: 15 minutes

Servings: 2

Ingredients:

¾-pound. chicken meat, diced

2 to 3 slices pancetta; diced

¾ cup risotto or Arborio rice

1 tsp. fresh thyme

2 tbsp. lemon zest

2 tbsp. unsalted butter

2 tbsp. olive oil

3 tbsp. parmesan; grated

2 garlic cloves; chopped

½ onion; chopped

⅓ cup white wine

½ cups chicken stock

Salt and pepper to taste

Directions:

Put oil and butter in Instant Pot and press the "Sauté" button (*Normal* preset), wait till you see Hot on display.

Add onion, cook for 1 to 2 minutes. Add pancetta, chicken, and garlic. Cook for another 2 to 3 minutes.

Add rice and mix well, the rice should be covered with an oil-butter mixture. Pour the wine and scrape the sides of the pot. Cook for 2 to 3 minutes, stirring constantly. Press the *Cancel* button.

Add chicken stock, thyme, lemon zest, salt, and pepper. Seal the lid and turn the vent to *Sealed*. Press the *Pressure Cook* (Manual) button, use the *+* or *-* button to set the timer for 6 minutes. Use the *Pressure level* button to set Pressure to *HIGH*.

When the timer is up, press the *Cancel* button and allow the pressure to be released naturally; until the float valve drops down.

Open the lid; Add parmesan cheese to the pot and stir well until it melts.

Serve topped with extra parmesan and lemon zest.

Nutrition: Calories: 586; Total Fat: 22.5 g; Total Carbohydrate: 23.6 g; Protein: 45 g.

714 SPINACH CHICKEN CHEESY BAKE

Preparation Time: 25 minutes

Cooking Time: 20 minutes

Servings: 6

Ingredients:

6 chicken breasts, skinless and boneless

½ tsp. mixed spice seasoning

Pink salt and black pepper to season

loose cups baby spinach

1 tsp. olive oil

¼ oz. cream cheese, cubed

¼ cups shredded mozzarella cheese

1 tbsp. water

Directions:

Preheat oven to 370°F.

Season chicken with spice mix, salt, and black pepper. Pat with your hands to have the seasoning stick on the chicken.

Put in the casserole dish and layer spinach over the chicken.

Mix the oil with cream cheese, mozzarella, salt, and black pepper and stir in water, a tablespoon at a time.

Pour the mixture over the chicken and cover the pot with aluminum foil.

Bake for at least 20 minutes. Take off the foil and continue cooking for 15 minutes until a nice golden-brown color is formed on top. Take out and allow sitting for 5 minutes. Serve warm with braised asparagus.

Nutrition: Calories: 340: Fat: 30.2 g; Net Carbs: 3.1 g; Protein: 15 g.

715 ROASTED WHOLE CHICKEN

Preparation Time: 20 minutes

Cooking Time: 1 hour, 32 minutes

Servings: 6

Ingredients:

10 tbsp. unsalted butter

3 garlic cloves, minced

1 (3-pounds) grass-fed whole chicken, neck, and giblets removed

Salt and ground black pepper, as required

Directions:

Preheat the oven to 400°F. Arrange an oven rack into the lower portion of the oven.

Grease a large baking dish.

Place the butter and garlic in a small pan over medium heat and cook for about 1-2 minutes.

Remove the pan from heat and let it cool for about 2 minutes.

Season the inside and outside of the chicken evenly with salt and black pepper.

Arrange the chicken into a prepared baking dish, breast side up.

Pour the garlic butter over and inside of the chicken.

Bake for about 1-1 ½ hours, basting with the pan juices every 20 minutes.

Remove from oven and place the chicken onto a cutting board for about 5-10 minutes before carving.

Cut into desired size pieces and serve.

Nutrition: Calories: 772; Fat: 39.1 g; Net Carbs: 0.7 g; Protein: 99 g.

716 BUFFALO PIZZA CHICKEN

Preparation Time: 5 minutes

Cooking Time: 5-6 minutes

Servings: 5

Ingredients:

Vegetable cooking spray

½ cup Buffalo-style hot sauce

(16-oz.) package prebaked Italian pizza crust

3 cups chopped deli-roasted whole chicken

cup (4 oz.) shredded Provolone cheese

¼ cup crumbled blue cheese

Directions:

Coat the grill with the spray and put it on the grill. Preheat grill to 350°F (medium heat).

Spread the hot sauce over the crust, and the next 3 ingredients above mentioned.

Place the crust on the cooking grate directly. Grill at 350°F (medium heat) for 4 minutes, covered with the grill lid.

Rotate 1-quarter turn pizza and grill, covered with grill top, for 5 to 6 minutes or until heated thoroughly. Serve right away.

Nutrition: Calories: 365; Fat: 11 g; Net Carbs: 42 g; Protein: 24 g.

717 HOT CHICKEN MEATBALLS

Preparation Time: 5 minutes

Cooking Time: 21 minutes

Servings: 2

Ingredients:

1 pound ground chicken

Salt and black pepper, to taste

1 tbsp. yellow mustard

½ cup almond flour

¼ cup mozzarella cheese, grated

¼ cup hot sauce

egg

Directions:

Preheat oven to 400°F and line a baking tray with parchment paper.

In a bowl, combine the chicken, black pepper, mustard, flour, mozzarella cheese, salt, and egg. Form meatballs and arrange them on the baking tray.

Cook for 16 minutes, then pour over the hot sauce and bake for 5 more minutes.

Nutrition: Calories: 487; Fat: 35 g; Net Carbs: 4.3 g; Protein: 31.5 g.

718 INTERMITTENT CHICKEN ENCHILADAS

Preparation Time: 10 minutes
Cooking Time: 25 minutes
Servings: 6
Ingredients:

2 cups gluten-free enchilada sauce
Chicken:

2 tbsp. avocado oil
4 cloves Garlic (minced)
2 cups shredded chicken (cooked)
¼ cup chicken broth
¼ cup fresh cilantro (chopped)
Assembly:

12 coconut tortillas
¾ cup Colby's jack cheese (shredded)
¼ cup green onions (chopped)
Directions:

Warm oil at medium to high heat in a large pan. Add the chopped garlic and cook until fragrant for about a minute.

Add rice, 1 cup of enchilada sauce (half the total), chicken, and coriander. Simmer for 5 minutes.

In the meantime, heat the oven to 375°F. Grease a 9x13 baking dish.

In the middle of each tortilla, place ¼ cup of chicken mixture. Roll up and place seam side down in the baking dish.

Pour the remaining cup of sauce over the enchiladas. Sprinkle with shredded cheese. Bake for 10 to 12 minutes Sprinkle with green onions.

Nutrition: Calories: 349; Fat: 19 g; Net Carbs: 9 g; Protein: 31 g.

719 HOME-STYLE CHICKEN KEBAB

Preparation Time: 10 minutes
Cooking Time: 10 minutes
Servings: 2
Ingredients:

2 Roma tomatoes, chopped
1 pound chicken thighs, boneless, skinless and halved
1 tbsp. olive oil
½ cup Greek-style yogurt

½-oz. Swiss cheese, sliced
Directions:

Place the chicken thighs, yogurt, tomatoes, and olive oil in a glass storage container. You can add mustard seeds, cinnamon, and sumac if desired.

Cover then place in the fridge to marinate for 3 to 4 hours.

Thread the chicken thighs onto skewers, creating a thick log shape. Grill the kebabs over medium-high heat for 3 or 4 minutes on each side.

Use an instant-read thermometer to check the doneness of the meat; it should read about 165°F.

Top with the cheese; continue cooking for 4 minutes or until cheesy is melted. Enjoy!

Nutrition: Calories: 498; Fat: 23.2 g; Carbs: 6.2 g; Protein: 61 g; Fiber: 1.7 g.

720 TRADITIONAL HUNGARIAN GULYÁS

Preparation Time: 10 minutes
Cooking Time: 1 hour, 10 minutes
Servings: 4
Ingredients:

½ cup celery ribs, chopped
ripe tomato, pureed
1 tbsp. spice mix for goulash
1 (1-oz.) slices bacon, chopped
½-pound duck legs, skinless and boneless
Directions:

Heat a heavy-bottomed pot over the medium-high flame; then, fry the bacon for about 3 minutes. Stir in the duck legs and continue cooking until they are nicely browned on all sides.

Shred the meat and discard the bones. Set aside.

In the pan drippings, sauté the celery for about 3 minutes, stirring with a wide spatula. Add in pureed tomatoes and spice mix for goulash; add in the reserved bacon and meat.

Pour 2 cups of water or chicken broth into the pot.

Place heat to medium-low, cover, and simmer for 50 minutes more or until everything is cooked thoroughly. Serve warm and enjoy!

Nutrition: Calories: 363; Fat: 22.3 g; Carbs: 5.1 g; Protein: 33.2 g; Fiber: 1.4 g.

721 GREEK CHICKEN STIFADO

Preparation Time: 10 minutes
Cooking Time: 35 minutes
Servings: 2

Ingredients:

2 oz. bacon, diced
½ tsp. poultry seasoning mix
vine-ripe tomatoes, pureed
¾-pound whole chicken, boneless and chopped
½ medium-sized leek, chopped
Directions:

Cook the bacon in the preheated skillet over medium-high heat. Fold in the chicken and continue cooking for 5 minutes more until it is no longer pink; set aside.

In the same skillet, sauté the leek until it has softened or about 4 minutes. Stir in the poultry seasoning mix and 2 cups of water or chicken broth.

Now, reduce the heat to medium-low and continue to simmer for 15 to 20 minutes.

Add in tomatoes, along with the reserved meat. Continue to cook for a further 13 minutes or until cooked through. Bon appétit!

Nutrition: Calories: 352; Fat: 14.3 g; Carbs: 5.9 g; Protein: 44.2 g; Fiber: 2.4 g.

722 TANGY CHICKEN WITH SCALLIONS

Preparation Time: 10 minutes
Cooking Time: 40 minutes
Servings: 4
Ingredients:

3 tbsp. butter, melted
1 pound chicken drumettes
2 tbsp. white wine
2 garlic clove, sliced
2 tbsp. fresh scallions, chopped
Directions:

Arrange the chicken drumettes on a foil-lined baking pan. Brush with melted butter.

Add in the garlic and wine. Spice with salt and black pepper to taste. Bake in the preheated oven at 400°F for about 30 minutes or until internal temperature reaches about 165°F.

Serve garnished with scallions and enjoy!

Nutrition: Calories: 209; Fat: 12.2 g; Carbs: 0.4 g; Protein: 23.2 g; Fiber: 1.9 g.

723 DOUBLE CHEESE ITALIAN CHICKEN

Preparation Time: 10 minutes
Cooking Time: 20 minutes
Servings: 2
Ingredients:

2 chicken drumsticks
2 cups baby spinach
1 tsp. Italian spice mix
½ cup cream cheese

½ cup Asiago cheese, grated

Directions:

In a saucepan, heat 1 tablespoon of oil over medium-high heat. Sear the chicken drumsticks for 7 to 8 minutes or until nicely browned on all sides; reserve.

Pour in ½ cup of chicken bone broth; add in spinach and continue cooking for 5 minutes more until spinach has wilted.

Add in the Italian spice mix, cream cheese, Asiago cheese, and reserved chicken drumsticks; partially cover and continue cooking for 5 more minutes. Serve warm.

Nutrition: Calories: 589; Fat: 46 g; Carbs: 5.8 g; Protein: 37.5 g; Fiber: 2 g.

724 MIDDLE EASTERN SHISH KEBAB

Preparation Time: 10 minutes
Cooking Time: 20 minutes
Servings: 5
Ingredients:

2 pounds chicken tenders, cut into bite-sized cubes
½ cup ajran
¼ tbsp. mustard
½ cup tomato sauce
Turkish spice mix

Directions:

Place chicken tenders with the remaining ingredients in a ceramic dish. Cover and let it marinate for 4 hours in your refrigerator.

Thread chicken tenders onto skewers and place them on the preheated grill until golden brown on all sides, approximately 15 minutes.

Serve immediately and enjoy!

Nutrition: Calories: 274; Fat: 10.7 g; Carbs: 3.3 g; Protein: 39.3 g; Fiber: 0.8 g.

725 CAPOCOLLO AND GARLIC CHICKEN

Preparation Time: 10 minutes
Cooking Time: 40 minutes
Servings: 5
Ingredients:

2 pounds chicken drumsticks, skinless and boneless, butterflied
10 thin slices of capocollo
garlic clove, peeled and halved
Coarse sea salt, to taste
Ground black pepper, to taste
½ tsp. smoked paprika

Directions:

Rub garlic halves over the surface of chicken drumsticks. Season with paprika, salt, and black pepper.

Place a slice of capocollo on each chicken drumsticks and roll them up; secure with kitchen twine.

Bake in the oven at 410°F for 30 to 35 minutes, until your chicken begins to brown. Bon appétit!

Nutrition: Calories: 485; Fat: 33.8 g; Carbs: 3.6 g; Protein: 39.2 g; Fiber: 1 g.

726 CHEESY MEXICAN-STYLE CHICKEN

Preparation Time: 10 minutes
Cooking Time: 25 minutes
Servings: 6
Ingredients:

½ pounds chicken breasts, cut into bite-sized cubes
ripe tomatoes, pureed
1 oz. sour cream
6 oz. Cotija cheese, crumbled
Mexican chili pepper, finely chopped

Directions:

Preheat your oven to 390°F.

In a saucepan, heat 2 tablespoons of olive oil over medium-high heat. Cook the chicken breasts for about 10 minutes, frequently stirring to ensure even cooking.

Then, add in Mexican chili pepper and cook until it has softened.

Add in the pureed tomatoes and continue cooking, partially covered, for 4 to 5 minutes—season with the Mexican spice mix. Transfer the mixture to a lightly greased baking dish.

Top with sour cream and Cotija cheese. Bake in the preheated oven for about 15 minutes or until hot and bubbly. Enjoy!

Nutrition: Calories: 354; Fat: 23.2 g; Carbs: 6 g; Protein: 29.3 g; Fiber: 0.6 g.

727 ASIAN SAUCY CHICKEN

Preparation Time: 10 minutes
Cooking Time: 15 minutes
Servings: 4
Ingredients:

2 tbsp. sesame oil
4 chicken legs
¼ cup Shaoxing wine
1 tbsp. brown erythritol
¼ cup spicy tomato sauce

Directions:

Heat the sesame oil in a wok at medium-high heat. Fry the chicken until golden in color; reserve.

Add Shaoxing wine to deglaze the pan.

Add in erythritol and spicy tomato sauce, and bring the mixture to a boil. Then, immediately reduce the heat to medium-low.

Let it simmer for about 10 minutes until the sauce coats the back of a spoon. Add the chicken back to the wok.

Continue to cook until the chicken is sticky and golden or about 4 minutes. Enjoy!

Nutrition: Calories: 367; Fat: 14.7 g; Carbs: 3.5 g; Protein: 51.2 g; Fiber: 1.1 g.

728 DUCK STEW OLLA TAPADA

Preparation Time: 15 minutes
Cooking Time: 30 minutes
Servings: 3
Ingredients:

1 red bell pepper, deveined and chopped
1 pound duck breasts, boneless, skinless, and chopped into small chunks
½ cup chayote, peeled and cubed
1 shallot, chopped
1 tsp. Mexican spice mix
2 tsp. canola oil
1 ½ cups water

Directions:

In a clay pot, heat 2 teaspoons of canola oil over a medium-high flame. Sauté the peppers and shallot until softened for about 4 minutes.

Add in the remaining ingredients; pour in 1 ½ cups of water or chicken bone broth. Once your mixture starts boiling, reduce the heat to medium-low.

Let it simmer, partially covered, for 18 to 22 minutes, until cooked through. Enjoy!

Nutrition: Calories: 228; Fat: 9.5 g; Carbs: 3.3 g; Protein: 30.6 g; Fiber: 1 g.

729 CHEESY RANCH CHICKEN

Preparation Time: 10 minutes
Cooking Time: 20 minutes
Servings: 4
Ingredients:

2 chicken breasts
½ tbsp. ranch seasoning mix
4 slices bacon, chopped
½ cup Monterey-Jack cheese, grated
4 oz. Ricotta cheese, room temperature

Directions:

Preheat your oven to 360°F.

Rub the chicken with ranch seasoning mix.

Heat a saucepan over medium-high flame. Now, sear the chicken for about 8 minutes. Lower the chicken into a lightly greased casserole dish.

Top with cheese and bacon and bake in the preheated oven for about 10 minutes until hot and bubbly.

Serve with freshly snipped scallions, if desired.

Nutrition: Calories: 295; Fat: 19.5 g; Carbs: 2.9 g; Protein: 25.5 g; Fiber: 0.4 g.

730 TURKEY CRUST MEATZA

Preparation Time: 15 minutes
Cooking Time: 35 minutes
Servings: 4
Ingredients:

½-pound ground turkey
2 slices Canadian bacon
1 tomato, chopped
2 tbsp. pizza spice mix
1 cup mozzarella cheese, grated

Directions:

Mix the ground turkey and cheese; season with salt and black pepper and mix until everything is well combined.

Press the mixture into a foil-lined baking pan. Bake in the preheated oven at 380°F for 25 minutes.

Top the crust with Canadian bacon, tomato, and pizza spice mix. Continue to bake for a further 8 minutes.

Let it rest for a few minutes before slicing and serving. Bon appétit!

Nutrition: Calories: 360; Fat: 22.7 g; Carbs: 5.9 g; Protein: 32.6 g; Fiber: 0.7 g.

731 SIMPLE TURKEY GOULASH

Preparation Time: 15 minutes
Cooking Time: 45 minutes
Servings: 4
Ingredients:

2 tbsp. olive oil
1 large-sized leek, chopped
2 cloves garlic, minced
1 ½ pounds turkey thighs, skinless, boneless and chopped
2 celery stalks, chopped

Directions:

In a clay pot, heat 2 olive oil over a medium-high flame. Then, cook the leeks until tender and translucent.

Then, continue to sauté the garlic for 30 seconds to 1 minute.

Stir in the turkey, celery, and 4 cups of water. Once your mixture starts boiling, let it simmer, partially covered, for about 40 minutes. Bon appétit!

Nutrition: Calories: 220; Fat: 7.4 g; Carbs: 2.7 g; Protein: 35.5 g; Fiber: 1 g.

732 CHICKEN FRITTATA WITH ASIAGO CHEESE AND HERBS

Preparation Time: 10 minutes
Cooking Time: 30 minutes

Servings: 4
Ingredients:

1 pound chicken breasts, chopped into small strips
4 slices of bacon
1 cup Asiago cheese, shredded
6 eggs
½ cup yogurt

Directions:

Preheat an oven-proof skillet. Then, fry the bacon until crisp and reserve. Then, in the pan drippings, cook the chicken for about 8 minutes or until no longer pink.

Add the reserved bacon back to the skillet.

In a mixing dish, thoroughly combine the eggs and yogurt; season with the Italian spice mix.

Pour the egg mixture over the chicken and bacon. Top with cheese and bake in the preheated oven at 380°F for 22 minutes until hot and bubbly.

Let it sit for 1-2 minutes before slicing and serving. Bon appétit!

Nutrition: Calories: 484; Fat: 31.8 g; Carbs: 5.8 g; Protein: 41.9 g; Fiber: 0.7 g.

733 STUFFED CHICKEN WITH SAUERKRAUT AND CHEESE

Preparation Time: 10 minutes
Cooking Time: 35 minutes
Servings: 4
Ingredients:

5 chicken cutlets
1 cup Romano cheese, shredded
2 garlic cloves, minced
5 Italian peppers, deveined and chopped
5 tbsp. sauerkraut, for serving
2 tbsp. of olive oil.
1 tbsp Italian spice mix
1 tsp Dijon mustard

Directions:

Spritz a baking pan with 1 tablespoon of olive oil. Brush the chicken with another tablespoon of olive oil.

Season the chicken with the Italian spice mix. You can spread Dijon mustard on one side of each chicken cutlet if desired.

Divide the garlic, peppers and Romano cheese between chicken cutlets; roll them up.

Bake at 360°F for 25 to 33 minutes until nicely brown on all sides. Serve with the sauerkraut and serve. Bon appétit!

Nutrition: Calories: 376; Fat: 16.7 g; Carbs: 5.8 g; Protein: 47 g; Fiber: 1 g.

734 CHICKEN BACON BURGER

Preparation Time: 10 minutes
Cooking Time: 15 minutes
Servings: 8
Ingredients:

4 chicken breasts
4 slices of bacon
¼ medium onion
2 cloves of garlic
¼ cup (60 ml.) avocado oil, to cook with

Directions:

Food process the chicken, bacon, onion, and garlic and form 8 patties. You need to do this in batches.

Fry patties in the avocado oil in batches. Make sure burgers are fully cooked.

Serve with guacamole (see recipe 838 for recipe).

Nutrition: Calories: 319; Fat: 24 g; Net Carbohydrates: 1 g; Protein: 25 g.

735 COUNTRY-STYLE CHICKEN STEW

Preparation Time: 20 minutes
Cooking Time: 1 hour
Servings: 6
Ingredients:

1 pound chicken thighs
2 tbsp. butter, room temperature
½-pound carrots, chopped
1 bell pepper, chopped
1 Chile pepper, deveined and minced
1 cup tomato puree
Kosher salt and ground black pepper, to taste
½ tsp. smoked paprika
1 onion, finely chopped
1 tsp. garlic, sliced
4 cups vegetable broth
1 tsp. dried basil
1 celery, chopped

Directions:

Melt the butter in a stockpot over medium-high flame. Sweat the onion and garlic until just tender and fragrant.

Reduce the heat to medium-low. Stir in the broth, chicken thighs, and basil; bring to a rolling boil.

Add in the remaining ingredients. Partially cover and let it simmer for 45 to 50 minutes. Shred the meat, discarding the bones; add the chicken back to the pot.

Nutrition: Calories: 280; Fat: 14.7 g; Carbs: 2.5 g; Protein: 25.6 g; Fiber: 2.5 g.

736 AUTUMN CHICKEN SOUP WITH ROOT VEGETABLES

Preparation Time: 10 minutes
Cooking Time: 25 minutes
Servings: 4
Ingredients:

4 cups chicken broth
1 cup full-fat milk
1 cup double cream
½ cup turnip, chopped
2 chicken drumsticks, boneless and cut into small pieces
Salt and pepper, to taste
1 tbsp. butter
1 tsp. garlic, finely minced
1 carrot, chopped
½ parsnip, chopped
½ celery
1 whole egg

Directions:

Melt the butter in a heavy-bottomed pot over medium-high heat; sauté the garlic until aromatic or about 1 minute. Add in the vegetables and continue cooking until they've softened.

Add in the chicken and cook until it is no longer pink for about 4 minutes. Season with salt and pepper.

Pour in the chicken broth, milk, and heavy cream and bring it to a boil. Reduce the heat too. Partially cover and continue to simmer for 20 to 25 minutes longer. Afterward, fold the beaten egg and stir until it is well incorporated.

Nutrition: Calories: 342; Fat: 22.4 g; Carbs: 6.3 g; Protein: 25.2 g; Fiber: 1.3 g.

737 PANNA COTTA WITH CHICKEN AND BLEU D' AUVERGNE

Preparation Time: 10 minutes
Cooking Time: 20 minutes
Servings:
Ingredients:

2 chicken legs, boneless and skinless
1 tbsp. avocado oil
2 tsp. granular erythritol
3 tbsp. water
1 cup Bleu d' Auvergne, crumbled
2 gelatin sheets
¾ cup double cream
Salt and cayenne pepper, to your liking

Directions:

Heat the oil in a frying pan over medium-high heat; fry the chicken for about 10 minutes.

Soak the gelatin sheets in cold water. Cook with the cream, erythritol, water, and Bleu d' Auvergne.

Season with salt and pepper and let it simmer over low heat, stirring for

about 3 minutes. Spoon the mixture into four ramekins.

Nutrition: Calories: 306; Fat: 18.3 g; Carbs: 4.7 g; Protein: 29.5 g; Fiber: 0 g.

738 BREADED CHICKEN FILLETS

Preparation Time: 15 minutes
Cooking Time: 30 minutes
Servings: 4
Ingredients:

1 pound chicken fillets
3 bell peppers, quartered lengthwise
⅓ cup Romano cheese
2 tsp. olive oil
1 garlic clove, minced
Kosher salt and ground black pepper, to taste
⅓ cup crushed pork rinds

Directions:

Start by preheating your oven to 410°F.

Mix the crushed pork rinds, Romano cheese, olive oil and minced garlic. Dredge the chicken into this mixture.

Place the chicken in a lightly greased baking dish. Season with salt and black pepper to taste.

Scatter the peppers around the chicken and bake in the preheated oven for 20 to 25 minutes or until thoroughly cooked.

Nutrition: Calories: 367; Fat: 16.9 g; Carbs: 6 g; Protein: 43 g; Fiber: 0.7 g.

739 CHICKEN DRUMSTICKS WITH BROCCOLI AND CHEESE

Preparation Time: 40 minutes
Cooking Time: 1 hour & 15 minutes
Servings: 4
Ingredients:

1 pound chicken drumsticks
1 pound broccoli, broken into florets
2 cups cheddar cheese, shredded
½ tsp. dried oregano
½ tsp. dried basil
3 tbsp. olive oil
1 celery, sliced
1 cup green onions, chopped
1 tsp. minced green garlic

Directions:

Roast the chicken drumsticks in the preheated oven at 380°F for 30 to 35 minutes. Add in the broccoli, celery, green onions, and green garlic.

Add in the oregano, basil and olive oil; roast an additional 15 minutes.

Nutrition: Calories: 533; Fat: 40.2 g; Carbs: 5.4 g; Protein: 35.1 g; Fiber: 3.5 g.

740 TURKEY HAM AND MOZZARELLA PATE

Preparation Time: 5 minutes
Cooking Time: 10 minutes

Servings: 6
Ingredients:

4 oz. turkey ham, chopped
2 tbsp. fresh parsley, roughly chopped
2 tbsp. flaxseed meal
4 oz. mozzarella cheese, crumbled
2 tbsp. sunflower seeds

Directions:

Thoroughly combine the ingredients, except for the sunflower seeds, in your food processor.

Spoon the mixture into a serving bowl and scatter the sunflower seeds over the top.

Nutrition: Calories: 212; Fat: 18.8 g; Carbs: 2 g; Protein: 10.6 g; Fiber: 1.6 g.

741 GREEK-STYLE SAUCY CHICKEN DRUMETTES

Preparation Time: 25 minutes
Cooking Time: 50 minutes
Servings: 6
Ingredients:

1 ½ pounds chicken drumettes
½ cup port wine
½ cup onions, chopped
2 garlic cloves, minced
1 tsp. tzatziki spice mix
1 cup double cream
2 tbsp. butter
Sea salt and crushed mixed peppercorns, to season

Directions:

Melt the butter in an oven-proof skillet over a moderate heat; then, cook the chicken for about 8 minutes.

Add in the onions, garlic, wine, tzatziki spice mix, double cream, salt, and pepper.

Bake in the preheated oven at 390°F for 35 to 40 minutes (a meat thermometer should register 165°F).

Nutrition: Calories: 333; Fat: 20.2 g; Carbs: 2 g; Protein: 33.5 g; Fiber: 0.2 g.

742 CHICKEN WITH AVOCADO SAUCE

Preparation Time: 10 minutes
Cooking Time: 20 minutes
Servings: 4
Ingredients:

8 chicken wings, boneless, cut into bite-size chunks
2 tbsp. olive oil
Sea salt and pepper, to your liking
2 eggs
1 tsp. onion powder
1 tsp. hot paprika
⅓ tsp. mustard seeds - ⅓ cup almond meal

For the Sauce:

½ cup mayonnaise
½ medium avocado

½ tsp. sea salt

1 tsp. green garlic, minced

Directions:

Pat dry the chicken wings with a paper towel.

Thoroughly combine the almond meal, salt, pepper, onion powder, paprika, and mustard seeds.

Whisk the eggs in a separate dish. Dredge the chicken chunks into the whisked eggs, then in the almond meal mixture.

In a frying pan, heat the oil over a moderate heat; once hot, fry the chicken for about 10 minutes, stirring continuously to ensure even cooking.

Make the sauce by whisking all of the sauce ingredients.

Nutrition: Calories: 370; Fat: 25 g; Carbs: 4.1 g; Protein: 31.4 g; Fiber: 2.6 g.

743 OLD-FASHIONED TURKEY CHOWDER

Preparation Time: 15 minutes

Cooking Time: 35 minutes

Servings: 4

Ingredients:

2 tbsp. olive oil

2 tbsp. yellow onions, chopped

2 cloves garlic, roughly chopped

½-pound leftover roast turkey, shredded and skin removed

1 tsp. Mediterranean spice mix

3 cups chicken bone broth

1 ½ cups milk

½ cup double cream

1 egg, lightly beaten

2 tbsp. dry sherry

Directions:

Heat the olive oil in a heavy-bottomed pot over a moderate flame. Sauté the onion and garlic until they've softened.

Stir in the leftover roast turkey, Mediterranean spice mix, and chicken bone broth; bring to a rapid boil. Partially cover and continue cooking for 20 to 25 minutes.

Turn the heat to simmer. Pour in the milk and double cream and continue cooking until it has reduced slightly.

Fold in the egg and dry sherry; continue to simmer, stirring frequently, for a further 2 minutes.

Nutrition: Calories: 350; Fat: 25.8 g; Carbs: 5.5 g; Protein: 20 g; Fiber: 0.1 g.

744 DUCK AND EGGPLANT CASSEROLE

Preparation Time: 10 minutes

Cooking Time: 45 minutes

Servings: 4

Ingredients:

1 pound ground duck meat

1 ½ tbsp. ghee, melted

⅓ cup double cream

½-pound eggplant, peeled and sliced

1 ½ cups almond flour

Salt and black pepper, to taste

½ tsp. fennel seeds

½ tsp. oregano, dried

8 eggs

Directions:

Mix the almond flour with salt, black, fennel seeds, and oregano. Fold in one egg and the melted ghee and whisk to combine well.

Press the crust into the bottom of a lightly-oiled pie pan. Cook the ground duck until no longer pink for about 3 minutes, stirring continuously.

Whisk the remaining eggs and double cream. Fold in the browned meat and stir until everything is well incorporated. Pour the mixture into the prepared crust. Top with the eggplant slices.

Bake for about 40 minutes. Cut into four pieces.

Nutrition: Calories: 562; Fat: 49.5 g; Carbs: 6.7 g; Protein: 22.5 g; Fiber: 2.1 g.

745 HERBED CHICKEN BREASTS

Preparation Time: 10 minutes

Cooking Time: 40 minutes

Servings: 8

Ingredients:

4 chicken breasts, skinless and boneless

1 Italian pepper, deveined and thinly sliced

10 black olives, pitted

1 ½ cups vegetable broth

2 garlic cloves, pressed

2 tbsp. olive oil

1 tbsp. Old Sub Sailor

Salt, to taste

Directions:

Rub the chicken with the garlic and Old Sub Sailor; salt to taste. Heat the oil in a frying pan over a moderately high heat.

Sear the chicken until it is browned on all sides, about 5 minutes.

Add in the pepper, olives, and vegetable broth and bring it to boil. Reduce the heat simmer and continue cooking, partially covered, for 30 to 35 minutes.

Nutrition: Calories: 306; Fat: 17.8 g; Carbs: 3.1 g; Protein: 31.7 g; Fiber: 0.2 g.

746 CHEESE AND PROSCIUTTO CHICKEN ROULADE

Preparation Time: 15 minutes

Cooking Time: 35 minutes

Servings: 2

Ingredients:

½ cup Ricotta cheese

4 slices of prosciutto

1 pound chicken fillet

1 tbsp. fresh coriander, chopped

Salt and ground black pepper, to taste pepper

1 tsp. cayenne pepper

Directions:

Season the chicken fillet with salt and pepper. Spread the Ricotta cheese over the chicken fillet; sprinkle with the fresh coriander.

Roll up and cut into 4 pieces. Wrap each piece with one slice of prosciutto; secure with a kitchen twine.

Place the wrapped chicken in a parchment-lined baking pan. Now, bake in the preheated oven at 385°F for about 30 minutes.

Nutrition: Calories: 499; Fat: 18.9 g; Carbs: 5.7 g; Protein: 41.6 g; Fiber: 0.6 g.

747 BOOZY GLAZED CHICKEN

Preparation Time: 40 minutes

Cooking Time: 1 hour + marinating time

Servings: 4

Ingredients:

2 pounds chicken drumettes

2 tbsp. ghee, at room temperature

Sea salt and ground black pepper, to taste

1 tsp. Mediterranean seasoning mix

2 vine-ripened tomatoes, pureed

¾ cup rum

3 tbsp. coconut aminos

A few drops of liquid Stevia

1 tsp. Chile peppers, minced

1 tbsp. minced fresh ginger

1 tsp. ground cardamom

2 tbsp. fresh lemon juice, plus wedges for serving

Directions:

Toss the chicken with the melted ghee, salt, black pepper, and Mediterranean seasoning mix until well coated on all sides.

In another bowl, thoroughly combine the pureed tomato puree, rum, coconut aminos, Stevia, Chile peppers, ginger, cardamom, and lemon juice.

Pour the tomato mixture over the chicken drumettes; let it marinate for 2 hours. Bake in the preheated oven at 410°F for about 45 minutes.

Add in the reserved marinade and place under the preheated broiler for 10 minutes.

Nutrition: Calories: 307; Fat: 12.1 g; Carbs: 2.7 g; Protein: 33.6 g; Fiber: 1.5 g.

748 FESTIVE TURKEY ROULADEN

Preparation Time: 15 minutes
Cooking Time: 30 minutes
Servings: 5
Ingredients:

  2 pounds turkey fillet, marinated and cut into 10 pieces
  10 strips prosciutto
  ½ tsp. chili powder
  1 tsp. marjoram
  1 sprig rosemary, finely chopped
  2 tbsp. dry white wine
  1 tsp. garlic, finely minced
  1 ½ tbsp. butter, room temperature
  1 tbsp. Dijon mustard
  Sea salt and freshly ground black pepper, to your liking

Directions:

  Start by preheating your oven to 430°F.
  Pat the turkey dry and cook in hot butter for about 3 minutes per side. Add in the mustard, chili powder, marjoram, rosemary, wine, and garlic.
  Continue cooking for 2 minutes more. Wrap each turkey piece into one prosciutto strip and secure with toothpicks.
  Roast in the preheated oven for about 30 minutes.

Nutrition: Calories: 286; Fat: 9.7 g; Carbs: 6.9 g; Protein: 39.9 g; Fiber: 0.3 g.

749 PAN-FRIED CHORIZO SAUSAGE

Preparation Time: 10 minutes
Cooking Time: 20 minutes
Servings: 4
Ingredients:

  16 oz. smoked turkey chorizo
  1 ½ cups Asiago cheese, grated
  1 tsp. oregano
  1 tsp. basil
  1 cup tomato puree
  4 scallion stalks, chopped
  1 tsp. garlic paste
  Sea salt and ground black pepper, to taste
  1 tbsp. dry sherry
  1 tbsp. extra-virgin olive oil
  2 tbsp. fresh coriander, roughly chopped

Directions:

  Heat the oil in a frying pan over moderately high heat. Now, brown the turkey chorizo, crumbling with a fork for about 5 minutes.
  Add in the other ingredients, except for cheese; continue cooking for 10

minutes more or until cooked through.

Nutrition: Calories: 330; Fat: 17.2 g; Carbs: 4.5 g; Protein: 34.4 g; Fiber: 1.6 g.

750 CHINESE BOK CHOY AND TURKEY SOUP

Preparation Time: 15 minutes
Cooking Time: 40 minutes
Servings: 8
Ingredients:

  ½-pound baby Bok choy, sliced into quarters lengthwise
  2 pounds turkey carcass
  1 tbsp. olive oil
  ½ cup leeks, chopped
  1 celery rib, chopped
  2 carrots, sliced
  6 cups turkey stock
  Himalayan salt and black pepper, to taste

Directions:

  In a heavy-bottomed pot, heat the olive oil until sizzling. Once hot, sauté the celery, carrots, leek and Bok choy for about 6 minutes.
  Add the salt, pepper, turkey, and stock; bring to a boil.
  Turn the heat to simmer. Continue to cook, partially covered, for about 35 minutes.

Nutrition: Calories: 211; Fat: 11.8 g; Carbs: 3.1 g; Protein: 23.7 g; Fiber: 0.9 g.

751 HERBY CHICKEN MEATLOAF

Preparation Time: 20 minutes
Cooking Time: 30 minutes
Servings: 6
Ingredients:

  2 ½ lb. ground chicken
  3 tbsp. flaxseed meal
  2 large eggs
  2 tbsp. olive oil
  1 lemon, 1 tbsp. juiced
  ¼ cup chopped parsley
  ¼ cup chopped oregano
  4 garlic cloves, minced
  Lemon slices to garnish

Directions:

  Preheat oven to 400°F. In a bowl, combine ground chicken and flaxseed meal; set aside. In a small bowl, whisk the eggs with olive oil, lemon juice, parsley, oregano, and garlic.
  Pour the mixture onto the chicken mixture and mix well. Spoon into a greased loaf pan and press to fit. Bake for 40 minutes.
  Remove the pan, drain the liquid, and let cool a bit. Slice, garnish with lemon slices and serve.

Nutrition: Calories: 362; Net Carbs: 1.3 g; Fat: 24 g; Protein: 35 g.

752 LOVELY PULLED CHICKEN EGG BITES

Preparation Time: 15 minutes
Cooking Time: 30 minutes
Servings: 4
Ingredients:

  2 tbsp. butter
  1 chicken breast
  2 tbsp. chopped green onions
  ½ tsp. red chili flakes
  12 eggs
  ¼ cup grated Monterey Jack

Directions:

  Preheat oven to 400°F. Line a 12-hole muffin tin with cupcake liners. Melt butter in a skillet over medium heat and cook the chicken until brown on each side, 10 minutes.
  Transfer to a plate and shred with 2 forks. Divide between muffin holes along with green onions and red chili flakes.
  Crack an egg into each muffin hole and scatter the cheese on top. Bake for 15 minutes until eggs set. Serve.

Nutrition: Calories: 393; Net Carbs: 0.5 g; Fat: 27 g; Protein: 34 g.

753 CREAMY MUSTARD CHICKEN WITH SHIRATAKI

Preparation Time: 20 minutes
Cooking Time: 30 minutes
Servings: 4
Ingredients:

  2 (8 oz.) packs angel hair shirataki
  4 chicken breasts, cut into strips
  1 cup chopped mustard greens
  1 yellow bell pepper, sliced
  1 tbsp. olive oil
  1 yellow onion, finely sliced
  1 garlic clove, minced
  1 tbsp. wholegrain mustard
  5 tbsp. heavy cream
  1 tbsp. chopped parsley

Directions:

  Boil 2 cups of water in a medium pot.
  Strain the shirataki pasta and rinse well under hot running water. Allow proper draining and pour the shirataki pasta into the boiling water.
  Cook for 3 minutes and strain again. Place a dry skillet and stir-fry the shirataki pasta until visibly dry, 1-2 minutes; set aside.
  Heat olive oil in a skillet, season the chicken with salt and pepper and cook for 8-10 minutes; set aside. Stir in onion, bell pepper, and garlic and cook until softened, 5 minutes.

Mix in mustard and heavy cream; simmer for 2 minutes and mix in the chicken and mustard greens for 2 minutes. Stir in shirataki pasta, garnish with parsley and serve.

Nutrition: Calories: 692; Net Carbs: 15 g; Fats 38 g; Protein: 65 g.

754 PARSNIP & BACON CHICKEN BAKE

Preparation Time: 10 minutes
Cooking Time: 50 minutes
Servings: 4
Ingredients:

6 bacon slices, chopped
2 tbsp. butter
½ lb. parsnips, diced
2 tbsp. olive oil
1 lb. ground chicken
2 tbsp. butter
1 cup heavy cream
2 oz. cream cheese, softened
1 ¼ cups grated Pepper Jack
¼ cup chopped scallions

Directions:

Preheat oven to 300°F. Put the bacon in a pot and fry it until brown and crispy, 6 minutes; set aside. Melt butter in a skillet and sauté parsnips until softened and lightly browned. Transfer to a greased baking sheet.

Heat olive oil in the same pan and cook the chicken until no longer pink, 8 minutes. Spoon onto a plate and set aside too.

Add heavy cream, cream cheese, and two-thirds of the Pepper Jack cheese to the pot. Melt the ingredients over medium heat, frequently stirring, for 7 minutes.

Spread the parsnips on the baking dish, top with chicken, pour the heavy cream mixture over, and scatter bacon and scallions.

Sprinkle the remaining cheese on top and bake until the cheese melts and is golden, 30 minutes. Serve warm.

Nutrition: Calories: 757; Net Carbs: 5.5 g; Fat: 66 g; Protein: 29 g.

755 CHICKEN BAKE WITH ONION & PARSNIP

Preparation Time: 15 minutes
Cooking Time: 30 minutes
Servings:
Ingredients:

3 parsnips, sliced
1 onion, sliced
4 garlic cloves, crushed
2 tbsp olive oil

2 lb. chicken breasts
½ cup chicken broth
¼ cup white wine
Salt and black pepper to taste

Directions:

Preheat oven to 360°F. Warm oils in a skillet over medium heat and brown chicken for a couple of minutes, and transfer to a baking dish.

Arrange the vegetables around the chicken and add in wine and chicken broth. Bake for 25 minutes, stirring once. Serve warm.

Nutrition: Calories: 278; Net Carbs: 5.1 g; Fat: 8.7 g; Protein: 35 g.

756 CARROT BROCCOLI STEW

Preparation Time: 10 minutes
Cooking Time: 45 minutes
Servings: 3
Ingredients:

1 cup broccoli, florets
1 cup carrots, sliced
Salt and black pepper to taste
3 cups chicken broth
1 cup heavy cream

Directions:

Add florets, cream, carrots, salt, and chicken broth; toss well. Seal the lid and cook on Meat/Stew mode for 40 minutes on High. When ready, do a quick pressure release.

Transfer into serving bowls and sprinkle black pepper on top.

Nutrition: Calories: 145; Protein: 1.5 g; Net Carbs: 1.2 g.

757 CHEESY BROCCOLI SOUP

Preparation Time: 5 minutes
Cooking Time: 20 minutes
Servings: 4
Ingredients:

1 cup broccoli, cut into florets
3 cup chicken broth
1 cup heavy whipping cream
1 cup shredded Cheddar cheese, plus more for topping

From the cupboard:

2 tbsp. butter
Salt and freshly ground black pepper, to taste

Directions:

Put the butter in a saucepan, and melt over medium heat.

Add and sauté the broccoli for 4 to 5 minutes or until soft.

Mix in the chicken broth and heavy whipping cream over the broccoli, and sprinkle with salt and black pepper. Cook for about 15 minutes or until the soup is

smooth and thickened. Keep stirring during the cooking.

Reduce the heat to low and gently fold in the Cheddar cheese. Keep stirring until well combined.

Spoon the soup into a large bowl. Scatter more cheese over the soup before serving.

Nutrition: Calories: 386; Total Fats: 37.3 g; Total Carbs: 3.8 g; Fiber: 1.1 g; Net Carbs: 2.7 g; Protein: 9.8 g.

758 INTERMITTENT RICH ONION AND BEEF STEW

Preparation Time: 5 minutes
Cooking Time: 10 hours
Servings: 6
Ingredients:

2 pounds (907 g.) boneless stewing beef, cut into cubes
beef stock cube
2 tsp. dried mixed herbs (such as Italian seasoning)
5 garlic cloves, crushed
2 onions, roughly chopped

From the cupboard:

2 tbsp. olive oil, divided
Salt and freshly ground black pepper, to taste
3 cups water

Directions:

Grease the inside of the slow cooker with 2 tbsp. of olive oil. Coat a nonstick skillet with the remaining olive oil.

Heat the oil in the skillet over medium-high heat, then put the beef in the skillet and sear for 2 minutes or until medium-rare. Shake the skillet constantly to sear the beef cubes evenly.

Arrange the cooked beef in the slow cooker, then add the stock cube, mixed herbs, garlic, onions, salt, black pepper, and water. Stir to mix well.

Put the slow cooker lid on and cook on LOW for 10 hours.

Spoon the stew in a large bowl and serve warm.

Nutrition: Calories: 199; Total Fats: 6.3 g; Carbs: 1.9 g; Protein: 33.8 g.

759 CHICKEN AND KALE SOUP

Preparation Time: 5 minutes
Cooking Time: 4 hours
Servings: 4
Ingredients:

2 large chicken breast, cut into small strips
6 cups chicken stock
1 (7-oz. / 198-g;) bunch kale, trimmed and chopped
1 tbsp. fresh ginger, grated

6 garlic cloves, finely chopped

From the cupboard:

1 tbsp. olive oil

Salt and freshly ground black pepper, to taste

Directions:

Grease the inside of the slow cooker with olive oil.

Mix the chicken breast, stock, kale, ginger, garlic, ginger, salt, and black pepper in the slow cooker.

Put the slow cooker lid on and cook on HIGH for 4 hours.

Spoon the stew in a large bowl and serve warm.

Nutrition: Calories: 168; Total Fats: 7.6 g; Total Carbs: 8.3 g; Fiber: 2.1 g; Net Carbs: 6.2 g; Protein: 18.7 g.

760 GARLIC MUSHROOM & BEEF SOUP

Preparation Time: 10 minutes
Cooking Time: 40 minutes
Servings: 6
Ingredients:

1 pound beef chuck, cubed

1 ½ cups cremini mushrooms

6 cups beef broth

½ cup heavy cream

½ cup whipped cream cheese

1 yellow onion, chopped

2 cloves garlic, chopped

Salt & pepper, to taste

2 tbsp. coconut oil, for cooking

Directions:

Add the coconut oil to a skillet and brown the beef.

Once cooked, add the beef to the base of a stockpot with all of the ingredients, minus the heavy cream. Mix well.

Bring to a simmer and whisk again until the cream cheese is mixed evenly into the soup.

Cook for 30 minutes.

Warm the heavy cream, and then add to the soup.

Nutrition: Calories: 315; Carbs: 5 g; Fiber: 1 g; Net Carbs: 4 g; Fat: 19 g; Protein: 30 g.

761 CREAMY CELERY AND CHICKEN BROTH

Preparation Time: 5 minutes
Cooking Time: 20 minutes
Servings: 4
Ingredients:

¼ cup celery, chopped

onion, chopped

chicken breasts, chopped

½ cup coconut cream

From the Cupboard:

tbsp. butter

Salt and freshly ground black pepper, to taste

cups water

Directions:

Put the butter in a saucepan, and melt over medium heat.

Add and sauté the celery and onion for 3 minutes or until the onion is translucent.

Add the chicken, salt, black pepper, and water, and simmer for 15 minutes. Keep stirring during the simmering.

Stir in the coconut cream. Pour the soup into a large bowl and serve warm.

Nutrition: Calories: 398; Total Fats: 24.4 g; Net Carbs 5.9 g; Protein: 29.3 g.

762 INTERMITTENT BUFFALO SAUCE AND TURKEY SOUP

Preparation Time: 5 minutes
Cooking Time: 10 minutes
Servings: 4
Ingredients:

⅓ cup buffalo sauce

4 oz. (113 g.) cream cheese

4 cups chicken broth

2 cups turkey, cooked, shredded

4 tbsp. cilantro, chopped

From the Cupboard:

3 tbsp. butter, melted

Salt and freshly ground black pepper, to taste

Directions:

Put the buffalo sauce, cream cheese, and melted butter in a blender, and process until smooth.

Pour the buffalo sauce mixture into a saucepan, and add the chicken broth. Heat the soup over high heat until hot and almost boil but not boil. Keep stirring during the heating.

Add the shredded turkey, and sprinkle with salt and black pepper. Cook for 5 minutes or until smooth. Stir constantly.

Ladle the soup into a large bowl and top with chopped cilantro before serving.

Nutrition: Calories: 409; Total Fats: 29.7 g; Net Carbs: 9.2 g; Protein: 26.4 g.

763 CROCK-POT TURKEY TACO SOUP

Preparation Time: 10 minutes
Cooking Time: 4 hours
Servings: 6
Ingredients:

pound ground turkey

5 cups chicken bone broth (you can also use regular chicken broth)

cup canned diced tomatoes (no sugar added)

cup whipped cream cheese

yellow onion, chopped

tbsp. chili powder

tsp. cumin

tsp. garlic powder

tsp. onion powder

Directions:

Add all the ingredients to the base of a Crock-Pot minus the cream cheese and cover with the chicken broth.

Set on high and cook for 4 hours adding in the cream cheese at the 3.5-hour mark.

Stir well before serving.

Nutrition: Calories: 335; Carbs: 6 g; Fiber: 1 g; Net Carbs: 5 g; Fat: 23 g; Protein: 28 g.

764 SLOW COOKER LAMB & CAULIFLOWER SOUP

Preparation Time: 10 minutes
Cooking Time: 4 hours
Servings: 6
Ingredients:

1 pound ground lamb

5 cups beef broth

cauliflower head, cut into florets

½ cup heavy cream

yellow onion, chopped

cloves garlic, chopped

½ tbsp. freshly chopped thyme

½ tsp. cracked black pepper

½ tsp. salt

Directions:

Add the ground lamb and cauliflower to the base of a stockpot.

Add in the remaining ingredients minus the heavy cream, and cook on high for 4 hours.

Warm the heavy cream before adding to the soup. Use an immersion blender to blend the soup until creamy.

Nutrition: Calories: 263; Carbs: 6 g; Fiber: 2 g; Net Carbs: 4 g; Fat: 14 g; Protein: 27 g.

765 BUFFALO SAUCE AND TURKEY SOUP

Preparation Time: 10 minutes
Cooking Time: 5 minutes
Servings: 4
Ingredients:

⅓ cup buffalo sauce

4 oz. (113 g.) cream cheese

4 cups chicken broth

2 cups turkey, cooked, shredded

4 tbsp. cilantro, chopped

3 tbsp. butter, melted

Salt and freshly ground black pepper, to taste

Directions:

Put the buffalo sauce, cream cheese, and melted butter in a blender, and process until smooth.

Pour the buffalo sauce mixture into a saucepan, and add the chicken broth. Heat the soup over high heat until hot and almost boil but not boil. Keep stirring during the heating.

Add the shredded turkey, and sprinkle with salt and black pepper. Cook for 5 minutes or until smooth. Stir constantly.

Ladle the soup into a large bowl and top with chopped cilantro before serving.

Nutrition: Calories: 409; Total Fat: 29.7 g; Net Carbs: 9.2 g; Protein: 26.4 g.

766 LEMON CHICKEN SOUP

Preparation Time: 10 minutes
Cooking Time: 4 hours
Servings: 4
Ingredients:

2 boneless, skinless chicken breasts
6 cups chicken broth
¼ cup freshly squeezed lemon juice
2 tbsp. chives, chopped
yellow onion, chopped
cloves garlic, chopped
Salt & pepper, to taste

Directions:

Add all the ingredients to a slow cooker and cook on high for 4 hours.

Once cooked, shred the chicken and stir back into the soup.

Nutrition: Calories: 171; Carbs: 6 g; Fiber: 1 g; Net Carbs: 5 g; Fat: 6 g; Protein: 22 g.

767 RICH ONION AND BEEF STEW

Preparation Time: 5 minutes
Cooking Time: 10 hours
Servings: 6
Ingredients:

2 pounds (907 g.) boneless stewing beef, cut into cubes
beef stock cube
2 tsp. dried mixed herbs (such as Italian seasoning)
5 garlic cloves, crushed
onions, roughly chopped
2 tbsp. olive oil, divided
Salt and freshly ground black pepper, to taste
1 ½ cups water

Directions:

Grease the inside of the slow cooker with 2 tablespoons of olive oil. Coat a nonstick skillet with the remaining olive oil.

Heat the oil in the skillet over medium-high heat, then put the beef in the skillet and sear for 2 minutes or until medium-rare. Shake the skillet constantly to sear the beef cubes evenly.

Arrange the cooked beef in the slow cooker, then add the stock cube, mixed herbs, garlic, onions, salt, black pepper, and water. Stir to mix well.

Put the slow cooker lid on and cook on LOW for 10 hours.

Spoon the stew in a large bowl and serve warm.

Nutrition: Calories: 199; Total fat: 6.3 g; Carbs: 1.9 g; Protein: 33.8 g.

768 HAMBURGER & TOMATO SOUP

Preparation Time: 10 minutes
Cooking Time: 4 hours
Servings: 6
Ingredients:

1-pound lean ground beef
½ cup no-sugar added marinara sauce
½ cup beef broth
½ cup shredded cheddar cheese
yellow onion, chopped
cloves garlic, chopped
Salt & pepper, to taste

Directions:

Add all the ingredients to a slow cooker minus the shredded cheese and cook on high for 4 hours.

Stir in the cheese and serve.

Nutrition: Calories: 209; Carbs: 5 g; Fiber: 1 g; Net Carbs: 4 g; Fat: 9 g; Protein: 26 g.

769 CREAMY CAULIFLOWER SOUP WITH BACON CHIPS

Preparation Time: 10 minutes
Cooking Time: 15 minutes
Servings: 4
Ingredients:

2 tbsp. ghee
1 onion, chopped
1 head cauliflower, cut into florets
3 cups water
Salt and black pepper to taste
2 cups almond milk
1 cup shredded white cheddar cheese
4 bacon strips

Directions:

Melt the ghee in a saucepan over medium heat and sauté the onion for 3 minutes until fragrant.

Include the cauli florets, sauté for 3 minutes to slightly soften, add the water, and season with salt and black pepper. Bring to a boil, and then reduce the heat to low. Cover and cook for 10 minutes. Puree cauliflower with an immersion blender until the ingredients are evenly combined and stir in the almond milk and cheese until the cheese melts. Adjust taste with salt and black pepper.

In a non-stick skillet over high heat, fry the bacon, until crispy. Divide soup between serving bowls, top with crispy bacon, and serve hot.

Nutrition: Calories: 402; Fat: 37 g; Net Carbs: 6; Protein: 8 g.

770 SPICY SAUSAGE SOUP

Preparation Time: 10 minutes
Cooking Time: 40 minutes
Servings: 4
Ingredients:

4 cups chicken broth
4 sausage links, sliced
½ cup cauliflower florets
yellow onion, chopped
1 tsp. paprika
Sea salt & pepper, to taste

Directions:

Add all the ingredients minus the salt and black pepper to a stockpot over medium heat and bring to a boil. Reduce to a simmer and cook for 40 minutes.

Season with salt and black pepper and serve.

Nutrition: Calories: 107; Carbs: 6 g; Fiber: 1 g; Net Carbs: 5 g; Fat: 6 g; Protein: 8 g.

771 VEGGIE BEEF SOUP

Preparation Time: 10 minutes
Cooking Time: 40 minutes
Servings: 6
Ingredients:

6 cups beef broth
2 cup heavy cream
2 pound lean ground beef
1 cup frozen mixed vegetables
1 yellow onion, chopped
Salt & black pepper, to taste

Directions:

Add all the ingredients, minus the salt, black pepper and heavy cream, and bring to a boil. Reduce the heat to a simmer and cook for 40 minutes.

Before the soup is done cooking, warm the heavy cream, and then add once the soup is cooked.

Season with salt and black pepper and serve.

Nutrition: Calories: 270; Carbs: 6 g; Fiber: 2 g; Net Carbs: 4 g; Fat: 14 g; Protein: 29 g.

772 PUMPKIN & MEAT PEANUT STEW

Preparation Time: 15 minutes
Cooking Time: 30-45 minutes
Servings: 6
Ingredients:

cup pumpkin puree
pounds chopped pork stew meat
tbsp. peanut butter
tbsp. chopped peanuts

garlic clove, minced

½ cup chopped onion

½ cup white wine

tbsp. olive oil

tsp lemon juice

¼ cup granulated sweetener

¼ tsp cardamom powder

¼ tsp allspice

cups water

cups chicken stock

Directions:

Heat the olive oil in a large pot and sauté onion for 3 minutes, until translucent. Add garlic and cook for 30 more seconds. Add the pork and cook until browned, about 5-6 minutes, stirring occasionally. Pour in the wine and cook for one minute.

Add in the remaining ingredients, except for the lemon juice and peanuts. Bring the mixture to a boil, and cook for 5 minutes. Reduce the heat to low, cover the pot, and let cook for about 30 minutes. Adjust seasonings and stir in the lemon juice before serving. Ladle into bowls and serve topped with peanuts.

Nutrition: Calories: 451; Fat: 33 g; Net Carbs: 4 g; Protein: 27.5 g.

773 SLOW COOKER BEER SOUP WITH CHEDDAR & SAUSAGE

Preparation Time: 20 minutes

Cooking Time: 8 hours

Servings: 8

Ingredients:

1 cup heavy cream

10 oz. sausages, sliced

1 cup celery, chopped

1 cup carrots, chopped

4 garlic cloves, minced

8 oz. cream cheese

1 tsp red pepper flakes

6 oz. beer

16 oz. beef stock

1 onion, diced

1 cup cheddar cheese, grated

Salt and black pepper, to taste

Fresh cilantro, chopped, to garnish

Directions:

Turn on the slow cooker. Add beef stock, beer, sausages, carrots, onion, garlic, celery, salt, red pepper flakes, and black pepper, and stir to combine. Pour in enough water to cover all the ingredients by roughly 2 inches. Close the lid and cook for 6 hours on Low.

Open the lid and stir in the heavy cream, cheddar, and cream cheese, and cook for 2 more

hours. Ladle the soup into bowls and garnish with cilantro before serving. Yummy!

Nutrition: Calories: 244; Fat, 17 g; Net Carbs: 4 g; Protein: 5 g.

774 CAULIFLOWER CHEESE SOUP

Preparation Time: 10 minutes

Cooking Time: 30 minutes

Servings: 4

Ingredients:

1 head cauliflower, chopped

½ onion, chopped

2 tbsp. olive oil

2 cups chicken stock

1 tsp. garlic powder

1 tsp. kosher salt

1 oz. cream cheese, cubed

1 cup cheddar cheese, grated

½ cup milk

Directions:

Heat the oil in a heavy stockpot over medium-high heat. Add onion and cook until softened, about 3 minutes.

Add cauliflower, stock, salt and garlic powder.

Bring to a low simmer and cook until the cauliflower is tender, about 20 minutes. Add water if necessary, during cooking.

Transfer cauliflower to a blender or food processor and blend to a smooth puree.

Return pureed cauliflower to the pot and add the cream cheese and cheddar cheese, stirring as the mixture heats over medium-low heat.

When the cheese has melted, add the milk and heat thoroughly.

Nutrition: Total Fat: 8 g; Carbohydrates: 17 g; Protein: 5 g.

775 CHEESY CAULIFLOWER SOUP

Preparation Time: 10 minutes

Cooking Time: 30 minutes

Servings: 8

Ingredients:

¼ cup butter

1 head cauliflower, chopped

½ onion, chopped

½ tsp. ground nutmeg

4 cups chicken stock

1 cup heavy whipping cream

Salt and freshly ground black pepper, to taste

1 cup Cheddar cheese, shredded

Directions:

Take a large stockpot and place it over medium heat.

Add butter to this pot and let it melt.

Add cauliflower and onion to the melted butter and sauté for 10

minutes until these veggies are soft.

Add nutmeg and chicken stock to the pot and bring to a boil.

Reduce the heat to low and allow it to simmer for 15 minutes.

Remove the stockpot from the heat and then add heavy cream.

Purée the cooked soup with an immersion blender until smooth.

Sprinkle this soup with salt and black pepper.

Garnish with Cheddar cheese and serve warm.

Nutrition: Calories: 224; Fat: 16.8 g; Total Carbs: 10.8 g; Fiber: 2.2 g; Protein: 9.6 g.

776 EGG BROTH

Preparation Time: 5 minutes

Cooking Time: 5 minutes

Servings: 4

Ingredients:

2 tbsp. unsalted butter

4 cups chicken broth

3 large eggs

Salt and black pepper, to taste

1 sliced green onion, for garnish

Directions:

Take a medium stockpot and place it over high heat.

Add butter and chicken broth to the pot and bring to a boil.

Break eggs into a bowl and beat them for 1 minute with a fork until frothy.

Once the broth boils, slowly pour in beaten eggs while stirring the broth with a spoon.

Cook for 1 minute with continuously stirring, then sprinkle salt and black pepper to season.

Garnish with sliced green onion, then serve warm.

Nutrition: Calories: 93; Fat: 7.8 g; Total Carbs: 1.8 g; Fiber: 0.1 g; Protein: 3.9 g.

777 BEEF REUBEN SOUP

Preparation Time: 10 minutes

Cooking Time: 20 minutes

Servings: 6

Ingredients:

1 onion, diced

6 cups beef stock

1 tsp caraway seeds

2 celery stalks, diced

3 garlic cloves, minced

2 cups heavy cream

1 cup sauerkraut, shredded

1 pound corned beef, chopped

2 tbsp. butter

½ cup Swiss cheese, shredded

Salt and black pepper, to taste

Directions:

Melt the butter in a large pot. Add onion and celery, and fry for 3 minutes until tender. Add garlic and cook for another minute.

Pour the beef stock over and stir in sauerkraut, salt, caraway seeds, and add a pinch of black pepper. Bring to a boil. Reduce the heat to low, and add the corned beef. Cook for about 15 minutes, adjust the seasoning. Stir in heavy cream and cheese and cook for 1 minute.

Nutrition: Calories: 450; Fat: 37 g; Net Carbs: 8 g; Protein: 23 g.

778 INTERMITTENT MEXICAN-STYLE SOUP

Preparation Time: 10 minutes
Cooking Time: 40 minutes
Servings: 8-10
Ingredients:

¼ cup onion, diced
4 cloves garlic, minced
2 tbsp. chili powder
2 tsp. cumin
20 oz. canned diced tomatoes
4 oz. canned green chilis
32 oz. beef stock
8 oz. cream cheese
½ cup heavy cream
2 tbsp. olive oil

Directions:

Heat the oil in a heavy stockpot over medium-high heat. When the oil is hot, add the onions and sauté until soft and translucent, about 5 minutes.

Add garlic and sauté for one minute more.

Add ground beef and sauté until the meat is thoroughly browned, stirring constantly with a wooden spoon or spatula. This should take about 10 minutes.

Add the rest of the ingredients, excluding the cream and cream cheese, and stir to combine.

Bring to a low simmer and cook until fragrant, about 30 minutes. Add water if necessary, during cooking.

Stir in cream and cream cheese, stirring constantly until cream cheese is melted and soup is thick and creamy. Transfer to serving bowls and serve hot.

Nutrition: Total Fat: 28 g; Carbohydrates: 8 g; Protein: 27 g.

779 CAULIFLOWER CREAM SOUP

Preparation Time: 15 minutes
Cooking Time: 4 hours, 10 minutes
Servings: 5

Ingredients:

10 slices bacon
3 small heads cauliflower, cored and cut into florets
4 cups chicken broth
¼ cup (½ stick) salted butter
3 cloves garlic, pressed
½ large yellow onion, chopped
1 cup heavy whipping cream
2 cups Cheddar cheese, shredded
Salt and black pepper, to taste
Freshly chopped chives or green onions, for garnish

Directions:

Take a large skillet and place it over medium heat.

Add bacon to the skillet and cook for about 8 minutes until brown and crispy.

Transfer the cooked bacon to a paper towel-lined plate to absorb the excess grease.

Allow the bacon to cool, then chop it. Wrap the plate of chopped bacon in plastic and refrigerate it.

Add the cauliflower florets to the food processor and pulse until chopped thoroughly.

Add chicken broth, butter, garlic, onion, and chopped cauliflower to the slow cooker.

Give all these ingredients a gentle stir, then put on the lid.

Cook the cauliflower soup for 4 hours on high heat.

Once the cauliflower is tender, purée the soup with an immersion blender until smooth.

Add chopped bacon, heavy cream, cheese, salt, and black pepper. Mix well and let the cheese melt in the hot soup.

Garnish with green onions or chives, then serve warm.

Nutrition: Calories: 627; Fat: 54.3 g; Total Carbs: 13.7 g; Fiber: 3.7 g; Protein: 24.6 g.

780 SHRIMP MUSHROOM CHOWDER

Preparation Time: 10 minutes
Cooking Time: 40 minutes
Servings: 6
Ingredients:

¼ cup refined avocado oil
⅓ cup diced yellow onions
1 ⅔ cups diced mushrooms
10½ oz. (298 g.) small raw shrimp, shelled and deveined
1 can (13 ½-oz. / 383-g.) unsweetened coconut milk
⅓ cup chicken bone broth
2 tbsp. apple cider vinegar
1 tsp. onion powder
1 tsp. paprika
1 bay leaf

¾ tsp. finely ground gray sea salt
½ tsp. dried oregano leaves
¼ tsp. ground black pepper
1 medium zucchini (7-oz. / 198-g.), cubed
12 radishes (6-oz. / 170-g.), cubed

Directions:

Add avocado oil to a large saucepan and place it over medium heat.

Add onions and mushrooms to the pan and sauté for 10 minutes or until onions are soft and mushrooms are lightly browned.

Stir in shrimp, coconut milk, chicken broth, apple cider vinegar, onion powder, paprika, bay leaf, sea salt, oregano leaves, and black pepper.

Cover the soup mixture with a lid and cook for 20 minutes on low heat.

Add zucchini and radishes to the soup and cook for 10 minutes.

Remove the bay leaf from the soup and divide the soup into 6 small serving bowls. Serve hot.

Nutrition: Calories: 311; Fat: 26.3 g; Total Carbs: 7.7 g; Fiber: 2.9 g; Protein: 13.7 g.

781 PORK TARRAGON SOUP

Preparation Time: 10 minutes
Cooking Time: 1 hour, 20 minutes
Servings: 6
Ingredients:

⅓ cup lard
1 pound (454 g.) pork loin, cut into ½-inch (1.25-cm) pieces
10 strips bacon (about 10-oz. / 284-g.), cut into ½-inch (1.25-cm) pieces
¾ cup sliced shallots
3 medium turnips (about 12 ½-oz. / 354-g.), cubed
1 tbsp. yellow mustard
¼ cup dry white wine
1 ¾ cups chicken bone broth
4 sprigs fresh thyme
2 tbsp. unflavored gelatin
2 tbsp. apple cider vinegar
½ cup unsweetened coconut milk
1 tbsp. dried tarragon leaves

Directions:

Take a large saucepan and place it over medium heat.

Add lard to the saucepan and allow it to melt.

Add pork pieces to the melted lard and sauté for 8 minutes until golden brown.

Add bacon pieces and sliced shallots and sauté for 5 minutes or until fragrant.

Add turnips, mustard, wine, bone broth, and thyme sprigs to the soup.

Mix these ingredients gently and cover this soup with a lid.

Bring the soup to a boil, then reduce the heat to medium-low. Cook this soup for 1 hour.

Remove and discard the thyme sprigs from the soup; then add gelatin, vinegar, coconut milk, and tarragon.

Increase the heat to medium and bring the soup to a boil. Cover to cook for 10 minutes.

Divide the cooked soup into 6 serving bowls and serve warm.

Nutrition: Calories: 566; Fat: 41.5 g; Total Carbs: 9.7 g; Fiber: 1.2 g; Protein: 39.6 g.

782 CHICKEN TURNIP SOUP

Preparation Time: 10 minutes
Cooking Time: 6 to 8 hours
Servings: 5
Ingredients:

12 oz. (340 g.) bone-in chicken
¼ cup turnip, chopped
¼ cup onions, chopped
4 garlic cloves, smashed
4 cups water
3 sprigs thyme
2 bay leaves
Salt, to taste
¼ tsp. freshly ground black pepper

Directions:

Put the chicken, turnip, onions, garlic, water, thyme springs, and bay leaves in a slow cooker.

Season with salt and pepper, then give the mixture a good stir.

Cover and cook on low for 6 to 8 hours until the chicken is cooked through.

When ready, remove the bay leaves and shred the chicken with a fork.

Divide the soup among five bowls and serve.

Nutrition: Calories: 186; Fat: 13.6 g; Total Carbs: 3.3 g; Fiber: 2.6 g; Protein: 15.2 g.

783 SPINACH MUSHROOM SOUP

Preparation Time: 10 minutes
Cooking Time: 5 minutes
Servings: 3

Ingredients:

1 tbsp. olive oil
1 tsp. garlic, finely chopped
1 cup spinach, torn into small pieces
½ cup mushrooms, chopped
Salt and freshly ground black pepper, to taste
½ tsp. tamari
3 cups vegetable stock
1 tsp. sesame seeds, roasted

Directions:

Place a saucepan over medium heat and add olive oil to heat.

Add garlic to the hot oil and sauté for 30 seconds or until fragrant.

Add spinach and mushrooms, then sauté for 1 minute or until lightly tender.

Add salt, black pepper, tamari, and vegetable stock. Cook for another 3 minutes. Stir constantly.

Garnish with sesame seeds and serve warm.

Nutrition: Calories: 80; Fat: 7.4 g; Total carbs: 3.2 g; Fiber: 1.1 g; Protein: 1.2 g.

784 GARLICKY CHICKEN SOUP

Preparation Time: 10 minutes
Cooking Time: 10 minutes
Servings: 4
Ingredients:

2 tbsp. butter
1 large chicken breast cut into strips
4 oz. (113 g.) cream cheese, cubed
2 tbsp. Garlic Gusto Seasoning
½ cup heavy cream
14½ oz. (411 g.) chicken broth
Salt, to taste

Directions:

Place a saucepan over medium heat and add butter to melt.

Add chicken strips and sauté for 2 minutes.

Add cream cheese and seasoning, and cook for 3 minutes, stirring occasionally.

Pour in the heavy cream and chicken broth. Bring the soup to a boil, then lower the heat.

Allow the soup to simmer for 4 minutes, then sprinkle with salt.

Let cool for 5 minutes and serve while warm.

Nutrition: Calories: 243; Fat: 22.5 g; Total carbs: 7.0 g; Fiber: 6.6 g; Protein: 9.6 g.

785 CAULIFLOWER CURRY SOUP

Preparation Time: 15 minutes
Cooking Time: 26 minutes
Servings: 4
Ingredients:

2 tbsp. avocado oil
1 white onion, chopped
4 garlic cloves, chopped
½ Serrano pepper, seeds removed and chopped
1-inch ginger, chopped
¼ tsp. turmeric powder
2 tsp. curry powder
½ tsp. black pepper
1 tsp. salt
1 cup of water
1 large cauliflower, cut into florets
1 cup chicken broth
1 can unsweetened coconut milk
Cilantro, for garnish

Directions:

Place a saucepan over medium heat and add oil to heat.

Add onions to the hot oil and sauté them for 3 minutes.

Add garlic, Serrano pepper, and ginger, then sauté for 2 minutes.

Add turmeric, curry powder, black pepper, and salt. Cook for 1 minute after a gentle stir.

Pour water into the pan, then add cauliflower.

Cover this soup with a lid and cook for 10 minutes. Stir constantly.

Remove the soup from the heat and allow it to cool at room temperature.

Transfer this soup to a blender and purée the soup until smooth.

Return the soup to the saucepan and add broth and coconut milk. Cook for 10 minutes more and stir frequently.

Divide the soup into four bowls and sprinkle the cilantro on top for garnish before serving.

Nutrition: Calories: 342; Fat: 29.1 g; Total Carbs: 18.3 g; Fiber: 5.5 g; Protein: 7.17 g.

786 ASPARAGUS CREAM SOUP

Preparation Time: 15 minutes
Cooking Time: 22 minutes
Servings: 6
Ingredients:

4 tbsp. butter
1 small onion, chopped
6 cups low-sodium chicken broth
Salt and black pepper, to taste
2 pounds (907 g.) asparagus, cut in half
½ cup sour cream

Directions:

Place a large pot over low heat and add butter to melt.

Add onion to the melted butter and sauté for 2 minutes or until soft.

Add chicken broth, salt, black pepper, and asparagus.

Bring the soup to a boil, then cover the lid and cook for 20 minutes.

Remove the pot from the heat and allow it to cool for 5 minutes.

Transfer the soup to a blender and blend until smooth.

Add sour cream and pulse again to mix well.

Serve fresh and warm.

Nutrition: Calories: 138; Fat: 10.5 g; Total Carbs: 10.2 g; Fiber: 3.5 g; Protein: 5.9 g.

787 RED GAZPACHO CREAM SOUP

Preparation Time: 15 minutes
Cooking Time: 20 minutes
Servings: 10
Ingredients:

1 large red bell pepper, halved

1 large green bell pepper, halved
2 tbsp. basil, freshly chopped
4 medium tomatoes
1 small red onion
1 large cucumber, diced
2 medium spring onions, diced
2 tbsp. apple cider vinegar
2 garlic cloves
2 tbsp. fresh lemon juice
1 cup extra virgin olive oil
Salt and black pepper, to taste
1 ¼ pounds (567 g.) feta cheese, shredded

Directions:

Preheat the oven to 400°F (205°C) and line a baking tray with parchment paper.

Place all the bell peppers in the baking tray and roast in the preheated oven for 20 minutes.

Remove the bell peppers from the oven. Allow to cool, then peel off their skin.

Transfer the peeled bell peppers to a blender along with basil, tomatoes, red onions, cucumber, spring onions, vinegar, garlic, lemon juice, olive oil, black pepper, and salt. Blend until the mixture smooth.

Add black pepper and salt to taste.

Garnish with feta cheese and serve warm.

Nutrition: Calories: 248; Fat: 21.6 g; Total Carbs: 8.3 g; Fiber: 4.1 g; Protein: 9.3 g.

788 BEEF TACO SOUP

Preparation Time: 15 minutes
Cooking Time: 24 minutes
Servings: 8
Ingredients:

2 garlic cloves, minced
½ cup onions, chopped
1 pound (454 g.) ground beef
1 tsp. chili powder
1 tbsp. ground cumin
1 (8-oz. / 227-g.) package cream cheese, softened
2 (10-oz. / 284-g.) cans diced tomatoes and green chilies
½ cup heavy cream
2 tsp. salt
2 (14 ½-oz. / 411-g.) cans beef broth

Directions:

Take a large saucepan and place it over medium-high heat.

Add garlic, onions, and ground beef to the soup and sauté for 7 minutes until beef is browned.

Add chili powder and cumin, then cook for 2 minutes.

Add cream cheese and cook for 5 minutes while mashing the cream cheese into the beef with a spoon.

Add diced tomatoes and green chilies, heavy cream, salt and broth then cook for 10 minutes.

Mix gently and serve warm.

Nutrition: Calories: 205; Fat: 13.3 g; Total Carbs: 4.4 g; Fiber: 0.8 g; Protein: 8.0 g.

789 CREAMY TOMATO SOUP

Preparation Time: 15 minutes
Cooking Time: 30 minutes
Servings: 4
Ingredients:

2 cups water
4 cups tomato juice
3 tomatoes, peeled, seeded and diced
14 leaves fresh basil
2 tbsp. butter
1 cup heavy whipping cream
Salt and black pepper, to taste

Directions:

Take a suitable cooking pot and place it over medium heat.

Add water, tomato juice, and tomatoes, then simmer for 30 minutes.

Transfer the soup to a blender, then add basil leaves.

Press the pulse button and blend the soup until smooth.

Return this tomato soup to the cooking pot and place it over medium heat.

Add butter, heavy cream, salt, and black pepper. Cook and mix until the butter melts.

Serve warm and fresh.

Nutrition: Calories: 203; Fat: 17.7 g; Total Carbs: 13.0 g; Fiber: 5.6 g; Protein: 3.7 g.

790 CREAMY BROCCOLI AND LEEK SOUP

Preparation Time: 5 minutes
Cooking Time: 25 minutes
Servings: 4
Ingredients:

10 oz. broccoli
1 leek
8 oz. cream cheese
3 oz. butter
3 cups water
1 garlic clove
½ cup fresh basil
salt and pepper

Directions:

Rinse the leek and chop both parts finely. Slice the broccoli thinly.

Place the veggies in a pot and cover with water and then season them. Boil the water until the broccoli softens.

Add the florets and garlic, while lowering the heat.

Add in the cheese, butter, pepper, and basil. Blend until desired

consistency: if too thick use water; if you want to make it thicker, use a little bit of heavy cream.

Nutrition: Calories: 451; Fats: 37 g; Protein: 10 g; Carbs: 4 g.

791 CHICKEN SOUP

Preparation Time: 25 minutes
Cooking Time: 80 minutes
Servings: 4
Ingredients:

6 cups water
1 chicken
1 medium carrot
1 yellow onion
1 bay leaf
1 leek
2 garlic cloves
1 tbsp. dried thyme
½ cup white wine, dry (no, not for drinking)
1 tsp. peppercorns
salt and pepper

Directions:

Peel and cut your veggies. Brown them in oil in a big pot.

Split your chicken in half, down in the middle. Pour water and spices into the pot. Let it simmer for one hour.

Take out the chicken save the meat, and toss away the bones.

Put the meat back in the pot, and let it simmer on medium heat for 20-25 minutes again, while seasoning to your liking.

Nutrition: Calories: 145; Fats: 12 g; Carbs: 1 g; Protein: 8 g.

792 GREEK EGG AND LEMON SOUP WITH CHICKEN

Preparation Time: 5 minutes
Cooking Time: 30 minutes
Servings: 4
Ingredients:

4 cups water
¾ lbs. cauli
1 lb. boneless chicken thighs
⅓ lb. butter
4 eggs
1 lemon
2 tbsp. fresh parsley
1 bay leaf
2 chicken bouillon cubes
salt and pepper

Directions:

Slice your chicken thinly and then place in a saucepan while adding cold water and the cubes and bay leaf. Let the meat simmer for 10 minutes before removing it and the bay leaf.

Grate your cauli and place it in a saucepan. Add butter and boil for a few minutes.

Beat your eggs and lemon juice in a bowl, while seasoning it.

Reduce the heat a bit and add the eggs, stirring continuously. Let simmer but don't boil.

Return the chicken.

Nutrition: Calories: 582; Carbs: 4 g; Fats: 49 g; Protein: 31 g.

793 WILD MUSHROOM SOUP

Preparation Time: 10 minutes
Cooking Time: 30 minutes
Servings: 4
Ingredients:

6 oz. mix of portabella mushrooms, oyster mushrooms, and shiitake mushrooms
3 cups water
1 garlic clove
1 shallot
4 oz. butter
1 chicken bouillon cube
½ lb. celery root
1 tbsp. white wine vinegar
1 cup heavy whipping cream
fresh parsley

Directions:

Clean, trim, and chop your mushrooms and celery. Do the same to your shallot and garlic.

Sauté your chopped veggies in butter over medium heat in a saucepan.

Add thyme, vinegar, chicken bouillon cube, and water as you bring to boil. Then let it simmer for 10-15 minutes.

Add cream to them with an immersion blender until your desired consistency. Serve with parsley on top.

Nutrition: Calories: 481; Fats: 47 g; Protein: 7 g; Carbs: 9 g.

794 ROASTED BUTTERNUT SQUASH SOUP

Preparation Time: 15 minutes
Cooking Time: 30 minutes
Servings: 4
Ingredients:

1 large butternut squash, cubed and peeled
1 stalk celery, sliced
2 potatoes, peeled, chopped
1 onion, chopped
1 large carrot, chopped
3 tbsp. olive oil
1 tbsp. fresh thyme

25 oz. chicken broth
1 tbsp. butter
salt and pepper

Directions:

Preheat your oven to 400°F. On a baking sheet, toss squash and potatoes with 2 tablespoons of oil and season to your taster. Roast for 20-25 minutes.

In the meantime, melt your butter and the rest of the oil in a large pot over medium heat. Add the onion, celery, carrot and cook for 5-8 minutes. Season them, too.

Add roasted squash and potatoes. Then pour over the chicken broth. Simmer it for 10 minutes using an immersion blender until the soup is creamy.

Garnish it with thyme.

Nutrition: Calories: 254; Fats: 15 g; Carbs: 19 g; Protein: 6 g.

795 ZUCCHINI CREAM SOUP

Preparation Time: 5 minutes
Cooking Time: 20 minutes
Servings: 4
Ingredients:

3 zucchinis
32 oz. chicken broth
2 cloves garlic
2 tbsp. sour cream
½ small onion
parmesan cheese (for topping if desired)

Directions:

Combine your broth, garlic, zucchini, and onion in a large pot over medium heat until boiling.

Lower the heat, cover, and let simmer for 15-20 minutes.

Remove from heat and purée with an immersion blender, while adding the sour cream and pureeing until smooth.

Season to taste and top with your cheese.

Nutrition: Calories: 117; Fats: 9 g; Carbs: 3 g; Protein: 4 g.

796 CAULI SOUP

Preparation Time: 5 minutes
Cooking Time: 25 minutes
Servings: 6
Ingredients:

32 oz. vegetable broth
1 head cauli, diced
2 garlic cloves, minced
1 onion, diced
½ tbsp. olive oil
salt and pepper

grated parmesan, sliced green onion for topping

Directions:

In a pot, heat oil over medium heat, while adding the onion and garlic. Then cook them for 4-5 minutes.

Add in the cauli and vegetable broth. Boil it and then cover for 15-20 minutes while covered.

Pour all contents of the pot into a blender and season it.

Blend until smooth. Top it with your cheese and green onion.

Nutrition: Calories: 37; Fats: 1 g; Carbs: 3 g; Protein: 3 g.

797 THAI COCONUT SOUP

Preparation Time: 10 minutes
Cooking Time: 35 minutes
Servings: 4
Ingredients:

3 chicken breasts
9 oz. coconut milk
9 oz. chicken broth
⅔ tbsp. chili sauce
18 oz. water
⅔ tbsp. coconut aminos
¾ oz. lime juice
⅔ tsp. ground ginger
¼ cup red boat fish sauce
salt and pepper

Directions:

Slice up the chicken breasts thinly. Make them bite-sized.

In a large stock pot, mix your coconut milk, water, fish sauce, chili sauce, lime juice, ginger, coconut aminos, and broth. Bring to a boil.

Stir in chicken pieces. Then reduce the heat and cover the pot, while simmering it for 30 minutes.

Remove the basil leaves and season it.

Nutrition: Calories: 227; Fats: 17 g; Carbs: 3 g; Protein: 19 g.

798 CHICKEN RAMEN SOUP

Preparation Time: 10 minutes
Cooking Time: 20 minutes
Servings: 2
Ingredients:

1 chicken breast
2 eggs
1 zucchini, made into noodles
4 cups chicken broth
2 cloves of garlic, peeled and minced
2 tbsp. coconut aminos
3 tbsp. avocado oil
1 tbsp. ginger

Directions:

Pan-fry the chicken in avocado oil in a pan until brown.

Hard boil your eggs and slice them in half.

Add chicken broth to a large pot and simmer with the garlic, coconut aminos, and ginger. Then add in the zucchini noodles for 4-5 minutes.

Put the broth into a bowl. Top it with eggs and chicken slices, and season to your liking.

Nutrition: Calories: 478; Fats: 39 g; Carbs: 3 g; Protein: 31 g.

799 CHICKEN BROTH AND EGG DROP SOUP

Preparation Time: 5 minutes
Cooking Time: 15 minutes
Servings: 2
Ingredients:

3 cups chicken broth
2 cups Swiss chard chopped
2 eggs, whisked
1 tsp. grated ginger
1 tsp. ground oregano
2 tbsp. coconut aminos
salt and pepper

Directions:

Heat your broth in a saucepan.
Slowly drizzle in the eggs while stirring slowly.
Add the Swiss chard, grated ginger, oregano, and coconut aminos. Next, season it and let it cook for 5-10 minutes.

Nutrition: Calories: 225; Fats: 19 g; Carbs: 4 g; Protein: 11 g.

800 OKRA AND BEEF STEW

Preparation Time: 15 minutes
Cooking Time: 25 minutes
Servings: 3
Ingredients:

6 oz. okra, chopped
8 oz. beef sirloin, chopped
1 cup of water
¼ cup coconut cream
1 tsp. dried basil
¼ tsp. cumin seeds
1 tbsp. avocado oil

Directions:

Sprinkle the beef sirloin with cumin seeds and dried basil and put it in the instant pot.
Add avocado oil and roast the meat in sauté mode for 5 minutes. Stir it occasionally.
Then add coconut cream, water, and okra.
Close the lid and cook the stew on manual mode (high pressure) for 25 minutes. Allow the natural pressure release for 10 minutes.

Nutrition: Calories: 216; Fat: 10.2; Fiber: 2.5; Carbs: 5.7; Protein: 24.6.

801 CHIPOTLE STEW

Preparation Time: 15 minutes
Cooking Time: 10 minutes
Servings: 3
Ingredients:

2 chipotle chilies in adobo sauce, chopped
1 oz. fresh cilantro, chopped
9 oz. chicken fillet, chopped
1 tsp. ground paprika
2 tbsp. sesame seeds
¼ tsp. salt
1 cup chicken broth

Directions:

In the mixing bowl mix up chipotle chili, cilantro, chicken fillet, ground paprika, sesame seeds, and salt.
Then transfer the ingredients to the instant pot and add chicken broth.
Cook the stew on manual mode (high pressure) for 10 minutes. Allow the natural pressure release for 10 minutes more.

Nutrition: Calories: 230; Fat: 10.6; Fiber: 2.6; Carbs: 4.5; Protein: 27.6.

802 INTERMITTENT CHILI

Preparation Time: 10 minutes
Cooking Time: 25 minutes
Servings: 2
Ingredients:

½ cup ground beef
½ tsp. chili powder
1 tsp. dried oregano
¼ cup crushed tomatoes
2 oz. scallions, diced
1 tsp. avocado oil
¼ cup of water

Directions:

Mix up ground beef, chili powder, dried oregano, and scallions.
Then add avocado oil and stir the mixture.
Transfer it to the instant pot and cook in sauté mode for 10 minutes.
Add water and crushed tomatoes. Stir the ingredients with the help of the spatula until homogenous.
Close and seal the lid and cook the chili for 15 minutes on manual mode (high pressure). Then make a quick pressure release.

Nutrition: Calories: 94; Fat: 4.6; Fiber: 2.4; Carbs: 5.6; Protein: 8.

803 PIZZA SOUP

Preparation Time: 10 minutes
Cooking Time: 22 minutes
Servings: 3

Ingredients:

¼ cup cremini mushrooms, sliced
1 tsp. tomato paste
4 oz. Mozzarella, shredded
½ jalapeno pepper, sliced
½ tsp. Italian seasoning
1 tsp. coconut oil
5 oz. Italian sausages, chopped
1 cup of water

Directions:

Melt the coconut oil in the instant pot on sauté mode.
Add mushrooms and cook them for 10 minutes.
After this, add chopped sausages, Italian seasoning, sliced jalapeno, and tomato paste.
Mix up the ingredients well and add water.
Close and seal the lid and cook the soup on manual mode (high pressure) for 12 minutes.
Then make a quick pressure release and ladle the soup in the bowls. Top it with Mozzarella.

Nutrition: Calories: 289; Fat: 23.2; Fiber: 0.2; Carbs: 2.5; Protein: 17.7.

804 LAMB SOUP

Preparation Time: 10 minutes
Cooking Time: 25 minutes
Servings: 4
Ingredients:

½ cup broccoli, roughly chopped
7 oz. lamb fillet, chopped
¼ tsp. ground cumin
¼ daikon, chopped
2 bell peppers, chopped
1 tbsp. avocado oil
5 cups beef broth

Directions:

Sauté the lamb fillet with avocado oil in the instant pot for 5 minutes.
Then add broccoli, ground cumin, and daikon, bell peppers, and beef broth.
Close and seal the lid.
Cook the soup on manual mode (high pressure) for 20 minutes.
Allow the natural pressure release.

Nutrition: Calories: 169; Fat: 6; Fiber: 1.3; Carbs: 6.8; Protein: 21.

805 MINESTRONE SOUP

Preparation Time: 10 minutes
Cooking Time: 25 minutes
Servings: 4
Ingredients:

1 ½ cup ground pork
½ bell pepper, chopped
2 tbsp. chives, chopped
2 oz. celery stalk, chopped
1 tsp. butter
1 tsp. Italian seasonings

4 cups chicken broth

½ cup mushrooms, sliced

Directions:

Heat up butter on the sauté mode for 2 minutes.

Add bell pepper. Cook the vegetable for 5 minutes.

Then stir them well and add mushrooms, celery stalk, and Italian seasonings. Stir well and cook for 5 minutes more.

Add ground pork, chives, and chicken broth.

Close and seal the lid.

Cook the soup on manual mode (high pressure) for 15 minutes. Make a quick pressure release.

Nutrition: Calories: 408; Fat: 27.2; Fiber: 0.6; Carbs: 3; Protein: 35.6.

806 CHORIZO SOUP

Preparation Time: 10 minutes

Cooking Time: 17 minutes

Servings: 3

Ingredients:

8 oz. chorizo, chopped

1 tsp. tomato paste

4 oz. scallions, diced

1 tbsp. dried cilantro

½ tsp. chili powder

1 tsp. avocado oil

2 cups beef broth

Directions:

Heat up avocado oil on sauté mode for 1 minute.

Add chorizo and cook it for 6 minutes, stir it from time to time.

Then add scallions, tomato paste, cilantro, and chili powder. Stir well.

Add beef broth.

Close and seal the lid.

Cook the soup on manual mode (high pressure) for 10 minutes. Make a quick pressure release.

Nutrition: Calories: 387; Fat: 30.2; Fiber: 1.3; Carbs: 5.5; Protein: 22.3.

807 RED FETA SOUP

Preparation Time: 10 minutes

Cooking Time: 25 minutes

Servings: 4

Ingredients:

1 cup broccoli, chopped

1 tsp. tomato paste

½ cup coconut cream

4 cups beef broth

1 tsp. chili flakes

6 oz. feta, crumbled

Directions:

Put broccoli, tomato paste, coconut cream, and beef broth in the instant pot.

Add chili flakes and stir the mixture until it is red.

Then close and seal the lid and cook the soup for 8 minutes on manual mode (high pressure).

Then make a quick pressure release and open the lid.

Add feta cheese and sauté the soup on sauté mode for 5 minutes more.

Nutrition: Calories: 229; Fat: 17.7; Fiber: 1.3; Carbs: 6.1; Protein: 12.3.

808 "RAMEN" SOUP

Preparation Time: 10 minutes

Cooking Time: 15 minutes

Servings: 2

Ingredients:

1 zucchini, trimmed

2 cups chicken broth

2 eggs, boiled, peeled

1 tbsp. coconut aminos

5 oz. beef loin, strips

1 tsp. chili flakes

1 tbsp. chives, chopped

½ tsp. salt

Directions:

Put the beef loin strips in the instant pot.

Add chili flakes, salt, and chicken broth.

Close and seal the lid. Cook the ingredients on manual mode (high pressure) for 15 minutes. Make a quick pressure release and open the lid.

Then make the s from zucchini with the help of the spiralizer and add them to the soup.

Add chives and coconut aminos.

Then ladle the soup in the bowls and top with halved eggs.

Nutrition: Calories: 254; Fat: 11.8; Fiber: 1.1; Carbs: 6.2; Protein: 30.6.

809 BEEF TAGINE

Preparation Time: 15 minutes

Cooking Time: 25 minutes

Servings: 6

Ingredients:

1-pound beef fillet, chopped

1 eggplant, chopped

6 oz. scallions, chopped

1 tsp. ground allspices

1 tsp. Erythritol

1 tsp. coconut oil

4 cups beef broth

Directions:

Put all ingredients in the instant pot.

Close and seal the lid.

Cook the meal on manual mode (high pressure) for 25 minutes.

Then allow the natural pressure release for 15 minutes.

Nutrition: Calories: 146; Fat: 5.3; Fiber: 3.5; Carbs: 8.8; Protein: 16.7.

810 CHILI VERDE SOUP

Preparation Time: 10 minutes

Cooking Time: 25 minutes

Servings: 4

Ingredients:

2 oz. chili Verde sauce

½ cup Cheddar cheese, shredded

5 cups chicken broth

1-pound chicken breast, skinless, boneless

1 tbsp. dried cilantro

Directions:

Put chicken breast and chicken broth in the instant pot.

Add cilantro, close and seal the lid.

Then cook the ingredients on manual (high pressure) for 15 minutes.

Make a quick pressure release and open the lid.

Shred the chicken breast with the help of the fork.

Add dried cilantro and chili Verde sauce to the soup and cook it in sauté mode for 10 minutes.

Then add dried cilantro and stir well.

Nutrition: Calories: 257; Fat: 10.2; Fiber: 0.2; Carbs: 4; Protein: 34.5.

811 PEPPER STUFFING SOUP

Preparation Time: 10 minutes

Cooking Time: 14 minutes

Servings: 4

Ingredients:

1 cup ground beef

½ cup cauliflower, shredded

1 tsp. dried oregano

½ tsp. salt

1 tsp. tomato paste

1 tsp. minced garlic

4 cups water

¼ cup coconut milk

Directions:

Put all ingredients in the instant pot bowl and stir well.

Then close and seal the lid.

Cook the soup on manual mode (high pressure) for 14 minutes.

When the time of cooking is finished, make a quick pressure release and open the lid.

Nutrition: Calories: 106; Fat: 7.7; Fiber: 0.9; Carbs: 2.2; Protein: 7.3.

812 STEAK SOUP

Preparation Time: 10 minutes

Cooking Time: 40 minutes

Servings: 5

Ingredients:

5 oz. scallions, diced

1 tbsp. coconut oil

1 oz. daikon, diced

1-pound beef round steak, chopped

1 tsp. dried thyme

5 cups water

½ tsp. ground black pepper

Directions:

Heat up coconut oil on sauté mode for 2 minutes.

Add daikon and scallions.

After this, stir them well and add chopped beef steak, thyme, and ground black pepper.

Sauté the ingredients for 5 minutes more and then add water.

Close and seal the lid.

Cook the soup on manual mode (high pressure) for 35 minutes. Make a quick pressure release.

Nutrition: Calories: 232; Fat: 11; Fiber: 0.9; Carbs: 2.5; Protein: 29.5.

813 MEAT SPINACH STEW

Preparation Time: 20 minutes

Cooking Time: 30 minutes

Servings: 4

Ingredients:

2 cups spinach, chopped

1-pound beef sirloin, chopped

1 tsp. allspices

3 cups chicken broth

1 cup coconut milk

1 tsp. coconut aminos

Directions:

Put all ingredients in the instant pot.

Close and seal the lid.

After this, set the manual mode (high pressure) and cook the stew for 30 minutes.

When the cooking time is finished, allow the natural pressure release for 10 minutes.

Stir the stew gently before serving.

Nutrition: Calories: 383; Fat: 22.2; Fiber: 1.8; Carbs: 5.1; Protein: 39.9.

814 LEEK SOUP

Preparation Time: 10 minutes

Cooking Time: 15 minutes

Servings: 4

Ingredients:

7 oz. leek, chopped

2 oz. Monterey Jack cheese, shredded

1 tsp. Italian seasonings

½ tsp. salt

4 tbsp. butter

2 cups chicken broth

Directions:

Heat up butter in the instant pot for 4 minutes.

Then add chopped leek, salt, and Italian seasonings.

Cook the leek on sauté mode for 5 minutes. Stir the vegetables from time to time.

After this, add chicken broth and close the lid.

Cook the soup on sauté mode for 10 minutes.

Then add shredded cheese and stir it till the cheese is melted.

The soup is cooked.

Nutrition: Calories: 208; Fat: 17; Fiber: 0.9; Carbs: 7.7; Protein: 6.8.

815 ASPARAGUS SOUP

Preparation Time: 10 minutes

Cooking Time: 17 minutes

Servings: 4

Ingredients:

1 cup asparagus, chopped

2 cups coconut milk

1 tsp. salt

½ tsp. cayenne pepper

3 oz. scallions, diced

1 tsp. olive oil

Directions:

Sauté the chopped asparagus, scallions, and olive oil in the instant pot for 7 minutes.

Then stir the vegetables well and add cayenne pepper, salt, and coconut milk

Cook the soup on manual mode (high pressure) for 10 minutes.

After this, make a quick pressure release and open the lid.

Blend the soup until you get the creamy texture.

Nutrition: Calories: 300; Fat: 29.9; Fiber: 4; Carbs: 9.6; Protein: 3.9.

816 BOK CHOY SOUP

Preparation Time: 5 minutes

Cooking Time: 2 minutes

Servings: 1

Ingredients:

1 bok choy stalk, chopped

¼ tsp. nutritional yeast

½ tsp. onion powder

¼ tsp. chili flakes

1 cup chicken broth

Directions:

Put all ingredients from the list above in the instant pot.

Close and seal the lid and cook the soup on manual (high pressure) for 2 minutes.

Make a quick pressure release.

Nutrition: Calories: 58; Fat: 1.7; Fiber: 1.3; Carbs: 4.5; Protein: 6.9.

817 CURRY KALE SOUP

Preparation Time: 10 minutes

Cooking Time: 15 minutes

Servings: 3

Ingredients:

2 cups kale

1 tbsp. fresh cilantro

1 tsp. curry paste

½ cup heavy cream

½ cup ground chicken

1 tsp. almond butter

½ tsp. salt 1 cup chicken stock

Directions:

Blend the kale until smooth and put it in the instant pot.

Add cilantro, almond butter, and ground chicken. Sauté the mixture for 5 minutes.

Meanwhile, in the shallow bowl, mix up curry paste and heavy cream. When the liquid is smooth, pour it into the instant pot.

Add chicken stock and salt, and close the lid.

Cook the soup on manual (high pressure) for 10 minutes. Make a quick pressure release.

Nutrition: Calories: 183; Fat: 13.3; Fiber: 1.2; Carbs: 7; Protein: 9.9.

818 TURMERIC RUTABAGA SOUP

Preparation Time: 15 minutes

Cooking Time: 15 minutes

Servings: 5

Ingredients:

3 turnips, chopped

1 tsp. ginger paste

2 oz. celery, chopped

1 tsp. ground turmeric

1 tsp. minced garlic

2 cups of coconut milk

1 cup beef broth

2 oz. bell pepper, chopped

Directions:

Place all ingredients in the instant pot and stir them gently.

Then close and seal the lid; set manual mode (high pressure) and cook the soup for 15 minutes.

Then allow the natural pressure release for 10 minutes and ladle the soup into the serving bowls.

Nutrition: Calories: 255; Fat: 23.2; Fiber: 3.6; Carbs: 11.4; Protein: 4.

819 CREAM OF MUSHROOMS SOUP

Preparation Time: 10 minutes

Cooking Time: 35 minutes

Servings: 6

Ingredients:

3 cups cremini mushrooms, sliced

1 cup coconut milk

1 tbsp. almond flour

1 tsp. salt

1 tsp. ground black pepper

4 cups chicken broth

3 tbsp. butter

Directions:

Melt the butter on sauté mode.

Add cremini mushrooms and sauté them for 10 minutes. Stir them with the help of the spatula from time to time.

After this, in the bowl mix up salt, almond flour, and ground black pepper. Add coconut milk and stir the liquid.

Pour the liquid over the mushrooms.

Add chicken broth. Close and seal the lid.

Cook the soup on sauté mode for 25 minutes.

Nutrition: Calories: 206; Fat: 18.6; Fiber: 1.7; Carbs: 5.5; Protein: 6.2.

820 FLU SOUP

Preparation Time: 10 minutes
Cooking Time: 15 minutes
Servings: 4
Ingredients:

1 cup mushrooms, chopped
1 cup spinach, chopped
3 oz. scallions, diced
2 oz. Cheddar cheese, shredded
1 tsp. cayenne pepper
1 cup organic almond milk
2 cups chicken broth
½ tsp. salt

Directions:

Put all ingredients in the instant pot and close the lid.

Set the manual mode (high pressure) and cook the soup for 15 minutes.

Make a quick pressure release.

Blend the soup with the help of the immersion blender.

When the soup will get a smooth texture – it is cooked.

Nutrition: Calories: 228; Fat: 19.9; Fiber: 2.3; Carbs: 6.6; Protein: 8.5.

821 JALAPENO SOUP

Preparation Time: 10 minutes
Cooking Time: 10 minutes
Servings: 4
Ingredients:

2 jalapeno peppers, sliced
3 oz. pancetta, chopped
½ cup heavy cream
2 cups water
½ cup Monterey jack cheese, shredded
½ tsp. garlic powder
1 tsp. coconut oil
½ tsp. smoked paprika

Directions:

Toss pancetta in the instant pot, add coconut oil, and cook it for 4 minutes on sauté mode. Stir it from time to time.

After this, add sliced jalapenos, garlic powder, and smoked paprika.

Stir the ingredients for 1 minute.

Add heavy cream and water.

Then add Monterey Jack cheese and stir the soup well.

Close and seal the lid; cook the soup for 5 minutes on manual mode (high pressure); make a quick pressure release.

Nutrition: Calories: 234; Fat: 20; Fiber: 0.4; Carbs: 1.7; Protein: 11.8.

822 GARDEN SOUP

Preparation Time: 20 minutes
Cooking Time: 29 minutes
Servings: 5
Ingredients:

½ cup cauliflower florets
1 cup kale, chopped
1 garlic clove, diced
1 tbsp. olive oil
1 tsp. sea salt
6 cups beef broth
2 tbsp. chives, chopped

Directions:

Heat up olive oil in the instant pot on sauté mode for 2 minutes and add clove.

Cook the vegetables for 2 minutes and stir well.

Add kale, cauliflower, and sea salt, chives, and beef broth.

Close and seal the lid.

Cook the soup on manual mode (high pressure) for 5 minutes.

Then make a quick pressure release and open the lid.

Ladle the soup into the bowls.

Nutrition: Calories: 80; Fat: 4.5; Fiber: 0.5; Carbs: 2.3; Protein: 6.5.

823 SHIRATAKI NOODLE SOUP

Preparation Time: 25 minutes
Cooking Time: 15 minutes
Servings: 2
Ingredients:

2 oz. shirataki noodles
2 cups water
6 oz. chicken fillet, chopped
1 tsp. salt
1 tbsp. coconut aminos

Directions:

Pour water into the instant pot bowl.

Add salt and chopped chicken fillet. Close and seal the lid.

Cook the ingredients on manual mode (high pressure) for 15 minutes. Allow the natural pressure release for 10 minutes.

After this, add shirataki noodles and coconut aminos.

Leave the soup for 10 minutes to rest.

Nutrition: Calories: 175; Fat: 6.3; Fiber: 3; Carbs: 1.5; Protein: 24.8.

824 CORDON BLUE SOUP

Preparation Time: 15 minutes

Cooking Time: 6 minutes
Servings: 4
Ingredients:

4 cups chicken broth
7 oz. ham, chopped
3 oz. Mozzarella cheese, shredded
1 tsp. ground black pepper
½ tsp. salt
2 tbsp. ricotta cheese
2 oz. scallions, chopped

Directions:

Put all ingredients in the instant pot bowl and stir gently.

Close and seal the lid; cook the soup on manual mode (high pressure) for 6 minutes.

Then allow the natural pressure release for 10 minutes and ladle the soup into the bowls.

Nutrition: Calories: 196; Fat: 10.1; Fiber: 1.2; Carbs: 5.3; Protein: 20.3.

825 BACON SOUP

Preparation Time: 10 minutes
Cooking Time: 20 minutes
Servings: 4
Ingredients:

3 oz. bacon, chopped
1 cup cheddar cheese, shredded
1 tbsp. scallions, chopped
3 cups beef broth 1 cup of coconut milk
1 tsp. curry powder

Directions:

Heat up the instant pot on sauté mode for 3 minutes and add bacon.

Cook it for 5 minutes. Stir it from time to time.

Then add scallions and curry powder. Cook the Ingredients for 5 minutes more. Stir them from time to time.

After this, add coconut milk and beef broth.

Add cheddar cheese and stir the soup well.

Cook it on manual mode (high pressure) for 10 minutes. Make a quick pressure release.

Mix up the soup well before serving.

Nutrition: Calories: 398; Fat: 33.6; Fiber: 1.5; Carbs: 5.1; Protein: 20.

826 INTERMITTENT CHINESE-STYLE SOUP

Preparation Time: 5 minutes
Cooking Time: 35 minutes
Servings: 8-10
Ingredients:

5 cups vegetable stock
4 lb. pork tenderloin or other lean pork, sliced into thin bite-sized pieces
1 cup fresh mushrooms, chopped

2 tbsp. soy sauce
2 tbsp. white vinegar
2 tbsp. rice vinegar
2 tsp. salt
1 tsp. freshly ground black pepper
4 tbsp. water
2 eggs, beaten
2 lb. tofu, extra firm, cubed

Directions:

Put all ingredients, excluding eggs and tofu, in a heavy stock pot.

Bring to a low simmer and cook until the meat is thoroughly cooked and the mushrooms are tender, about 30 minutes. Add water if necessary, during cooking.

Slowly and carefully, stir in the tofu and beaten eggs. Allow the warm soup to sit for at least 3 minutes to allow the eggs to cook.

Transfer to serving bowls and serve hot.

Nutrition: Total Fat: 5 g; Carbohydrates: 5 g; Protein: 20 g.

827 SALSA VERDE CHICKEN SOUP

Preparation Time: 5 minutes
Cooking Time: 10 minutes
Servings: 4
Ingredients:

½ cup salsa Verde
2 cups cooked and shredded chicken
2 cups chicken broth
¼ cup shredded cheddar cheese
4 oz. cream cheese
½ tsp chili powder
½ tsp ground cumin
½ tsp fresh cilantro, chopped
Salt and black pepper, to taste

Directions:

Combine the cream cheese, salsa Verde, and broth, in a food processor; pulse until smooth. Transfer the mixture to a pot and place over medium heat. Cook until hot, but do not bring to a boil. Add chicken, chili powder, and cumin and cook for about 3-5 minutes, or until it is heated through.

Stir in cheddar cheese and season with salt and pepper to taste. If it is very thick, add a few tbsp. of water and boil for 1-3 more minutes. Serve hot in bowls sprinkled with fresh cilantro.

Nutrition: Calories: 346; Fat: 23 g; Net Carbs: 3 g; Protein: 25 g.

828 CUCUMBER-TURKEY CANAPES

Preparation Time: 10 minutes
Cooking Time: 5 minutes
Servings: 6
Ingredients:

2 cucumbers, sliced
2 cups dice leftover turkey
¼ jalapeño pepper, minced
1 tbsp Dijon mustard
¼ cup mayonnaise
Salt and black pepper to taste

Directions:

Cut mid-level holes in cucumber slices with a knife and set aside.

Mix turkey, jalapeno pepper, mustard, mayonnaise, salt, and black pepper in a bowl.

Carefully fill cucumber holes with turkey mixture and serve.

Nutrition: Calories: 170; Net Carbs: 1.3 g; Fat: 14 g; Protein: 10 g.

829 BAKED CHICKEN SKEWERS WITH RUTABAGA FRIES

Preparation Time: 20 minutes
Cooking Time: 45 minutes
Servings: 6
Ingredients:

2 chicken breasts, halved
Salt and black pepper to taste
4 tbsp. olive oil
¼ cup chicken broth
1 lb. rutabaga
2 tbsp. olive oil

Directions:

Set oven to 400°F. Grease and line a baking sheet. In a bowl, mix 2 tablespoons of the olive oil, salt, and pepper and add in the chicken; toss to coat. Set in the fridge for 20 minutes.

Peel and chop rutabaga to form fry shapes and place into a separate bowl. Coat with the remaining olive oil and season with salt and pepper. Arrange the rutabaga shapes on the baking sheet and bake for 10 minutes.

Take the chicken from the refrigerator and thread onto the skewers. Place over the rutabaga, pour in the chicken broth and bake for 30 minutes. Serve immediately.

Nutrition: Calories: 579; Net Carbs: 6 g; Fat: 53 g; Protein: 39 g.

830 LOUISIANA CHICKEN FETTUCCINE

Preparation Time: 10 minutes
Cooking Time: 45 minutes
Servings: 4
Ingredients:

1 medium red bell pepper, deseeded and thinly sliced
1 medium green bell pepper, deseeded and thinly sliced
2 cups grated mozzarella
½ cup grated Parmesan
1 cup shredded mozzarella

1 egg yolk
2 tbsp. olive oil
4 chicken breasts, cubed
1 yellow onion, thinly sliced
4 garlic cloves, minced
4 tsp. Cajun seasoning
1 cup Alfredo sauce
½ cup marinara sauce
2 tbsp. chopped fresh parsley

Directions:

Microwave mozzarella cheese for 2 minutes. Take out the bowl and allow cooling for 1 minute.

Mix in egg yolk until well-combined. Lay a parchment paper on a flat surface, pour the cheese mixture on top and cover with another parchment paper.

Flatten the dough into ⅛-inch thickness. Take off the parchment paper and cut the dough into thick fettuccine strands. Place in a bowl and refrigerate overnight.

Bring 2 cups of water to a boil and add fettuccine. Cook for 1 minute and drain; set aside.

Preheat oven to 350 F. Heat olive oil in a skillet and cook chicken for 6 minutes. Transfer to a plate. Add onion, garlic and bell peppers to the skillet and cook for 5 minutes. Return the chicken to the pot and stir in Cajun seasoning, Alfredo sauce, and marinara sauce.

Cook for 3 minutes. Stir in fettuccine and transfer to a greased baking dish. Cover with the mozzarella and Parmesan cheeses and bake for 15 minutes. Garnish with parsley and serve.

Nutrition: Calories: 778; Net Carbs: 4 g; Fats 38 g; Protein: 93 g.

831 FRIED EGGS WITH BACON

Preparation Time: 5 minutes
Cooking Time: 10 minutes
Servings: 4

Ingredients:

8 medium eggs
5 oz. bacon
2 medium tomatoes
1 tsp. chopped parsley
1 tbsp. ghee butter
Salt to taste

Directions:

Heat the ghee butter in a skillet over medium-high heat.

Slice the bacon and fry it until crispy for 3-4 minutes, then set aside on a paper towel.

Meanwhile, cut the tomatoes into small cubes.

Crack the eggs in the same skillet, add tomatoes, season with salt, and cook till the desired readiness.

Top with bacon and parsley. Serve hot.

Nutrition: Carbs: 1 g; Fat: 22 g; Protein: 15 g; Calories: 273.

832 CLASSIC STEAK 'N EGGS

Preparation Time: 5 minutes
Cooking Time: 15 minutes
Servings: 4
Ingredients:

8 eggs
16-oz. sirloin steak
4 tbsp. butter
ripe avocado
Salt and pepper to taste

Directions:

Melt 2 tablespoons of butter in a huge skillet.

Fry eggs, 4 at a time, until the edges are crispy.

While the second batch of eggs are cooking, cook the sirloin in another skillet (with the other 2 tablespoons of butter) until it's at least 160°F.

Season eggs and steak well with salt and pepper.

Serve with slices of avocado.

Nutrition: Total Calories: 480; Protein: 37; Carbs: 4; Fat: 37; Fiber: 3.

833 SAUSAGE STUFFED BELL PEPPERS

Preparation Time: 15 minutes
Cooking Time: 4-5 hours
Servings: 4
Ingredients:

1 cup breakfast sausage, crumbled
4 bell peppers, seedless and cut the top
½ cup coconut milk
6 eggs
1 cup cheddar cheese, shredded

From the cupboard:

1 tbsp. extra-virgin olive oil
½ tsp. freshly ground black pepper

Directions:

Add the coconut milk, eggs, and black pepper in a medium bowl, whisking until smooth. Set aside.

Line your slow cooker inserts with aluminum foil. Grease the aluminum foil with 1 tablespoon of olive oil.

Evenly stuff four bell peppers with the crumbled sausage, and spoon the egg mixture into the peppers.

Arrange the stuffed peppers in the slow cooker. Sprinkle the cheese on top.

Cook covered on LOW for 4 t0 5 hours, or until the peppers are

browned and the eggs are completely set.

Divide into 4 serving plates and serve warm.

Nutrition: Calories: 459; Fat: 36.3 g; Protein: 25.2 g; Net carbs: 7.9 g; Fiber: 3 g; Cholesterol: 376 mg.

834 INTERMITTENT TACOS WITH GUACAMOLE AND BACON

Preparation Time: 5 minutes
Cooking Time: 10 minutes
Servings: 2

Ingredients:

¼ cup organic romaine lettuce (chopped)
3 tbsp. organic sweet potatoes (diced and cooked)
2 tbsp. Brain Octane Oil
1 tbsp. ghee (grass-fed)
2 pieces eggs (pasture-raised)
1 piece medium avocado (organic)
2 slices pastured bacon (cooked)
¼ tsp. Himalayan pink salt
organic micro cilantro (for garnish)

Directions:

In a skillet over medium heat, heat up the ghee.

Crack the egg in the middle of the skillet. Poke the egg yolk.

Let the egg cook until solid for about 2 minutes per side. Transfer the cooked egg onto a plate lined with paper towels to absorb the excess oil.

Cook the other egg in a similar way. The 2 cooked eggs will serve as the taco shells.

In a mixing bowl, put in the avocado, pink salt, and octane oil. Mash the avocado and mix well.

Equally, divide the avocado mixture into 2 portions. Spread each avocado mixture onto each egg taco. Arrange the romaine lettuce on top of each taco shell.

Put a bacon slice on each taco. Top each taco with the cooked sweet potatoes.

Garnish the tacos with micro cilantro and sprinkle some pink salt for added taste.

Fold each taco in half. Serve.

Nutrition: Calories: 387; Carbs: 9 g; Fats: 35 g; Proteins: 11 g; Fiber: 5 g.

835 SPINACH AND EGGS MIX

Preparation Time: 5 minutes
Cooking Time: 20 minutes
Servings: 4
Ingredients:

2 tbsp. olive oil
½ tsp. smoked paprika

12 eggs, whisked
1 ½ cups baby spinach
Salt and black pepper to the taste

Directions:

Combine all ingredients in a bowl except the oil and whisk them well.

Heat up your air fryer at 360°F. Add the oil, heat it up, add the eggs and spinach mix and cover. Cook for 20 minutes, divide between plates and serve.

Nutrition: Calories: 220; Fat: 11; Fiber: 3; Carbohydrates: 4; Protein: 6.

836 CLASSIC SPANAKOPITA FRITTATA

Preparation Time: 10 minutes
Cooking Time: 3-4 hours
Servings: 8
Ingredients:

12 eggs, beaten
½ cup feta cheese
2 cup heavy whipping cream
1 cups spinach, chopped
2 tsp. garlic, minced

From the cupboard:

1 tbsp. extra-virgin olive oil

Directions:

Grease the bottom of the slow cooker, put with the olive oil lightly.

Stir together the beaten eggs, feta cheese, heavy cream, spinach, and garlic until well combined.

Slowly pour the mixture into the slow cooker. Cook covered on LOW for 3 to 4 hours, or until a knife inserted in the center comes out clean.

Take off from the slow cooker and cool for about 3 minutes before slicing.

Nutrition: Calories: 254; Fat: 22.3 g; Protein: 11.1 g; Net carbs: 2.1 g; Fiber: 0 g; Cholesterol: 364 mg.

837 SAVORY HAM AND CHEESE WAFFLES

Preparation Time: 10 minutes
Cooking Time: 10 minutes
Servings: 2
Ingredients:

2 oz. (57 g.) ham steak, chopped
2 oz. (57 g.) Cheddar cheese, grated
8 eggs
¼ tsp. baking powder
Basil, to taste

From the cupboard:

12 tbsp. butter, melted
Olive oil, as needed
1-tsp. sea salt
Special Equipment:
A waffle irons

Directions:

Preheat the waffle iron and set aside.

Crack the eggs and keep the egg yolks and egg whites in two separate bowls.

Add the butter, baking powder, basil, and salt to the egg yolks. Whisk well. Fold in the chopped ham and stir until well combined. Set aside.

Lightly season the egg whites with salt and beat until it forms stiff peaks.

Add the egg whites into the bowl of the egg yolk mixture. Allow to sit for about 5 minutes.

Lightly coat the waffle iron with olive oil. Slowly pour half of the mixture into the waffle iron and cook for about 4 minutes. Repeat with the remaining egg mixture.

Take off from the waffle iron and serve warm on two serving plates.

Nutrition: Calories: 636; Fat: 50.2 g; Protein: 45.1 g; Net carbs: 1.1 g.

838 HOMEMADE SAUSAGE, EGG, AND CHEESE SANDWICH

Preparation Time: 5 minutes
Cooking Time: 30 minutes
Servings: 1
Ingredients:
Muffin:
- 1 egg
- 1 tbsp. coconut flour
- 1 tbsp. almond milk
- ½ tbsp. olive oil
- ½-tsp. baking powder
- Pinch of salt

Filling:
- 1 egg
- ¼-pound breakfast sausage
- 1 slice cheddar cheese

Directions:

Preheat oven to 400°F.

Begin by mixing your muffin batter together first by cracking an egg in a bowl, then mixing in the rest of the ingredients.

Grease a ramekin and pour in the batter.

Bake for 15 minutes.

To get an egg that's the same size as your muffin, crack an egg in a ramekin and whisk.

Flavor with salt and pepper, then bake for 10 minutes.

For your sausage, just form the meat into a patty.

Heat a skillet, and then cook patty for 4-5 minutes per side.

When the muffins are ready, remove from the oven and carefully slice in half.

For a toasty muffin, stick in a toaster for a few minutes.

Build sandwich and top with a slice of cheese.

Eat!

Nutrition: Total Calories: 460; Protein: 29; Carbs: 3; Fat: 37; Fiber: 0.

839 CHICKEN SAUSAGE BREAKFAST CASSEROLE

Preparation Time: 10 minutes
Cooking Time: 40 minutes
Servings: 4
Ingredients:
- 1-pound chicken sausage
- 3 big eggs
- 2 cups chopped tomatoes
- 2 cups diced zucchini
- ½ cups cheddar cheese
- ½ cup diced onion
- ½ cup plain Greek yogurt
- 1 tsp. dried sage
- 1 tsp. dried mustard

Directions:

Preheat oven to 375°F.

Preheat a skillet until warm, then add sausage.

When nearly all the pink is gone, put the zucchini and onion.

Cook until the veggies are softened.

Move skillet contents to a greased casserole dish.

In a separate bowl, mix eggs, yogurt, and seasonings together.

Lastly, mix one cup of cheese into eggs.

Pour into the casserole dish on top of the sausage and veggies.

Bake for at least 30 minutes until cheese has melted and starts browning.

Serve right away!

Nutrition: Total calories: 487; Protein: 19; Carbs: 4.8; Fat: 42; Fiber: 1.3.

840 CHEDDAR-CHIVE OMELET FOR ONE

Preparation Time: 8 minutes
Cooking Time: 5 minutes
Servings: 1
Ingredients:
- 2 slices cooked bacon
- 2 big eggs
- 2 stalks chives
- 2 tbsp. sharp cheddar cheese
- 2 tsp. olive oil
- Salt and pepper to taste

Directions:

Heat oil in a skillet.

While it heats, chop chives.

Pour in eggs and sprinkle chives, salt, and pepper on top.

Wait until edges are beginning to set.

Crumble bacon on top and wait another 25 seconds.

Remove skillet from heat.

Sprinkle on cheese and carefully fold the omelet over.

Enjoy!

Nutrition: Total Calories: 463; Protein: 24; Carbs: 1; Fat: 39; Fiber: 1.

841 HOMEMADE COLD GAZPACHO SOUP

Preparation Time: 15 minutes + chilling time
Cooking Time: 0 minutes
Servings: 6
Ingredients:
- 2 small green peppers, roasted
- 2 large red peppers, roasted
- 2 medium avocados, flesh scoped out
- 2 garlic cloves
- 2 spring onions, chopped
- 1 cucumber, chopped
- 1 cup olive oil
- 2 tbsp. lemon juice
- 2 tomatoes, chopped
- 7 oz. goat cheese
- 1 small red onion, chopped
- 2 tbsp. apple cider vinegar
- Salt to taste

Directions:

Place the peppers, tomatoes, avocados, red onion, garlic, lemon juice, olive oil, vinegar, and salt, in a food processor. Pulse until your desired consistency is reached. Taste and adjust the seasoning.

Transfer the mixture to a pot. Stir in cucumber and spring onions. Cover and chill in the fridge for at least 2 hours. Divide the soup between 6 bowls. Serve topped with goat cheese and an extra drizzle of olive oil.

Nutrition: Calories: 528; Fat: 45.8 g; Net Carbs: 6.5 g; Protein: 7.5 g.

842 BREAKFAST-STUFFED BELL PEPPERS

Preparation Time: 25 minutes
Cooking Time: 10 minutes
Servings: 4
Ingredients:
- 4 large yellow bell peppers
- 4 eggs
- 4 bacon strips
- 4-oz. pork breakfast sausage
- cup shredded mozzarella cheese
- ½ cup diced onion
- 1 tbsp. minced garlic
- Couple tsp. olive oil
- Salt and pepper to taste

Directions:

Preheat your oven to 275°F.

Chop the tops off the peppers and hollow out the insides.

Set on a baking sheet and brush insides with a little olive oil.

Stick peppers in the oven.

Heat a skillet and cook bacon and sausage until nearly done.

Add onions and garlic.

Cook until onions have softened.

Take out the peppers and stuff.

Top with cheese and press down with a spoon, creating a little hollow.

Crack in an egg.

Turn oven up to 325-degrees and put stuffed peppers in the oven for 10 minutes, or until eggs have reached the doneness you like. Serve!

Nutrition: Total calories: 372; Protein: 27; Carbs: 15 Fat: 24; Fiber: 2.

843 SMALL INTERMITTENT PIES

Preparation Time: 10 minutes
Cooking Time: 30 minutes
Servings: 6
Ingredients:

3 eggs
5 bacon slices
½ red bell pepper
leek
½ cup broccoli
¼ oz. ground cheese
½ cup yogurt
¼ pack baking powder
2 tbsp. olive oil
Salt, pepper, powdered garlic, parsley to taste

Directions:

Whisk and blend the eggs with baking powder.

Cook the broccoli in water.

Cut bacon, leek and pepper into smaller pieces to taste.

Mix cheese with yogurt well. Then, add bacon, leek, pepper, and spices to taste.

Join the 2 mixtures together and then pour into cupcake or muffin molds.

Bake for 30 minutes at 200°F.

Nutrition: Calories: 121; Total Fats: 2.1 g; Net Carbs: 2 g; Protein: 1.3 g; Fiber: 6 g.

844 INTERMITTENT WRAPS

Preparation Time: 30 minutes
Cooking Time: 0 minutes
Servings: 6
Ingredients:

10 oz. turkey meat
3 oz. bacon
1 tomato
½ oz. mozzarella
Cabbage leaves for wrapping

For coating:

1 cup mayonnaise
6 basil leaves
1 tsp. lemon juice
1 tsp. powdered garlic

1 tsp. salt
1 tsp. pepper

Directions:

Mix all ingredients listed for coating in one bowl. You should get a dense mixture.

Prepare bacon in a frying pan.

Coat cabbage leaves with coating mixture. Pile ingredients over (turkey, tomatoes, bacon and cheese).

Wrap the cabbage like tortillas and serve.

Nutrition: Calories: 121; Total Fats: 6.9 g; Net Carbs: 4 g; Protein: 2.4 g; Fiber: 5.6 g.

845 CHICKEN OMELET

Preparation Time: 5 minutes
Cooking Time: 10 minutes
Servings: 2
Ingredients:

½ oz. of rotisserie chicken, shredded
1 tsp. of mustard
1 tbsp. of mayonnaise
1 tomato, cored and chopped
bacon slices, cooked and crumbled
eggs
1 small avocado, pitted, peeled and chopped
Salt and ground black pepper, to taste

Directions:

Heat up a pan over medium heat, grease lightly with cooking oil.

Mix the eggs with some salt and pepper in a bowl and whisk.

Add the eggs to the pan and cook the omelet for 5 minutes.

Add the chicken, avocado, tomato, bacon, mayonnaise and mustard on one half of the omelet.

Fold the omelet, cover the pan, cook for 5 minutes and serve.

Nutrition: Calories: 400; Total Fats: 32 g; Net Carbs: 4 g; Protein: 25 g; Fiber: 6 g.

FISH AND SEAFOOD RECIPES

846 QUINOA AND SCALLOPS SALAD

Preparation Time: 10 minutes
Cooking Time: 35 minutes
Servings: 6
Ingredients:

12 oz. dry sea scallops
4 tbsp. canola oil
2 tsp. canola oil
4 tsp. low sodium soy sauce
1 ½ cup quinoa, rinsed
2 tsp. garlic, minced
3 cups water
1 cup snow peas, sliced diagonally
1 tsp. sesame oil
⅓ cup rice vinegar
1 cup scallions, sliced

⅓ cup red bell pepper, chopped
¼ cup cilantro, chopped

Directions:

In a bowl, mix scallops with 2 teaspoons of soy sauce. Stir gently and leave aside for now.

Heat a pan with 1 tablespoon of canola oil over medium-high heat. Add the quinoa, stir and cook for 8 minutes. Put garlic, stir and cook within 1 more minute.

Put the water, boil over medium heat, stir, cover, and cook for 15 minutes. Remove from heat and leave aside covered for 5 minutes. Add snow peas, cover again and leave for 5 more minutes.

Meanwhile, in a bowl, mix 3 tablespoons of canola oil with 2 teaspoons of soy sauce, vinegar, and sesame oil and stir well. Add quinoa and snow peas to this mixture and stir again. Add scallions, bell pepper, and stir again.

Pat dries the scallops and discard the marinade. Heat another pan with 2 teaspoons of canola oil over high heat. Add scallops, and cook for 1 minute on each side. Add them to the quinoa salad, stir gently, and serve with chopped cilantro.

Nutrition: Calories: 181; Carbs: 12 g; Fat: 6 g; Protein: 13 g; Sodium: 153 mg.

847 AVOCADO STUFFED WITH TUNA

Preparation Time: 20 minutes
Cooking Time: 0 minutes
Servings: 2
Ingredients:

1 avocado
1 can of tuna
1 tomato
½ onion
Parsley to taste

Directions:

Cut the avocado into halves. Remove the middle parts so that you can have a room for stuffing. (Keep the "meat" parts)

Cut the tomato and onion into tiny circles.

Mix meat parts with tuna, tomato, and onion.

Stuff the avocado halves with the mixture, decorate with parsley to taste and serve!

Nutrition: Calories: 132; Fats: 3 g; Net Carbs: 6 g; Protein: 1.2 g; Fiber: 7 g.

848 COD TACOS WITH SALSA

Preparation Time: 5 minutes
Cooking Time: 15 minutes
Servings: 4
Ingredients:

- 2 eggs
- 1 ¼ cups Mexican beer
- 1 ½ cups coconut flour
- 1 ½ cups almond flour
- ½ tbsp. chili powder
- 1 tbsp. cumin
- Salt, to taste
- 1 pound (454 g.) cod fillet, slice into large pieces
- 4 toasted corn tortillas
- 4 large lettuce leaves, chopped
- ¼ cup salsa
- Cooking spray

Directions:

Spritz the air fry basket with cooking spray.

Break the eggs in a bowl, then pour in the beer. Whisk to combine well.

Combine the almond flour, coconut flour, cumin, chili powder, and salt in a separate bowl. Stir to mix well.

Dunk the cod pieces in the egg mixture, then shake the excess off and dredge into the flour mixture to coat well. Arrange the cod in the basket.

Place the basket on the air fry position.

Select Air Fry, set temperature to 375°F (190°C) and Time to 15 minutes. Flip the cod halfway through the cooking time.

When cooking is complete, the cod should be golden brown.

Unwrap the toasted tortillas on a large plate, then divide the cod and lettuce leaves on top. Baste with salsa and wrap to serve.

Nutrition: Calories: 133; Fat: 19 g; Protein: 8 g.

849 DILL SALMON SALAD WRAPS

Preparation Time: 20 minutes
Cooking Time: 60 minutes
Servings: 2
Ingredients:

- 1-pound salmon filet, cooked and flaked, or 3 (5-oz.) cans salmon
- ½ cup diced carrots (about 1 carrot)
- ½ cup diced celery (about 1 celery stalk)
- 3 tbsp. chopped fresh dill
- 3 tbsp. diced red onion (a little less than ⅛ onion)
- 2 tbsp. capers
- 1 ½ tbsp. extra-virgin olive oil
- 1 tbsp. aged balsamic vinegar
- ½ tsp. freshly ground black pepper
- ¼ tsp. kosher or sea salt
- 4 whole-wheat flatbread wraps or soft whole-wheat tortillas

Directions:

In a large bowl, mix together the salmon, carrots, celery, dill, red onion, capers, oil, vinegar, pepper, and salt.

Divide the salmon salad among the flatbreads. Fold up the bottom of the wrap and serve.

Nutrition: Calories: 336; Total Fat: 16 g; Saturated Fat: 2 g; Cholesterol: 67 mg; Sodium: 628 mg; Total Carbohydrates: 23 g; Fiber: 5 g; Protein: 32 g.

850 CABBAGE AND PRAWN WRAPS

Preparation Time: 20 minutes
Cooking Time: 18 minutes
Servings: 4
Ingredients:

- 2 tbsp. olive oil
- 1 carrot, cut into strips
- 1-inch piece fresh ginger, grated
- 1 tbsp. minced garlic
- 2 tbsp. soy sauce
- ¼ cup chicken broth
- 1 tbsp. sugar
- 1 cup shredded Napa cabbage
- 1 tbsp. sesame oil
- 8 cooked prawns, minced
- 8 egg roll wrappers
- 1 egg, beaten
- Cooking spray

Directions:

Spritz the perforated pan with cooking spray. Set aside.

Heat the olive oil in a nonstick skillet over medium heat until shimmering.

Add the carrot, ginger, and garlic and sauté for 2 minutes or until fragrant.

Pour in the soy sauce, broth, and sugar. Bring to a boil. Keep stirring.

Add the cabbage and simmer for 4 minutes or until the cabbage is tender.

Turn off the heat and mix in the sesame oil. Let sit for 15 minutes.

Use a strainer to remove the vegetables from the liquid, then combine with the minced prawns.

Unfold the egg roll wrappers on a clean work surface, then divide the prawn mixture in the center of the wrappers.

Dab the edges of a wrapper with the beaten egg, then fold a corner over the filling and tuck the corner under the filling. Fold the left and right corner into the center. Roll the wrapper up and press to seal. Repeat with remaining wrappers.

Arrange the wrappers in the pan and spritz with cooking spray.

Select Air Fry. Set temperature to 370°Fahrenheit (188°Celsius) and Time to 12 minutes. Press Start to begin preheating.

Once the oven has preheated, place the pan into the oven. Flip the wrappers halfway through the cooking time.

When cooking is complete, the wrappers should be golden.

Serve immediately.

Nutrition: Calories: 339; Total Fat: 15.9 g; Total Carbohydrates: 27.5 g; Protein: 24.2 g.

851 TUNA AND LETTUCE WRAPS

Preparation Time: 10 minutes
Cooking Time: 4 to 7 minutes
Servings: 4
Ingredients:

- 1 pound (454 g.) fresh tuna steak, cut into 1-inch cubes
- 1 tbsp. grated fresh ginger
- 2 garlic cloves, minced
- ½ tsp. toasted sesame oil
- 2 low-sodium whole-wheat tortillas
- ¼ cup low-fat mayonnaise
- 1 cup shredded romaine lettuce
- 1 red bell pepper, thinly sliced

Directions:

In a medium bowl, mix the tuna, ginger, garlic, and sesame oil. Let it stand for 10 minutes.

Transfer the tuna to the air fryer basket.

Select the Air Fry function and cook at 390°Fahrenheit (199°Celsius) for 4 to 7 minutes, or until lightly browned.

Make the wraps with tuna, tortillas, mayonnaise, lettuce, and bell pepper.

Serve immediately.

Nutrition: Calories: 485; Carbohydrates: 6.3 g; Protein: 47.6 g; Fat: 29.9 g.

852 TUNA IN CUCUMBER

Preparation Time: 15 minutes
Cooking Time: 0 minutes
Servings: 6
Ingredients:

- 1 cucumber
- ½ celery leaf
- ½ red bell pepper
- 1 can of tuna
- Pepper and salt to taste

Directions:

Peel the cucumber and cut it into thicker circles. Make a hole in each piece.

Cut the celery and pepper into tiny cubes. Mix them with tuna.

Put 1 tablespoon of tuna mixture into cucumbers.

Add spices to taste and serve.

Enjoy!

Nutrition: Calories: 109; Total Fats: 1.6 g; Net Carbs: 4 g; Protein: 1 g; Fiber: 5.4 g.

853 EASY LUNCH SALMON STEAKS

Preparation Time: 10 minutes
Cooking Time: 20 minutes
Servings: 4
Ingredients:

- 1 big salmon fillet, cut into 4 steaks
- 3 garlic cloves, minced
- 1 yellow onion, chopped
- Black pepper to the taste
- 2 tbsp. olive oil
- ¼ cup parsley, chopped
- Juice of 1 lemon
- 1 tbsp. thyme, chopped
- 4 cups water

Directions:

Heat a pan with the oil on medium-high heat, cook onion and garlic within 3 minutes.

Add black pepper, parsley, thyme, water, and lemon juice. Stir, bring to a gentle boil, add salmon steaks and cook them for 15 minutes. Drain, divide between plates and serve with a side salad for lunch.

Nutrition: Calories: 110; Carbs: 3 g; Fat: 4 g; Protein: 15 g; Sodium: 330 mg.

854 COD SOUP

Preparation Time: 10 minutes
Cooking Time: 25 minutes
Servings: 4
Ingredients:

- 1 yellow onion, chopped
- 12 cups low-sodium fish stock
- 1-pound carrots, sliced
- 1 tbsp. olive oil
- Black pepper to the taste
- 2 tbsp. ginger, minced
- 1 cup of water
- 1-pound cod, skinless, boneless, and cut into medium chunks

Directions:

Heat-up a pot with the oil over medium-high heat, add onion, stir and cook for 4 minutes. Add water, stock, ginger, and carrots, stir and cook for 10 minutes more.

Blend soup using an immersion blender, add the fish and pepper, stir, cook for 10 minutes more, ladle into bowls and serve. Enjoy!

Nutrition: Calories: 344; Carbs: 35 g; Fat: 4 g; Protein: 46 g; Sodium: 334 mg.

855 TUNA CROQUETTES

Preparation Time: 40 minutes
Cooking Time: 25 minutes
Servings: 36
Ingredients:

- 6 tbsp. extra-virgin olive oil, plus 1 to 2 cups
- 5 tbsp. almond flour, plus 1 cup, divided
- 1 ¼ cups heavy cream
- 1 (4-oz.) can olive oil-packed yellowfin tuna
- 1 tbsp. chopped red onion
- 2 tsp. minced capers
- ½ tsp. dried dill
- ¼ tsp. freshly ground black pepper
- 2 large eggs
- 1 cup panko breadcrumbs (or a gluten-free version)

Directions:

In a large skillet, warm up 6 tablespoons of olive oil over medium-low heat. Add 5 tablespoons of almond flour and cook, stirring constantly, until a smooth paste forms and the flour browns slightly, 2 to 3 minutes.

Select the heat to medium-high and gradually mix in the heavy cream, whisking constantly until completely smooth and thickened, another 4 to 5 minutes. Remove and add in the tuna, red onion, capers, dill, and pepper.

Transfer the mixture to an 8-inch square baking dish that is well coated with olive oil and set aside at room temperature.

Wrap and cool for 4 hours or up to overnight. To form the croquettes, set out three bowls. In one, beat together the eggs.

In another, add the remaining almond flour. In the third, add the panko. Line a baking sheet with parchment paper.

Scoop about 1 tablespoon of cold prepared dough into the flour mixture and roll to coat. Shake off excess and, using your hands, roll into an oval.

Dip the croquette into the beaten egg, then lightly coat in panko. Set on the lined baking sheet and repeat with the remaining dough.

In a small saucepan, warm up the remaining 1 to 2 cups of olive oil, over medium-high heat.

Once the oil is heated, fry the croquettes 3 or 4 at a time, depending on the size of your pan, removing with a slotted spoon when golden brown.

You will need to adjust the temperature of the oil occasionally to prevent burning. If the croquettes get dark brown very quickly, lower the temperature.

Nutrition: Calories: 245; Fat: 22 g; Carbohydrates: 1 g; Protein: 6 g.

856 SHRIMP COCKTAIL

Preparation Time: 10 minutes
Cooking Time: 5 minutes
Servings: 8
Ingredients:

- 2 pounds big shrimp, deveined
- 4 cups water
- 2 bay leaves
- 1 small lemon, halved
- Ice for cooling the shrimp
- Ice for serving
- 1 medium lemon sliced for serving
- ¾ cup tomato passata
- 2 ½ tbsp. horseradish, prepared
- ¼ tsp. chili powder
- 2 tbsp. lemon juice

Directions:

Pour the 4 cups of water into a large pot. Add lemon and bay leaves. Boil over medium-high heat, reduce temperature and boil for 10 minutes. Put shrimp, stir and cook within 2 minutes. Move the shrimp to a bowl filled with ice and leave aside for 5 minutes.

In a bowl, mix tomato passata with horseradish, chili powder, and lemon juice and stir well. Place shrimp in a serving bowl filled with ice, and lemon slices. Serve with the cocktail sauce you've prepared.

Nutrition: Calories: 276; Carbs: 0 g; Fat: 8 g; Protein: 25 g; Sodium: 182 mg.

857 SQUID AND SHRIMP SALAD

Preparation Time: 10 minutes
Cooking Time: 15 minutes
Servings: 4
Ingredients:

- 8 oz. squid, cut into medium pieces
- 8 oz. shrimp, peeled and deveined
- 1 red onion, sliced
- 1 cucumber, chopped
- 2 tomatoes, cut into medium wedges
- 2 tbsp. cilantro, chopped
- 1 hot jalapeno pepper, cut in rounds
- 3 tbsp. rice vinegar
- 3 tbsp. dark sesame oil
- Black pepper to the taste

Directions:

In a bowl, mix the onion with cucumber, tomatoes, pepper, cilantro, shrimp, and squid and stir well. Cut a big parchment paper in half, fold it in half heart shape and open. Place the seafood mixture in this parchment piece, fold over, seal edges, place on a baking sheet, and introduce in the oven at 400°F for 15 minutes.

Meanwhile, in a small bowl, mix sesame oil with rice vinegar and black pepper and stir very well. Take the salad out of the oven, leave to cool down for a few minutes, and transfer to a serving plate. Put the dressing over the salad and serve right away.

Nutrition: Calories: 235; Carbs: 9 g; Fat: 8 g; Protein: 30 g; Sodium: 165 mg.

858 PARSLEY SEAFOOD COCKTAIL

Preparation Time: 2 hours, 10 minutes
Cooking Time: 1 hour, 30 minutes
Servings: 4
Ingredients:

1 big octopus, cleaned
1-pound mussels
2 pounds clams
1 big squid cut in rings
3 garlic cloves, chopped
1 celery rib, cut crosswise into thirds
½ cup celery rib, sliced
1 carrot, cut crosswise into 3 pieces
1 small white onion, chopped
1 bay leaf
¾ cup white wine
2 cups radicchio, sliced
1 red onion, sliced
1 cup parsley, chopped
1 cup olive oil
1 cup red wine vinegar
Black pepper to the taste

Directions:

Put the octopus in a pot with celery rib cut in thirds, garlic, carrot, bay leaf, white onion, and white wine. Add water to cover the octopus, cover with a lid, bring to a boil over high heat, reduce to low, and simmer within 1 and ½ hours.

Drain octopus, reserve boiling liquid, and leave aside to cool down. Put ¼ cup of octopus cooking liquid in another pot, add mussels, heat up over medium-high heat, cook until they open, transfer to a bowl, and leave aside.

Add clams to the pan, cover, cook over medium-high heat until they open, transfer to the bowl with mussels, and leave aside. Add squid to the pan, cover and cook over medium-high heat for 3 minutes, transfer to the bowl with mussels and clams.

Meanwhile, slice octopus into small pieces and mix with the rest of the seafood. Add sliced celery, radicchio, red onion, vinegar, olive oil, parsley, salt, and pepper. Stir gently and leave aside in the fridge within 2 hours before serving.

Nutrition: Calories: 102; Carbs: 7 g; Fat: 1 g; Protein: 16 g; Sodium: 0 mg.

859 SHRIMP AND ONION GINGER DRESSING

Preparation Time: 10 minutes
Cooking Time: 5 minutes
Servings: 2
Ingredients:

8 medium shrimp, peeled and deveined
12 oz. package mixed salad leaves
10 cherry tomatoes, halved
2 green onions, sliced
2 medium mushrooms, sliced
⅓ cup rice vinegar
¼ cup sesame seeds, toasted
1 tbsp. low-sodium soy sauce
2 tsp. ginger, grated
2 tsp. garlic, minced
⅔ cup canola oil
⅓ cup sesame oil

Directions:

In a bowl, mix rice vinegar with sesame seeds, soy sauce, garlic, ginger, and stir well. Pour this into your kitchen blender, add canola oil and sesame oil, pulse very well, and leave aside. Brush shrimp with 3 tbsp. of the ginger dressing you've prepared.

Heat your kitchen grill over high heat. Add shrimp and cook for 3 minutes, flipping once. In a salad bowl, mix salad leaves with grilled shrimp, mushrooms, green onions, and tomatoes. Drizzle ginger dressing on top and serve right away!

Nutrition: Calories: 360; Carbs: 14 g; Fat: 11 g; Protein: 49 g; Sodium: 469 mg.

860 SALMON AND CABBAGE MIX

Preparation Time: 5 minutes
Cooking Time: 25 minutes
Servings: 4
Ingredients:

4 salmon fillets, boneless
1 yellow onion, chopped
2 tbsp. olive oil
1 cup red cabbage, shredded
1 red bell pepper, chopped
1 tbsp. rosemary, chopped
1 tbsp. coriander, ground
1 cup tomato sauce
A pinch of sea salt
black pepper

Directions:

Bring the pan to medium heat. Add the onion and sauté for 5 minutes. Put the fish and sear it within 2 minutes on each side. Add the cabbage and the remaining ingredients. Toss, cook over medium heat for 20 minutes more. Divide between plates and serve.

Nutrition: Calories: 130; Carbs: 8 g; Fat: 6 g; Protein: 12 g; Sodium: 345 mg.

861 FRUIT SHRIMP SOUP

Preparation Time: 10 minutes
Cooking Time: 25 minutes
Servings: 6
Ingredients:

8 oz. shrimp, peeled and deveined
1 stalk lemongrass, smashed
2 small ginger pieces, grated
6 cup chicken stock
2 jalapenos, chopped
4 lime leaves
1 ½ cups pineapple, chopped
1 cup shiitake mushroom caps, chopped
1 tomato, chopped
½ bell pepper, cubed
2 tbsp. fish sauce
1 tsp. sugar
¼ cup lime juice
⅓ cup cilantro, chopped
2 scallions, sliced

Directions:

In a pot, mix ginger with lemongrass, stock, jalapenos, and lime leaves. Stir, boil over medium heat and cook within 15 minutes. Strain liquid in a bowl and discard solids.

Return soup to the pot again. Add pineapple, tomato, mushrooms, bell pepper, sugar, and fish sauce. Stir, boil over medium heat and cook for 5 minutes. Add shrimp and cook for 3 more minutes. Remove from heat, add lime juice, cilantro, and scallions. Stir, ladle into soup bowls and serve.

Nutrition: Calories: 290; Carbs: 39 g; Fat: 12 g; Protein: 7 g; Sodium: 21 mg.

862 MUSSELS AND CHICKPEA SOUP

Preparation Time: 10 minutes
Cooking Time: 10 minutes
Servings: 6
Ingredients:

3 garlic cloves, minced
2 tbsp. olive oil
A pinch of chili flakes
1 ½ tbsp. fresh mussels, scrubbed
1 cup white wine
1 cup chickpeas, rinsed
1 small fennel bulb, sliced

Black pepper to the taste
Juice of 1 lemon
3 tbsp. parsley, chopped

Directions:

Heat a big saucepan with the olive oil over medium-high heat. Add garlic and chili flakes, stir and cook within a couple of minutes. Add white wine and mussels. Stir, cover, and cook for 3-4 minutes until mussels open.

Transfer mussels to a baking dish. Add some of the cooking liquid over them and fridge until they are cold enough. Take mussels out of the fridge and discard shells.

Heat another pan over medium-high heat. Add mussels, reserved cooking liquid, chickpeas, and fennel. Stir well, and heat them. Add black pepper to the taste, lemon juice, and parsley, stir again. Divide between plates and serve.

Nutrition: Calories: 286; Carbs: 49 g; Fat: 4 g; Protein: 14 g; Sodium: 145 mg.

863 SHRIMP AND BROCCOLI SOUP

Preparation Time: 5 minutes
Cooking Time: 25 minutes
Servings: 4
Ingredients:

2 tbsp. olive oil
1 yellow onion, chopped
4 cups chicken stock
Juice of 1 lime
1-pound shrimp, peeled and deveined
½ cup coconut cream
½-pound broccoli florets
1 tbsp. parsley, chopped

Directions:

Heat a pot with the oil over medium heat. Add the onion and sauté for 5 minutes. Add the shrimp and the other ingredients. Simmer over medium heat for 20 minutes more. Ladle the soup into bowls and serve.

Nutrition: Calories: 220; Carbs: 12 g; Fat: 7 g; Protein: 26 g; Sodium: 577 mg.

864 LIME SHRIMP AND KALE

Preparation Time: 10 minutes
Cooking Time: 20 minutes
Servings: 4
Ingredients:

1-pound shrimp, peeled and deveined
4 scallions, chopped
1 tsp. sweet paprika
1 tbsp. olive oil
Juice of 1 lime
Zest of 1 lime, grated
A pinch of salt and black pepper
2 tbsp. parsley, chopped

Directions:

Bring the pan to medium heat. Add the scallions and sauté for 5 minutes. Add the shrimp and the other ingredients. Toss, cook over medium heat for 15 minutes more. Divide into bowls and serve.

Nutrition: Calories: 149; Carbs: 12 g; Fat: 4 g; Protein: 21 g; Sodium: 250 mg.

865 PARSLEY COD MIX

Preparation Time: 10 minutes
Cooking Time: 20 minutes
Servings: 4
Ingredients:

1 tbsp. olive oil
2 shallots, chopped
4 cod fillets, boneless and skinless
2 garlic cloves, minced
2 tbsp. lemon juice
1 cup chicken stock
A pinch of salt and black pepper

Directions:

Bring the pan to medium heat -high heat, add the shallots and the garlic and sauté for 5 minutes. Add the cod and the other ingredients. Cook everything for 15 minutes more. Divide between plates and serve for lunch.

Nutrition: Calories: 216; Carbs: 7 g; Fat: 5 g; Protein: 34 g; Sodium: 380 mg.

866 SHRIMP WITH GARLIC AND MUSHROOMS

Preparation Time: 15 minutes
Cooking Time: 15 minutes
Servings: 4

Ingredients:

1 pound (454 g.) peeled and deveined fresh shrimp
1 tsp. salt
1 cup extra-virgin olive oil
8 large garlic cloves, thinly sliced
4 oz. (113 g.) sliced mushrooms (shiitake, baby bella, or button)
½ tsp. red pepper flakes
¼ cup chopped fresh flat-leaf Italian parsley
Zucchini noodles or riced cauliflower, for serving

Directions:

Rinse the shrimp and pat dry. Place in a small bowl and sprinkle with salt. In a large rimmed, thick skillet, heat the olive oil over medium-low heat.

Add the garlic and heat until very fragrant, 3 to 4 minutes, reducing the heat if the garlic starts to burn.

Add the mushrooms and sauté for 5 minutes, until softened. Add the shrimp and red pepper flakes and sauté until the shrimp begins to turn pink, another 3 to 4 minutes.

Remove from the heat and stir in the parsley. Serve over zucchini noodles or riced cauliflower.

Nutrition: Calories: 620; Fat: 56 g; Protein: 24 g; Carbs: 4 g.

867 PISTACHIO-CRUSTED WHITEFISH

Preparation Time: 10 minutes
Cooking Time: 20 minutes
Servings: 2
Ingredients:

¼ cup shelled pistachios
1 tbsp. fresh parsley
1 tbsp. grated Parmesan cheese
1 tbsp. panko bread crumbs
2 tbsp. olive oil
¼ tsp. salt
10 oz. skinless whitefish (1 large piece or 2 smaller ones)

Directions:

Preheat the oven to 350°F and set the rack to the middle position. Line a sheet pan with foil or parchment paper.

Combine all of the ingredients, except the fish, in a mini food processor, and pulse until the nuts are finely ground.

Alternatively, you can mince the nuts with a chef's knife and combine the ingredients by hand in a small bowl.

Place the fish on the sheet pan. Spread the nut mixture evenly over the fish and pat it down lightly.

Bake the fish for 20 to 30 minutes, depending on the thickness, until it flakes easily with a fork.

Keep in mind that a thicker cut of fish takes a bit longer to bake. You'll know it's done when it's opaque, flakes apart easily with a fork, or reaches an internal temperature of 145°F.

Nutrition: Calories: 185; Carbs: 23.8 g; Protein: 10.1 g; Fat: 5.2 g.

868 CRISPY HOMEMADE FISH STICKS RECIPE

Preparation Time: 10 minutes
Cooking Time: 15 minutes
Servings: 2
Ingredients:

½ cup of flour
1 beaten egg
1 cup of flour
½ cup of parmesan cheese
½ cup of bread crumbs.

Zest of 1 lemon juice
Parsley
Salt
1 tsp. of black pepper
1 tbsp. of sweet paprika
1 tsp. of oregano
1 ½ lb. of salmon
Extra virgin olive oil

Directions:

Preheat your oven to about 450°F. Get a bowl, dry your salmon and season its two sides with the salt.

Then chop into small sizes of 1½ inch length each. Get a bowl and mix black pepper with oregano.

Add paprika to the mixture and blend it. Then spice the fish stick with the mixture you have just made. Get another dish and pour your flours.

You will need a different bowl again to pour your egg wash into. Pick yet the fourth dish; mix your breadcrumb with your parmesan and add lemon zest to the mixture.

Return to the fish sticks and dip each fish into flour such that both sides are coated with flour. As you dip each fish into flour, take it out and dip it into the egg wash and lastly, dip it in the breadcrumb mixture.

Do this for all fish sticks and arrange on a baking sheet. Ensure you oil the baking sheet before arranging the stick and drizzle the top of the fish sticks with extra virgin olive oil.

Caution: allow excess flours to fall off a fish before dipping it into other ingredients.

Also, ensure that you do not let the coating peel while you add extra virgin olive oil on top of the fish.

Fix the baking sheet in the middle of the oven and allow it to cook for 13 minutes. By then, the fishes should be golden brown and you can remove them from the oven. Serve immediately.

Top it with your lemon zest, parsley and fresh lemon juice.

Nutrition: Calories: 119; Fat: 3.4 g; of Sodium: 293.1 mg; Carbs: 9.3 g; Protein: 13.5 g.

869 SAUCED SHELLFISH IN WHITE WINE

Preparation Time: 10 minutes
Cooking Time: 10 minutes
Servings: 2
Ingredients:

2-lbs fresh cuttlefish

½-cup olive oil
1-pc large onion, finely chopped
1-cup of Robola white wine
¼-cup lukewarm water
1-pc bay leaf
½-bunch parsley, chopped
4-pcs tomatoes, grated
Salt and pepper

Directions:

Take out the hard centerpiece of cartilage (cuttlebone), the bag of ink, and the intestines from the cuttlefish.

Wash the cleaned cuttlefish with running water. Slice it into small pieces, and drain excess water. Heat the oil in a saucepan placed over medium-high heat and sauté the onion for 3 minutes until tender.

Add the sliced cuttlefish and pour in the white wine. Cook for 5 minutes until it simmers.

Pour in the water, and add the tomatoes, bay leaf, parsley, tomatoes, salt, and pepper. Simmer the mixture over low heat until the cuttlefish slices are tender and left with their thick sauce. Serve them warm with rice.

Be careful not to overcook the cuttlefish as its texture becomes very hard. A safe rule of thumb is grilling the cuttlefish over a ragingly hot fire for 3 minutes before using it in any recipe.

Nutrition: Calories: 308; Fats: 18.1 g; Dietary Fiber: 1.5 g; Carbohydrates: 8 g; Protein: 25.6 g.

870 PISTACHIO SOLE FISH

Preparation Time: 5 minutes
Cooking Time: 10 minutes
Servings: 2
Ingredients:

4 (5 oz.) boneless sole fillets
½ cup pistachios, finely chopped
Juice of 1 lemon
1 tsp. extra virgin olive oil

Directions:

Preheat your oven to 350°F.

Wrap baking sheet using parchment paper and keep it aside.

Pat fish dry with kitchen towels and lightly season with salt and pepper.

Take a small bowl and stir in pistachios.

Place sol on the prepped sheet and press 2 tablespoons of pistachio mixture on top of each fillet.

Rub the fish with lemon juice and olive oil.

Bake for 10 minutes until the top is golden and fish flakes with a fork.

Nutrition: Calories: 166; Fat: 6 g; Carbohydrates: 2 g.

871 SPEEDY TILAPIA WITH RED ONION AND AVOCADO

Preparation Time: 10 minutes
Cooking Time: 5 minutes
Servings: 2
Ingredients:

1 tbsp. extra-virgin olive oil
1 tbsp. freshly squeezed orange juice
¼ tsp. kosher or sea salt
4 (4-oz.) tilapia fillets, more oblong than square, skin-on or skinned
¼ cup chopped red onion (about ⅛ onion)
1 avocado, pitted, skinned, and sliced

Directions:

In a 9-inch glass pie dish, use a fork to mix together the oil, orange juice, and salt. Working with one fillet at a time, place each in the pie dish and turn to coat on all sides.

Arrange the fillets in a wagon-wheel formation, so that one end of each fillet is in the center of the dish and the other end is temporarily draped over the edge of the dish.

Top each fillet with 1 tablespoon of onion, then fold the end of the fillet that's hanging over the edge in half over the onion.

When finished, you should have 4 folded-over fillets with the fold against the outer edge of the dish and the ends all in the center.

Cover the dish with plastic wrap, leaving a small part open at the edge to vent the steam. Microwave on high for about 3 minutes.

The fish is done when it just begins to separate into flakes (chunks) when pressed gently with a fork. Top the fillets with the avocado and serve.

Nutrition: Carbohydrates: 4 g; Fiber: 3 g; Protein: 22 g.

872 STEAMED MUSSELS IN WHITE WINE SAUCE

Preparation Time: 5 minutes
Cooking Time: 10 minutes
Servings: 2
Ingredients:

2 pounds small mussels
1 tbsp. extra-virgin olive oil
1 cup thinly sliced red onion
3 garlic cloves, sliced - 1 cup dry white wine
2 (¼-inch-thick) lemon slices
¼ tsp. freshly ground black pepper
¼ tsp. kosher or sea salt

Fresh lemon wedges, for serving (optional)

Directions:

In a large colander in the sink, run cold water over the mussels (but don't let the mussels sit in standing water).

All the shells should be closed tight; discard any shells that are a little bit open or cracked. Leave the mussels in the colander until you're ready to use them.

In a large skillet over medium-high flame, heat the oil. Add the onion and cook for 4 minutes, stirring occasionally.

Add the garlic and cook for 1 minute, stirring constantly. Add the wine, lemon slices, pepper, and salt, and bring to a simmer. Cook for 2 minutes.

Add the mussels and cover. Cook for 3 minutes, or until the mussels open their shells. Gently shake the pan two or three times while they are cooking.

All the shells should now be wide open. Using a slotted spoon, discard any mussels that are still closed. Spoon the opened mussels into a shallow serving bowl, and pour the broth over the top. Serve with additional fresh lemon slices, if desired.

Nutrition: Calories: 22, Total Fat: 7 g; Fiber: 1 g; Protein: 18 g.

873 ORANGE AND GARLIC SHRIMP

Preparation Time: 20 minutes
Cooking Time: 10 minutes
Servings: 2
Ingredients:

1 large orange
3 tbsp. extra-virgin olive oil, divided
1 tbsp. chopped fresh Rosemary
1 tbsp. chopped fresh thyme
3 garlic cloves, minced (about 1½ tsp.)
¼ tsp. freshly ground black pepper
¼ tsp. kosher or sea salt
1 ½ pounds fresh raw shrimp, shells, and tails removed

Directions:

Zest the entire orange using a citrus grater. In a large zip-top plastic bag, combine the orange zest and 2 tablespoons of oil with the rosemary, thyme, garlic, pepper, and salt.

Add the shrimp, seal the bag, and gently massage the shrimp until all the ingredients are combined and the shrimp is completely covered with the seasonings. Set aside.

Heat a grill, grill pan, or a large skillet over medium heat. Brush on or swirl in the remaining 1 tablespoon of oil.

Add half the shrimp, and cook for 4 to 6 minutes, or until the shrimp turns pink and white, flipping halfway through if on the grill, or stirring every minute if in a pan. Transfer the shrimp to a large serving bowl.

Repeat with the remaining shrimp, and add them to the bowl.

While the shrimp cooks, peel the orange and cut the flesh into bite-size pieces. Add to the serving bowl, and toss with the cooked shrimp. Serve immediately or refrigerate and serve cold.

Nutrition: Calories: 190; Total Fat: 8 g; Fiber: 1 g; Protein: 24 g.

874 ROASTED SHRIMP-GNOCCHI BAKE

Preparation Time: 10 minutes
Cooking Time: 20 minutes
Servings: 2
Ingredients:

1 cup chopped fresh tomato
2 tbsp. extra-virgin olive oil
2 garlic cloves, minced
½ tsp. freshly ground black pepper
¼ tsp. crushed red pepper
1 (12-oz.) jar roasted red peppers
1-pound fresh raw shrimp, shells and tails removed
1-pound frozen gnocchi (not thawed)
½ cup cubed feta cheese
⅓ cup fresh torn basil leaves

Directions:

Preheat the oven to 425°F. In a baking dish, mix the tomatoes, oil, garlic, black pepper, and crushed red pepper. Roast in the oven for 10 minutes.

Stir in the roasted peppers and shrimp. Roast for 10 more minutes, until the shrimp turns pink and white.

While the shrimp cooks, cook the gnocchi on the stovetop according to the package directions.

Drain in a colander and keep warm. Remove the dish from the oven. Mix in the cooked gnocchi, feta, and basil, and serve.

Nutrition: Calories: 227; Total Fat: 7 g; Fiber: 1 g; Protein: 20 g.

875 TUNA SANDWICH

Preparation Time: 15 minutes
Cooking Time: 0 minutes
Servings: 1
Ingredients:

2 slices whole-grain bread
1 6-oz. can low sodium tuna in water, in its juice
2 tsp Yogurt (1.5% fat) or low-fat mayonnaise
1 medium tomato, diced
½ small sweet onion, finely diced
Lettuce leaves

Directions:

Toast whole grain bread slices. Mix tuna, yogurt, or mayonnaise, diced tomato, and onion. Cover a toasted bread with lettuce leaves and spread the tuna mixture on the sandwich. Spread tuna mixed on toasted bread with lettuce leaves. Place another disc as a cover on top. Enjoy the sandwich.

Nutrition: Calories: 235; Fat: 3 g; Protein: 27.8 g; Sodium: 350 mg; Carbohydrates: 25.9 g.

876 DILL CHUTNEY SALMON

Preparation Time: 5 minutes
Cooking Time: 3 minutes
Servings: 2
Ingredients:
Chutney:

¼ cup fresh dill
¼ cup extra virgin olive oil
Juice from ½ lemon
Sea salt, to taste

Fish:

2 cups water
2 salmon fillets
Juice from ½ lemon
¼ tsp. paprika
Salt and freshly ground pepper to taste

Directions:

Pulse all the chutney ingredients in a food processor until creamy. Set aside.

Add the water and steamer basket to the Instant Pot. Place salmon fillets, skin-side down, on the steamer basket. Drizzle the lemon juice over salmon and sprinkle with the paprika.

Secure the lid. Select the Manual mode and set the cooking time for 3 minutes at High pressure.

Once cooking is complete, do a quick pressure release. Carefully open the lid.

Season the fillets with pepper and salt to taste. Serve topped with the dill chutney.

Nutrition: Calories: 636; Fat: 41 g; Protein: 65 g.

877 BAKED COD FILLETS WITH GHEE SAUCE

Preparation Time: 10 minutes
Cooking Time: 15 minutes
Servings: 2
Ingredients:

- Pepper and salt to taste
- 2 tbsp. minced parsley
- 1 lemon, sliced into ¼-inch-thick circles
- 1 lemon, juiced and zested
- 4 garlic cloves, crushed, peeled, and minced
- ¼ cup melted ghee
- 4 cod fillets

Directions:

- Bring the oven to 425°F.
- Mix parsley, lemon juice, lemon zest, garlic, and melted ghee in a small bowl. Mix well and then season with pepper and salt to taste.
- Prepare a large baking dish by greasing it with cooking spray.
- Evenly lay the cod fillets on the greased dish. Season generously with pepper and salt.
- Pour the bowl of garlic-ghee sauce from step 2 on top of cod fillets. Top the cod fillets with the thinly sliced lemon.
- Pop in the preheated oven and bake until flaky, around 13 to 15 minutes. Remove from oven, transfer to dishes, serve, and enjoy.

Nutrition: Calories: 200; Fat: 12 g; Protein: 21 g; Carbs: 2 g.

878 AVOCADO PEACH SALSA ON GRILLED SWORDFISH

Preparation Time: 15 minutes
Cooking Time: 12 minutes
Servings: 2
Ingredients:

- 1 garlic clove, minced
- 1 lemon juice
- 1 tbsp. apple cider vinegar
- 1 tbsp. coconut oil
- 1 tsp. honey
- 2 swordfish fillets (around 4oz. each)
- Pinch cayenne pepper
- Pinch of pepper and salt

Salsa Ingredients:

- ¼ red onion, finely chopped
- ½ cup cilantro, finely chopped
- 1 avocado, halved and diced
- 1 garlic clove, minced
- 2 peaches, seeded and diced
- Juice of 1 lime
- Salt to taste

Directions:

- In a shallow dish, mix all swordfish marinade ingredients, except fillet. Mix well then add fillets to marinate. Place in refrigerator for at least an hour.
- Meanwhile, create salsa by mixing all salsa ingredients in a medium bowl. Put in the refrigerator to cool.
- Preheat grill and grill fish on medium fire after marinating until cooked, around 4 minutes per side.
- Place each cooked fillet on one serving plate. Top with half of the salsa, serve and enjoy.

Nutrition: Calories: 416; Carbs: 21 g; Protein: 30 g; Fat: 23.5 g.

879 BREADED AND SPICED HALIBUT

Preparation Time: 10 minutes
Cooking Time: 15 minutes
Servings: 4
Ingredients:

- ¼ cup chopped fresh chives
- ¼ cup chopped fresh dill
- ¼ tsp. ground black pepper
- ¾ cup panko breadcrumbs
- 1 tbsp. extra-virgin olive oil
- 1 tsp. finely grated lemon zest
- 1 tsp. sea salt
- ⅓ cup chopped fresh parsley
- 4 pieces of 6-oz. halibut fillets

Directions:

- Line a baking sheet with foil. Grease with cooking spray and preheat the oven to 400°F.
- In a small bowl, mix black pepper, sea salt, lemon zest, olive oil, chives, dill, parsley and breadcrumbs. If needed, add more salt to taste. Set aside.
- Meanwhile, wash halibut fillets on cold tap water. Dry with paper towels and place on prepared baking sheet.
- Generously spoon crumb mixture onto halibut fillets. Ensure that fillets are covered with crumb mixture. Press down on crumb mixture onto each fillet.
- Pop into the oven and bake for 10-15 minutes or until fish is flaky and crumb topping is already lightly browned.

Nutrition: Calories: 336.4; Protein: 25.3 g; Fat: 25.3 g; Carbs: 4.1 g.

880 BERRIES AND GRILLED CALAMARI

Preparation Time: 10 minutes
Cooking Time: 5 minutes
Servings: 4
Ingredients:

- ¼ cup dried cranberries
- ¼ cup extra virgin olive oil
- ¼ cup olive oil
- ¼ cup sliced almonds
- ½ lemon, juiced
- ¾ cup blueberries
- 1 ½ lb. calamari tube, cleaned
- 1 granny smith apple, sliced thinly
- 1 tbsp. fresh lemon juice
- 2 tbsp. apple cider vinegar
- 6 cups fresh spinach
- Freshly grated pepper to taste
- Sea salt to taste

Directions:

- In a small bowl, make the vinaigrette by mixing well the tablespoon of lemon juice, apple cider vinegar, and extra virgin olive oil. Season with pepper and salt to taste. Set aside.
- Turn on the grill to medium fire and let the grates heat up for a minute or two.
- In a large bowl, add olive oil and the calamari tube. Season calamari generously with pepper and salt.
- Place seasoned and oiled calamari onto heated grate and grill until cooked or opaque. This is around two minutes per side.
- As you wait for the calamari to cook, you can combine almonds, cranberries, blueberries, spinach, and the thinly sliced apple in a large salad bowl. Toss to mix.
- Remove cooked calamari from the grill and transfer on a chopping board. Cut into ¼-inch-thick rings and throw into the salad bowl.
- Drizzle with vinaigrette and toss well to coat the salad.
- Serve and enjoy!

Nutrition: Calories: 567; Fat: 24.5 g; Protein: 54.8 g; Carbs: 30.6 g.

881 COCONUT SALSA ON CHIPOTLE FISH TACOS

Preparation Time: 10 minutes
Cooking Time: 10 minutes
Servings: 4
Ingredients:

- ¼ cup chopped fresh cilantro
- ½ cup seeded and finely chopped plum tomato
- 1 cup peeled and finely chopped mango
- 1 lime cut into wedges
- 1 tbsp. chipotle Chile powder
- 1 tbsp. safflower oil
- ⅓ cup finely chopped red onion
- 10 tbsp. fresh lime juice, divided
- 4 6-oz. boneless, skinless cod fillets
- 5 tbsp. dried unsweetened shredded coconut
- 8 pcs of 6-inch tortillas, heated

Directions:

Whisk well Chile powder, oil, and 4 tablespoons of lime juice in a glass baking dish. Add cod and marinate for 12 – 15 minutes. Turning once halfway through the marinating time.

Make the salsa by mixing coconut, 6 tablespoons of lime juice, cilantro, onions, tomatoes and mangoes in a medium bowl. Set aside.

On high, heat a grill pan. Place cod and grill for four minutes per side turning only once.

Once cooked, slice cod into large flakes and evenly divide onto tortilla.

Evenly divide salsa on top of cod and serve with a side of lime wedges.

Nutrition: Calories: 477; Protein: 35.0 g; Fat: 12.4 g; Carbs: 57.4 g.

882 BAKED COD CRUSTED WITH HERBS

Preparation Time: 5 minutes
Cooking Time: 10 minutes
Servings: 4
Ingredients:

¼ cup honey
¼ tsp. salt
½ cup panko
½ tsp. pepper
1 tbsp. extra virgin olive oil
1 tbsp. lemon juice
1 tsp. dried basil
1 tsp. dried parsley
1 tsp. rosemary
4 pieces of 4-oz. cod fillets

Directions:

With olive oil, grease a 9 x 13-inch baking pan and preheat the oven to 375F.

In a zip-top bag mix panko, rosemary, salt, pepper, parsley and basil.

Evenly spread cod fillets in prepped dish and drizzle with lemon juice.

Then brush the fillets with honey on all sides. Discard remaining honey if any.

Then evenly divide the panko mixture on top of cod fillets.

Pop in the oven and bake for ten minutes or until fish is cooked.

Serve and enjoy.

Nutrition: Calories: 137; Protein: 5 g; Fat: 2 g; Carbs: 21 g.

883 CAJUN GARLIC SHRIMP NOODLE BOWL

Preparation Time: 10 minutes
Cooking Time: 15 minutes
Servings: 2
Ingredients:

½ tsp. salt
1 onion, sliced

1 red pepper, sliced
1 tbsp. butter
1 tsp. garlic granules
1 tsp. onion powder
1 tsp. paprika
2 large zucchinis, cut into noodle strips
20 jumbo shrimps, shells removed and deveined
3 cloves garlic, minced
3 tbsp. ghee
A dash of cayenne pepper
A dash of red pepper flakes

Directions:

Prepare the Cajun seasoning by mixing the onion powder, garlic granules, pepper flakes, cayenne pepper, paprika and salt. Toss in the shrimp to coat in the seasoning.

In a skillet, heat the ghee and sauté the garlic. Add in the red pepper and onions and continue sautéing for 4 minutes.

Add the Cajun shrimp and cook until opaque. Set aside.

In another pan, heat the butter and sauté the zucchini noodles for three minutes.

Assemble by placing the Cajun shrimps on top of the zucchini noodles.

Nutrition: Calories: 712; Fat: 30.0 g; Protein: 97.8 g; Carbs: 20.2 g.

884 CRAZY SAGANAKI SHRIMP

Preparation Time: 10 minutes
Cooking Time: 10 minutes
Servings: 4
Ingredients:

¼ tsp. salt
½ cup Chardonnay
½ cup crumbled Greek feta cheese
1 medium bulb. fennel, cored and finely chopped
1 small Chile pepper, seeded and minced
1 tbsp. extra virgin olive oil
12 jumbo shrimps, peeled and deveined with tails left on
2 tbsp. lemon juice, divided
5 scallions sliced thinly
Pepper to Taste

Directions:

In a medium bowl, mix salt, lemon juice and shrimp.

On medium fire, place a saganaki pan (or large nonstick saucepan) and heat oil.

Sauté Chile pepper, scallions, and fennel for 4 minutes or until starting to brown and is already soft.

Add wine and sauté for another minute.

Place shrimps on top of the fennel, cover, and cook for 4 minutes or until shrimps are pink.

Remove just the shrimp and transfer to a plate.

Add pepper, feta and 1 tablespoon of lemon juice to pan and cook for a minute or until cheese begins to melt.

To serve, place cheese and fennel mixture on a serving plate and top with shrimps.

Nutrition: Calories: 310; Protein: 49.7 g; Fat: 6.8 g; Carbs: 8.4 g.

885 CREAMY BACON-FISH CHOWDER

Preparation Time: 10 minutes
Cooking Time: 30 minutes
Servings: 8
Ingredients:

1 ½ lbs. cod
1 ½ tsp. dried thyme
1 large onion, chopped
1 medium carrot, coarsely chopped
1 tbsp. butter, cut into small pieces
1 tsp. salt, divided
3 ½ cups baking potato, peeled and cubed
3 slices uncooked bacon
¼ tsp. freshly ground black pepper, divided
4 ½ cups water
4 bay leaves
4 cups 2% reduced-fat milk

Directions:

In a large skillet, add the water and bay leaves and let it simmer. Add the fish. Cover and let it simmer some more until the flesh flakes easily with a fork. Remove the fish from the skillet and cut into large pieces. Set aside the cooking liquid.

Place Dutch oven on medium heat and cook the bacon until crisp. Remove the bacon and reserve the bacon drippings. Crush the bacon and set aside.

Stir potato, onion and carrot in the pan with the bacon drippings, cook over medium heat for 10 minutes. Add the cooking liquid, bay leaves, ½ teaspoon of salt, ¼ teaspoon of pepper and thyme; let it boil. Lower the heat and let simmer for 10 minutes. Add the milk and butter, simmer until the potatoes become tender, but do not boil. Add the fish, ½ teaspoon of salt, and ½ teaspoon of pepper. Remove the bay leaves.

Serve sprinkled with the crushed bacon.

Nutrition: Calories: 400; Carbs: 34.5 g; Protein: 20.8 g; Fat: 19.7 g.

886 TROUT AND PEPPERS MIX

Preparation Time: 10 minutes
Cooking Time: 20 minutes
Servings: 4
Ingredients:
- 4 trout fillets, boneless
- 2 tbsp. kalamata olives, pitted and chopped
- 1 tbsp. capers, drained
- 2 tbsp. olive oil
- A pinch of salt and black pepper
- 1 ½ tsp. chili powder
- 1 yellow bell pepper, chopped
- 1 red bell pepper, chopped
- 1 green bell pepper, chopped

Directions:
Heat up a pan with the oil over medium-high heat. Add the trout, salt and pepper and cook for 10 minutes.

Flip the fish. Add the peppers and the rest of the ingredients and cook for 10 minutes more. Divide the whole mix between plates and serve.

Nutrition: Calories: 572; Fat: 17.4 g, Fiber: 6 g, Carbs: 71 g, Protein: 33.7 g.

887 CRISPED COCO SHRIMP WITH MANGO DIP

Preparation Time: 10 minutes
Cooking Time: 20 minutes
Servings: 4
Ingredients:
- 1 cup shredded coconut
- 1 lb. raw shrimp, peeled and deveined
- 2 egg whites
- 4 tbsp. tapioca starch
- Pepper and salt to taste

Mango Dip Ingredients:
- 1 cup mango, chopped
- 1 jalapeño, thinly minced
- 1 tsp. lime juice - ⅓ cup coconut milk
- 3 tsp. raw honey

Directions:
Preheat oven to 400°F. Ready a pan with a wire rack on top.

In a medium bowl, add tapioca starch and season with pepper and salt.

In a second medium bowl, add egg whites and whisk.

In a third medium bowl, add coconut.

To ready shrimps, dip first in tapioca starch, then egg whites, and then coconut. Place dredged shrimp on a wire rack. Repeat until all shrimps are covered.

Pop shrimps in the oven and roast for 10 minutes per side.

Meanwhile, make the dip by adding all ingredients to a blender. Puree until smooth and creamy. Transfer to a dipping bowl.

Once shrimps are golden brown, serve with mango dip.

Nutrition: Calories: 294.2; Protein: 26.6 g; Fat: 7 g; Carbs: 31.2 g.

888 CUCUMBER-BASIL SALSA ON HALIBUT POUCHES

Preparation Time: 10 minutes
Cooking Time: 17 minutes
Servings: 4
Ingredients:
- 1 lime, thinly sliced into 8 pieces
- 2 cups mustard greens, stems removed
- 2 tsp. olive oil
- 4 – 5 radishes trimmed and quartered
- 4 (4-oz.) skinless halibut filets
- 4 large fresh basil leaves
- Cayenne pepper to taste – optional
- Pepper and salt to taste

Salsa Ingredients:
- 1 ½ cups diced cucumber
- 1 ½ finely chopped fresh basil leaves
- 2 tsp. fresh lime juice
- Pepper and salt to taste

Directions:
Preheat oven to 400°F.

Prepare parchment papers by making 4 pieces of 15 x 12-inch rectangles. Lengthwise, fold in half and unfold pieces on the table.

Season halibut fillets with pepper, salt and cayenne—if using cayenne.

Just to the right of the fold going lengthwise, place ½ cup of mustard greens. Add a basil leaf to the center of mustard greens and topped with 1 lime slice. Around the greens, layer ¼ of the radishes. Drizzle with ½ teaspoon of oil, season with pepper and salt. Top it with a slice of halibut fillet.

Just as you would make a calzone, fold the parchment paper over your filling and crimp the edges of the parchment paper beginning from one end to the other end. To seal the end of the crimped parchment paper, pinch it.

Repeat the process to the remaining ingredients until you have 4 pieces of parchment paper filled with halibut and greens.

Place pouches in a baking pan and bake in the oven until halibut is flaky, around 15 to 17 minutes.

While waiting for halibut pouches to cook, make your salsa by mixing all salsa ingredients in a medium bowl.

Once halibut is cooked, remove from the oven and make a tear on top. Be careful of the steam as it is very hot. Equally, divide salsa and spoon ¼ of salsa on top of halibut through the slit you have created.

Nutrition: Calories: 335.4; Protein: 20.2 g; Fat: 16.3 g; Carbs: 22.1 g.

889 CURRY SALMON WITH MUSTARD

Preparation Time: 10 minutes
Cooking Time: 8 minutes
Servings: 4
Ingredients:
- ¼ tsp. ground red pepper or chili powder
- ¼ tsp. ground turmeric
- ¼ tsp. salt
- 1 tsp. honey
- ⅛ tsp. garlic powder or 1 clove garlic minced
- 2 tsp. whole grain mustard
- 4 pcs 6-oz. salmon fillets

Directions:
In a small bowl mix well salt, garlic powder, red pepper, turmeric, honey and mustard.

Preheat the oven to broil and grease a baking dish with cooking spray.

Place salmon on a baking dish with skin side down and spread evenly mustard mixture on top of salmon.

Pop in the oven and broil until flaky around 8 minutes.

Nutrition: Calories: 324; Fat: 18.9 g; Protein: 34 g; Carbs: 2.9 g.

890 DIJON MUSTARD AND LIME MARINATED SHRIMP

Preparation Time: 10 minutes
Cooking Time: 10 minutes
Servings: 8
Ingredients:
- ½ cup fresh lime juice, plus lime zest as garnish
- ½ cup rice vinegar
- ½ tsp. hot sauce
- 1 bay leaf
- 1 cup water
- 1 lb. uncooked shrimp, peeled and deveined
- 1 medium red onion, chopped
- 2 tbsp. capers
- 2 tbsp. Dijon mustard
- 3 whole cloves

Directions:
Mix hot sauce, mustard, capers, lime juice and onion in a shallow baking dish and set aside.

Bring to a boil in a large saucepan bay leaf, cloves, vinegar and water.

Once boiling, add shrimps and cook for a minute while stirring continuously.

Drain shrimps and pour shrimps into the onion mixture.

For an hour, refrigerate while covered the shrimps.

Then serve shrimps cold and garnished with lime zest.

Nutrition: Calories: 232.2; Protein: 17.8 g; Fat: 3 g; Carbs: 15 g.

891 DILL RELISH ON WHITE SEA BASS

Preparation Time: 10 minutes
Cooking Time: 12 minutes
Servings: 4
Ingredients:

1 ½ tbsp. chopped white onion
1 ½ tsp. chopped fresh dill
1 lemon, quartered
1 tsp. Dijon mustard
1 tsp. lemon juice
1 tsp. pickled baby capers, drained
4 pieces of 4-oz. white sea bass fillets

Directions:

Preheat oven to 375°F.

Mix lemon juice, mustard, dill, capers and onions in a small bowl.

Prepare four aluminum foil squares and place 1 fillet per foil.

Squeeze a lemon wedge per fish.

Evenly divide into 4 the dill spread and drizzle over the fillet.

Close the foil over the fish securely and pop in the oven.

Bake for 10 to 12 minutes or until fish is cooked through.

Remove from foil and transfer to a serving platter, serve and enjoy.

Nutrition: Calories: 115; Protein: 7 g; Fat: 1 g; Carbs: 12 g.

892 GARLIC ROASTED SHRIMP WITH ZUCCHINI PASTA

Preparation Time: 10 minutes
Cooking Time: 10 minutes
Servings: 2
Ingredients:

2 medium-sized zucchinis, cut into thin strips or spaghetti noodles
Salt and pepper to taste
1 lemon, zested and juiced
2 garlic cloves, minced
2 tbsp. ghee, melted
2 tbsp. olive oil
8 oz. shrimps, cleaned and deveined

Directions:

Preheat the oven to 400°F.

In a mixing bowl, mix all ingredients, except the zucchini noodles. Toss to coat the shrimp.

Bake for 10 minutes until the shrimps turn pink.

Add the zucchini pasta; then toss.

Nutrition: Calories: 299; Fat: 23.2 g; Protein: 14.3 g; Carbs: 10.9 g.

893 EASY SEAFOOD FRENCH STEW

Preparation Time: 10 minutes
Cooking Time: 45 minutes
Servings: 12

Ingredients:

Pepper and salt
½ lb. littleneck clams
½ lb. mussels
1 lb. shrimp, peeled and deveined
1 large lobster
2 lbs. assorted small whole fresh fish, scaled and cleaned
2 tbsp. parsley, finely chopped
2 tbsp. garlic, chopped
1 cup fennel, julienned
Juice and zest of one orange
3 cups tomatoes, peeled, seeded, and chopped
1 cup leeks, julienned
Pinch of Saffron

Stew Ingredients:

1 cup white wine
Water
1 lb. fish bones
2 sprigs thyme
8 peppercorns
1 bay leaf
3 cloves garlic
Salt and pepper
½ cup chopped celery
½ cup chopped onion
2 tbsp. olive oil

Directions:

Do the stew:

Heat oil in a large saucepan. Sauté the celery and onions for 3 minutes. Season with pepper and salt. Stir in the garlic and cook for about a minute. Add the thyme, peppercorns, and bay leaves. Stir in the wine, water and fish bones. Let it boil then before reducing to a simmer. Take the pan off the fire and strain the broth into another container.

For the Bouillabaisse:

Bring the strained broth to a simmer and stir in the parsley, leeks, orange juice, orange zest, garlic, fennel, tomatoes and saffron. Sprinkle with pepper and salt. Stir in the lobsters and fish. Let it simmer for eight minutes before stirring in the clams, mussels and shrimps. For six minutes, allow to cook while covered before seasoning again with pepper and salt.

Assemble in a shallow dish all the seafood and pour the broth over it.

Nutrition: Calories: 348; Carbs: 20.0 g; Protein: 31.8 g; Fat: 15.2 g.

894 FRESH AND NO-COOK OYSTERS

Preparation Time: 10 minutes
Cooking Time: 5 minutes
Servings: 4
Ingredients:

2 lemons
24 medium oysters
tabasco sauce

Directions:

If you are a newbie when it comes to eating oysters, then I suggest that you blanch the oysters before eating.

For some, eating oysters raw is a great way to enjoy this dish because of the consistency and juiciness of raw oysters. Plus, adding lemon juice prior to eating the raw oysters, cooks it a bit.

To blanch oysters, bring a big pot of water to a rolling boil. Add oysters in batches of 6-10 pieces. Leave on the boiling pot of water between 3-5 minutes and remove oysters right away. To eat oysters, squeeze lemon juice on oyster on the shell, add tabasco as desired.

Nutrition: Calories: 247; Protein: 29 g; Fat: 7 g; Carbs: 17 g.

895 EASY BROILED LOBSTER TAILS

Preparation Time: 10 minutes
Cooking Time: 10 minutes
Servings: 2
Ingredients:

1 6-oz. frozen lobster tails
1 tbsp. olive oil
1 tsp. lemon pepper seasoning

Directions:

Preheat oven broiler.

With kitchen scissors, cut thawed lobster tails in half lengthwise.

Brush with oil the exposed lobster meat. Season with lemon pepper.

Place lobster tails on a baking sheet with exposed meat facing up.

Place on top broiler rack and broil for 10 minutes until lobster meat is lightly browned on the sides and center meat is opaque. Serve and enjoy.

Nutrition: Calories: 175.6; Protein: 23 g; Fat: 10 g; Carbs: 18.4 g.

896 GINGER SCALLION SAUCE OVER SEARED AHI

Preparation Time: 10 minutes
Cooking Time: 6 minutes
Servings: 4
Ingredients:

- 1 bunch scallions, bottoms removed, finely chopped
- 1 tbsp. rice wine vinegar
- 1 tbsp. bragg's liquid amino
- 16-oz. ahi tuna steaks
- 2 tbsp. fresh ginger, peeled and grated
- 3 tbsp. coconut oil, melted
- Pepper and salt to taste

Directions:

In a small bowl mix together vinegar, 2 tablespoons of oil, soy sauce, ginger and scallions. Put aside.

On medium fire, place a large saucepan and heat the remaining oil. Once the oil is hot and starts to smoke, sear tuna until deeply browned or for two minutes per side.

Place seared tuna on a serving platter and let it stand for 5 minutes before slicing into 1-inch-thick strips.

Drizzle ginger-scallion mixture over seared tuna, serve and enjoy.

Nutrition: Calories: 247; Protein: 29 g; Fat: 1 g; Carbs: 8 g.

897 HEALTHY POACHED TROUT

Preparation Time: 10 minutes
Cooking Time: 10 minutes
Servings: 2
Ingredients:

- 1 8-oz. boneless, skin on trout fillet
- 2 cups chicken broth or water
- 2 leeks, halved
- 6-8 slices lemon
- salt and pepper to taste

Directions:

On medium fire, place a large nonstick skillet and arrange leeks and lemons on the pan in a layer. Cover with soup stock or water and bring to a simmer.

Meanwhile, season trout on both sides with pepper and salt. Place trout on the simmering pan of water. Cover and cook until trout are flaky, around 8 minutes.

In a serving platter, spoon leek and lemons on the bottom of the plate, top with trout and spoon sauce into the plate. Serve and enjoy.

Nutrition: Calories: 360.2; Protein: 13.8 g; Fat: 7.5 g; Carbs: 51.5 g.

898 LEFTOVER SALMON SALAD POWER BOWLS

Preparation Time: 10 minutes
Cooking Time: 10 minutes
Servings: 1
Ingredients:

- ½ cup raspberries
- ½ cup zucchini, sliced
- 1 lemon, juice squeezed
- 1 tbsp. balsamic glaze
- 2 sprigs of thyme, chopped
- 2 tbsp. olive oil
- 4 cups seasonal greens
- 4 oz. leftover grilled salmon
- Salt and pepper to taste

Directions:

Heat oil in a skillet over medium flame and sauté the zucchini. Season with salt and pepper to taste.

In a mixing bowl, mix all ingredients together.

Toss to combine everything.

Sprinkle with nut cheese.

Nutrition: Calories: 450.3; Fat: 35.5 g; Protein: 23.4g; Carbs: 9.3 g.

899 LEMON-GARLIC BAKED HALIBUT

Preparation Time: 10 minutes
Cooking Time: 15 minutes
Servings: 2
Ingredients:

- 1 large garlic clove, minced
- 1 tbsp. chopped flat leaf parsley
- 1 tsp. olive oil
- 2 5-oz. boneless, skin-on halibut fillets
- 2 tsp. lemon zest
- Juice of ½ lemon, divided
- Salt and pepper to taste

Directions:

Grease a baking dish with cooking spray and preheat the oven to 400°F.

Place halibut with skin touching the dish and drizzle with olive oil.

Season with pepper and salt.

Pop into the oven and bake until flaky around 12-15 minutes.

Remove from oven and drizzle with remaining lemon juice, serve and enjoy with a side of salad greens.

Nutrition: Calories: 315.3; Protein: 14.1 g; Fat: 10.5 g; Carbs: 36.6 g.

900 MINTY-CUCUMBER YOGURT TOPPED GRILLED FISH

Preparation Time: 10 minutes
Cooking Time: 2 minutes
Servings: 4
Ingredients:

- ¼ cup 2% plain Greek yogurt
- ¼ tsp. + ⅛ tsp. salt
- ¼ tsp. black pepper
- ½ green onion, finely chopped
- ½ tsp. dried oregano
- 1 tbsp. finely chopped fresh mint leaves
- 3 tbsp. finely chopped English cucumber
- 4 5-oz. cod fillets
- Cooking oil as needed

Directions:

Brush grill grate with oil and preheat grill to high.

Season cod fillets on both sides with pepper, ¼ teaspoon of salt and oregano.

Grill cod for 3 minutes per side or until cooked to desired doneness.

Mix thoroughly ⅛ teaspoon of salt, onion, mint, cucumber and yogurt in a small bowl. Serve cod with a dollop of the dressing. This dish can be paired with salad greens or brown rice.

Nutrition: Calories: 253.5; Protein: 25.5 g; Fat: 1 g; Carbs: 5 g.

901 ONE-POT SEAFOOD CHOWDER

Preparation Time: 10 minutes
Cooking Time: 10 minutes
Servings: 3
Ingredients:

- 3 cans coconut milk
- 1 tbsp. garlic, minced
- Salt and pepper to taste
- 3 cans clams, chopped
- 2 cans shrimps, canned
- 1 package fresh shrimps, shelled and deveined
- 1 can corn, drained
- 4 large potatoes, diced
- 2 carrots, peeled and chopped
- 2 celery stalks, chopped

Directions:

Place all ingredients in a pot and give a good stir to mix everything.

Close the lid and turn on the heat to medium.

Bring to a boil and allow to simmer for 10 minutes.

Place in individual containers.

Put a label and store in the fridge.

Allow to warm at room temperature before heating in the microwave oven.

Nutrition: Calories: 532; Carbs: 92.5 g; Protein: 25.3 g; Fat: 6.7 g.

902 ORANGE ROSEMARY SEARED SALMON

Preparation Time: 10 minutes
Cooking Time: 10 minutes
Servings: 4
Ingredients:

- ½ cup chicken stock
- 1 cup fresh orange juice
- 1 tbsp. coconut oil
- 1 tbsp. tapioca starch

2 garlic cloves, minced
2 tbsp. fresh lemon juice
2 tsp. fresh rosemary, minced
2 tsp. orange zest
4 salmon fillets, skins removed
Salt and pepper to taste

Directions:

Season the salmon fillet on both sides.

In a skillet, heat coconut oil over medium-high heat. Cook the salmon fillets for 5 minutes on each side. Set aside.

In a mixing bowl, combine the orange juice, chicken stock, lemon juice and orange zest.

In the skillet, sauté the garlic and rosemary for 2 minutes and pour the orange juice mixture. Bring to a boil. Lower the heat to medium-low and simmer. Season with salt and pepper to taste.

Pour the sauce all over the salmon fillet then serve.

Nutrition: Calories: 493; Fat: 17.9 g; Protein: 66.7 g; Carbs: 12.8 g.

903 ORANGE HERBED SAUCED WHITE BASS

Preparation Time: 10 minutes
Cooking Time: 33 minutes
Servings: 6
Ingredients:

¼ cup thinly sliced green onions
½ cup orange juice
1 ½ tbsp. fresh lemon juice
1 ½ tbsp. olive oil
1 large onion, halved, thinly sliced
1 large orange, unpeeled, sliced
3 tbsp. chopped fresh dill
6 3-oz. skinless white bass fillets
Additional unpeeled orange slices

Directions:

Grease a 13 x 9-inch glass baking dish and preheat the oven to 400F.

Arrange orange slices in a single layer on a baking dish, top with onion slices, seasoned with pepper and salt plus drizzled with oil.

Pop in the oven and roast for 25 minutes or until onions are tender and browned.

Remove from oven and increased oven temperature to 450F.

Push onion and orange slices on sides of the dish and place bass fillets in middle of the dish. Season with 1 ½ tablespoon of dill, pepper and salt. Arrange onions and orange slices on top of fish and pop into the oven.

Roast for 8 minutes or until salmon is opaque and flaky.

In a small bowl, mix 1 ½ tablespoon of dill, lemon juice, green onions and orange juice.

Transfer salmon to a serving plate, discard roasted onions, drizzle with the newly made orange sauce and garnish with fresh orange slices. Serve and enjoy.

Nutrition: Calories: 312.42; Protein: 84.22 g; Fat: 23.14 g; Carbs: 33.91 g.

904 PAN FRIED TUNA WITH HERBS AND NUT

Preparation Time: 10 minutes
Cooking Time: 5 minutes
Servings: 4
Ingredients:

¼ cup almonds, chopped finely
¼ cup fresh tangerine juice
½ tsp. fennel seeds, chopped finely
½ tsp. ground pepper, divided
½ tsp. sea salt, divided
1 tbsp. olive oil
2 tbsp. fresh mint, chopped finely
2 tbsp. red onion, chopped finely
4 pieces of 6-oz. Tuna steak cut in half

Directions:

Mix fennel seeds, olive oil, mint, onion, tangerine juice and almonds in a small bowl. Season with ¼ each of pepper and salt.

Season fish with the remaining pepper and salt.

On medium-high fire, place a large nonstick fry pan and grease with cooking spray.

Pan fry tuna until the desired doneness is reached or for one minute per side.

Transfer cooked tuna to a serving plate, drizzle with dressing and serve.

Nutrition: Calories: 272; Fat: 9.7 g; Protein: 42 g; Carbs: 4.2 g.

905 PAPRIKA SALMON AND GREEN BEANS

Preparation Time: 10 minutes
Cooking Time: 20 minutes
Servings: 3
Ingredients:

¼ cup olive oil
½ tbsp. onion powder
½ tsp. bouillon powder
½ tsp. cayenne pepper
1 tbsp. smoked paprika
1-lb. green beans
2 tsp. minced garlic
3 tbsp. fresh herbs
6 oz. of salmon steak
Salt and pepper to taste

Directions:

Preheat the oven to 400°F.
Grease a baking sheet and set aside.

Heat a skillet over medium-low heat and add the olive oil. Sauté the garlic, smoked paprika, fresh herbs, cayenne pepper and onion powder. Stir for a minute; then let the mixture sit for 5 minutes. Set aside.

Put the salmon steaks in a bowl and add salt and the paprika spice mixture. Rub to coat the salmon well.

Place the salmon on the baking sheet and cook for 18 minutes.

Meanwhile, blanch the green beans in boiling water with salt.

Serve the beans with the salmon.

Nutrition: Calories: 945.8; Fat: 66.6 g; Protein: 43.5 g; Carbs: 43.1 g.

906 PECAN CRUSTED TROUT

Preparation Time: 10 minutes
Cooking Time: 12 minutes
Servings: 4
Ingredients:

½ cup crushed pecans
½ tsp. grated fresh ginger
1 egg, beaten
1 tsp. crush dried rosemary
1 tsp. salt
4 4-oz. trout fillets
Black pepper to taste
Cooking spray
Whole wheat flour, as needed

Directions:

Grease baking sheet lightly with cooking spray and preheat oven to 400°F.

In a shallow bowl, combine black pepper, salt, rosemary and pecans. In another shallow bowl, add whole wheat flour. In a third bowl, add beaten egg.

To prepare fish, dip in flour until covered well. Shake off excess flour. Then dip into beaten egg until coated well. Let excess egg drip off before dipping trout fillet into pecan crumbs. Press the trout lightly onto pecan crumbs to make it stick to the fish.

Place breaded fish onto prepared pan. Repeat process for remaining fillets.

Pop into the oven and bake for 10 to 12 minutes or until the fish is flaky.

Nutrition: Calories: 329; Fat: 19 g; Protein: 26.95 g; Carbs: 3 g.

907 PESTO AND LEMON HALIBUT

Preparation Time: 10 minutes
Cooking Time: 10 minutes
Servings: 4
Ingredients:

1 tbsp. fresh lemon juice
1 tbsp. lemon rind, grated
2 garlic cloves, peeled
2 tbsp. olive oil
¼ cup Parmesan Cheese, freshly grated
⅔ cups firmly packed basil leaves
⅛ tsp. freshly ground black pepper
¼ tsp. salt, divided
4 pcs 6-oz. halibut fillets

Directions:

Preheat grill to medium fire and grease grate with cooking spray.

Season fillets with pepper and ⅛ teaspoon of salt. Place on grill and cook until halibut is flaky, around 4 minutes per side.

Meanwhile, make your lemon pesto by combining lemon juice, lemon rind, garlic, olive oil, Parmesan cheese, basil leaves and remaining salt in a blender. Pulse mixture until finely minced but not pureed.

Once fish is done cooking, transfer to a serving platter, pour over the lemon pesto sauce, serve and enjoy.

Nutrition: Calories: 277.4; Fat: 13 g; Protein: 38.7 g; Carbs: 1.4 g.

908 RED PEPPERS & PINEAPPLE TOPPED MAHI-MAHI

Preparation Time: 10 minutes
Cooking Time: 30 minutes
Servings: 4
Ingredients:

¼ tsp. black pepper
¼ tsp. salt
1 cup whole wheat couscous
1 red bell pepper, diced
2 ⅓ cups low sodium chicken broth
2 cups chopped fresh pineapple
2 tbsp. chopped fresh chives
2 tsp. olive oil
4 pieces of skinless, boneless Mahi midsolo (dolphin fish) fillets (around 4-oz. each)

Directions:

On high fire, add 1 ⅓ cups of broth to a small saucepan and heat until boiling. Once boiling, add couscous. Turn off fire, cover and set aside to allow liquid to be fully absorbed around 5 minutes.

On medium-high fire, place a large nonstick saucepan and heat oil.

Season fish on both sides with pepper and salt. Add Mahi midsolo to a hot pan and pan fry until golden around one minute on each side. Once cooked, transfer to plate.

On the same pan, sauté bell pepper and pineapples until soft, around 2 minutes on a medium high fire.

Add couscous to the pan along with chives, and remaining broth.

On top of the mixture in the pan, place fish. With foil, cover the pan and continue cooking until fish is steaming and tender underneath the foil, around 3-5 minutes.

Nutrition: Calories: 302; Protein: 43.1 g; Fat: 4.8 g; Carbs: 22.0 g.

909 ROASTED HALIBUT WITH BANANA RELISH

Preparation Time: 10 minutes
Cooking Time: 12 minutes
Servings: 4
Ingredients:

¼ cup cilantro
½ tsp. freshly grated orange zest
½ tsp. kosher salt, divided
1 lb. halibut or any deep-water fish
1 tsp. ground coriander, divided into half
2 oranges (peeled, segmented and chopped)
2 ripe bananas, diced
2 tbsp. lime juice

Directions:

In a pan, prepare the fish by rubbing ½ teaspoon of coriander and ¼ teaspoon of kosher salt.

Place in a baking sheet with cooking spray and bake for 8 to 12 minutes inside a 450°F preheated oven.

Prepare the relish by stirring the orange zest, bananas, chopped oranges, lime juice, cilantro and the rest of the salt and coriander in a medium bowl.

Spoon the relish over the roasted fish. Serve and enjoy.

Nutrition: Calories: 245.7; Protein: 15.3 g; Fat: 6 g; Carbs: 21 g.

910 ROASTED POLLOCK FILLET WITH BACON AND LEEKS

Preparation Time: 10 minutes
Cooking Time: 30 minutes
Servings: 2
Ingredients:

¼ cup olive oil
½ cup white wine
1 ½ lbs. Pollock fillets
1 sprig fresh thyme
1 tbsp. chopped fresh thyme
2 tbsp. olive oil
4 leeks, sliced

Directions:

Grease a 9x13 baking dish and preheat the oven to 400°F.

In the baking pan add olive oil and leeks. Toss to combine.

Pop into the oven and roast for 10 minutes.

Remove from oven; add white wine and 1 teaspoon of chopped thyme. Return to oven and roast for another 10 minutes.

Remove pan from oven and add fish on top. Apply olive oil mixture onto fish until coated fully. Return to oven and roast for another ten minutes.

Remove from oven, garnish with a sprig of thyme and serve.

Nutrition: Calories: 442; Carbs: 13.6 g; Protein: 42.9 g; Fat: 24 g.

911 SCALLOPS IN WINE 'N OLIVE OIL

Preparation Time: 10 minutes
Cooking Time: 8 minutes
Servings: 4
Ingredients:

¼ tsp. salt
½ cup dry white wine
1 ½ lbs. large sea scallops
1 ½ tsp. chopped fresh tarragon
2 tbsp. olive oil
Black pepper – optional

Directions:

On medium-high fire, place a large nonstick fry pan and heat oil.

Add scallops and fry for 3 minutes per side or until edges are lightly browned. Transfer to a serving plate.

On the same pan, add salt, tarragon and wine while scraping the pan to loosen browned bits.

Turn off the fire.

Pour sauce over scallops and serve.

Nutrition: Calories: 205.2; Fat: 8 g; Protein: 28.6 g; Carbs: 4.7 g.

912 SEAFOOD STEW CIOPPINO

Preparation Time: 10 minutes
Cooking Time: 40 minutes
Servings: 6
Ingredients:

¼ cup Italian parsley, chopped
¼ tsp. dried basil
¼ tsp. dried thyme
½ cup dry white wine like pinot grigio
½ lb. King crab legs, cut at each joint
½ onion, chopped
½ tsp. red pepper flakes (adjust to the desired spiciness)
1 28-oz. can crush tomatoes
1 lb. Mahi midsolo, cut into ½-inch cubes
1 lb. raw shrimp
1 tbsp. olive oil
2 bay leaves
2 cups clam juice
50 live clams, washed
6 cloves garlic, minced

Pepper and salt to taste

Directions:

On medium fire, place a stockpot and heat oil.

Add onion and for 4 minutes sauté until soft.

Add bay leaves, thyme, basil, red pepper flakes and garlic. Cook for a minute while stirring a bit.

Add clam juice and tomatoes. Once simmering, place fire to medium-low and cook for 20 minutes uncovered.

Add white wine and clams. Cover and cook for 5 minutes or until clams have slightly opened.

Stir pot; then add fish pieces, crab legs and shrimps. Do not stir the soup to maintain the fish shape. Cook, while covered for 4 minutes, or until clams are fully opened and fish and shrimps are opaque and cooked.

Season with pepper and salt to taste.

Transfer Cioppino to serving bowls and garnish with parsley before serving.

Nutrition: Calories: 371; Carbs: 15.5 g; Protein: 62 g; Fat: 6.8 g.

913 SIMPLE COD PICCATA

Preparation Time: 10 minutes
Cooking Time: 15 minutes
Servings: 3
Ingredients:

¼ cup capers, drained
½ tsp. salt
¾ cup chicken stock
⅓ cup almond flour
1-lb. cod fillets, patted dry
2 tbsp. fresh parsley, chopped
2 tbsp. grapeseed oil
3 tbsp. extra-virgin oil
3 tbsp. lemon juice

Directions:

In a bowl, combine the almond flour and salt.

Dredge the fish in the almond flour to coat. Set aside.

Heat a little bit of olive oil to coat a large skillet. Heat the skillet over medium-high heat. Add grapeseed oil. Cook the cod for 3 minutes on each side to brown. Remove from the plate and place on a paper towel-lined plate.

In a saucepan, mix together the chicken stock, capers and lemon juice. Simmer to reduce the sauce to half. Add the remaining grapeseed oil.

Drizzle the fried cod with the sauce and sprinkle with parsley.

Nutrition: Calories: 277.1; Fat: 28.3 g; Protein: 21.9 g; Carbs: 3.7 g.

914 SMOKED TROUT TARTINE

Preparation Time: 10 minutes
Cooking Time: 0 minutes
Servings: 4
Ingredients:

½ 15-oz. can cannellini beans
½ cup diced roasted red peppers
¾ lb. smoked trout, flaked into bite-sized pieces
1 stalk celery, finely chopped
1 tbsp. extra virgin olive oil
1 tsp. chopped fresh dill
1 tsp. Dijon mustard
2 tbsp. capers, rinsed and drained
2 tbsp. freshly squeezed lemon juice
2 tsp. minced onion
4 large whole-grain bread, toasted
Dill sprigs – for garnish
Pinch of sugar

Directions:

Mix sugar, mustard, olive oil and lemon juice in a big bowl.

Add the rest of the ingredients, except for toasted bread.

Toss to mix well.

Evenly divide fish mixture on top of bread slices and garnish with dill sprigs.

Serve and enjoy.

Nutrition: Calories: 348.1; Protein: 28.2 g; Fat: 10.1 g; Carbs: 36.1 g.

915 STEAMED MUSSELS THAI STYLE

Preparation Time: 10 minutes
Cooking Time: 15 minutes
Servings: 4
Ingredients:

¼ cup minced shallots
½ tsp. Madras curry
1 cup dry white wine
1 small bay leaf
1 tbsp. chopped fresh basil
1 tbsp. chopped fresh cilantro
1 tbsp. chopped fresh mint
2 lbs. mussel, cleaned and debearded
2 tbsp. butter
4 medium garlic cloves, minced

Directions:

In a large heavy-bottomed pot, on medium-high fire add to the pot the curry powder, bay leaf, wine plus minced garlic and shallots. Bring to a boil and simmer for 3 minutes.

Add the cleaned mussels. Stir, cover, and cook for 3 minutes.

Stir mussels again. Cover, and cook for another 2 or 3 minutes. Cooking is done when the majority of shells have opened.

With a slotted spoon, transfer cooked mussels to a large bowl. Discard any unopened mussels.

Continue heating the pot with sauce. Add butter and the chopped herbs.

Season with pepper and salt to taste.

Once good, pour over mussels, serve and enjoy.

Nutrition: Calories: 407.2; Protein: 43.4 g; Fat: 21.2 g; Carbs: 10.8 g.

916 TASTY TUNA SCALOPPINE

Preparation Time: 10 minutes
Cooking Time: 10 minutes
Servings: 4

Ingredients:

¼ cup chopped almonds
¼ cup fresh tangerine juice
½ tsp. fennel seeds
½ tsp. ground black pepper, divided
½ tsp. salt
1 tbsp. extra virgin olive oil
2 tbsp. chopped fresh mint
2 tbsp. chopped red onion
4 6-oz. sushi-grade Yellowfin tuna steaks, each split in half horizontally
Cooking spray

Directions:

In a small bowl, mix fennel seed, olive oil, mint, onion, tangerine juice, almonds, ¼ teaspoon of pepper and ¼ teaspoon of salt. Combine thoroughly.

Season fish with remaining salt and pepper.

On medium-high fire, place a large nonstick pan and grease with cooking spray. Pan fry fish in two batches cooking each side for a minute.

Fish is best served with a side of salad greens or a half cup of cooked brown rice.

Nutrition: Calories: 405; Protein: 27.5 g; Fat: 11.9 g; Carbs: 27.5 g.

917 THYME AND LEMON ON BAKED SALMON

Preparation Time: 10 minutes
Cooking Time: 25 minutes
Servings: 2
Ingredients:

1 (32-oz.) salmon fillet
1 lemon, sliced thinly
1 tbsp. capers
1 tbsp. fresh thyme
Olive oil for drizzling
Pepper and salt to taste

Directions:

In a foil line baking sheet, place a parchment paper on top.

Place salmon with skin side down on parchment paper.

Season generously with pepper and salt.

Place capers on top of the fillet. Cover with thinly sliced lemon.

Garnish with thyme.

Pop in a cold oven and bake for 25 minutes at 400°F settings.

Serve right away and enjoy.

Nutrition: Calories: 684.4; Protein: 94.3 g; Fat: 32.7 g; Carbs: 4.3 g.

918 WARM CAPER TAPENADE ON COD

Preparation Time: 10 minutes
Cooking Time: 30 minutes
Servings: 4
Ingredients:

¼ cup chopped cured olives
¼ tsp. freshly ground pepper
1 ½ tsp. chopped fresh oregano
1 cup halved cherry tomatoes
1 lb. cod fillet
1 tbsp. capers, rinsed and chopped
1 tbsp. minced shallot
1 tsp. balsamic vinegar
3 tsp. extra virgin olive oil, divided

Directions:

Grease baking sheet with cooking spray and preheat oven to 450°F.

Place cod on a prepared baking sheet. Rub with 2 teaspoons of oil and season with pepper.

Roast in the oven for 15 to 20 minutes or until the cod is flaky.

While waiting for cod to cook, on medium fire, place a small fry pan and heat 1 teaspoon of oil.

Sauté shallots for a minute.

Add tomatoes and cook for two minutes or until soft.

Add capers and olives. Sauté for another minute.

Add vinegar and oregano. Turn off fire and stir to mix well.

Evenly divide cod into 4 servings and place on a plate.

To serve, top cod with Caper-Olive-Tomato Tapenade and enjoy.

Nutrition: Calories: 107; Fat: 2.9 g; Protein: 17.6 g; Carbs: 2.0 g.

919 YUMMY SALMON PANZANELLA

Preparation Time: 10 minutes
Cooking Time: 10 minutes
Servings: 4
Ingredients:

¼ cup thinly sliced fresh basil
¼ cup thinly sliced red onion
¼ tsp. freshly ground pepper, divided
½ tsp. salt

1 lb. center cut salmon, skinned and cut into 4 equal portions
1 medium cucumber, peeled, seeded, and cut into 1-inch slices
1 tbsp. capers, rinsed and chopped
2 large tomatoes, cut into 1-inch pieces
2 thick slices day old whole grain bread, sliced into 1-inch cubes
3 tbsp. extra virgin olive oil
3 tbsp. red wine vinegar
8 Kalamata olives, pitted and chopped

Directions:

Grease grill grate and preheat grill to high.

In a large bowl, whisk ⅛ teaspoon of pepper, capers, vinegar, and olives. Add oil and whisk well.

Stir in basil, onion, cucumber, tomatoes, and bread.

Season both sides of salmon with remaining pepper and salt.

Grill on high for 4 minutes per side.

Into 4 plates, evenly divide salad, top with grilled salmon, and serve.

Nutrition: Calories: 383; Fat: 20.6 g; Protein: 34.8 g; Carbs: 13.6 g.

920 FISH AND ORZO

Preparation Time: 10 minutes
Cooking Time: 35 minutes
Servings: 4
Ingredients:

1 tsp. garlic, minced
1 tsp. red pepper, crushed
2 shallots, chopped
1 tbsp. olive oil
1 tsp. anchovy paste
1 tbsp. oregano, chopped
2 tbsp. black olives, pitted and chopped
2 tbsp. capers, drained
15 oz. canned tomatoes, crushed
A pinch of salt and black pepper
4 cod fillets, boneless
1 oz. feta cheese, crumbled
1 tbsp. parsley, chopped
3 cups chicken stock
1 cup orzo pasta
Zest of 1 lemon, grated

Directions:

Heat up a pan with the oil over medium heat. Add the garlic, red pepper and the shallots and sauté for 5 minutes.

Add the anchovy paste, oregano, black olives, capers, tomatoes, salt and pepper, stir and cook for 5 minutes more.

Add the cod fillets, sprinkle the cheese and the parsley on top. Introduce in the oven and bake at 375°F for 15 minutes more.

Meanwhile, put the stock in a pot. Bring to a boil over medium heat, add the orzo and the lemon zest.

Bring to a simmer and cook for 10 minutes, fluff with a fork, and divide between plates.

Top each serving with the fish mix and serve.

Nutrition: Calories: 402; Fat: 21 g; Fiber: 8 g; Carbs: 21 g; Protein: 31 g.

921 BAKED SEA BASS

Preparation Time: 10 minutes
Cooking Time: 12 minutes
Servings: 4
Ingredients:

4 sea bass fillets, boneless
Sal and black pepper to the taste
2 cups potato chips, crushed
1 tbsp. mayonnaise

Directions:

Season the fish fillets with salt and pepper. Brush with the mayonnaise and dredge each in the potato chips.

Arrange the fillets on a baking sheet lined with parchment paper and bake at 400°F for 12 minutes.

Divide the fish between plates and serve with a side salad.

Nutrition: Calories: 228; Fat: 8.6 g; Fiber: 0.6 g; Carbs: 9.3 g; Protein: 25 g.

922 FISH AND TOMATO SAUCE

Preparation Time: 10 minutes
Cooking Time: 30 minutes
Servings: 4
Ingredients:

4 cod fillets, boneless
2 garlic cloves, minced
2 cups cherry tomatoes, halved
1 cup chicken stock
A pinch of salt and black pepper
¼ cup basil, chopped

Directions:

Put the tomatoes, garlic, salt and pepper in a pan, heat up over medium heat and cook for 5 minutes.

Add the fish and the rest of the ingredients, bring to a simmer, cover the pan and cook for 25 minutes.

Divide the mix between plates and serve.

Nutrition: Calories: 180; Fat: 1.9 g; Fiber: 1.4 g; Carbs: 5.3 g; Protein: 33.8 g.

923 HALIBUT AND QUINOA MIX

Preparation Time: 10 minutes
Cooking Time: 12 minutes
Servings: 4
Ingredients:

4 halibut fillets, boneless
2 tbsp. olive oil
1 tsp. rosemary, dried
2 tsp. cumin, ground

1 tbsp. coriander, ground
2 tsp. cinnamon powder
2 tsp. oregano, dried
A pinch of salt and black pepper
2 cups quinoa, cooked
1 cup cherry tomatoes, halved
1 avocado, peeled, pitted and sliced
1 cucumber, cubed
½ cup black olives, pitted and sliced
Juice of 1 lemon

Directions:

In a bowl, combine the fish with the rosemary, cumin, coriander, cinnamon, oregano, salt and pepper and toss.

Heat up a pan with the oil over medium heat. Add the fish, and sear for 2 minutes on each side. Introduce the pan in the oven and bake the fish at 425°F for 7 minutes.

Meanwhile, in a bowl, mix the quinoa with the remaining ingredients, toss and divide between plates.

Add the fish next to the quinoa mix and serve right away.

Nutrition: Calories: 364; Fat: 15.4 g; Fiber: 11.2 g; Carbs: 56.4 g; Protein: 24.5 g.

924 LEMON AND DATES BARRAMUNDI

Preparation Time: 10 minutes
Cooking Time: 12 minutes
Servings: 2
Ingredients:

2 barramundi fillets, boneless
1 shallot, sliced
4 lemon slices
Juice of ½ lemon
Zest of 1 lemon, grated
2 tbsp. olive oil
6 oz. baby spinach
¼ cup almonds, chopped
4 dates, pitted and chopped
¼ cup parsley, chopped
Salt and black pepper to the taste

Directions:

Season the fish with salt and pepper and arrange on 2 parchment paper pieces.

Top the fish with the lemon slices, drizzle the lemon juice, and then top with the other ingredients except for the oil.

Drizzle 1 tablespoon of oil over each fish mix, wrap the parchment paper around the fish shaping to packets and arrange them on a baking sheet.

Bake at 400°F for 12 minutes. Cool the mix a bit, unfold, divide everything between plates and serve.

Nutrition: Calories: 232; Fat: 16.5 g; Fiber: 11.1 g; Carbs: 24.8 g; Protein: 6.5 g.

925 FISH CAKES

Preparation Time: 10 minutes
Cooking Time: 10 minutes
Servings: 6
Ingredients:

20 oz. canned sardines, drained and mashed well
2 garlic cloves, minced
2 tbsp. dill, chopped
1 yellow onion, chopped
1 cup panko breadcrumbs
1 egg, whisked
A pinch of salt and black pepper
2 tbsp. lemon juice
5 tbsp. olive oil

Directions:

In a bowl, combine the sardines with the garlic, dill and the rest of the ingredients, except the oil. Stir well and shape medium cakes out of this mix.

Heat up a pan with the oil over medium-high heat. Add the fish cakes, cook for 5 minutes on each side.

Serve the cakes with a side salad.

Nutrition: Calories: 288; Fat: 12.8 g; Fiber: 10.2 g; Carbs: 22.2 g; Protein: 6.8 g.

926 CATFISH FILLETS AND RICE

Preparation Time: 10 minutes
Cooking Time: 55 minutes
Servings: 2
Ingredients:

2 catfish fillets, boneless
2 tbsp. Italian seasoning
2 tbsp. olive oil
For the rice:
1 cup brown rice
2 tbsp. olive oil
1 ½ cups water
½ cup green bell pepper, chopped
2 garlic cloves, minced
½ cup white onion, chopped
2 tsp. Cajun seasoning
½ tsp. garlic powder
Salt and black pepper to the taste

Directions:

Heat up a pot with 2 tablespoons of oil over medium heat. Add the onion, garlic, garlic powder, salt and pepper, and sauté for 5 minutes.

Add the rice, water, bell pepper and the seasoning. Bring to a simmer, and cook over medium heat for 40 minutes.

Heat up a pan with 2 tablespoons of oil over medium heat. Add the fish and the Italian seasoning. Cook for 5 minutes on each side.

Divide the rice between plates. Add the fish on top and serve.

Nutrition: Calories: 261; Fat: 17.6 g; Fiber: 12.2 g; Carbs: 24.8 g; Protein: 12.5 g.

927 HALIBUT PAN

Preparation Time: 10 minutes
Cooking Time: 20 minutes
Servings: 4
Ingredients:

4 halibut fillets, boneless
1 red bell pepper, chopped
2 tbsp. olive oil
1 yellow onion, chopped
4 garlic cloves, minced
½ cup chicken stock
1 tsp. basil, dried
½ cup cherry tomatoes, halved
⅓ cup kalamata olives, pitted and halved
Salt and black pepper to the taste

Directions:

Heat up a pan with the oil over medium heat. Add the fish, cook for 5 minutes on each side and divide between plates.

Add the onion, bell pepper, garlic and tomatoes to the pan. Stir and sauté for 3 minutes.

Add salt, pepper and the rest of the ingredients. Toss, cook for 3 minutes more, divide next to the fish and serve.

Nutrition: Calories: 253; Fat: 8 g; Fiber: 1 g; Carbs: 5 g; Protein: 28 g.

928 BAKED SHRIMP MIX

Preparation Time: 10 minutes
Cooking Time: 32 minutes
Servings: 4
Ingredients:

4 gold potatoes, peeled and sliced
2 fennel bulbs, trimmed and cut into wedges
2 shallots, chopped
2 garlic cloves, minced
3 tbsp. olive oil
½ cup kalamata olives, pitted and halved
2 lb. shrimp, peeled and deveined
1 tsp. lemon zest, grated
2 tsp. oregano, dried
4 oz. feta cheese, crumbled
2 tbsp. parsley, chopped

Directions:

In a roasting pan, combine the potatoes with 2 tablespoons of oil, garlic and the rest of the ingredients except the shrimp. Toss, introduce in the oven and bake at 450°F for 25 minutes.

Add the shrimp. Toss, bake for 7 minutes more, divide between plates and serve.

186

Nutrition: Calories: 341; Fat: 19 g; Fiber: 9 g; Carbs: 34 g; Protein: 10 g.

929 SHRIMP AND LEMON SAUCE

Preparation Time: 10 minutes
Cooking Time: 15 minutes
Servings: 4
Ingredients:

- 1 lb. shrimp, peeled and deveined
- ⅓ cup lemon juice
- 4 egg yolks
- 2 tbsp. olive oil
- 1 cup chicken stock
- Salt and black pepper to the taste
- 1 cup black olives, pitted and halved
- 1 tbsp. thyme, chopped

Directions:

In a bowl, mix the lemon juice with the egg yolks and whisk well.

Heat up a pan with the oil over medium heat. Add the shrimp and cook for 2 minutes on each side and transfer to a plate.

Heat up a pan with the stock over medium heat. Add some of this over the egg yolks and lemon juice mix and whisk well.

Add this over the rest of the stock. Also add salt and pepper. Whisk well and simmer for 2 minutes.

Add the shrimp and the rest of the ingredients. Toss and serve right away.

Nutrition: Calories: 237; Fat: 15.3 g; Fiber: 4.6 g; Carbs: 15.4 g; Protein: 7.6 g.

930 SHRIMP AND BEANS SALAD

Preparation Time: 10 minutes
Cooking Time: 4 minutes
Servings: 4
Ingredients:

- 1 lb. shrimp, peeled and deveined
- 30 oz. canned cannellini beans, drained and rinsed
- 2 tbsp. olive oil
- 1 cup cherry tomatoes, halved
- 1 tsp. lemon zest, grated
- ½ cup red onion, chopped
- 4 handfuls baby arugula
- A pinch of salt and black pepper

For the dressing:

- 3 tbsp. red wine vinegar
- 2 garlic cloves, minced
- ½ cup olive oil

Directions:

Heat up a pan with 2 tablespoons of oil over medium-high heat. Add the shrimp and cook for 2 minutes on each side.

In a salad bowl, combine the shrimp with the beans and the rest of the ingredients, except the ones for the dressing and toss.

In a separate bowl, combine the vinegar with ½ cup of oil and the garlic and whisk well.

Pour over the salad, toss and serve right away.

Nutrition: Calories: 207; Fat: 12.3 g; Fiber: 6.6 g; Carbs: 15.4 g; Protein: 8.7 g.

931 PECAN SALMON FILLETS

Preparation Time: 10 minutes
Cooking Time: 15 minutes
Servings: 6
Ingredients:

- 3 tbsp. olive oil
- 3 tbsp. mustard
- 5 tsp. honey
- 1 cup pecans, chopped
- 6 salmon fillets, boneless
- 1 tbsp. lemon juice
- 3 tsp. parsley, chopped
- Salt and pepper to the taste

Directions:

In a bowl, mix the oil with the mustard and honey and whisk well.

Put the pecans and the parsley in another bowl.

Season the salmon fillets with salt and pepper. Arrange them on a baking sheet lined with parchment paper. Brush with the honey and mustard mix. Top with the pecans mix.

Introduce in the oven at 400°F. Bake for 15 minutes and divide between plates. Drizzle the lemon juice on top and serve.

Nutrition: Calories: 282; Fat: 15.5 g; Fiber: 8.5 g; Carbs: 20.9 g; Protein: 16.8 g.

932 SALMON AND BROCCOLI

Preparation Time: 10 minutes
Cooking Time: 20 minutes
Servings: 4
Ingredients:

- 2 tbsp. balsamic vinegar
- 1 broccoli head, florets separated
- 4 pieces salmon fillets, skinless
- 1 big red onion, roughly chopped
- 1 tbsp. olive oil
- Sea salt and black pepper to the taste

Directions:

In a baking dish. Combine the salmon with the broccoli and the rest of the ingredients. Introduce in the oven and bake at 390°F for 20 minutes.

Divide the mix between plates and serve.

Nutrition: Calories: 302; Fat: 15.5 g; Fiber: 8.5 g; Carbs: 18.9 g; Protein: 19.8 g.

933 SALMON AND PEACH PAN

Preparation Time: 10 minutes
Cooking Time: 11 minutes

Servings: 4
Ingredients:

- 1 tbsp. balsamic vinegar
- 1 tsp. thyme, chopped
- 1 tbsp. ginger, grated
- 2 tbsp. olive oil
- Sea salt and black pepper to the taste
- 3 peaches, cut into medium wedges
- 4 salmon fillets, boneless

Directions:

Heat up a pan with the oil over medium-high heat. Add the salmon and cook for 3 minutes on each side.

Add the vinegar, the peaches and the rest of the ingredients. Cook for 5 minutes more; divide everything between plates and serve.

Nutrition: Calories: 293; Fat: 17.1 g; Fiber: 4.1 g; Carbs: 26.4 g; Protein: 24.5 g.

934 TARRAGON COD FILLETS

Preparation Time: 10 minutes
Cooking Time: 12 minutes
Servings: 4
Ingredients:

- 4 cod fillets, boneless
- ¼ cup capers, drained
- 1 tbsp. tarragon, chopped
- Sea salt and black pepper to the taste
- 2 tbsp. olive oil
- 2 tbsp. parsley, chopped
- 1 tbsp. olive oil
- 1 tbsp. lemon juice

Directions:

Heat up a pan with the oil over medium-high heat. Add the fish and cook for 3 minutes on each side.

Add the rest of the ingredients. Cook everything for 7 minutes more, divide between plates and serve.

Nutrition: Calories: 162; Fat: 9.6 g; Fiber: 4.3 g; Carbs: 12.4 g; Protein: 16.5 g.

935 SALMON AND RADISH MIX

Preparation Time: 10 minutes
Cooking Time: 15 minutes
Servings: 4
Ingredients:

- 2 tbsp. olive oil
- 1 tbsp. balsamic vinegar
- 1 ½ cups chicken stock
- 4 salmon fillets, boneless
- 2 garlic cloves, minced
- 1 tbsp. ginger, grated
- 1 cup radishes, grated
- ¼ cup scallions, chopped

Directions:

Heat up a pan with the oil over medium-high heat. Add the salmon, cook for 4 minutes on each side and divide between plates

Add the vinegar and the rest of the
ingredients to the pan. Toss
gently and cook for 10 minutes.
Pour over the salmon and serve.
Nutrition: Calories: 274; Fat: 14.5 g; Fiber:
3.5 g; Carbs: 8.5 g; Protein: 22.3 g.

936 SMOKED SALMON AND WATERCRESS SALAD

Preparation Time: 5 minutes
Cooking Time: 0 minutes
Servings: 4
Ingredients:
- 2 bunches watercress
- 1 lb. smoked salmon, skinless, boneless and flaked
- 2 tsp. mustard
- ¼ cup lemon juice
- ½ cup Greek yogurt
- Salt and black pepper to the taste
- 1 big cucumber, sliced
- 2 tbsp. chives, chopped

Directions:
In a salad bowl, combine the salmon
with the watercress and the rest
of the ingredients. Toss and serve
right away.
Nutrition: Calories: 244; Fat: 16.7 g; Fiber:
4.5 g; Carbs: 22.5 g; Protein: 15.6 g.

937 SALMON AND CORN SALAD

Preparation Time: 5 minutes
Cooking Time: 0 minutes
Servings: 4
Ingredients:
- ½ cup pecans, chopped
- 2 cups baby arugula
- 1 cup corn
- ¼ lb. smoked salmon, skinless, boneless and cut into small chunks
- 2 tbsp. olive oil
- 2 tbsp. lemon juice
- Sea salt and black pepper to the taste

Directions:
In a salad bowl, combine the salmon
with the corn and the rest of the
ingredients. Toss and serve right
away.
Nutrition: Calories: 284; Fat: 18.4 g; Fiber:
5.4 g; Carbs: 22.6 g; Protein: 17.4 g.

938 COD AND MUSHROOMS MIX

Preparation Time: 10 minutes
Cooking Time: 25 minutes
Servings: 4
Ingredients:
- 2 cod fillets, boneless
- 4 tbsp. olive oil
- 4 oz. mushrooms, sliced
- Sea salt and black pepper to the taste
- 12 cherry tomatoes, halved
- 8 oz. lettuce leaves, torn
- 1 avocado, pitted, peeled and cubed
- 1 red chili pepper, chopped
- 1 tbsp. cilantro, chopped
- 2 tbsp. balsamic vinegar
- 1 oz. feta cheese, crumbled

Directions:
Put the fish in a roasting pan. Brush it
with 2 tablespoons of oil, sprinkle
salt and pepper all over and broil
under medium-high heat for 15
minutes. Meanwhile, heat up a
pan with the rest of the oil over
medium heat. Add the
mushrooms, stir and sauté for 5
minutes.
Add the rest of the ingredients. Toss,
cook for 5 minutes more and
divide between plates.
Top with the fish and serve right away.
Nutrition: Calories: 257; Fat: 10 g; Fiber: 3.1
g; Carbs: 24.3 g; Protein: 19.4 g.

939 SESAME SHRIMP MIX

Preparation Time: 10 minutes
Cooking Time: 0 minutes
Servings: 4
Ingredients:
- 2 tbsp. lime juice
- 3 tbsp. teriyaki sauce
- 2 tbsp. olive oil
- 8 cups baby spinach
- 14 oz. shrimp, cooked, peeled and deveined
- 1 cup cucumber, sliced
- 1 cup radish, sliced
- ¼ cup cilantro, chopped
- 2 tsp. sesame seeds, toasted

Directions:
In a bowl, mix the shrimp with the lime
juice, spinach and the rest of the
ingredients. Toss and serve cold.
Nutrition: Calories: 177; Fat: 9 g; Fiber: 7.1
g; Carbs: 14.3 g; Protein: 9.4 g.

940 CREAMY CURRY SALMON

Preparation Time: 10 minutes
Cooking Time: 20 minutes
Servings: 2
Ingredients:
- 2 salmon fillets, boneless and cubed
- 1 tbsp. olive oil
- 1 tbsp. basil, chopped
- Sea salt and black pepper to the taste
- 1 cup Greek yogurt
- 2 tsp. curry powder
- 1 garlic clove, minced
- ½ tsp. mint, chopped

Directions:
Heat up a pan with the oil over
medium-high heat. Add the
salmon and cook for 3 minutes.
Add the rest of the ingredients. Toss,
cook for 15 minutes more. Divide
between plates and serve.

Nutrition: Calories: 284; Fat: 14.1 g; Fiber:
8.5 g; Carbs: 26.7 g; Protein: 31.4 g.

941 MAHI MIDSOLO AND POMEGRANATE SAUCE

Preparation Time: 10 minutes
Cooking Time: 10 minutes
Servings: 4
Ingredients:
- 1 ½ cups chicken stock
- 1 tbsp. olive oil
- 4 Mahi midsolo fillets, boneless
- 4 tbsp. tahini paste
- Juice of 1 lime
- Seeds from 1 pomegranate
- 1 tbsp. parsley, chopped

Directions:
Heat up a pan with the oil over
medium-high heat. Add the fish
and cook for 3 minutes on each
side.
Add the rest of the ingredients. Flip the
fish again, cook for 4 minutes
more. Divide everything between
plates and serve.
Nutrition: Calories: 224; Fat: 11.1; Fiber: 5.5;
Carbs: 16.7 g; Protein: 11.4 g.

942 SMOKED SALMON AND VEGGIES MIX

Preparation Time: 10 minutes
Cooking Time: 20 minutes
Servings: 4
Ingredients:
- 3 red onions, cut into wedges
- ¼ cup green olives, pitted and halved
- 3 red bell peppers, roughly chopped
- ½ tsp. smoked paprika
- Salt and black pepper to the taste
- 3 tbsp. olive oil
- 4 salmon fillets, skinless and boneless
- 2 tbsp. chives, chopped

Directions:
In a roasting pan, combine the salmon
with the onions and the rest of
the ingredients. Introduce in the
oven and bake at 390°F for 20
minutes.
Divide the mix between plates and
serve.
Nutrition: Calories: 301; Fat: 5.9 g; Fiber:
11.9 g; Carbs: 26.4 g; Protein: 22.4 g.

943 SALMON AND MANGO MIX

Preparation Time: 10 minutes
Cooking Time: 25 minutes
Servings: 2
Ingredients:
- 2 salmon fillets, skinless and boneless
- Salt and pepper to the taste
- 2 tbsp. olive oil
- 2 garlic cloves, minced
- 2 mangos, peeled and cubed
- 1 red chili, chopped

1 small piece ginger, grated
Juice of 1 lime
1 tbsp. cilantro, chopped

Directions:

In a roasting pan, combine the salmon with the oil, garlic and the rest of the ingredients, except the cilantro. Toss, introduce in the oven at 350°F and bake for 25 minutes.

Divide everything between plates and serve with the cilantro sprinkled on top.

Nutrition: Calories: 251; Fat: 15.9 g; Fiber: 5.9 g; Carbs: 26.4 g; Protein: 12.4 g.

944 SALMON AND CREAMY ENDIVES

Preparation Time: 10 minutes
Cooking Time: 15 minutes
Servings: 4
Ingredients:

4 salmon fillets, boneless
2 endives, shredded
Juice of 1 lime
Salt and black pepper to the taste
¼ cup chicken stock
1 cup Greek yogurt
¼ cup green olives pitted and chopped
¼ cup fresh chives, chopped
3 tbsp. olive oil

Directions:

Heat up a pan with half of the oil over medium heat. Add the endives and the rest of the ingredients, except the chives and the salmon. Toss, cook for 6 minutes and divide between plates.

Heat up another pan with the rest of the oil. Add the salmon, season with salt and pepper and cook for 4 minutes on each side. Add the creamy endives mix; sprinkle the chives on top and serve.

Nutrition: Calories: 266; Fat: 13.9 g; Fiber: 11.1 g; Carbs: 23.8 g; Protein: 17.5 g.

945 TROUT AND TZATZIKI SAUCE

Preparation Time: 10 minutes
Cooking Time: 10 minutes
Servings: 4
Ingredients:

Juice of ½ lime
Salt and black pepper to the taste
1 and ½ tsp. coriander, ground
1 tsp. garlic, minced
4 trout fillets, boneless
1 tsp. sweet paprika
2 tbsp. avocado oil

For the sauce:

1 cucumber, chopped
4 garlic cloves, minced
1 tbsp. olive oil
1 tsp. white vinegar
1 ½ cups Greek yogurt

A pinch of salt and white pepper

Directions:

1. Heat up a pan with the avocado oil over medium-high heat. Add the fish, salt, pepper, lime juice, 1 teaspoon of garlic and the paprika. Rub the fish gently and cook for 4 minutes on each side.
2. In a bowl, combine the cucumber with 4 garlic cloves and the rest of the ingredients for the sauce. Whisk well.
3. Divide the fish between plates. Drizzle the sauce all over and serve with a side salad.

Nutrition: Calories: 393; Fat: 18.5 g; Fiber: 6.5 g; Carbs: 18.3 g; Protein: 39.6 g.

946 PARSLEY TROUT AND CAPERS

Preparation Time: 10 minutes
Cooking Time: 10 minutes
Servings: 4
Ingredients:

4 trout fillets, boneless
3 oz. tomato sauce
A handful parsley, chopped
2 tbsp. olive oil
Salt and black pepper to the taste 3 oz. tomato sauce

Directions:

1. Heat up a pan with the oil over medium-high heat. Add the fish, salt and pepper and cook for 3 minutes on each side.
2. Add the rest of the ingredients. Cook everything for 4 minutes more.
3. Divide everything between plates and serve.

Nutrition: Calories: 308; Fat: 17 g; Fiber: 1 g; Carbs: 3 g; Protein: 16 g.

947 BAKED TROUT AND FENNEL

Preparation Time: 10 minutes
Cooking Time: 22 minutes
Servings: 4
Ingredients:

1 fennel bulb, sliced
2 tbsp. olive oil
1 yellow onion, sliced
3 tsp. Italian seasoning
4 rainbow trout fillets, boneless
¼ cup panko breadcrumbs
½ cup kalamata olives, pitted and halved
Juice of 1 lemon

Directions:

1. Spread the fennel the onion and the rest of the ingredients, except the trout and the breadcrumbs, on a baking sheet lined with parchment paper. Toss them and cook at 400°F for 10 minutes.

2. Add the fish dredged in breadcrumbs and seasoned with salt and pepper. Cook it at 400°F for 6 minutes on each side.
3. Divide the mix between plates and serve.

Nutrition: Calories: 306; Fat: 8.9 g; Fiber: 11.1 g; Carbs: 23.8 g; Protein: 14.5 g.

948 LEMON RAINBOW TROUT

Preparation Time: 10 minutes
Cooking Time: 15 minutes
Servings: 2
Ingredients:

2 rainbow trout
Juice of 1 lemon
3 tbsp. olive oil
4 garlic cloves, minced
A pinch of salt and black pepper

Directions:

1. Line a baking sheet with parchment paper. Add the fish and the rest of the ingredients and rub.
2. Bake at 400°F for 15 minutes. Divide between plates and serve with a side salad.

Nutrition: Calories: 321; Fat: 19 g; Fiber: 5 g; Carbs: 6 g; Protein: 35 g.

949 FAVORITE GREEK SALMON

Preparation Time: 10 minutes
Cooking Time: 7 hours
Servings: 6
Ingredients:

1 cup homemade chicken broth
2 tbsp. fresh lemon juice
¼ cup fresh dill, chopped
6 (4-oz.) salmon fillets
Salt and freshly ground black pepper, to taste
2 cups water

Directions:

1. In the pot of crockpot, mix together the 2 cups. of water, broth, lemon juice and dill.
2. Arrange the salmon fillets on top, skin side down and sprinkle with cayenne pepper, salt and black pepper.
3. Set the crockpot on "Low" and cook, covered for about 1-2 hours.
4. Uncover the crockpot and serve hot.

Nutrition: Calories: 164; Carbohydrates: 1.6 g; Protein: 23.3 g; Fat: 7.4 g; Sugar: 0 g.

950 CITRUS FLAVORED SALMON

Preparation Time: 10 minutes
Cooking Time: 7 hours
Servings: 6
Ingredients:

¾ cup fresh cilantro leaves, chopped

2 garlic cloves, chopped finely
2-3 tbsp. fresh lime juice
Salt, to taste
1 lb. salmon fillets

Directions:
1. In a medium bowl, add all the ingredients, except for salmon fillets and mix well.
2. In the bottom of a greased crockpot, place the salmon fillets and top with garlic mixture.
3. Set the crockpot on "Low" and cook, covered, for about 2-2 ½ hours.
4. Uncover the crockpot and serve.

Nutrition: Calories: 154; Carbohydrates: 0.7 g; Protein: 22.2 g; Fat: 7 g; Sugar: 0.1 g; Fiber: 0.1g.

951 LIVELY FLAVORED SALMON

Preparation Time: 10 minutes
Cooking Time: 4 hours
Servings: 8
Ingredients:
2 (4-oz.) salmon fillets
½ cup scallions, thinly sliced
1 cup fresh mushrooms, sliced
Salt and freshly ground black pepper, to taste
3 cup homemade fish broth

Directions:
1. In the pot of crockpot, place the ingredients and stir to combine.
2. Set the crockpot on "Low" and cook, covered, for about 1-2 hours.
3. Uncover the crockpot and serve hot.

Nutrition: Calories: 225; Carbohydrates: 1.5 g; Protein: 54.7 g; Fat: 10 g; Sugar: 1.2 g; Fiber: 1 g.

952 SIMPLY DELICIOUS TILAPIA

Preparation Time: 10 minutes
Cooking Time: 7 hours
Servings: 6
Ingredients:
4 tilapia fillets
Salt and freshly ground black pepper, to taste
2 tbsp. unsalted butter, cubed
1 lemon, cut into slices

Directions:
1. In the pot of crockpot, place the tilapia fillets and sprinkle with salt and black pepper.
2. Top with butter, followed by the lemon.
3. Set the crockpot on "Low" and cook, covered for about 1 ½ hours.
4. Uncover the crockpot and serve hot.

Nutrition: Calories: 169; Carbohydrates: 0.4 g; Protein: 26.5 g; Fat: 7.1 g; Sugar: 0.1 g; Fiber: 0.1 g.

953 AROMATIC TILAPIA

Preparation Time: 10 minutes
Cooking Time: 7 hours
Servings: 6
Ingredients:
6 (4-oz.) tilapia fillets
Sea salt and freshly ground black pepper, to taste
½ cup onion, chopped
¼ cup fresh parsley, chopped
2 tbsp. unsalted butter, melted

Directions:
1. Grease a crockpot.
2. Sprinkle the tilapia fillets with salt and black pepper generously.
3. Place onion and parsley over fillets evenly.
4. Drizzle with melted butter.
5. Set the crockpot on "Low" and cook, covered for about 1 ½ hours.
6. Uncover the crockpot and serve hot.

Nutrition: Calories: 133; Carbohydrates: 1.3 g; Protein: 21.3 g; Fat: 5 g; Sugar: 0 g; Fiber: 0 g.

954 RICHLY DELICIOUS TILAPIA

Preparation Time: 10 minutes
Cooking Time: 7 hours
Servings: 6
Ingredients:
½ cup Parmesan cheese, grated
¼ cup mayonnaise
¼ cup fresh lemon juice
Salt and freshly ground black pepper, to taste
4 (4-oz.) tilapia fillets

Directions:
1. In a bowl, mix together all ingredients, except tilapia fillets and cilantro.
2. Coat the fillets with the mayonnaise mixture evenly.
3. Place the filets over a large piece of foil.
4. Wrap the foil around fillets to seal them.
5. Arrange the foil packet in the bottom of the crockpot.
6. Set the crockpot on "Low" and cook, covered, for about 3-4 hours.
7. Uncover the crockpot and transfer the foil parcel onto a platter.
8. Carefully, open the parcel and serve hot

Nutrition: Calories: 190; Carbohydrates: 3.9 g; Protein: 25.4 g; Fat: 8.5 g; Sugar: 1.3 g; Fiber: 0.1 g.

955 NO-FUSS SARDINE

Preparation Time: 10 minutes
Cooking Time: 7 hours
Servings: 6
Ingredients:
2 lb. fresh sardines, cubed
4 plum tomatoes, chopped finely
1 large onion, sliced
1 cup sugar-free tomato puree
Salt and freshly ground black pepper, to taste

Directions:
1. Grease the crockpot
2. In the prepared crockpot, place the sardine cubes and top with remaining all ingredients.
3. Set the crockpot on "Low" and cook, covered for about 8 hours.
4. Uncover the crockpot and serve hot.

Nutrition: Calories: 269; Carbohydrates: 0 g; Protein: 7.7 g; Fat: 13.2 g; Sugar: 4 g; Fiber: 1.7 g.

956 SPANISH STYLE SARDINE

Preparation Time: 10 minutes
Cooking Time: 7 hours
Servings: 6
Ingredients:
3 large carrots peeled, cut into thin discs
2 ¼ lb. sardine, heads, tails, and gut removed
1 cup olive oil
1 cup homemade fish broth
Salt and freshly ground black pepper, to taste

Directions:
1. In the pot of a crockpot, place the carrots and top with sardine.
2. Drizzle with oil and sprinkle with salt and black pepper.
3. Set the crockpot on "Low" and cook, covered for about 8 hours.
4. Uncover the crockpot and serve hot.

Nutrition: Calories: 425; Carbohydrates: 7 g; Protein: 29.4 g; Fat: 21.5 g; Sugar: 4.8 g; Fiber: 1.7 g.

957 MOUTH-WATERING TUNA

Preparation Time: 10 minutes
Cooking Time: 7 hours
Servings: 6
Ingredients:
2 tbsp. olive oil
4-5 garlic cloves, chopped finely
1 small jalapeño pepper, chopped finely
Salt and freshly ground black pepper, to taste

¾ lb. fresh tuna, cut into 1-inch cubes

Directions:

1. In the pot of crockpot, add all the ingredients, except for tuna and stir to combine.
2. Set the crockpot on "Low" and cook, covered, for about 4 hours.
3. Uncover the crockpot and stir in the tuna cubes.
4. Set the crockpot on "High" and cook, covered, for about 15 minutes.
5. Uncover the crockpot and stir the mixture.
6. Serve hot.

Nutrition: Calories: 326; Carbohydrates: 2 g; Protein: 43.8 g; Fat: 15.4 g; Sugar: 0.1 g.

958 SATISFYING HALIBUT MEAL

Preparation Time: 10 minutes
Cooking Time: 7 hours
Servings: 6
Ingredients:

1 ½ lb. halibut, cubed
¾ cup yellow onion, sliced thinly
½ cup homemade chicken broth
Salt and ground black pepper, as required
1 ½ cup Kalamata olives, pitted and halved

Directions:

1. In the pot of crockpot, add all the ingredients, except for olives, and stir to combine.
2. Set the crockpot on "Low" and cook, covered, for about 1 ½ hours.
3. Uncover the crockpot and stir in the olives.
4. Set the crockpot on "Low" and cook, covered, for about 30 minutes.
5. Uncover the crockpot and serve hot.

Nutrition: Calories: 196; Carbohydrates: 3.5 g; Protein: 31.9 g; Fat: 6.4 g; Sugar: 0.7 g.

959 BOLD FLAVORED HALIBUT

Preparation Time: 10 minutes
Cooking Time: 7 hours
Servings: 6
Ingredients:

12 oz. halibut fillet
Salt and freshly ground black pepper, to taste
1 tbsp. balsamic vinegar
1 tbsp. butter, melted
1 ½ tsp. dried parsley

Directions:

1. Arrange a large 18-inch piece of greased piece foil onto a smooth surface.
2. Season the halibut fillet with salt and black pepper.
3. In a small bowl, add the lemon juice, oil and dill and mix well.
4. Place the halibut fillet in the center of foil and drizzle with the oil mixture.
5. Carefully bring up the edges of the foil and crimp them together, leaving plenty of air inside of the foil packet.
6. Place the foil packet in the bottom of a crockpot.
7. Set the crockpot on "High" and cook, covered, for about 1 ½-2 hours.
8. Uncover the crockpot and remove the foil packet.
9. Carefully open the foil packet and serve.

Nutrition: Calories: 242; Carbohydrates: 0.1 g; Protein: 35.9 g; Fat: 9.8 g; Sugar: 0 g.

960 MIDWEEK DINNER HALIBUT

Preparation Time: 10 minutes
Cooking Time: 5 hours
Servings: 8
Ingredients:

1 (15-oz.) can diced tomatoes
1 large green bell pepper, seeded and chopped
1 lb. halibut fillets
Salt and freshly ground black pepper, to taste
⅓ cup homemade chicken broth

Directions:

1. Grease the pot of crockpot.
2. In the pot of crockpot, place the tomatoes and bell pepper.
3. Place the fish fillets on top of the tomato mixture and sprinkle with salt and black pepper.
4. Place the broth on top evenly.
5. Set the crockpot on "High" and cook, covered, for about 3-4 hours.
6. Uncover the crockpot and serve hot.

Nutrition: Calories: 156; Carbohydrates: 3 g; Protein: 25.6 g; Fat: 3 g; Sugar: 3.8 g.

961 DELICATE COD DISH

Preparation Time: 10 minutes
Cooking Time: 7 hours
Servings: 6
Ingredients:

1 lb. cod fillets, cubed
1 small onion, sliced
½ cup fish broth
Salt and black pepper, to taste
2 large tomatoes, cut into quarters

Directions:

1. In the pot of a crockpot, add cod cubes, onion, garlic and broth and stir to combine.

2. Set the crockpot on "Low" and cook, covered, for about 2 hours.
3. During the last 30 minutes of cooking, stir in the tomatoes.

Nutrition: Calories: 119; Carbohydrates: 5.2 g; Protein: 21.9 g; Fat: 1.5 g; Sugar: 3.1 g.

962 VERSATILE COD

Preparation Time: 10 minutes
Cooking Time: 7 hours
Servings: 6
Ingredients:

1 lb. cod fillets, cubed
1 medium onion, chopped
2 red bell peppers, seeded and cubed
½ cup homemade fish broth
Salt and freshly ground black pepper, to taste

Directions:

1. In the pot of crockpot, add all the ingredients and stir to combine.
2. Set the crockpot on "Low" and cook, covered, for about 6 hours.
3. Uncover the crockpot and serve hot.

Nutrition: Calories: 119; Carbohydrates: 5 g; Protein: 21.7 g; Fat: 1.4 g; Sugar: 2.6 g.

963 FANCY BRAESIDE SHRIMP

Preparation Time: 10 minutes
Cooking Time: 2 hours
Servings: 6
Ingredients:

1 lb. raw shrimp, peeled and deveined
¼ cup homemade chicken broth
3 tbsp. olive oil
1 tbsp. fresh lime juice
Salt and freshly ground black pepper, to taste

Directions:

1. In a crockpot, place all the ingredients and stir to combine.
2. Set the crockpot on "High" and cook, covered, for about 1½ hours.
3. Uncover the crockpot and stir the mixture.
4. Serve hot.

Nutrition: Calories: 227; Carbohydrates: 1.8 g; Protein: 26.1 g; Fat: 12.5 g; Sugar: 0 g.

964 ENJOYABLE SHRIMP

Preparation Time: 10 minutes
Cooking Time: 7 hours
Servings: 6
Ingredients:

3 cups green bell pepper, seeded and sliced
2 cups tomatoes, chopped finely
1 cup sugar-free tomato sauce
Salt and freshly ground black pepper, to taste
1 ¾ lb. large shrimp, peeled and deveined

Directions:

1. In a crockpot, add all ingredients, except shrimp, and stir to combine.
2. Set the crockpot on "High" and cook, covered, for about 2-3 hours.
3. Uncover the crockpot and stir in the shrimp.
4. Set the crockpot on "High" and cook, covered, for about 30 minutes.
5. Uncover the crockpot and serve hot.

Nutrition: Calories: 118; Carbohydrates: 3 g; Protein: 22.5 g; Fat: 0.2 g; Sugar: 3.3 g.

965 OUTSTANDING SHRIMP MEAL

Preparation Time: 10 minutes
Cooking Time: 7 hours
Servings: 6
Ingredients:

- 1 (14-oz.) can sugar-free peeled tomatoes, chopped finely
- 4 oz. canned sugar-free tomato paste
- 2 tbsp. fresh parsley, chopped
- Salt and ground black pepper, as required
- 2 lb. cooked shrimp, peeled and deveined

Directions:

1. In the pot of crockpot, add all the ingredients except for shrimp and stir to combine.
2. Set the crockpot on "Low" and cook, covered for about 6-7 hours.
3. Uncover the crockpot and stir in the shrimp.
4. Set the crockpot on "High" and cook, covered, for about 15 minutes.
5. Uncover the crockpot and serve hot.

Nutrition: Calories: 199; Carbohydrates: 2.5 g; Protein: 35.4 g; Fat: 2.7 g; Sugar: 2.7 g.

966 BUTTERED SHRIMP

Preparation Time: 10 minutes
Cooking Time: 15 minutes
Servings: 6
Ingredients:

- 8 garlic cloves, chopped
- ¼ cup fresh cilantro, chopped
- ⅓ cup unsalted butter
- Salt and freshly ground black pepper, to taste
- 2 lb. extra-large shrimp, peeled and deveined

Directions:

1. In a crockpot, add all ingredients except shrimp and stir to combine.

2. Set the crockpot on "High" and cook, covered, for about 30 minutes.
3. Uncover the crockpot and stir in shrimp.
4. Set the crockpot on "High" and cook, covered, for about 20 minutes.
5. Uncover the crockpot and serve hot.

Nutrition: Calories: 276; Carbohydrates: 0 g; Protein: 34.8 g; Fat: 12.8 g; Sugar: 0.1 g.

967 FLAVORFUL SHRIMP CURRY

Preparation Time: 10 minutes
Cooking Time: 2 hours
Servings: 6
Ingredients:

- 3 cups tomatoes, chopped finely
- 1 ½ cups small cauliflower florets
- 1 cup unsweetened coconut milk
- Salt and freshly ground black pepper, to taste
- 1 ½ lb. shrimp, peeled and deveined

Directions:

1. In the pot of crockpot, add all the ingredients, except for shrimp, and stir to combine.
2. Set the crockpot on "High" and cook, covered, for about 80 minutes.
3. Uncover the crockpot and stir in shrimp.
4. Set the crockpot on "High" and cook, covered, for about 40 minutes.
5. Uncover the crockpot and serve hot.

Nutrition: Calories: 165; Carbohydrates: 6.9 g; Protein: 27.1 g; Fat: 2.8 g; Sugar: 3 g.

968 MAHI TACO WRAPS

Preparation Time: 5 minutes
Cooking Time: 2 hours
Servings: 6
Ingredients:

- 1 pound Mahi, wild-caught
- ½ cup cherry tomatoes
- 1 small green bell pepper, cored and sliced
- ¼ of a medium red onion, thinly sliced
- ½ tsp. garlic powder
- 1 tsp. sea salt
- ½ tsp. ground black pepper
- 1 tsp. chipotle pepper
- ½ tsp. dried oregano
- 1 tsp. cumin
- 1 tbsp. avocado oil
- ¼ cup chicken stock
- 1 medium avocado, diced
- 1 cup sour cream
- 6 large lettuce leaves

Directions:

1. Grease a 6-quarts slow cooker with oil. Place fish in it and then pour in chicken stock.
2. Stir together garlic powder, salt, black pepper, chipotle pepper, oregano and cumin; and then season fish with half of this mixture.
3. Layer fish with tomatoes, pepper and onion. Season with remaining spice mixture and shut with lid.
4. Plug in the slow cooker and cook fish for 2 hours at a high heat setting or until cooked through.
5. When done, evenly spoon fish among lettuce. Top with avocado and sour cream and serve.

Nutrition: Calories: 260; Fat: 15.1 g; Protein: 27.8 g; Carbs: 1.9 g; Fiber: 2.2 g; Sugar: 3 g.

969 SALMON

Preparation Time: 5 minutes
Cooking Time: 5 minutes
Servings: 4
Ingredients:

- 3 lemons, sliced
- ¼ cup water
- 4 Salmon fillets
- 1 bunch of dill weed, fresh
- 1 tbsp. butter, unsalted
- ¼ tsp. salt
- ¼ tsp. ground black pepper

Directions:

1. Switch on the instant pot. Pour in water, stir in lemon juice, and insert a steel steamer rack.
2. Place salmon on the steamer rack. Sprinkle with dill and then top with lemon slices.
3. Press the 'keep warm' button. Shut the instant pot with its lid in the sealed position. Then press the 'manual' button. Press '+/-' to set the cooking time to 5 minutes, and cook at a high-pressure setting; when the pressure builds in the pot, the cooking timer will start.
4. When the instant pot buzzes, press the 'keep warm' button. Do a quick pressure release and open the lid.
5. Remove and discard the lemon slices. Transfer salmon to a dish. Season with salt and black pepper, garnish with more dill and serve with lemon wedges and cauliflower rice.

Nutrition: Calories: 199.2; Fat: 8.1 g; Protein: 29.2 g; Carbs: 0.8 g; Fiber: 0.1 g.

970 SHRIMP TACOS

Preparation Time: 5 minutes
Cooking Time: 3 hours
Servings: 6
Ingredients:

- 1 pound medium wild-caught shrimp, peeled and tails off
- 12-oz. fire-roasted tomatoes, diced
- 1 small green bell pepper, chopped
- ½ cup chopped white onion
- 1 tsp. minced garlic
- ½ tsp. sea salt
- ½ tsp. ground black pepper
- ½ tsp. red chili powder
- ½ tsp. cumin
- ¼ tsp. cayenne pepper
- 2 tbsp. avocado oil
- ½ cup salsa
- 4 tbsp. chopped cilantro
- 1 ½ cup sour cream
- 2 medium avocados, diced

Directions:

1. Rinse shrimps, layer into a 6-quarts slow cooker and drizzle with oil.
2. Add tomatoes. Stir until mixed. Then add peppers and remaining ingredients, except for sour cream and avocado, and stir until combined.
3. Plug in the slow cooker. Shut with lid, and cook for 2 to 3 hours at low heat setting or 1 hour and 30 minutes to 2 hours at high heat setting, or until shrimps turn pink.
4. When done, serve shrimps with avocado and sour cream.

Nutrition: Calories: 324; Fat: 12 g; Protein: 28 g; Carbs: 4.2 g; Fiber: 13 Sugar: 2 g.

971 FISH CURRY

Preparation Time: 5 minutes
Cooking Time: 4 hours
Servings: 6
Ingredients:

- 2.2 pounds wild-caught white fish fillet, cubed
- 18-oz. spinach leaves
- 4 tbsp. red curry paste, organic
- 14-oz. coconut cream, unsweetened and full-fat
- 14-oz. water

Directions:

1. Plug in a 6-quart slow cooker and let preheat at a high heat setting.
2. In the meantime, whisk together coconut cream and water until smooth.
3. Place fish into the slow cooker. Spread with curry paste and then pour in coconut cream mixture.
4. Shut with lid and cook for 2 hours at high heat setting or 4 hours at low heat setting until tender.
5. Then add spinach and continue cooking for 20 to 30 minutes, or until spinach leaves wilt.
6. Serve straightaway.

Nutrition: Calories: 129; Fat: 6 g; Protein: 12 g; Carbs: 4.8 g; Fiber: 10 g; Sugar: 6 g.

972 SALMON WITH CREAMY LEMON SAUCE

Preparation Time: 5 minutes
Cooking Time: 2 hours
Servings: 6
Ingredients:
For the Salmon:

- 2 pounds wild-caught salmon fillet, skin-on
- 1 tsp. garlic powder
- 1 ½ tsp. salt
- 1 tsp. ground black pepper
- ½ tsp. red chili powder
- 1 tsp. Italian Seasoning
- 1 lemon, sliced
- 1 lemon, juiced
- 2 tbsp. avocado oil
- 1 cup chicken broth

For the Creamy Lemon Sauce:

- Chopped parsley, for garnish
- ⅛ tsp. lemon zest
- ¼ cup heavy cream
- ¼ cup grated parmesan cheese

Directions:

1. Line a 6-quart slow cooker with a parchment sheet. Spread its bottom with lemon slices, then top with salmon and drizzle with oil.
2. Stir together garlic powder, salt, black pepper, red chili powder, Italian seasoning, and oil until combined and rub this mixture all over salmon.
3. Pour lemon juice and broth around the fish and shut with lid.
4. Plug in the slow cooker and cook for 2 hours at a low heat setting.
5. In the meantime, set the oven at 400°F and let preheat.
6. When fish is done, lift out an inner pot of slow cooker. Place into the oven and cook for 5 to 8 minutes, or until the top is nicely browned.
7. Lift out fish using a parchment sheet and keep it warm.
8. Transfer juices from slow cooker to a medium skillet pan. Place it over medium-high heat; then bring to boil and cook for 1 minute.
9. Turn heat to a low level. Whisk the cream into the sauce along with lemon zest and parmesan cheese and cook for 2 to 3 minutes or until thickened.
10. Cut salmon in pieces. Then top each piece with lemon sauce and serve.

Nutrition: Calories: 364; Fat: 19 g; Protein: 12.9 g; Carbs: 3.8 g; Fiber: 7 g; Sugar: 9 g.

973 SALMON WITH LEMON-CAPER SAUCE

Preparation Time: 5 minutes
Cooking Time: 1 hour
Servings: 4
Ingredients:

- 1 pound wild-caught salmon fillet
- 2 tsp. capers, rinsed and mashed
- 1 tsp. minced garlic
- 1 tsp. salt
- ½ tsp. ground black pepper
- ½ tsp. dried oregano
- 1 tsp. lemon zest
- 2 tbsp. lemon juice
- 4 tbsp. unsalted butter

Directions:

1. Cut salmon into 4 pieces. Then season with salt and black pepper and sprinkle lemon zest on top.
2. Line a 6-quart slow cooker with parchment paper. Place seasoned salmon pieces on it and shut with a lid.
3. Plug in the slow cooker and cook for 1 hour and 30 minutes, or until salmon is cooked through.
4. When 10 minutes of cooking time is left, prepare lemon-caper sauce. For this, place a small saucepan over low heat; add butter and let it melt.
5. Then add capers, garlic, and lemon juice. Stir until mixed and simmer for 1 minute.
6. Remove saucepan from heat and stir in oregano.
7. When salmon is cooked, spoon lemon-caper sauce on it and serve.

Nutrition: Calories: 421; Fat: 11 g; Protein: 13.8 g; Carbs: 2.4 g; Fiber: 7 g; Sugar: 8 g.

974 SPICY BARBECUE SHRIMP

Preparation Time: 5 minutes
Cooking Time: 1 hour
Servings: 6
Ingredients:

- 1 ½ pounds large wild-caught shrimp, unpeeled
- 1 green onion, chopped
- 1 tsp. minced garlic
- 1 ½ tsp. salt
- ¾ tsp. ground black pepper

1 tsp. Cajun seasoning
1 tbsp. hot pepper sauce
¼ cup Worcestershire Sauce
1 lemon, juiced
2 tbsp. avocado oil
½ cup unsalted butter, chopped

Directions:
1. Place all the ingredients, except for shrimps, in a 6-quart slow cooker and whisk until mixed.
2. Plug in the slow cooker, then shut with lid and cook for 30 minutes at high heat setting.
3. Then take out ½ cup of this sauce and reserve.
4. Add shrimps to the slow cooker.

Nutrition: Calories: 313; Fat: 15 g; Protein: 13.8 g; Carbs: 2.6 g; Fiber: 7 g; Sugar: 7 g.

975 LEMON DILL HALIBUT

Preparation Time: 5 minutes
Cooking Time: 2 hours
Servings: 6
Ingredients:

12-oz. wild-caught halibut fillet
1 tsp. salt
½ tsp. ground black pepper
1 ½ tsp. dried dill
1 tbsp. fresh lemon juice
3 tbsp. avocado oil

Directions:
1. Cut an 18-inch piece of aluminum foil. Place halibut fillet in the middle and then season with salt and black pepper.
2. Whisk together remaining ingredients. Drizzle this mixture over halibut, then crimp the edges of foil and place it into a 6-quart slow cooker.
3. Plug in the slow cooker. Shut with lid and cook for 1 hour and 30 minutes, or 2 hours at high heat setting or until cooked through.
4. When done, carefully open the crimped edges and check the fish. It should be tender and flaky.
5. Serve straightaway.

Nutrition: Calories: 312; Fat: 15 g; Protein: 13.8 g; Carbs: 0 g; Fiber: 7 g; Sugar: 0 g.

976 COCONUT CILANTRO CURRY SHRIMP

Preparation Time: 5 minutes
Cooking Time: 2 hours
Servings: 4
Ingredients:

1 pound wild-caught shrimp, peeled and deveined
2 ½ tsp. lemon garlic seasoning
2 tbsp. red curry paste
4 tbsp. chopped cilantro
30 oz. coconut milk, unsweetened

16 oz. water

Directions:
1. Whisk together all the ingredients, except for shrimps, and 2 tablespoons of cilantro and add to a 4-quart slow cooker.
2. Plug in the slow cooker. Shut with lid, and cook for 2 hours at high heat setting, or 4 hours at low heat setting.
3. Then add shrimps. Toss until evenly coated and cook for 20 to 30 minutes at high heat settings, or until shrimps are pink.
4. Garnish shrimps with remaining cilantro and serve.

Nutrition: Calories: 213; Fat: 12 g; Protein: 15 g; Carbs: 1.9 g; Fiber: 7 g; Sugar: 1.4 g.

977 SHRIMP IN MARINARA SAUCE

Preparation Time: 5 minutes
Cooking Time: 5 hours
Servings: 5
Ingredients:

1 pound cooked wild-caught shrimps, peeled and deveined
14.5 oz. crushed tomatoes
½ tsp. minced garlic
1 tsp. salt
½ tsp. seasoned salt
¼ tsp. ground black pepper
½ tsp. crushed red pepper flakes
½ tsp. dried basil
½ tsp. dried oregano
½ tbsp. avocado oil
6-oz. chicken broth
2 tbsp. minced parsley
½ cup grated Parmesan cheese

Directions:
1. Place all the ingredients, except for shrimps, parsley, and cheese, in a 4-quart slow cooker and stir well.
2. Then plug in the slow cooker. Shut with lid and cook for 4 to 5 hours at low heat setting.
3. Then add shrimps and parsley. Stir until mixed and cook for 10 minutes at high heat setting.
4. Garnish shrimps with cheese and serve.

Nutrition: Calories: 213; Fat: 12 g; Protein: 15 g; Carbs: 3.9 g; Fiber: 7 g; Sugar: 3.6 g.

978 GARLIC SHRIMP

Preparation Time: 5 minutes
Cooking Time: 5 hours
Servings: 5
Ingredients:
For the Garlic Shrimp:
1 ½ pounds large wild-caught shrimp, peeled and deveined
¼ tsp. ground black pepper
⅛ tsp. ground cayenne pepper

2 ½ tsp. minced garlic
¼ cup avocado oil
4 tbsp. unsalted butter
For the Seasoning:
1 tsp. onion powder
1 tbsp. garlic powder
1 tbsp. salt
2 tsp. ground black pepper
1 tbsp. paprika
1 tsp. cayenne pepper
1 tsp. dried oregano
1 tsp. dried thyme

Directions:
1. Stir together all the ingredients for seasoning, garlic, oil, and butter, and add to a 4-quart slow cooker.
2. Plug in the slow cooker. Shut with lid, and cook for 25 to 30 minutes at high heat setting, or until cooked.
3. Then add shrimps. Toss until evenly coated, and continue cooking for 20 to 30 minutes at high heat setting or until shrimps are pink.
4. When done, transfer shrimps to a serving plate. Top with sauce and serve.

Nutrition: Calories: 227; Fat: 13 g; Protein: 21 g; Carbs: 1.2 g; Fiber: 7 g; Sugar: 5 g.

979 POACHED SALMON

Preparation Time: 5 minutes
Cooking Time: 3 hours
Servings: 4
Ingredients:

4 steaks of wild-caught salmon
1 medium white onion, peeled and sliced
2 tsp. minced garlic
½ tsp. salt
⅛ tsp. ground white pepper
½ tsp. dried dill weed
2 tbsp. avocado oil
2 tbsp. unsalted butter
2 tbsp. lemon juice
1 cup water

Directions:
1. Place butter in a 4-quart slow cooker. Then add salmon and drizzle with oil.
2. Place remaining ingredients in a medium saucepan. Stir until mixed and bring the mixture to boil over high heat.
3. Then pour this mixture all over salmon and shut with a lid.
4. Plug in the slow cooker and cook salmon for 3 hours and 30 minutes at low heat setting, or until salmon is tender.
5. Serve straightaway.

Nutrition: Calories: 338; Fat: 11 g; Protein: 13 g; Carbs: 2.8 g; Fiber: 7 g; Sugar: 1.2 g.

980 LEMON PEPPER TILAPIA

Preparation Time: 5 minutes
Cooking Time: 3 hours
Servings: 6
Ingredients:

- 6 wild-caught Tilapia fillets
- 4 tsp. lemon-pepper seasoning, divided
- 6 tbsp. unsalted butter, divided
- ½ cup lemon juice, fresh

Directions:

1. Cut a large piece of aluminum foil for each fillet and then arrange them in a clean working space.
2. Place each fillet in the middle of the foil, then season with lemon-pepper seasoning. Drizzle with lemon juice and top with 1 tbsp. of butter.
3. Gently crimp the edges of foil to form a packet and place it into a 6-quart slow cooker.
4. Plug in the slow cooker. Shut with lid, and cook for 3 hours at high heat setting, or until cooked through.
5. When done, carefully remove packets from the slow cooker and open the crimped edges and check the fish. It should be tender and flaky.
6. Serve straightaway.

Nutrition: Calories: 321; Fat: 10 g; Protein: 21 g; Carbs: 1.2 g; Fiber: 7 g; Sugar: 1.8 g.

981 CLAM CHOWDER

Preparation Time: 5 minutes
Cooking Time: 6 hours
Servings: 6
Ingredients:

- 20-oz. wild-caught baby clams, with juice
- ½ cup chopped scallion
- ½ cup chopped celery
- 1 tsp. salt
- 1 tsp. ground black pepper
- 1 tsp. dried thyme
- 1 tbsp. avocado oil
- 2 cups coconut cream, full-fat
- 2 cups chicken broth

Directions:

1. Grease a 6-quart slow cooker with oil, then add ingredients and stir until mixed.
2. Plug in the slow cooker, shut with lid, and cook for 4 to 6 hours at low heat setting, or until cooked through.
3. Serve straightaway.

Nutrition: Calories: 190; Fat: 14 g; Protein: 12 g; Carbs: 4.1 g; Fiber: 17 g; Sugar: 3.9 g.

982 SOY-GINGER STEAMED POMPANO

Preparation Time: 5 minutes
Cooking Time: 1 hour
Servings: 6
Ingredients:

- 1 wild-caught whole pompano, gutted and scaled
- 1 bunch scallion, diced
- 1 bunch cilantro, chopped
- 3 tsp. minced garlic
- 1 tbsp. grated ginger
- 1 tbsp. swerve sweetener
- ¼ cup soy sauce
- ¼ cup white wine
- ¼ cup sesame oil

Directions:

1. Place scallions in a 6-quart slow cooker and top with fish.
2. Whisk together remaining ingredients, except for cilantro, and pour the mixture all over the fish.
3. Plug in the slow cooker, shut with lid, and cook for 1 hour at high heat setting or until cooked through.
4. Garnish with cilantro and serve.

Nutrition: Calories: 129; Fat: 13 g; Protein: 18 g; Carbs: 4 g; Fiber: 17 g; Sugar: 3.1 g.

983 VIETNAMESE BRAISED CATFISH

Preparation Time: 5 minutes
Cooking Time: 6 hours
Servings: 3
Ingredients:

- 1 fillet of wild-caught catfish, cut into bite-size pieces
- 1 scallion, chopped
- 3 red chilies, chopped
- 1 tbsp. grated ginger
- ½ cup swerve sweetener
- 2 tbsp. avocado oil
- ¼ cup fish sauce, unsweetened

Directions:

1. Place a small saucepan over medium heat. Add sweetener and cook until it melts.
2. Then add scallion, chilies, ginger and fish sauce and stir until mixed.
3. Transfer this mixture to a 4-quart slow cooker. Add fish and toss until coated.
4. Plug in the slow cooker, shut with lid, and cook for 6 hours at low heat setting until cooked.
5. Drizzle with avocado oil and serve straightaway.

Nutrition: Calories: 156; Fat: 21 g; Protein: 19 g; Carbs: 0.2 g; Fiber: 17 g; Sugar: 0.1 g.

984 CHILI PRAWNS

Preparation Time: 5 minutes
Cooking Time: 1 hour
Servings: 6
Ingredients:

- 18-oz. wild-caught prawns, shell-on
- ½ cup sliced scallions
- 1 thumb-sized ginger, minced
- 1 bulb. of garlic, peeled and minced
- 1 tbsp. swerve sweetener
- 2 tbsp. apple cider vinegar
- 2 tbsp. Sambal Oelek
- 1 tbsp. fish sauce, unsweetened
- 4 tbsp. sesame oil
- ½ cup tomato ketchup, keto and unsweetened
- 1 egg, beaten

Directions:

1. Place all the ingredients, except for prawns, oil, and egg, in a 6-quart slow cooker and stir until mixed.
2. Plug in the slow cooker. Shut with lid, and cook for 1 hour at high heat setting.
3. Then add prawns and continue cooking for 15 minutes at a high heat setting, or until prawns turn pink.
4. Stir in oil and egg and cook for 10 minutes.
5. Drizzle with more fish sauce and serve.

Nutrition: Calories: 154; Fat: 13 g; Protein: 15 g; Carbs: 3.6 g; Fiber: 17 g; Sugar: 1.7 g.

985 TUNA SALPICAO

Preparation Time: 5 minutes
Cooking Time: 3 hours
Servings: 2
Ingredients:

- 8 oz. cooked wild-caught tuna, cut into inch cubes
- 4 jalapeno peppers, chopped
- 5 red chili, chopped
- 1 bulb. of garlic, peeled and minced
- 1 tsp. salt
- 1 tsp. ground black pepper
- 1 cup avocado oil

Directions:

1. Place all the ingredients, except for tuna, in a 4-quart slow cooker and stir until mixed.
2. Plug in the slow cooker. Shut with lid, and cook for 4 hours at low heat setting.
3. Then add tuna and continue cooking for 10 minutes at a high heat setting.
4. Serve straightaway.

Nutrition: Calories: 154; Fat: 13 g; Protein: 15 g; Carbs: 1.8 g; Fiber: 17 g; Sugar: 1.0 g.

986 SOY-GINGER BRAISED SQUID

Preparation Time: 5 minutes
Cooking Time: 8 hours
Servings: 6
Ingredients:
- 18-oz. wild-caught squid, cut into rings
- 2 scallions, chopped
- 2 bay leaves
- 1 tbsp. grated ginger
- 1 bulb. of garlic, peeled and minced
- ½ cup swerve sweetener
- ¼ cup soy sauce
- ¼ cup oyster sauce
- ¼ cup avocado oil
- ¼ cup white wine

Directions:
1. Plug in a 6-quart slow cooker. Add all the ingredients and stir until mixed.
2. Shut with lid and cook for 8 hours at low heat setting or until cooked through.
3. Serve straightaway.

Nutrition: Calories: 154; Fat: 13 g; Protein: 15 g; Carbs: 3.4 g; Fiber: 17 g; Sugar: 1.9 g.

987 SEA BASS IN COCONUT CREAM SAUCE

Preparation Time: 5 minutes
Cooking Time: 1 hour
Servings: 3
Ingredients:
- 18-oz. wild-caught sea bass
- 5 jalapeno peppers
- 4 stalks of bock Choy
- 2 stalks of scallions, sliced
- 1 tbsp. grated ginger
- 1 ½ tsp. salt
- 1 tbsp. fish sauce, unsweetened
- 2 cups coconut cream

Directions:
1. Stir together all the ingredients, except for bok choy and fish, in a bowl and add this mixture to a 6-quarts slow cooker.
2. Plug in the slow cooker. Then add fish, top with bok choy and shut with lid.
3. Cook sea bass for 1 hour and 30 minutes, or until cooked.
4. Serve straightaway.

Nutrition: Calories: 315; Fat: 17 g; Protein: 15 g; Carbs: 2.4 g; Fiber: 17 g; Sugar: 3.2 g.

988 COD CHOWDER

Preparation Time: 20 minutes
Cooking Time: 3 hours
Servings: 6
Ingredients:
- yellow onion
- 10 oz. cod
- 3 oz. bacon, sliced
- 1 tsp. sage
- 5 oz. potatoes
- 1 carrot, grated
- 5 cups water
- 1 tbsp. almond milk
- 1 tsp. ground coriander
- 1 tsp. salt

Directions:
1. Peel the onion and chop it.
2. Put the chopped onion and grated carrot in the slow cooker bowl. Add the sage, almond milk, ground coriander, and water. After this, chop the cod into 6 pieces.
3. Add the fish to the slow cooker bowl too. Then chop the sliced bacon and peel the potatoes.
4. Cut the potatoes into cubes.
5. Add the ingredients to the slow cooker bowl and close the slow cooker lid.
6. Cook the chowder for 3 hours on HIGH. Ladle the prepared cod chowder in the serving bowls.
7. Sprinkle the dish with the chopped parsley if desired. Enjoy!

Nutrition: Calories: 108; Fat: 4.5; Fiber: 2; Carbs: 3.02; Protein: 10.

989 TUNA IN POTATOES

Preparation Time: 16 minutes
Cooking Time: 4 hours
Servings: 8
Ingredients:
- 4 large potatoes
- 8 oz. tuna, canned
- ½ cup cream cheese
- 4 oz. Cheddar cheese
- 1 garlic clove
- 1 tsp. onion powder
- ½ tsp. salt
- 1 tsp. ground black pepper
- 1 tsp. dried dill

Directions:
1. Wash the potatoes carefully and cut them into halves.
2. Wrap the potatoes in the foil and place in the slow cooker. Close the slow cooker lid and cook the potatoes on HIGH for 2 hours.
3. Meanwhile, peel the garlic clove and mince it. Combine the minced garlic clove with the cream cheese, tuna, salt, ground black pepper, onion powder, and dill.
4. Then shred Cheddar cheese and add it to the mixture.
5. Mix it carefully until homogenous.
6. When the time is over – remove the potatoes from the slow cooker and discard the foil only from the flat surface of the potatoes.
7. Then take the fork and mash the flesh of the potato halves gently. Add the tuna mixture in the potato halves and return them back to the slow cooker.
8. Cook the potatoes for 2 hours more on HIGH. Enjoy!

Nutrition: Calories: 247; Fat: 5.9; Fiber: 4; Carbs: 3.31; Protein: 14.

990 SHRIMP SCAMPI

Preparation Time: 15 minutes
Cooking Time: 3 hours
Servings: 4
Ingredients:
- ¼ cup chicken bone broth
- ½ cup white cooking wine
- 2 tbsp. olive oil
- 2 tbsp. butter
- 1 tbsp. garlic, minced
- 2 tbsp. parsley, chopped
- 1 tbsp. lemon juice
- Salt and pepper to taste
- 1 lb. shrimp, peeled and deveined

Directions:
1. Mix all the ingredients in your slow cooker.
2. Cover the pot.
3. Cook on low for 3 hours.

Nutrition: Calories: 256; Fat: 14.7 g; Sodium: 466 mg; Carbohydrate 2.1 g; Fiber: 0.1 g; Protein: 23.3 g; Sugars: 2 g.

991 SHRIMP BOIL

Preparation Time: 15 minutes
Cooking Time: 4 hours
Servings: 4
Ingredients:
- 1 ½ lb. potatoes, sliced into wedges
- 2 cloves garlic, peeled
- 2 ears corn
- 1 lb. sausage, sliced
- ¼ cup Old Bay seasoning
- 1 tbsp. lemon juice
- 2 cups water
- 2 lb. shrimp, peeled

Directions:
1. Put the potatoes in your slow cooker. Add the garlic, corn and sausage in layers.
2. Season with the Old Bay seasoning.
3. Drizzle lemon juice on top.
4. Pour in the water.
5. Do not mix.
6. Cover the pot.
7. Cook on high for 4 hours.
8. Add the shrimp on top.
9. Cook for 15 minutes.

Nutrition: Calories: 585; Fat: 25.1 g; Sodium: 2242 mg; Potassium 1166 mg; Carbohydrate

3.7 g; Fiber: 4.9 g; Protein: 53.8 g; Sugars: 3.9 g.

992 SHRIMP & SAUSAGE GUMBO

Preparation Time: 15 minutes
Cooking Time: 1 hour & 15 minutes
Servings: 4
Ingredients:

- 2 tbsp. olive oil
- 2 lb. chicken thigh fillet, sliced into cubes
- 2 cloves garlic, crushed and minced
- 1 onion, sliced
- 2 stalks celery, chopped
- 1 green bell pepper, chopped
- 1 tsp. Cajun seasoning
- Salt to taste
- 2 cups beef broth
- 28 oz. canned crushed tomatoes
- 4 oz. sausage
- 2 tbsp. butter
- 1 lb. shrimp, peeled and deveined

Directions:

1. Pour the olive oil into a pan over medium heat.
2. Cook the garlic and chicken for 5 minutes.
3. Add the onion, celery and bell pepper.
4. Cook until tender.
5. Season with the Cajun seasoning and salt.
6. Cook for 2 minutes.
7. Stir in the sausage, broth and tomatoes.
8. Cover and cook on low for 1 hour.
9. Add the butter and shrimp to the last 10 minutes of cooking.

Nutrition: Calories: 467; Fat: 33 g; Sodium: 1274 mg; Potassium 658 mg; Carbohydrate 5 g; Fiber: 2 g; Protein: 33 g; Sugars: 5 g.

993 FISH STEW

Preparation Time: 15 minutes
Cooking Time: 1 hour, 24 minutes
Servings: 2
Ingredients:

- 1 lb. white fish
- 1 tbsp. lime juice
- 1 onion, sliced
- 2 cloves garlic, sliced
- 1 red pepper, sliced
- 1 jalapeno pepper, sliced
- 1 tsp. paprika
- 2 cups chicken broth
- 2 cups tomatoes, chopped
- Salt and pepper to taste
- 2 oz. coconut milk

Directions:

1. Marinate the fish in lime juice for 10 minutes.
2. Pour the olive oil into a pan over medium heat.
3. Add the onion, garlic and peppers.
4. Cook for 4 minutes.
5. Add the rest of the ingredients except the coconut milk.
6. Cover the pot.
7. Cook on low for 1 hour.
8. Stir in the coconut milk and simmer for 10 minutes

Nutrition: Calories: 323; Fat: 28.6 g; Sodium: 490 mg; Carbohydrate 1.1 g; Protein: 9.3 g; Fiber: 3.2 g; Sugars: 6.2 g.

994 SALMON WITH LEMON & DILL

Preparation Time: 15 minutes
Cooking Time: 2 hours
Servings: 4
Ingredients:

- Cooking spray
- 1 tsp. olive oil
- 2 lb. salmon
- 1 tbsp. fresh dill, chopped
- Salt and pepper to taste
- 1 clove garlic, minced
- 1 lemon, sliced

Directions:

1. Spray your slow cooker with oil.
2. Brush both sides of salmon with olive oil.
3. Season the salmon with salt, pepper, dill and garlic.
4. Add to the slow cooker.
5. Put the lemon slices on top.
6. Cover the pot and cook on high for 2 hours.

Nutrition: Calories: 313; Fat: 15.2 g; Sodium: 102 mg; Carbohydrate 0.7 g; Fiber: 0.1 g; Protein: 44.2; Sugars: 0 g.

995 ASPARAGUS SMOKED SALMON

Preparation Time: 15 minutes
Cooking Time: 5 hours
Servings: 6
Ingredients:

- 1 tbsp. extra-virgin olive oil
- 6 large eggs
- 1 cup heavy (whipping) cream
- 2 tsp. chopped fresh dill, plus additional for garnish
- ½ tsp. kosher salt
- ¼ tsp. freshly ground black pepper
- 1 ½ cups shredded Havarti or Monterey Jack cheese
- 12 oz. asparagus, trimmed and sliced
- 6 oz. smoked salmon, flaked

Directions:

1. Brush butter into a cooker.
2. Whisk in the heavy cream with eggs, dill, salt, and pepper.
3. Stir in the cheese and asparagus.
4. Gently fold in the salmon and then pour the mixture into the prepared insert.
5. Cover and cook on low or 3 hours on high.
6. Serve warm, garnished with additional fresh dill.

Nutrition: Calories: 388; Fat: 19; Carbs: 1.0; Protein: 21.

996 SALMON WITH CAPER SAUCE

Preparation Time: 5 minutes
Cooking Time: 45 minutes.
Servings: 4
Ingredients:

- ½ cup dry white wine
- ½ cup water
- 1 yellow onion, thin sliced
- ½ tsp. salt
- ¼ tsp. black pepper
- 4 salmon steaks
- 2 tbsp. butter
- 2 tbsp. flour
- 1 cup chicken broth
- 2 tsp. lemon juice
- 3 tbsp. capers

Directions:

1. Combine wine, water, onion, salt and black pepper in a crock pot; cover and cook on high for 20 minutes.
2. Add salmon steaks; cover and cook on high until salmon is tender or about 20 minutes.
3. To make the sauce, in a small skillet, melt butter over medium flame. Stir in flour and cook for 1 minute.
4. Pour in chicken broth and lemon juice; whisk for 1 to 2 minutes. Add capers; serve the sauce with salmon.

Nutrition: Calories: 234; Fat: 15 g; Carbs: 2 g; Protein: 12 g.

997 HERBED SALMON LOAF WITH SAUCE

Preparation Time: 5 minutes
Cooking Time: 5 hours.
Servings: 4
Ingredients:
For the Salmon Meatloaf:

- 1 cup fresh bread crumbs
- 1 can (7 ½ oz.) salmon, drained
- ¼ cup scallions, chopped
- ⅓ cup whole milk
- 1 egg
- 1 tbsp. fresh lemon juice
- 1 tsp. dried rosemary
- 1 tsp. ground coriander
- ½ tsp. fenugreek
- 1 tsp. mustard seed
- ½ tsp. salt
- ¼ tsp. white pepper

½ cup cucumber, chopped
½ cup reduced-fat plain yogurt
½ tsp. dill weed
Salt, to taste

Directions:

1. Line your crock pot with a foil.
2. Mix all ingredients for the salmon meatloaf until everything is well incorporated; form into loaf and place in the crock pot.
3. Cover with a suitable lid and cook on a low heat setting for 5 hours.
4. Combine all of the ingredients for the sauce; whisk well.
5. Serve your meatloaf with prepared sauce.

Nutrition: Calories: 145; Fat: 11 g; Carbs: 2 g; Protein: 11 g.

998 CAULIFLOWER, COCONUT MILK, AND SHRIMP SOUP

Preparation Time: 5 minutes
Cooking Time: 2 hours, 15 minutes
Servings: 4

Ingredients:

2 cups riced cauliflower
2 tbsp. red curry paste
1 (13.5-oz. / 383-g.) can unsweetened full-fat coconut milk
1 tbsp. chopped fresh cilantro leaves, divided
1 cup shrimp, peeled, deveined, tail off, and cooked

From the cupboard:

2 cup water
Salt and freshly ground black pepper, to taste

Directions:

1. Add the rice cauliflower, red curry paste, coconut milk, 1 tablespoon of cilantro, water, then sprinkle with salt and black pepper. Blend the mixture to combine well.
2. Put the slow cooker lid on and cook on HIGH for 2 hours.
3. Put the shrimp on a clean working surface; then sprinkle salt and black pepper to season.
4. Put the shrimp in the slow cooker and cook for 15 minutes more.
5. Transfer the soup into a large bowl and top with the remaining cilantro leaves before serving.

Nutrition: Calories: 268; Total Fats: 21.3 g; Total Carbs: 7.8 g; Fiber: 3.2 g; Net Carbs: 4.6 g; Protein: 16.1 g.

999 BRAZILIAN MOQUECA (SHRIMP STEW)

Preparation Time: 10 minutes
Cooking Time: 15 minutes
Servings: 6

Ingredients:

4 cup coconut milk
2 tbsp. lime juice
¼ cup diced roasted peppers
½ pounds shrimp, peeled and deveined
¼ cup olive oil
2 garlic clove, minced
14 oz. diced tomatoes
1 tbsp. sriracha sauce
2 chopped onion
¼ cup chopped cilantro
Fresh dill, chopped to garnish
Salt and black pepper, to taste

Directions:

1. Heat the olive oil in a pot over medium heat. Add onion and cook for 3 minutes or until translucent. Add the garlic and cook for another minute, until soft. Add tomatoes, shrimp, and cilantro. Cook until the shrimp becomes opaque, about 3-4 minutes.
2. Stir in sriracha sauce and coconut milk, and cook for 2 minutes. Do not bring to a boil. Stir in the lime juice and season with salt and pepper. Spoon the stew in bowls, garnish with fresh dill to serve.

Nutrition: Calories: 324; Fat: 21 g; Net Carbs: 5 g; Protein: 23.1 g.

1000 COCONUT, GREEN BEANS & SHRIMP CURRY SOUP

Preparation Time: 10 minutes
Cooking Time: 15 minutes
Servings: 4

Ingredients:

2 tbsp. ghee
1 lb. jumbo shrimp, peeled and deveined
2 tsp ginger-garlic puree
1 tbsp. red curry paste
6 oz. coconut milk
Salt and chili pepper to taste
bunch green beans, halved

Directions:

1. Melt ghee in a medium saucepan over medium heat. Add the shrimp, season with salt and black pepper, and cook until they are opaque, 2 to 3 minutes. Remove shrimp to a plate. Add the ginger-garlic puree and red curry paste to the ghee and sauté for 2 minutes until fragrant.
2. Stir in the coconut milk; add the shrimp, salt, chili pepper, and green beans. Cook for 4 minutes. Reduce the heat to a simmer and cook an additional 3 minutes, occasionally stirring. Adjust taste with salt, fetch soup into serving bowls, and serve with cauli rice.

Nutrition: Calories 375; Fat: 35.4 g; Net Carbs: 2 g; Protein: 9 g.

1001 CAULIFLOWER AND CLAM CHOWDER

Preparation Time: 10 minutes
Cooking Time: 10 minutes
Servings: 6

Ingredients:

3 (6.5-oz. / 184-g.) cans chopped clams
1 small yellow onion
4 cups chopped cauliflower
1 ½ cups heavy whipping cream
½ tsp. dried thyme

From the cupboard:

1 tbsp. butter
Salt and freshly ground black pepper, to taste

Directions:

1. Divide the clams and clam juice into two bowls. Thin the clam juice with water to make 2 cups of juice.
2. Put the onion and butter in an instant pot and press the Sauté button; then sauté for 2 minutes or until the onion is translucent.
3. Add the clam juice and cauliflower into the instant pot. Put the lid on and press the Manual button, and set the temperature to 375°F (190°C). Then cook for 5 minutes.
4. Quick Release the pressure. Open the lid and mix in the heavy cream and clams.
5. Press the Sauté button and cook for 3 minutes or until the clams are opaque and firm. Sprinkle with thyme, salt, and black pepper. Stir to mix well.
6. Spoon the chowder in a large bowl and serve warm.

Nutrition: Calories: 252; Total Fats: 17.3 g; Total Carbs: 8.9 g; Fiber: 2.1 g; Net Carbs: 6.8 g; Protein: 17.1 g.

1002 GRILLED RED LOBSTER TAILS

Preparation Time: 15 minutes
Cooking Time: 12 minutes
Servings: 2

Ingredients:

1 tbsp. freshly squeezed lemon juice
½ cup extra virgin olive oil
½ tbsp. salt
Pinch of garlic powder
½ tbsp. paprika
Pinch of white pepper
1 (10-oz. / 284-g.) red lobster tails
2 tsp. olive oil, for greasing the grill grates

Directions:

1. Preheat the grill to high heat.

2. In a bowl, whisk together the lemon juice, olive oil, salt, garlic powder, paprika, and white pepper.

3. Using a large knife, cut open lobster tails and slice lengthwise. Brush the flesh side of the lobster tail with the marinade.

4. Lightly grease the grill grates with olive oil. Place the tails on the preheated grill, flesh-side down. Grill for about 10 minutes, flipping once, or until the lobster is opaque. Frequently baste tails with the marinade.

5. Let cool for 5 minutes before serving.

Nutrition: Calories: 416; Fat: 20.1 g; Total Carbs: 1.7 g; Fiber: 0.7 g; Protein: 57.8 g.

1003 INTERMITTENT TACO FISHBOWL

Preparation Time: 5 minutes
Cooking Time: 10 minutes
Servings: 4
Ingredients:
Dressing:

½ cup intermittent-friendly mayonnaise
2 tbsp. lime juice
tsp. hot sauce
½ tsp. garlic powder
salt and freshly ground black pepper, to taste

Main meal:

½ pound (227 g.) green cabbage or red cabbage
½ yellow onion
1 tomato
1 avocado
salt and ground black pepper, to taste
tbsp. olive oil, divided
10 oz. (284 g;) white fish, patted dry
1 tbsp. tex-mex seasoning
fresh cilantro, for garnish
lime, for garnish

Directions:

1. In a bowl, mix the ingredients for the dressing before frying the fish, so the flavors have time to develop. Allow to sit at room temperature or keep in the refrigerator.

2. With a sharp knife or mandolin, shred or slice all vegetables finely, except the avocado. Split the avocado in half and remove the pit. Slice the avocado thinly and use a spoon to scoop the avocado slices out of the skin. Season the vegetables and avocado slices with salt and pepper on a plate, then drizzle with 2 tablespoons of olive oil. Toss well and set aside.

3. Rub both sides of white fish with salt, pepper, and Tex-Mex seasoning.

4. In a skillet, add the remaining olive oil. Fry the fish in olive oil over medium heat for 3 to 4 minutes on both sides, or until the fish flakes easily with a fork.

5. Transfer the vegetable mixture to a serving bowl. Top with the fish and pour over the dressing. Garnish with fresh cilantro and lime before serving.

Nutrition: Calories: 489; Fat: 42.9 g; Total Carbs: 14.2 g; Fiber: 5.6 g; Protein: 15.1 g.

1004 LOW CARB POACHED EGGS WITH TUNA SALAD

Preparation Time: 10 minutes
Cooking Time: 20 minutes
Servings: 4
Ingredients:
Tuna salad:

4 oz. (113 g;) tuna in olive oil, rinsed and drained
⅓ cup chopped celery stalks
½ red onion
½ cup mayonnaise, intermittent-friendly
tsp. Dijon mustard
juice and zest of ½ lemon
salt and freshly ground black pepper, to taste

Poached eggs:

4 eggs
tsp. salt
tsp. white wine vinegar or white vinegar
tbsp. olive oil
oz. (57 g.) leafy greens or lettuce
oz. (57 g;). cherry tomatoes, chopped

Directions:

1. Chop the tuna and mix it in a bowl with the other ingredients for the salad. You can make it ahead of time and keep it in the refrigerator. The flavor will enhance with time.

2. Bring a pot of water to a boil over medium heat. Add the vinegar and salt, then stir the water in circles to create a swirl using a spoon. Crack the eggs into the pot, one at a time.

3. Let simmer for 3 minutes and use a slotted spoon to remove it from the water.

4. Transfer the eggs to the bowl of tuna salad and drizzle with olive oil. Gently toss until everything is combined.

5. Serve them with leafy greens and cherry tomatoes on the side.

Nutrition: Calories: 534; Fat: 40.5 g; Total Carbs: 7.2 g; Fiber: 1.4 g; Protein: 34.0 g.

1005 SMOKED SALMON AND LETTUCE BITES

Preparation Time: 20 minutes
Cooking Time: 0
Servings: 6
Ingredients:

7 oz. (198 g.) smoked salmon, cut into small pieces
8 oz. (227 g.) cream cheese
⅓ tbsp. mayonnaise, intermittent-friendly
4 tbsp. chopped fresh dill or fresh chives
½ lemon, zested
¼ tsp. ground black pepper
2 oz. (57 g.) lettuce, for serving

Directions:

1. Add the cream cheese, mayonnaise, fresh dill, lemon zest, and pepper in a bowl. Stir to combine well.

2. Lay the lettuce on a clean work surface. Top with the salmon pieces and pour the cream cheese mixture over. Serve immediately.

Nutrition: Calories: 179; Fat: 15.0 g; Total Carbs: 3.3 g; Fiber: 1.1 g; Protein: 8.6.

1006 LOW CARB SEAFOOD CHOWDER

Preparation Time: 10 minutes
Cooking Time: 20 minutes
Servings: 4
Ingredients:

4 tbsp. butter
5 oz. (142 g.) celery stalks, sliced
2 garlic cloves, minced
4 oz. (113 g.) cream cheese
1 cup clam juice
1 ½ cups heavy whipping cream
tsp. dried sage or dried thyme
½ lemon, juiced and zested
pound (454 g.) salmon fillets, cut into 1-inch pieces
8 oz. (227 g.) shrimp, peeled and deveined
1 oz. (57 g.) baby spinach
Salt and freshly ground black pepper, to taste
Fresh sage, for garnish

Directions:

1. Melt the butter in a large pot over medium heat. Add celery and garlic. Cook for about 5 minutes, stirring occasionally. Add clam juice, cream, cream cheese, sage, lemon juice and lemon zest. Let it simmer for about 10 minutes without a lid.

2. Add the salmon and shrimp. Simmer for 3 minutes or until salmon is opaque. Add the baby

spinach and stir until wilted. Season with salt and pepper.

3. Garnish with fresh sage before serving for extra flavor.

Nutrition: Calories: 622; Fat: 46.7 g; Total Carbs: 12.5 g; Fiber: 1.6 g; Protein: 38.8 g.

1007 CHEESY BROCCOLI WITH INTERMITTENT FRIED SALMON

Preparation Time: 10 minutes
Cooking Time: 25 minutes
Servings: 4
Ingredients:

1 pound (454 g;) broccoli, cut into florets
3 oz. (85 g;) butter
Salt and freshly ground black pepper, to taste
5 oz. (142 g.) grated Cheddar cheese
1 ½ pound (680 g.) salmon
lime

Directions:

1. Preheat the oven to 400°F (205°C).
2. Put the broccoli florets into a pot of lightly salted water. Bring to a simmer. Make sure the broccoli maintains its chewy texture and delicate color.
3. Drain the broccoli and discard the boiling water. Set aside, uncovered, for a minute or two to allow the steam to evaporate.
4. Place the drained broccoli in a well-greased baking dish. Add pepper and butter to taste.
5. Sprinkle cheese on top of the broccoli and bake in the oven for 15 to 20 minutes or until the cheese turns a golden color.
6. In the meantime, season the salmon with salt and pepper and fry in plenty of butter, a few minutes on each side. The lime can be fried in the same pan or be served raw.

Nutrition: Calories: 580; Fat: 39.2 g; Total Carbs: 9.0 g; Fiber: 3.0 g; Protein: 48.2 g.

1008 INTERMITTENT CHILI-COVERED SALMON WITH SPINACH

Preparation Time: 5 minutes
Cooking Time: 20 minutes
Servings: 4
Ingredients:

¼ cup olive oil
1 ½ pounds (680 g.) salmon, in pieces
Salt and freshly ground black pepper, to taste
1 oz. (28 g;) Parmesan cheese, grated finely
1 tbsp. chili paste
½ cup sour cream
1 pound (454 g.) fresh spinach

Directions:

1. Preheat oven to 400°F (205°C).
2. Grease the baking dish with half of the olive oil. Season the salmon with pepper and salt. Put in the baking dish, skin-side down.
3. Combine Parmesan cheese, chili paste and sour cream. Then spread them on the salmon fillets.
4. Bake for 20 minutes, or until the salmon flakes easily with a fork or it becomes opaque.
5. Heat the remaining olive oil in a nonstick skillet. Sauté the spinach until it's wilted, about a couple of minutes, and season with pepper and salt.
6. Serve with the oven-baked salmon immediately.

Nutrition: Calories: 461; Fat: 28.5 g; Total Carbs: 8.0 g; Fiber: 2.8 g; Protein: 42.6 g.

1009 INTERMITTENT EGG BUTTER WITH AVOCADO AND SMOKED SALMON

Preparation Time: 5 minutes
Cooking Time: 15 minutes
Servings: 4
Ingredients:

4 eggs
½ tsp. sea salt
¼ tsp. ground black pepper
5 oz. (142 g;) butter, at room temperature
4 oz. (113 g;) smoked salmon
1 tbsp. fresh parsley, chopped finely
avocados
2 tbsp. olive oil

Directions:

1. Put the eggs in a pot and cover them with cold water. Then put the pot on the stove without a lid and bring it to a boil.
2. Lower the heat and let it simmer for 6 to 9 minutes. Then remove eggs from the water and put them in a bowl with cold water.
3. Peel the eggs and cut them finely. Use a fork to mix the eggs and butter. Then season to taste with pepper, salt.
4. Serve the egg butter with slices of smoked salmon, finely chopped parsley, and a side of diced avocado tossed in olive oil.

Nutrition: Calories: 638; Fats: 61.1 g; Total Carbs: 9.8 g; Fiber: 6.8 g; Protein: 16.5 g.

1010 INTERMITTENT BAKED SALMON WITH BUTTER AND LEMON SLICES

Preparation Time: 10 minutes
Cooking Time: 25 minutes

Servings: 6
Ingredients:

2 tbsp. olive oil
2 pounds (907 g.) salmon
½ tsp. sea salt
Freshly ground black pepper, to taste
7 oz. (198 g.) butter
lemon

Directions:

1. Start by preheating the oven to 425°F (220°C).
2. In a large baking dish, spray it with olive oil. Then add the salmon, skin-side down. Season with salt and pepper.
3. Cut the lemon into thin slices and place them on the upper side of the salmon. Cut the butter into thin slices and spread them on top of the lemon slices.
4. Put the dish in the heated oven and bake on the middle rack for about 25 to 30 minutes, or until the salmon flakes easily with a fork.
5. Melt the rest of the butter in a small saucepan until it bubbles. Then remove from heat and let cool a little. Consider adding some lemon juice to the melted cool butter.
6. Serve the fish with lemon butter.

Nutrition: Calories: 474; Fats: 37.6 g; Total Carbs: 0.7 g; Fiber: 0.1 g; Protein: 32.6 g.

1011 GRILLED TUNA SALAD WITH GARLIC SAUCE

Preparation Time: 10 minutes
Cooking Time: 15 minutes
Servings: 4
Ingredients:
Garlic dressing:

⅔ cup intermittent-friendly mayonnaise
2 tbsp. water
2 tsp. garlic powder
salt and freshly ground black pepper, to taste

Tuna salad:

2 eggs
8 oz. (227 g;) green asparagus
tbsp. olive oil
¼ pound (340 g;) fresh tuna, in slices
4 oz. (113 g;) leafy greens
oz. (57 g;) cherry tomatoes
½ red onion
tbsp. pumpkin seeds
Salt and freshly ground black pepper, to taste

Directions:

1. Mix the ingredients together for the garlic dressing. Set them aside.
2. Put the eggs in boiling water for 8 to 10 minutes. Cooling in cold water would facilitate the peeling.

3. Slice the asparagus into lengths and rapidly fry them inside a hot pan with no oil or butter. Then set them aside.
4. Rub the tuna with oil and fry or grill for 2 to 3 minutes on each side. Season with salt and pepper.
5. Put the leafy greens, asparagus, peeled eggs cut in halves, tomatoes and thinly sliced onion into a plate.
6. Finally, cut the tuna into slices and spread the slices evenly over the salad. Pour the dressing on top and add some pumpkin seeds.

Nutrition: Calories: 397; Fats: 27.1 g; Total Carbs: 8.3 g; Fiber: 2.8 g; Protein: 30.0 g.

1012 CRISPY INTERMITTENT CREAMY FISH CASSEROLE

Preparation Time: 25 minutes
Cooking Time: 30 minutes
Servings: 4
Ingredients:

1 head broccoli, cut into florets
2 1tbsp. olive oil
tsp. salt
¼ tsp. freshly ground black pepper
6 scallions, chopped
oz. (28 g.) melted butter, for greasing the casserole dish
2 tbsp. parsley, finely chopped
1 ¼ cups heavy whipping cream
1 tbsp. Dijon mustard
1 ½ pounds (680 g.) white fish, in serving- pieces
oz. (85 g.) butter slices, under room temperature

Directions:

1. Preheat the oven to 400°F (205°C).
2. Heat the olive oil in a nonstick skillet over medium heat.
3. Add the broccoli to the skillet and sauté for 5 to 7 minutes or until tender. Then season the broccoli with salt and ground black pepper. Add the finely chopped scallions, and sauté for 1 to 2 minutes more.
4. Prepare a casserole dish and grease it with butter to add a tasty level of flavors to the meal. Then pour the sautéed broccoli and scallions in the casserole dish. Stir them well until they have a delicious butter smell.
5. In a bowl, mix finely chopped parsley with cream and Dijon mustard and pour the mixture over the casserole dish. Stir until fully incorporated. Then nestle the white fish in the casserole

dish. Top them with the butter slices.
6. Cook in the preheated oven for 20 to 30 minutes, or until the fish exudes tender and takes in the flavor from the delicious butter.
7. Remove the casserole dish from the oven and serve the fish and vegetables warm.

Nutrition: Calories: 611; Fats: 48.3 g; Total Carbs: 13.2 g; Fiber: 4.8 g; Protein: 34.4 g.

1013 COCONUT INTERMITTENT SALMON AND NAPA CABBAGE

Preparation Time: 10 minutes
Cooking Time: 20 minutes
Servings: 4
Ingredients:

1 ¼ pounds (567 g.) salmon
2 tbsp. coconut oil
1 tsp. sea salt
½ tsp. onion powder
1tsp. turmeric
oz. (57 g.) unsweetened shredded coconut
tbsp. olive oil, for frying
1¼ pounds (567 g.) Napa cabbage
Salt and freshly ground black pepper, to taste
oz. (113 g.) butter
Lemon, for serving

Directions:

1. On a wooden board, cut the salmon into 1×1-inch pieces. Then rub coconut oil on salmon pieces. Place the pieces in a medium bowl and set aside.
2. Prepare a mixture of salt, onion powder, turmeric, and unsweetened shredded coconut. Meanwhile, put the salmon pieces into this creamy mixture to get a good coating.
3. In a nonstick frying pan with 4 tablespoons of olive oil on medium heat, fry the seasoned salmon pieces with coconut mixture for about 4 to 7 minutes, stirring every 2 minutes. Leave it in the pan until golden brown, or until soft.
4. Meanwhile, prepare and cut the cabbage into wedges. Fry the cabbage in a saucepan with butter until it turns into a light creamy liquid. On a platter, pour the cabbage liquid and generously season with salt and pepper.
5. In a dish decorated with lemon slices, place the fried salmon and pour the creamy cabbage liquid and top with wedges of lemon. Serve warm!

Nutrition: Calories: 628; Fats: 52.9 g; Total Carbs: 7.1 g; Fiber: 1.6 g; Protein: 32.7 g.

1014 GRILLED WHITE FISH WITH ZUCCHINI AND KALE PESTO

Preparation Time: 10 minutes
Cooking Time: 15 minutes
Servings: 4
Ingredients:
Kale pesto:

3 oz. (85 g.) kale, chopped
2 garlic clove
1 tbsp. lemon juice
oz. (57 g.) walnuts, shelled
½ tsp. salt - ¼ tsp. ground black pepper
2 tsp. olive oil

Fish and Zucchini:

2 zucchinis, rinsed and drained, cut into slices
2 tbsp. olive oil, divided
salt and freshly ground black pepper, to taste
1 tsp. lemon juice
1 ½ pounds (680 g.) white fish (such as cod), thawed at room temperature, if frozen

Directions:

1. Make the kale pesto: Add the kale to the food processor with the garlic, lemon juice, and walnuts and blend, then sprinkle with salt and pepper for seasoning, and then add the olive oil and blend until the mixture becomes creamy. Set aside until ready to serve.
2. Rub the zucchini slices with 1 tablespoon of olive oil, salt, pepper, and lemon juice. Set aside.
3. Grease a nonstick skillet with remaining olive oil, and heat over medium-high heat.
4. Grill the fish in the skillet for 3 minutes on each side. Sprinkle with salt and black pepper, and serve with zucchini and kale pesto immediately.

Nutrition: Calories: 321; Fats: 19.5 g; Total Carbs: 8.1 g; Fiber: 2.8 g; Protein: 30.3 g.

1015 CHEESY VERDE SHRIMP

Preparation Time: 10 minutes
Cooking Time: 10 minutes
Servings: 4
Ingredients:

2 tbsp. olive oil
2 garlic cloves, minced
¼ cup scallions, chopped
1 pound (454 g.) fresh shrimps, deveined, and peeled
½ cup parsley, chopped
½ cup Parmesan cheese, grated

Directions:

1. In a large skillet, heat the olive oil over medium heat.
2. Add the garlic and chopped scallions and sauté briefly, making sure the garlic does not turn brown.
3. Add the shrimps and cook until they become opaque. Sprinkle chopped parsley over the shrimp.
4. Remove cooked shrimps from heat. Serve on a dish and sprinkle with grated cheese.

Nutrition: Calories: 215; Fats: 10.9 g; Total Carbs: 3.2 g; Fiber: 0.4 g; Protein: 26.8 g.

1016 BEST MARINATED GRILLED SHRIMP

Preparation Time: 15 minutes
Cooking Time: 6 minutes
Servings: 4
Ingredients:

⅓ cup olive oil
3 cloves garlic, minced
2 tbsp. chopped fresh basil
2 tbsp. red wine vinegar
½ tsp. salt - ¼ tsp. cayenne pepper
2 pounds (907 g.) fresh shrimp, peeled and deveined
2 tbsp. olive oil, for greasing
6 wooden skewers, soaked for at least 30 minutes

Directions:

1. Mix the olive oil, garlic, basil, red wine vinegar, salt, and cayenne in a large bowl. Stir in the shrimp and toss to coat well.
2. Cover the bowl with plastic wrap, then place in the refrigerator to marinate for 1 hour.
3. Preheat the grill to medium heat and lightly spray the grill grates with olive oil spray.
4. Thread the shrimp onto skewers, piercing once near the tail and once near the head, discarding the marinade.
5. Grill for 6 minutes, flipping occasionally, or until the shrimp is opaque.
6. Allow to cool for about 3 minutes and serve hot.

Nutrition: Calories: 278; Fats: 14.6 g; Total Carbs: 0.9 g; Fiber: 0.1 g; Protein: 36.4 g.

1017 SALMON FILLETS BAKED WITH DIJON

Preparation Time: 10 minutes
Cooking Time: 15 minutes
Servings: 4
Ingredients:

4 (4-oz. / 113-g.) salmon fillets
¼ cup butter, melted
3 tbsp. Dijon mustard

Salt and freshly ground black pepper, to taste
⅛ cup coconut flour

Directions:

1. Preheat the oven to 400°F (205°C) and line a baking pan with aluminum foil.
2. In a bowl, mix the salmon fillets, butter, mustard, salt and pepper. Stir well until the salmon is fully coated.
3. Place the salmon in the baking pan, then evenly sprinkle the coconut flour on top.
4. Transfer the pan into the preheated oven and bake until the salmon easily flakes when tested with a fork, about 15 minutes.
5. Remove from the oven and cool for 5 minutes before serving.

Nutrition: Calories: 484; Fats: 21.6 g; Total Carbs: 2.7 g; Fiber: 0.5 g; Protein: 70.1 g.

1018 SALMON WITH GARLIC DIJON MUSTARD

Preparation Time: 15 minutes
Cooking Time: 20 minutes
Servings: 4
Ingredients:

2 tbsp. olive oil
⅓ cup Dijon mustard
4 (6-oz. / 170-g.) salmon fillets
1 red onion, thinly sliced
4 large cloves garlic, thinly sliced
Salt and freshly ground black pepper, to taste
1 tsp. dried tarragon

Directions:

1. Preheat the oven to 400°F (205°C) and grease a baking pan with olive oil.
2. Generously rub the Dijon mustard all over the salmon. Then place the salmon in the pan, skin-side down.
3. Put the onion slices and garlic cloves on the salmon fillets. Sprinkle with salt, pepper, and tarragon.
4. Arrange the pan in the preheated oven and bake for 20 minutes, or until the salmon easily flakes when tested with a fork.
5. Remove from the heat and serve on a plate.

Nutrition: Calories: 265; Fats: 11.6 g; Total Carbs: 2.8 g; Fiber: 1.1 g; Protein: 36.0 g.

1019 BLACKENED TROUT

Preparation Time: 20 minutes
Cooking Time: 10 minutes
Servings: 6
Ingredients:

2 tsp. dry mustard

1 tbsp. paprika
1 tsp. ground cumin
1 tsp. cayenne pepper
1 tsp. white pepper
1 tsp. black pepper
1 tsp. dried thyme
1 tsp. salt
¾ cup unsalted butter, melted
6 (4-oz. / 113-g.) trout fillets
1 tbsp. olive oil

Directions:

1. Combine the dry mustard, paprika, cumin, cayenne pepper, white pepper, black pepper, thyme, and salt in a medium bowl. Stir to combine and set aside.
2. Put ¼ cup of butter on a platter, then dredge the trout fillets into the butter to coat evenly. Sprinkle with the spicy mixture, gently pressing the mixture into the fillets.
3. Heat the olive oil in a skillet over medium-high heat, then add the fillets. Cook the fish for about 2 to 3 minutes per side, turning occasionally, or until the fish is lightly browned on the edges.
4. Remove from the heat and serve warm.

Nutrition: Calories: 328; Fat: 25.0 g; Total Carbs: 1.7 g; Fiber: 0.8 g; Protein: 24.0 g.

1020 TROUT FILLETS WITH LEMONY YOGURT SAUCE

Preparation Time: 12 minutes
Cooking Time: 8 to 10 minutes
Servings: 4
Ingredients:

1 cup plain Greek yogurt
1 cucumber, shredded
1 tsp. lemon zest
1 tbsp. extra-virgin olive oil
Salt and freshly ground black pepper, to taste
1 tbsp. fresh dill weed, chopped
pinch lemon pepper
(6-oz. / 170-g.) rainbow trout fillets

Directions:

1. Mix the yogurt, cucumber, lemon zest, olive oil, salt, and pepper in a bowl. Stir thoroughly and set aside.
2. Preheat the oven to 400°F (205°C).
3. Sprinkle the lemon pepper on top and arrange the fillets in a greased baking dish.
4. Bake in the preheated oven for about 8 to 10 minutes or until fork-tender.

5. Remove from the oven and serve the fish alongside the yogurt sauce.

Nutrition: Calories: 281; Fats: 11.4 g; Total Carbs: 5.3 g; Fiber: 0.7 g; Protein: 37.6 g.

1021 CLASSIC SHRIMP SCAMPI

Preparation Time: 30 minutes
Cooking Time: 15 minutes
Servings: 4
Ingredients:

2 cloves garlic, minced
½ cup butter, melted
½ cup dry white wine
2 pounds (907 g.) medium shrimp, peeled and deveined
3 green onions, chopped

Directions:

1. Preheat the oven to 400°F (205°C).
2. In a bowl, combine the garlic, butter, wine, and shrimp. Stir thoroughly.
3. Arrange the shrimp in a greased baking dish. Put it in the oven and bake for about 8 minutes until the shrimp is opaque.
4. Remove from the oven and serve the shrimp with green onions on top.

Nutrition: Calories: 209; Fats: 2.2 g; Total Carbs: 1.6 g; Fiber: 0.2 g; Protein: 45.9 g.

1022 SNOW CRAB CLUSTERS WITH GARLIC BUTTER

Preparation Time: 5 minutes
Cooking Time: 15 minutes
Servings: 2
Ingredients:

1 pound (454 g.) snow crab clusters, thawed if necessary
¼ cup butter
clove garlic, minced
1 ½ tsp. dried parsley
⅛ tsp. salt
¼ tsp. ground black pepper

Directions:

1. On the cutting board, cut a split lengthwise into the shell of each crab. Set aside.
2. In a skillet, melt the butter over medium heat. Add the garlic and cook for 2 minutes until tender. Add the parsley, salt, and pepper, then cook for 1 minute more. Stir in the crab and simmer for 5 to 6 minutes.
3. Remove from the heat and serve on a plate.

Nutrition: Calories: 222; Fats: 4.0 g; Total Carbs: 0.8 g; Fiber: 0.1 g; Protein: 45.7 g.

1023 CREAMY SALMON SAUCE ZOODLES

Preparation Time: 15 minutes
Cooking Time: 15 minutes
Servings: 4
Ingredients:

2 pounds (907 g.) zucchini
Salt and freshly ground black pepper, to taste
4 oz. (113 g.) cream cheese
½ cup heavy whipping cream
¼ cup chopped fresh basil
1 pound (454 g.) smoked salmon
lime, juiced
2 tbsp. olive oil

Directions:

1. Cut the zucchini after washing it thoroughly into thin slices with a sharp knife.
2. Prepare a colander to filter the zucchini. Add a little salt and toss to coat well. Leave them to sit for 7 to 12 minutes. Gently press the mixture to get rid of excess salted water.
3. Meanwhile, mix the cream cheese with lemon juice, and chopped fresh basil in a bowl. Set aside until ready to serve.
4. Cut the salmon into thin slices and sprinkle with salt and pepper. Add the salmon to an oiled skillet and fry over medium-high heat for 8 minutes, or until the salmon is opaque and tender on both sides. Then add zucchini spirals and cook for 2 minutes until soft.
5. Serve the recipe on a large plate with the cream sauce.

Nutrition: Calories: 444; Fats: 33.4 g; Total Carbs: 10.1 g; Fiber: 2.6 g; Protein: 29.3 g.

1024 DELICIOUS INTERMITTENT CEVICHE

Preparation Time: 15 minutes
Cooking Time: 0 minutes
Servings: 4
Ingredients:

pound (454 g.) skinless white fish, cut into ½-inch cubes
½ red onion, thinly sliced
fresh jalapeño, deseeded and thinly sliced
¼ red bell pepper, thinly sliced
tbsp. salt
¾ cup lime juice, plus more as needed

For Servings:

2 tbsp. lime juice
1 lime, cut into wedges
2 tbsp. olive oil
1 tbsp. fresh cilantro, minced

Directions:

1. Prepare a dish with a lid to put the skinless white fish, then add the onions, jalapeño, thinly sliced bell pepper, and salt. Toss to coat the fish well. Pour the lime juice over.
2. Leave the fish in the fridge for about 3 hours for infusing.
3. Take the fish and vegetables out of the fridge and discard the marinade. Rinse the fish and vegetables thoroughly with cold water.
4. Place the fish on a serving dish, then drizzle with olive oil and lemon juice. Spread the fresh cilantro for topping. Serve cold with lime.

Nutrition: Calories: 174; Fats: 7.6 g; Total Carbs: 6.3 g; Fiber: 0.6 g; Protein: 20.7 g.

1025 BAKED SALMON WITH ORANGE JUICE

Preparation Time: 10 minutes
Cooking Time: 10 minutes
Servings: 2
Ingredients:

½ pound salmon steak
1 cup orange juice
Pinch of ginger powder
black pepper, to taste
salt, to taste
½ lemon juice
1-oz. coconut milk

Directions:

1. Rub salmon steak with spices and let it sit for 15 minutes.
2. Take a bowl and squeeze an orange.
3. Squeeze lemon juice as well and mix.
4. Pour milk into the mixture and stir.
5. Take a baking dish and line with aluminum foil.
6. Place teak on it and pour the sauce over the steak.
7. Cover with another sheet and bake for 10 minutes at 350°F.
8. Serve and enjoy!

Nutrition: Calories: 300; Fat: 3 g; Carbohydrates: 1 g; Protein: 7 g; Fiber: 1 g; Net Carbohydrates: 0 g.

1026 SALMON AND SHRIMP MIX

Preparation Time: 5 minutes
Cooking Time: 20 minutes
Servings: 4
Ingredients:

4 salmon fillets, boneless
1 pound shrimp, peeled and deveined
2tsp. Cajun seasoning
A pinch of salt and black pepper
2 tbsp. olive oil

Juice of 1 lemon

½ cup chicken stock

2 tbsp. tomato passata

Directions:

1. Set the instant pot on Sauté mode. Put the oil and heat it. Add the rest of the ingredients, except the salmon and shrimp, and cook for 3 minutes.
2. Add the salmon and cook for 2 minutes on each side.
3. Put the shrimp, set the lid on, and cook on High for 10 minutes.
4. Release the pressure fast for 5 minutes, divide the mix between plates and serve.

Nutrition: Calories: 393; Fat: 20; Fiber: 0.1; Carbs: 2.2; Protein: 25.

1027 AVOCADO & SALMON OMELET WRAP

Preparation Time: 10 minutes

Cooking Time: 20 minutes

Servings: 2

Ingredients:

3 large eggs

oz. smoked salmon

½ of 1 average size avocado

2 tbsp spring onion

2 tbsp. cream cheese - full-fat

2 tbsp. chives - freshly chopped

3 tbsp. butter or ghee

pepper and salt (as desired)

Directions:

1. Add a sprinkle of pepper and salt to the eggs. Use a fork or whisk—mixing them well. Blend in the chives and cream cheese.
2. Prepare the salmon and avocado (peel and slice or chop).
3. Combine the butter/ghee and the egg mixture in a frying pan. Continue cooking on low heat until done.
4. Place the omelet on a serving dish with a portion of cheese over it. Sprinkle the onion, prepared avocado, and salmon into the wrap.
5. Close and serve!

Nutrition: Calories: 765; Net Carbs: 6 g; Total Fat Content: 67 g; Protein: 37 g.

1028 BAKED TILAPIA WITH CHERRY TOMATOES

Preparation Time: 10 minutes

Cooking Time: 25-30 minutes

Servings: 2

Ingredients:

2 tsp. butter

1-4 oz. tilapia fillets

8 cherry tomatoes

¼ cup pitted black olives

½ tsp. salt

¼ tsp. paprika

¼ tsp. black pepper

2 tsp. garlic powder

2 tbsp. freshly squeezed lemon juice

1 tbsp. optional: balsamic vinegar

Directions:

1. Warm the oven to reach 375° F.
2. Grease a roasting pan and add the butter, along with the olives and tomatoes.
3. Season the tilapia with spices. Lastly, add the fish fillets into the pan with a spritz of lemon juice.
4. Add a piece of foil over the pan. Bake until the fish easily flakes (25 to 30 minutes).
5. Garnish with vinegar if desired.

Nutrition: Calories: 180; Net Carbs: 4 g; Total Fat Content: 8 g; Protein: 23 g.

1029 GARLIC & LEMON SHRIMP PASTA

Preparation Time: 10 minutes

Cooking Time: 30 minutes

Servings: 4

Ingredients:

2 pkg. miracle noodle angel hair pasta

4 garlic cloves

2 tbsp. olive oil

2 tbsp. butter

1 lb. large raw shrimp

½ of 1 lemon

½ tsp. paprika

fresh basil (as desired)

pepper and salt (to taste)

Directions:

1. Drain the water from the package of noodles and rinse them in cold water. Toss into a pot of boiling water for two minutes. Transfer to a hot skillet over medium heat to remove the excess liquid (dry roast). Set them aside.
2. Use the same pan to warm the butter, oil, and mashed garlic. Sauté for a few minutes but don't brown.
3. Slice the lemon into rounds and add them to the garlic along with the shrimp. Sauté for approximately three minutes on each side.
4. Fold in the noodles and spices and stir to blend the flavors.

Nutrition: Calories: 360; Net Carbs: 3.5 g; Total Fat Content: 21 g; Protein: 36 g.

1030 SESAME GINGER SALMON

Preparation Time: 10 minutes

Cooking Time: 20 minutes

Servings: 2

Ingredients:

1-10 oz. salmon fillet

1-2 tsp. minced ginger

2 tbsp. white wine

2 tsp. sesame oil

2 tbsp. rice vinegar

1 1tbsp. Intermittent-friendly soy sauce substitute

1 tbsp. sugar-free ketchup

1tbsp. fish sauce – Red Boat

Directions:

1. Combine all fixings in a plastic canister with a tight-fitting lid (omit the ketchup, oil, and wine for now). Marinade them for about 1o to 15 minutes.
2. On the stovetop, prepare a skillet using the high-heat temperature setting. Pour in the oil. Add the fish when it's hot, skin side down.
3. Brown each side for 3-5 minutes.
4. Pour in the marinated juices to the pan to simmer when the fish is flipped. Arrange the fish on two dinner plates.
5. Pour in the wine and ketchup to the pan and simmer for 5 minutes until it's reduced. Serve with your favorite vegetable.

Nutrition: Calories: 370; Net Carbs: 2.5 g; Total Fat Content: 24 g; Protein: 33 g.

1031 SALMON ROLLS

Preparation Time: 15 minutes

Cooking Time: 10 minutes

Servings: 3

Ingredients:

2 tbsp. butter

½ cup cream cheese

1 tbsp. oregano

1 tsp. cilantro

1tsp. salt

1 tbsp. dill

½ tsp. garlic, minced

1 oz. walnuts, crushed

1 tsp. nutmeg

10 oz. smoked salmon, sliced

Directions:

1. In a medium bowl, using a mixer, put butter and cream cheese, then mix until smooth and fluffy.
2. Add oregano, cilantro, salt, dill, garlic, and walnuts, stir carefully.
3. Add nutmeg and stir until you get a homogenous mass.
4. Put this cream mixture on each salmon slice and roll them.
5. Place salmon rolls in the fridge and wait for 10 minutes.
6. Take out rolls from the fridge and serve.

Nutrition: Calories: 349; Carbs: 3.98 g; Fat: 26.9 g; Protein: 23.1 g.

1032 CRAB RISSOLES

Preparation Time: 10 minutes
Cooking Time: 45 minutes
Servings: 5
Ingredients:

- 12 oz. crab meat
- 2 eggs, beaten
- 2 tbsp. flax meal
- 1 tsp. onion powder
- 2 tbsp. butter
- 2 tsp. salt
- 1 tsp. ground black pepper
- 1 tsp. chives
- 1 tsp. nutmeg
- ¼ cup almond milk
- 2 tbsp. coconut flour
- 2 tbsp. almond flour
- 2 tbsp. coconut oil

Directions:

1. Cut crab meat into tiny pieces.
2. In a bowl, combine eggs with crab meat, stir to get a homogenous mass.
3. Add flax meal, onion powder, butter, salt, and black pepper, stir.
4. Add chives and nutmeg. Mix carefully.
5. Make medium rissoles and dip in almond milk.
6. In a bowl, mix coconut flour and almond flour.
7. Season rissoles with flour mixture.
8. Heat skillet with coconut oil over medium heat.
9. Fry rissoles for 4 minutes on both sides.
10. Let them cool for 2-3 minutes and serve.

Nutrition: Calories: 229; Carbs: 5.98 g; Fat: 18 g; Protein: 12.95 g.

1033 MACKEREL BOMBS

Preparation Time: 15 minutes
Cooking Time: 10 minutes
Servings: 4
Ingredients:

- 10 oz. mackerel, chopped
- white onion, peeled and diced
- tsp. garlic, minced
- ⅓ cup almond flour
- 1 egg, beaten
- ½ tsp thyme
- 1 tsp. salt
- 1 tsp. mustard
- 1 tsp. chili flakes
- ¼ cup spinach, chopped
- 4 tbsp. coconut oil

Directions:

1. Place mackerel in blender or food processor and blend until texture is smooth.
2. In a bowl, combine onion with mackerel.
3. Add garlic, flour, egg, thyme, salt, and mustard, stir well.
4. Add chili flakes and mix up until getting a homogenous mass.
5. Add spinach and stir.
6. Heat a pan at medium heat then add oil.
7. Shape fish mixture into bombs 1 ½-inch in diameter.
8. Put bombs on a pan and cook for 5 minutes on all sides.
9. Transfer to paper towels and drain grease. Serve.

Nutrition: Calories: 318; Carbs: 3.45 g; Fat: 26.5 g; Protein: 20.1 g.

1034 SARDINE FRITTERS

Preparation Time: 25 minutes
Cooking Time: 35 minutes
Servings: 6
Ingredients:

- 2 lbs. sardines, minced
- 1 tsp salt
- 1 tsp cilantro
- ½ tbsp. ground ginger
- ¼ cup spinach, chopped roughly
- 2 tbsp. butter
- 1 tbsp. fish stock
- 2 tbsp. coconut milk

Directions:

1. In a bowl, combine sardines, salt, cilantro, and ginger. Stir gently.
2. Place spinach in a blender and blend for 1 minute.
3. Add spinach to the sardine mixture and mix well.
4. Shape fish mixture into balls and flatten them.
5. Heat pans over medium heat and melt butter.
6. Place fish fritters on a pan and fry for 2 minutes on one side.
7. Flip on the other side; pour in fish stock and coconut milk.
8. Then close the lid and simmer fritters for 10 minutes.
9. Serve hot.

Nutrition: Calories: 369; Carbs: 1 g; Fat: 24 g; Protein: 38 g.

1035 GRILLED SQUID WITH GUACAMOLE

Preparation Time: 15 minutes
Cooking Time: 15 minutes
Servings: 3
Ingredients:

- 2 medium squids
- Salt and ground black pepper to taste
- ½ tsp. olive oil
- Juice from 1 lime

For the guacamole:

- 2 avocados, pitted
- 2 tomato, cored and chopped
- Juice from 2 limes
- 1 tsp 1 Fresh coriander, chopped
- 1 onion, peeled and chopped
- 1 red chilies, chopped

Directions:

1. Separate tentacles from squid and score tubes lengthwise.
2. Rub squid and tentacles with black pepper, salt, and olive oil.
3. Heat grill over medium-high heat and put squid and tentacles score side down.
4. Cook for 2 minutes, flip, and cook for 2 minutes more.
5. Transfer to bowl and sprinkle all parts with lime juice.
6. Peel and chop avocado.
7. In a medium bowl, mash avocado using a fork.
8. Add tomato, the juice from 2 limes, coriander, onion, and chilies. Mix well.
9. Serve squid with guacamole.

Nutrition: Calories: 498; Carbs: 6.95 g; Fat: 44.5 g; Protein: 19.9 g.

1036 FISH MEATBALLS

Preparation Time: 12 minutes
Cooking Time: 15 minutes
Servings: 6
Ingredients:

- 15 oz. salmon, chopped roughly
- ½ tsp chili flakes
- 1 tsp. parsley, chopped
- 1 tbsp. dill, chopped
- 1 tsp. kosher salt
- 1 tsp. garlic, minced
- 2 eggs, beaten
- 8 oz. almond flour
- 2 tbsp. butter
- ¼ cup fish stock

Directions:

1. Place salmon in blender or food processor and blend until smooth.
2. In a medium bowl, mix chili flakes, parsley, dill, and salt.
3. Add blended salmon to spice mixture and stir well.
4. Add garlic and eggs, stir carefully until getting a homogeneous mass.
5. Shape mixture into meatballs 1½ inch in diameter and set aside.
6. Sprinkle meatballs with almond flour.
7. Preheat the pan on medium heat and melt butter.
8. Put fish meatballs in the pan and cook on high heat for 1 minute on both sides.

9. Then, add fish stock and close the lid. Simmer for 10 minutes on medium heat.
10. Serve hot.

Nutrition: Calories: 209; Carbs: 1.75 g; Fat: 16.1 g; Protein: 16.8 g.

1037 DELICIOUS OYSTERS AND PICO DE GALLO

Preparation Time: 10 minutes
Cooking Time: 10 minutes
Servings: 6
Ingredients:
- 18 oysters; scrubbed
- 2 tomatoes; chopped.
- jalapeno pepper; chopped.
- ¼ cup red onion; finely chopped.
- ½ cup Monterey Jack cheese; shredded
- limes; cut into wedges
- Handful cilantro; chopped.
- Juice from 1 lime
- Salt and black pepper to the taste.

Directions:
1. In a bowl, mix the onion with jalapeno, cilantro, tomatoes, salt, pepper, and lime juice and stir well.
2. Place oysters on preheated grill over medium-high heat; cover grill and cook for 7 minutes until they open.
3. Transfer opened oysters to a heatproof dish and discard unopened ones.
4. Top oysters with cheese then put on the preheated broiler for 1 minute.
5. Arrange oysters on a platter. Top each with tomatoes mix you've made earlier, and serve with lime wedges on the side.

Nutrition: Calories: 70; Fat: 2; Fiber: 0; Carbs: 1; Protein: 1.

1038 SPECIAL OYSTERS

Preparation Time: 10 minutes
Cooking Time: 0 minutes
Servings: 4
Ingredients:
- 12 oysters; shucked
- Juice of 1 lemon
- 2 tbsp. ketchup
- Serrano chili pepper; chopped.
- Juice from 1 orange
- Zest from 1 orange
- ¼ cup cilantro; chopped.
- ¼ cup scallions; chopped.
- Juice from 1 lime
- Zest from 1 lime
- ½ cup tomato juice
- ½ tsp. ginger; grated
- ¼ cup olive oil
- ¼ tsp. garlic; minced
- Salt to the taste.

Directions:
1. In a bowl, mix lemon juice, orange juice, orange zest, lime juice and zest, ketchup, chili pepper, tomato juice, ginger, garlic, oil, scallions, cilantro and salt and stir well.
2. Spoon this into oysters and serve them.

Nutrition: Calories: 100; Fat: 1; Fiber: 0; Carbs: 2; Protein: 5.

1039 OCTOPUS SALAD

Preparation Time: 10 minutes
Cooking Time: 40 minutes
Servings: 2
Ingredients:
- 21 oz. octopus; rinsed
- Juice of 1 lemon
- 4 celery stalks; chopped.
- 4 tbsp. parsley; chopped.
- 3 oz. olive oil
- Salt and black pepper to the taste.

Directions:
1. Put the octopus in a pot, add water to cover, cover the pot, bring to a boil over medium heat; cook for 40 minutes, drain and leave aside to cool down.
2. Chop octopus and put it in a salad bowl.
3. Add celery stalks, parsley, oil, and lemon juice and toss well.
4. Spice with salt and pepper, toss again and serve

Nutrition: Calories: 140; Fat: 10; Fiber: 3; Carbs: 6; Protein: 23.

1040 IRISH STYLE CLAMS

Preparation Time: 5 minutes
Cooking Time: 15 minutes
Servings: 4
Ingredients:
- 2 pounds clams; scrubbed
- 3 oz. pancetta
- 1 small green apple; chopped.
- 1 thyme springs; chopped.
- 2 tbsp. olive oil
- 1 tbsp. ghee
- 2 garlic cloves; minced
- ½ bottle infused cider
- Juice of ½ lemon
- Salt and black pepper to the taste.

Directions:
1. Heat a pan with the oil over medium-high heat; add pancetta, brown for 3 minutes and reduce temperature to medium.
2. Add ghee, garlic, salt, pepper, and shallot; stir and cook for 3 minutes.
3. Increase the heat again. Add cider; stir well and cook for 1 minute.
4. Add clams and thyme. Cover the pan and simmer for 5 minutes.
5. Discard unopened clams. Add lemon juice and apple pieces; stir and divide into bowls. Serve hot.

Nutrition: Calories: 100; Fat: 2; Fiber: 1; Carbs: 1; Protein: 20.

1041 GRILLED SWORDFISH

Preparation Time: 10 minutes
Cooking Time: 10 minutes
Servings: 3
Ingredients:
- 4 swordfish steaks
- 3 garlic cloves; minced
- 1 tbsp. parsley; chopped.
- ¼ cup lemon juice
- lemon; cut into wedges
- ⅓ cup chicken stock
- ½ tsp. marjoram; dried
- 2 tbsp. olive oil
- ½ tsp. rosemary; dried
- ½ tsp. sage; dried
- Salt and black pepper to the taste.

Directions:
1. In a bowl, mix chicken stock with garlic, lemon juice, olive oil, salt, pepper, sage, marjoram, and rosemary and whisk well.
2. Put swordfish steaks, toss to coat and keep in the fridge for 3 hours.
3. Place marinated fish steaks on preheated grill over medium-high heat and cook for 5 minutes on each side.
4. Arrange on plates, top with parsley, then serve with lemon wedges on the side.

Nutrition: Calories: 136; Fat: 5; Fiber: 0; Carbs: 1; Protein: 20.

1042 SALMON PATTIES

Preparation Time: 5 minutes
Cooking Time: 15 minutes
Servings: 4
Ingredients:
- 1 egg
- 14 oz. canned salmon, drained
- 4 tbsp. intermittent almond flour
- 4 tbsp. cup cornmeal
- 4 tbsp. onion, minced
- ½ tsp. garlic powder
- 2 tbsp. mayonnaise
- Salt and pepper to taste

Directions:
1. Flake apart the salmon with a fork.
2. Put the flakes in a bowl and combine with the garlic powder, mayonnaise, intermittent almond flour, cornmeal, egg, onion, pepper, and salt.

3. Use your hands to shape equal portions of the mixture into small patties and put each one in the Air Fryer basket.
4. Air fry the salmon patties at 350°F for 15 minutes. Serve hot.

Nutrition: Calories: 319; Protein: 22 g; Carbohydrates: 49 g; Fat: 13 g.

1043 CHEESE TILAPIA

Preparation Time: 10 minutes
Cooking Time: 10 minutes
Servings: 4
Ingredients:

1 lb. tilapia fillets
¼ cup parmesan cheese, grated
2 tbsp. parsley, chopped
1 tsp. paprika
2 tbsp. olive oil
Pepper and salt to taste

Directions:

1. Preheat the Air Fryer to 400°F.
2. In a shallow dish, combine the paprika, grated cheese, pepper, salt, and parsley.
3. Put a light drizzle of olive oil at the tilapia fillets. Cover the fillets with the paprika and cheese mixture.
4. Lay the fillets on a sheet of aluminum foil and transfer to the Air Fryer basket. Fry for 10 minutes. Serve hot.

Nutrition: Calories: 246; Protein: 30.12 g; Fat: 12.22 g; Carbohydrates: 4.35 g.

1044 PARMESAN CRUSTED TILAPIA

Preparation Time: 10 minutes
Cooking Time: 5 minutes
Servings: 4
Ingredients:

¾ cup grated parmesan cheese
4 tilapia fillets
2 tbsp. olive oil
2 tbsp. chopped parsley
2 tsp. paprika
Pinch garlic powder

Directions:

1. Preheat your Air Fryer at 350°F.
2. Coat each of the tilapia fillets with a light brushing of olive oil.
3. Combine all of the other ingredients in a bowl.
4. Cover the fillets with the parmesan mixture.
5. Line the base of a baking dish with a sheet of parchment paper and place the fillets in the dish.
6. Moved to the Air Fryer and cook for 5 minutes. Serve hot.

Nutrition: Calories: 244; Protein: 30.41 g; Fat: 12.24 g; Carbohydrates: 3.29 g.

1045 SALMON CROQUETTES

Preparation Time: 8 minutes
Cooking Time: 7 minutes
Servings: 4

Ingredients:

1 lb. can red salmon, drained and mashed
⅓ cup olive oil
2 eggs, beaten
1 cup intermittent-friendly bread crumbs
½ bunch parsley, chopped

Directions:

1. Preheat the Air Fryer to 400°F.
2. In a mixing bowl, combine the drained salmon, eggs, and parsley.
3. In a shallow dish, stir together the bread crumbs and oil to combine well.
4. Mold equal-sized amounts of the mixture into small balls and coat each one with bread crumbs.
5. Put the croquettes in the fryer's basket and air fry for 7 minutes.

Nutrition: Calories: 442; Protein: 30.48 g; Fat: 32.64 g; Carbohydrates: 5.31 g.

1046 CHUNKY FISH

Preparation Time: 10 minutes
Cooking Time: 8 minutes
Servings: 4
Ingredients:

2 cans canned fish
2 celery stalks, trimmed and finely chopped
1 egg, whisked
1 cup intermittent-friendly bread crumbs
2 tsp. whole-grain mustard
½ tsp. sea salt
¼ tsp. freshly cracked black peppercorns
1 tsp. paprika

Directions:

1. Combine all of the ingredients in which they appear. Mold the mixture into four equal-sized cakes. Leave to chill in the refrigerator for 50 minutes.
2. Put on an Air Fryer grill pan. Spritz all sides of each cake with cooking spray.
3. Grill at 360°F for 5 minutes. Turn the cakes over and resume cooking for an additional 3 minutes.
4. Serve with mashed potatoes if desired.

Nutrition: Calories: 245; Protein: 40.31 g; Fat: 5.67 g; Carbohydrates: 5.64 g.

1047 CRAB STUFFED SALMON

Preparation Time: 10 minutes
Cooking Time: 30 minutes
Servings: 8
Ingredients:

2 lbs. salmon (wider filet works best)
2 tsp lemon zest
2 tbsp. Butter (melted)
Sea salt
Black pepper
Crab Filling:
8 oz. lump crab meat
½ large onion (chopped)
2 tbsp. mayonnaise
2 tbsp. fresh parsley (chopped)
2 cloves garlic (minced)
2 tbsp. lemon juice
1 tsp Old Bay seasoning

Directions:

1. Preheat the oven to 400°F. Line a baking sheet using foil or parchment paper.
2. In a pan at medium heat, sauté onion for about 7-10 minutes, until translucent and browned (or cook longer to caramelize if desired).
3. On the other hand, whisk together the mayonnaise, minced garlic, fresh parsley, lemon juice, and Old Bay seasoning.
4. Stir in the sautéed onion. Carefully fold in the lump crab meat, without breaking up the lumps.
5. Place the salmon fillet on the baking sheet. Organize the crab mixture lengthwise down the middle of the salmon. Starting from the thinner sides of the filet, fold over the long way.
6. Mix together the melted butter and lemon zest. Brush the lemon butter at the top of the salmon. Dust lightly with sea salt and black pepper.
7. Bake for at least 16-20 minutes, until the fish flakes easily with a fork. Sprinkle with additional fresh parsley. Cut crosswise into individual filets to serve.

Nutrition: Calories: 243; Fat: 13 g; Carbs: 1 g; Protein: 29 g.

1048 GLAZED HALIBUT STEAK

Preparation Time: 10 minutes
Cooking Time: 15 minutes
Servings: 3
Ingredients:

lb. halibut steak
⅔ cup low-sodium soy sauce
½ cup mirin
tbsp. lime juice
¼ cup stevia
¼ tsp. crushed red pepper flakes
¼ cup orange juice
garlic clove, smashed

¼ tsp. ginger, ground

Directions:

1. Make the teriyaki glaze by mixing all of the ingredients except for the halibut in a saucepan.
2. Place it to a boil and lower the heat, continually stirring until the mixture reduces by half. Take off from the heat and leave to cool.
3. Pour half of the cooled glaze into a Ziploc bag. Add in the halibut, making sure to coat it well in the sauce. Place in the refrigerator for 30 minutes.
4. Preheat the Air Fryer to 390°F.
5. Put the marinated halibut in the fryer and allow it to cook for 10 – 12 minutes.
6. Use any remaining glaze to brush the halibut steak lightly.
7. Serve with white rice or shredded vegetables.

Nutrition: Calories: 357; Protein: 29.34 g; Fat: 23.16 g; Carbohydrates: 7.15 g.

1049 TOMATILLOS FISH STEW

Preparation Time: 15 minutes
Cooking Time: 12 minutes
Servings: 2
Ingredients:

2 tomatillos, chopped
10 oz. salmon fillet, chopped
1 tsp. ground paprika
½ tsp. ground turmeric
1 cup coconut cream
½ tsp. salt

Directions:

Put all ingredients in the instant pot.
Close and seal the lid.
Cook the fish stew on manual mode (high pressure) for 12 minutes.
Then allow the natural pressure release for 10 minutes.

Nutrition: Calories: 479; Fat: 37.9; Fiber: 3.8; Carbs: 9.6; Protein: 30.8.

BREAKFAST RECIPES

1050 BREAKFAST FRITTATA

Preparation Time: 10 minutes
Cooking Time: 30 minutes
Servings: 2
Ingredients:

2 eggs, beaten
2 tbsp. liquid egg whites
2 tbsp. whole ricotta cheese
Pinch sea salt
Pinch ground mustard spice
Pinch black pepper
¼ cup fresh spinach, chopped
2 slices bacon, cooked and crumbled
2 slices tomato
2 tbsp. grated cheese

Directions:

1. Preheat the oven to 400F. Grease a pie dish.
2. In a bowl, combine beaten eggs, egg whites, ricotta, sea salt, mustard, and black pepper. Whisk and beat well.
3. Add the crumbled bacon and spinach to the mixture and mix.
4. Pour the egg mixture into the prepared pie dish. Place the tomato slices on top.
5. Bake for 30 minutes.
6. Remove from oven and sprinkle with cheese.
7. Cool, slice, and serve.

Nutrition: Calories: 116; Fat: 9 g; Carb: 1 g; Protein: 0 g.

1051 INTERMITTENT WAFFLES

Preparation Time: 5 minutes
Cooking Time: 10 minutes
Servings: 2
Ingredients:

¼ cup almond milk, unsweetened
¼ tsp. apple cider vinegar
1 egg
½ tbsp. olive oil
¼ tsp. vanilla extract
½ cup almond flour
1 tbsp. coconut flour
1 tsp. baking powder
1 tsp. erythritol

Directions:

1. Preheat the waffle iron and grease it.
2. In a bowl, mix apple cider vinegar and almond milk.
3. Add vanilla extract, olive oil, and egg to this mixture. Whisk to combine and set aside.
4. In another bowl, combine baking powder, coconut flour, almond flour, and erythritol. Whisk the dry ingredients together.
5. Combine the dry flour mixture with the wet mixture and whisk to mix.
6. Pour about ¼ cup of batter in the waffle iron.
7. Cook about three to five minutes until steam stops rising from the waffle iron.
8. Repeat and serve.

Nutrition: Calories: 211; Fat: 16 g; Carb: 6.5 g; Protein: 8 g.

1052 PUMPKIN PANCAKES

Preparation Time: 5 minutes
Cooking Time: 12 to 15 minutes
Servings: 2

Ingredients:

1 egg - 1 egg white

1 tbsp. cream cheese
1 ½ tbsp. canned pumpkin, unsweetened
½ tbsp. vanilla extract
⅓ cup almond flour
1 tbsp. coconut flour
½ tbsp. Swerve sweetener
½ tsp. pumpkin pie spice
Pinch of salt
½ tsp. baking powder
Pinch of baking soda
¼ tsp. xanthan gum
Water as needed

Directions:

1. Preheat a griddle to 350°F. Add all the wet pancake ingredients except the water to a blender and blend. Now add the dry ingredients.
2. Continue to blend until smooth.
3. Add water until pancake batter has the right consistency.
4. Into the preheated, oiled griddle, pour a small amount of batter.
5. Cook until browned and the edges almost to the center are dry, about 3 to 4 minutes.
6. Then flip and heat for 2 to 3 minutes.
7. Repeat to finish the batter and serve.

Nutrition: Calories: 230; Fat: 16 g; Carb: 9.5 g; Protein: 8 g.

1053 BUTTERMILK PANCAKES

Preparation Time: 5 minutes
Cooking Time: 8 minutes
Servings: 2
Ingredients:

1 ½ tbsp. coconut flour
1 ½ tbsp. almond flour
1 egg
2 tbsp. almond milk + ¼ tsp. apple cider vinegar, mixed in a bowl
¼ tsp. vanilla extract
Pinch of baking powder
½ tsp. erythritol
1 tsp. butter, melted
Pinch of sea salt

Directions:

1. Mix all the ingredients in a bowl.
2. Heat a lightly greased skillet over medium-high heat. Make sure the skillet is hot.
3. Spoon batter onto the skillet and cook until the batter starts to bubble, about 2 minutes. Then flip and cook until the middle is done. Adjust the heat if needed.
4. Repeat with the remaining batter.
5. Serve with condiments of choice.

Nutrition: Calories: 81; Fat: 6 g; Carb: 4 g; Protein: 3 g.

1054 RICOTTA OMELET WITH SWISS CHARD

Preparation Time: 10 minutes
Cooking Time: 15 minutes
Servings: 2
Ingredients:

6 eggs
2 tbsp. almond milk
½ tsp. kosher salt
½ tsp. ground black pepper
6 tbsp. unsalted butter, divided
2 bunch Swiss chard, cleaned and stemmed
⅔ cup ricotta

Directions:

1. Add the eggs and milk. Season with salt and pepper then whisk. Set aside.
2. In a skillet, melt 4 tablespoons of butter. Add the veggie leaves and sauté until just wilted. Remove from pan. Set aside.
3. Now melt 1 tablespoon of butter in the skillet.
4. Add half of the egg mixture. Spread the mixture. Cook for about 2 minutes.
5. Add half of the ricotta when the edges are firm, but the center is still a bit runny.
6. Bend ⅓ of the omelet over the ricotta filling. Transfer to a plate.
7. Repeat with the remaining butter and egg mixture.
8. Serve with Swiss chard.

Nutrition: Calories: 693; Fat: 60 g; Carb: 8 g; Protein: 2 g.

1055 OMELET WITH GOAT CHEESE AND HERB

Preparation Time: 5 minutes
Cooking Time: 12 minutes
Servings: 2
Ingredients:

6 eggs, beaten
2 tbsp. chopped herbs (basil, parsley or cilantro)
Kosher salt and black pepper to taste
2 tbsp. unsalted butter
4 oz. fresh goat cheese

Directions:

1. Whisk together the eggs, herbs, salt, and pepper.
2. Melt 1 tbsp. butter in a skillet.
3. Put half of the egg mixture and cook for 4 to 5 minutes, or until just set.
4. Crumble half the goat cheese over the eggs and fold in half.
5. Cook for 1 minute, or until cheese is melted. Transfer to a plate.

6. Repeat process with the remaining butter, egg mixture, and goat cheese.
7. Serve.

Nutrition: Calories: 523; Fat: 43 g; Carb: 3 g; Protein: 31 g.

1056 BACON AND ZUCCHINI EGG BREAKFAST

Preparation Time: 10 minutes
Cooking Time: 10 minutes
Servings: 2
Ingredients:

2 cups zucchini noodles
2 slices of raw bacon
¼ cup grated Asiago cheese
2 eggs
Salt and pepper to taste

Directions:

1. Cut the bacon slices into ¼ inch thick strips.
2. Cook the bacon in a pan for 3 minutes.
3. Add the zucchini and mix well.
4. Season with salt and pepper.
5. Flatten slightly with a spatula and make 2 depressions for the eggs.
6. Sprinkle with the cheese.
7. Break one egg into each dent.
8. Cook 3 minutes more, then cover and cook for 2 to 4 minutes, or until the eggs are cooked.
9. Serve.

Nutrition: Calories: 242; Fat: 19 g; Carb: 4 g; Protein: 14 g.

1057 TURKEY AND SCRAMBLED EGGS BREAKFAST

Preparation Time: 10 minutes
Cooking Time: 15 minutes
Servings: 2
Ingredients:

4 slices avocado
Salt and pepper to taste
4 slices bacon, diced
4 turkey breast slices, cooked
4 tbsp. coconut oil
4 eggs, whisked

Directions:

1. Heat a pan over medium heat.
2. Add bacon slices and brown all over.
3. Heat oil in another pan.
4. Add eggs, salt, and pepper, and scramble.
5. Divide turkey breast slices, bacon, scrambled eggs, and avocado slices on 2 plates and serve.

Nutrition: Calories: 791; Fat: 64.3 g; Carb: 8.8 g; Protein: 41.8 g.

1058 CHIA BREAKFAST BOWL

Preparation Time: 10 minutes
Cooking Time: 0 minutes

Servings: 2
Ingredients:

¼ cup whole chia seeds
2 cups almond milk, unsweetened
2 tbsp. sugar-free maple syrup
1 tsp. vanilla extract

Toppings:

Cinnamon and extra maple syrup
Nuts and berries

Directions:

1. Combine the syrup, milk, chia seeds, and vanilla extract in a bowl and stir to mix.
2. Let stand for 30 minutes, then whisk.
3. Transfer to an airtight container.
4. Cover and refrigerate overnight.
5. Serve in the morning.

Nutrition: Calories: 298; Fat: 15 g; Carb: 5 g; Protein: 14 g.

1059 CINNAMON ROLL OATMEAL

Preparation Time: 10 minutes
Cooking Time: 10 minutes
Servings: 2
Ingredients:

⅓ cup crushed pecans
1 tbsp. flaxseed meal
1 tbsp. chia seeds
2 tbsp. cauliflower, riced
1 cup plus 1 tbsp. coconut milk
1 tbsp. heavy cream
1 oz. cream cheese
1 tbsp. butter
½ tsp. cinnamon
½ tsp. maple flavor
¼ tsp. vanilla essence
Pinch of nutmeg
Pinch of allspice
1 tbsp. erythritol, powdered
5 drops liquid stevia
Pinch of xanthan gum

Directions:

1. In a bowl, add flax seeds and chia seeds and set aside.
2. Heat the coconut milk in a saucepan. Once warm, add the cauliflower and cook until it starts to boil.
3. Lower the heat and add allspice, nutmeg, vanilla, maple flavor, and cinnamon.
4. Add stevia and erythritol to the pan and stir well.
5. Add the chia seed and flaxseed mixture to the pan and mix well.
6. Once the mixture is hot, add the cream, cream cheese, butter, and pecans.
7. Mix well and serve.

Nutrition: Calories: 398; Fat: 37.8 g; Carb: 3.1 g; Protein: 8.8 g.

1060 BREAKFAST CEREAL

Preparation Time: 5 minutes
Cooking Time: 3 minutes
Servings: 2
Ingredients:

- ½ cup shredded coconut, unsweetened
- 4 tsp. butter
- 2 cups almond milk, unsweetened
- 1 tbsp. stevia
- Pinch of salt
- 2 tbsp. macadamia nuts, chopped
- 2 tbsp. walnuts, chopped
- ⅓ cup flaxseed

Directions:

1. Melt the butter in a pan.
2. Add the coconut, milk, salt, nuts, flaxseed, and stevia, and stir well.
3. Cook for 3 minutes and stir again.
4. Remove from heat. Set aside for 10 minutes.
5. Serve.

Nutrition: Calories: 588; Fat: 48 g; Carb: 6.8 g; Protein: 16.5 g.

1061 BEST INTERMITTENT BREAD

Preparation Time: 10 minutes
Cooking Time: 30 minutes
Servings: 20
Ingredients:

- 1 ½ cups almond flour
- 6 drops liquid stevia
- 1 pinch pink Himalayan salt
- ¼ tsp. cream of tartar
- 3 tsp. baking powder
- ¼ cup butter, melted
- 6 large eggs, separated

Directions:

1. Preheat the oven to 375°F.
2. To the egg whites, add cream of tartar and beat until soft peaks are formed.
3. In a food processor, combine stevia, salt, baking powder, almond flour, melted butter, ⅓ of the beaten egg whites, and egg yolks. Mix well.
4. Then add the remaining ⅔ of the egg whites and gently process until fully mixed. Don't over mix.
5. Put a grease on a (8 x 4) loaf pan and pour the mixture into it.
6. Bake for 30 minutes.
7. Enjoy.

Nutrition: Calories: 90; Fat: 7; Carb: 2 g; Protein: 3 g.

1062 BREAD DE SOUL

Preparation Time: 10 minutes
Cooking Time: 45 minutes
Servings: 16
Ingredients:

- ¼ tsp. cream of tartar
- 2 ½ tsp. baking powder
- 1 tsp. xanthan gum
- ⅓ tsp. baking soda
- ½ tsp. salt
- ⅔ cup unflavored whey protein
- ¼ cup olive oil
- ¼ cup heavy whipping cream
- drops of sweet leaf stevia
- eggs - ¼ cup butter
- 12 oz. softened cream cheese

Directions:

1. Preheat the oven to 325°F.
2. In a bowl, microwave cream cheese and butter for 1 minute.
3. Remove and blend well with a hand mixer.
4. Add olive oil, eggs, heavy cream, and few drops of sweetener and blend well.
5. Put together the dry ingredients in a separate bowl.
6. Combine the dry ingredients with the wet ingredients and mix with a spoon. Don't use a hand blender to avoid whipping it too much.
7. Grease a bread pan and pour the mixture into the pan.
8. Bake in the oven until golden brown for about 45 minutes.
9. Cool and serve.

Nutrition: Calories: 200; Fat: 15.2 g; Carb: 1.8 g; Protein: 10 g.

1063 CHIA SEED BREAD

Preparation Time: 10 minutes
Cooking Time: 4 minutes
Servings: 16
Ingredients:

- ½ tsp. xanthan gum
- ½ cup butter
- 2 tbsp. coconut oil
- tbsp. baking powder
- tbsp. sesame seeds
- tbsp. chia seeds
- ½ tsp. salt
- ¼ cup sunflower seeds
- 2 cups almond flour
- 7 eggs

Directions:

1. Preheat the oven to 350°F.
2. Beat eggs in a bowl for 1 to 2 minutes.
3. Beat in the xanthan gum and combine coconut oil and melted butter into eggs, beating continuously.
4. Set aside the sesame seeds, but add the rest of the ingredients.
5. Get a loaf pan with baking paper and place the mixture in it. Top the mixture with sesame seeds.
6. Bake in the oven for about 35 to 40 minutes.

Nutrition: Calories: 405; Fat: 37 g; Carb: 4 g; Protein: 14 g.

1064 SPECIAL INTERMITTENT BREAD

Preparation Time: 15 minutes
Cooking Time: 40 minutes
Servings: 14
Ingredients:

- 2 tsp. baking powder
- ½ cup water
- tbsp. poppy seeds
- cups fine ground almond meal
- 5 large eggs
- ½ cup olive oil
- ½ tsp. fine Himalayan salt

Directions:

1. Preheat oven to 400°F.
2. In a bowl, combine salt, almond meal, and baking powder.
3. Drip in oil while mixing, until it forms a crumbly dough.
4. Make a little round hole in the middle of the dough and pour eggs into the middle of the dough.
5. Pour water and whisk eggs together with the mixer in the small circle until it is frothy.
6. Start making larger circles to combine the almond meal mixture with the dough until you have a smooth and thick batter.
7. Line your loaf pan with parchment paper.
8. Pour batter into the loaf pan and sprinkle poppy seeds on top.
9. Bake in the oven for 40 minutes in the center rack until firm and golden brown.
10. Cool in the oven for 30 minutes.
11. Slice and serve.

Nutrition: Calories: 227; Fat: 21 g; Carb: 4 g; Protein: 7 g.

1065 INTERMITTENT FLUFFY CLOUD BREAD

Preparation Time: 25 minutes
Cooking Time: 25 minutes
Servings: 3
Ingredients:

- pinch salt
- ½ tbsp. ground psyllium husk powder
- ½ tbsp. baking powder
- ¼ tsp. cream of tartar
- eggs, separated
- ½ cup, cream cheese

Directions:

1. Preheat oven to 300°F.
2. Whisk egg whites in a bowl until soft peaks are formed.
3. Mix egg yolks with cream cheese, salt, cream of tartar, psyllium

husk powder, and baking powder in a bowl.

4. Fold in the egg whites carefully and transfer to the baking tray.
5. Place in the oven and bake for 25 minutes.
6. Remove from the oven and serve.

Nutrition: Calories: 185; Fat: 16.4 g; Carb: 3.9 g; Protein: 6.6 g.

1066 SPLENDID LOW-CARB BREAD

Preparation Time: 15 minutes
Cooking Time: 60 to 70 minutes
Servings: 12
Ingredients:

½ tsp. herbs, such as basil, rosemary, or oregano
½ tsp. garlic or onion powder
tbsp. baking powder
5 tbsp. psyllium husk powder
½ cup almond flour
½ cup coconut flour
¼ tsp. salt
1 ½ cup egg whites
tbsp. oil or melted butter
tbsp. apple cider vinegar
⅓ to ¾ cup hot water

Directions:

1. Put a grease on a loaf pan and preheat the oven to 350°F.
2. In a bowl, whisk the salt, psyllium husk powder, onion or garlic powder, coconut flour, almond flour, and baking powder.
3. Stir in egg whites, oil, and apple cider vinegar. Slowly, add the hot water, stirring until dough increases in size. Do not add too much water.
4. Mold the dough into a rectangle and transfer to a grease loaf pan.
5. Bake in the oven for 60 to 70 minutes, or until the crust feels firm and brown on top.
6. Cool and serve.

Nutrition: Calories: 97; Fat: 5.7 g; Carb: 7.5 g; Protein: 4.1 g.

1067 COCONUT FLOUR ALMOND BREAD

Preparation Time: 10 minutes
Cooking Time: 30 minutes
Servings: 4
Ingredients:

tbsp. butter, melted
1 tbsp. coconut oil, melted
6 eggs
1 tsp. baking soda
tbsp. ground flaxseed
1 ½ tbsp. psyllium husk powder
5 tbsp. coconut flour
1 ½ cups almond flour

Directions:

1. Preheat the oven to 400°F.

2. Mix the eggs in a bowl for a few minutes.
3. Add in the butter and coconut oil and mix once more for 1 minute.
4. Add the almond flour, coconut flour, baking soda, psyllium husk, and ground flaxseed to the mixture. Let sit for 15 minutes.
5. Grease the loaf pan with coconut oil. Pour the mixture into the pan.
6. Put in the oven. Bake until a toothpick in it comes out dry, about 25 minutes.

Nutrition: Calories: 475; Fat: 38 g; Carb: 7 g; Protein: 19 g.

1068 QUICK LOW-CARB BREAD LOAF

Preparation Time: 45 minutes
Cooking Time: 40 to 45 minutes
Servings: 16
Ingredients:

⅔ cup coconut flour
½ cup butter, melted
3 tbsp. coconut oil, melted
⅓ cup almond flour
½ tsp. xanthan gum
½ tsp. baking powder
6 large eggs
½ tsp. salt

Directions:

1. Preheat the oven to 350°F. Cover the bread loaf pan with baking paper.
2. Beat the eggs until creamy.
3. Add in the coconut flour and almond flour, mixing them for 1 minute. Next, add the xanthan gum, coconut oil, baking powder, butter, and salt and mix them until the dough turns thick.
4. Put the completed dough into the prepared line of the bread loaf pan.
5. Put in oven and bake for 40 to 45 minutes. Check with a knife.
6. Slice and serve.

Nutrition: Calories: 174; Fat: 15 g; Carb: 5 g; Protein: 5 g.

1069 INTERMITTENT BAKERS BREAD

Preparation Time: 10 minutes
Cooking Time: 20 minutes
Servings: 12
Ingredients:

Pinch of salt
4 tbsp. light cream cheese, softened
½ tsp. cream of tartar
4 eggs, yolks, and whites separated

Directions:

1. Heat 2 racks in the middle of the oven at 350F.

2. Line 2 baking pan with parchment paper, then grease with cooking spray.
3. Separate egg yolks from the whites. Put in separate mixing bowls.
4. Beat the egg whites and cream of tartar with a hand mixer until stiff, about 3 to 5 minutes. Do not over-beat.
5. Whisk the cream cheese, salt, and egg yolks until smooth.
6. Slowly fold the cheese mix into the whites until fluffy.
7. Spoon ¼ cup measure of the batter onto the baking sheets, 6 mounds on each sheet.
8. Bake for 20 to 22 minutes, alternating racks halfway through.
9. Cool and serve.

Nutrition: Calories: 41; Fat: 3.2 g; Carb: 1 g; Protein: 2.4 g.

1070 CHEESE GARLIC BREAD

Preparation Time: 10 minutes
Cooking Time: 15 minutes
Servings: 10
Ingredients:

170g mozzarella cheese, shredded
85g almond meal
tbsp. crushed garlic
tbsp. full fat cream cheese
1 tsp. baking powder
1 tbsp. dried parsley
1 medium egg
1 pinch salt

Directions:

1. Add every ingredient into a bowl, excluding the egg.
2. Lightly stir the mixture until combined.
3. Place bowl in a microwave and microwave for 1 minute on high.
4. Stir mixture and microwave for 30 seconds more.
5. Add the egg into the dough and gently stir until incorporated.
6. Add mixture onto a prepared baking tray and mold into a loaf shape.
7. Sprinkle any leftover cheese over the bread.
8. Bake loaf for 15 minutes at 425°F, or until golden brown.

Nutrition: Calories: 117.4; Fat: 9.8 g; Carb: 2.4 g; Protein: 6.2 g.

1071 ALMOND FLOUR LEMON BREAD

Preparation Time: 15 minutes
Cooking Time: 45 minutes
Servings: 2
Ingredients:

1 tsp. French herbs

1 tsp. lemon juice
1 tsp. salt
1 tsp. cream of tartar
½ tsp. baking powder
¼ cup melted butter
5 large eggs, divided
¼ cup coconut flour
1 ½ cup almond flour

Directions:
1. Preheat the oven to 350°F.Beat the whites and cream of tartar until soft peaks form.
2. In a bowl, combine salt, egg yolks, melted butter, and lemon juice. Mix well.
3. Add coconut flour, almond flour, herbs, and baking powder. Mix well.
4. To the dough, add ⅓ of the egg whites and mix until well-combined.
5. Add the remaining egg white mixture and slowly mix to incorporate everything. Do not over mix.
6. Put a grease on a loaf pan with butter or coconut oil.
7. Pour mixture into the loaf pan and bake for 30 minutes.

Nutrition: Calories: 115; Fat: 9.9 g; Carb: 3.3 g; Protein: 5.2 g.

1072 SEED AND NUT BREAD

Preparation Time: 10 minutes
Cooking Time: 40 minutes
Servings: 24
Ingredients:
3 eggs
¼ cup avocado oil
½ tsp. psyllium husk powder
1 tsp. apple cider vinegar
¾ tsp. salt
5 drops liquid stevia
1 ½ cups raw unsalted almonds
½ cup raw unsalted pepitas
½ cup raw unsalted sunflower seeds
½ cup flaxseeds

Directions:
1. Preheat the oven to 325°F. Line a loaf pan with parchment paper.
2. In a huge bowl, whisk together the oil, eggs, psyllium husk powder, vinegar, salt, and liquid stevia.
3. Stir in the pepitas, almonds, sunflower seeds, and flaxseeds until well combined.
4. Pour the batter into the prepared loaf pan, smooth it out and let it rest for 2 minutes.
5. Bake for 40 minutes.
6. Cool, slice, and serve.

Nutrition: Calories: 131; Fat: 12 g; Carb: 4 g; Protein: 5 g.

1073 PURI BREAD

Preparation Time: 10 minutes
Cooking Time: 5 minutes
Servings: 6
Ingredients:
cup almond flour, sifted
½ cup of warm water
tbsp. clarified butter
1 cup olive oil for frying
Salt to taste

Directions:
1. Salt the water and add the flour.
2. Create a hole in the center of the dough and pour warm butter.
3. Knead the dough and let stand for 15 minutes, covered.
4. Shape into 6 balls.
5. Flatten the balls into 6 thin rounds using a rolling pin.
6. Heat enough oil to completely cover a round frying pan.
7. Place a puri in it when hot.
8. Fry for 20 seconds on each side.
9. Place on a paper towel.
10. Repeat with the rest of the puri and serve.

Nutrition: Calories: 106; Fat: 3 g; Carb: 6 g; Protein: 3 g.

1074 CRANBERRY BREAD

Preparation Time: 10 minutes
Cooking Time: 1 hour & 15 minutes
Servings: 12
Ingredients:
½ cup coconut milk
½ tsp baking soda
½ cup powdered erythritol
½ tsp. powdered stevia
½ tsp. salt
bag (6-oz.) cranberries
1 ½ tsp. baking powder
cups almond flour
eggs
tbsp. unsalted melted butter

Directions:
1. Preheat the oven to 350°F.
2. Add the flour, erythritol, baking powder, stevia, salt, and baking soda into a bowl and combine.
3. In another bowl, add in the butter, coconut milk, eggs, and mix well.
4. Combine the erythritol mixture with the butter mixture. Then add in the cranberries and fold them. Transfer into the loaf pan.
5. Bake in the oven for 1 hour and 15 minutes.
6. Cool, slice, and serve.

Nutrition: Calories: 179; Fat: 15 g; Carb: 7 g; Protein: 6.4 g.

1075 AVOCADO SALAD DISH

Preparation Time: 8 minutes

Cooking Time: 5 minutes
Servings: 2
Ingredients:
½ of a medium avocado, sliced
1 tbsp. apple cider vinegar
1 tbsp olive oil
4 oz. chopped lettuce
4 slices of bacon, chopped

Directions:
1. Prepare bacon. For this, put a skillet pan over medium heat and when hot, put chopped bacon and let it cook for 5 to 8 minutes until golden brown.
2. Then distribute lettuce and avocado between two plates, top with bacon, drizzle with olive oil and apple cider and serve.

Nutrition: Calories: 14; Fats: 6; Protein: 2; Carbohydrates: 1.

1076 POWER CREAM WITH STRAWBERRY

Preparation Time: 5 minutes
Cooking Time: 0
Servings: 2
Ingredients:
1 tbsp. coconut oil
1 tsp. vanilla extract, unsweetened
2 oz. coconut cream, full-fat
1 oz. fresh strawberries

Directions:
1. Bring out a large bowl, put all the ingredients in it and then mix by using a blender until smooth.
2. Distribute evenly between two bowls and then serve.

Nutrition: Calories: 214; Fats: 3; Protein: 4; Carbohydrates: 2.

1077 SAVORY INTERMITTENT PANCAKE

Preparation Time: 5 minutes
Cooking Time: 5 minutes
Servings: 2
Ingredients:
¼ cup almond flour
½ tbsp unsalted butter
eggs
oz. cream cheese, softened

Directions:
1. Bring out a bowl, crack eggs in it, whisk well until fluffy, and then whisk in flour and cream cheese until well combined.
2. Bring out a skillet pan, put it over medium heat, add butter and when it melts, drop pancake batter in four segments, spread it evenly, and cook for 2 minutes per side until brown.

Nutrition: Calories: 167; Fats: 15; Protein: 2; Carbohydrates: 1.

1078 MIX VEGGIE FRITTERS

Preparation Time: 5 minutes
Cooking Time: 7 minutes
Servings: 2
Ingredients:

½ tsp. nutritional yeast
1 oz. chopped broccoli
1 zucchini, grated, squeezed
2 eggs
1 tbsp. almond flour

Directions:

1. Wrap grated zucchini in a cheesecloth, twist it well to remove excess moisture, and then Put zucchini in a bowl.
2. Add remaining ingredients, except for oil, and then whisk well until combined.
3. Bring out a skillet pan. Put it over medium heat, add oil and when hot, drop zucchini mixture in four portions, shape them into flat patties and cook for 4 minutes per side until thoroughly cooked.

Nutrition: Calories: 191; Fats: 10; Protein: 1; Carbohydrate: 1.

1079 ZUCCHINI PANCAKES

Preparation Time: 5 minutes
Cooking Time: 10 minutes
Servings: 3
Ingredients:

1,5 oz. zucchini
½ cup almond flour
2 tbsp. coconut flour
1 oz. full-fat milk
2 eggs
½ tsp baking powder
1 tsp cinnamon
1 tbsp. ghee butter
Salt and erythritol to taste

Directions:

1. Grate the zucchini, season with salt and place into a sieve to drain.
2. Put into a blender. Add other ingredients, pulse well.
3. Melt the butter in a pan in medium heat.
4. Form the pancakes and put into the skillet.
5. Close the lid and cook for 3 minutes on each side.

Nutrition: Carbs: 0 7 g; Fats: 7 g; Protein: 7 5 g; Calories: 130.

THE BEST EXERCISE TO DO WITH YOUR INTERMITTENT FASTING DIET

A STRENGTH TRAINING EXERCISE FOR WOMEN OVER 50

Strength training is significant for everybody, except after 50, it turns out to be more critical than any other time in recent memory. It stops being about huge biceps or ripped abs, yet rather takes on a tone of maintenance. The accompanying exercise will give you 10 fantastic activities that ladies more than 50 can focus on during their workout.

A cardiovascular workout is best for the heart and lungs. It improves oxygen delivery to particular parts of your body, reduces stress, improves sleep, burns fat, and improves sex drive. A few of the more common cardio exercises are running, brisk strolling, and swimming. Within the exercise center, machines such as the elliptical, treadmill, and Stairmaster are utilized to assist with cardio.

Some people are satisfied and feel like they've done after 20 minutes on the treadmill, but if you need to continue to be strong and self-sufficient as you get older, you should consider including quality training in your workout. After 50, quality training for a lady is now not about getting six-pack abs, building biceps, or posturing muscles. Instead, it has changed to maintaining a body that's sound, solid, and is less inclined to develop injury and sickness.

SQUAT TO CHAIR

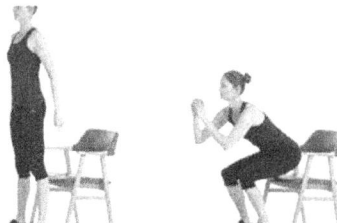

Seat squats are a beginner-friendly exercise extraordinary for building significant leg muscles like your quads, hamstrings, and glutes while offering the help of a strong surface.

Stand tall with your feet hip-distance apart. Your hips, knees, and toes should all point forward. (Hold free weights in your hands to make it harder).

Curve your knees and expand your bum backward as though you are going to sit once again onto a seat.

FOREARM PLANK

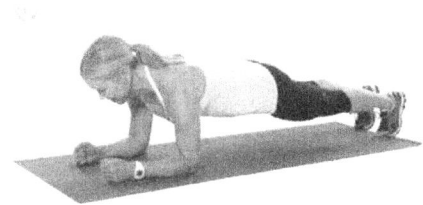

Although it's a challenge to do it correctly, once you get command of it, the Forearm Plank fortifies the abs, legs, and core. It is additionally useful for extending the curves of your feet just as your calves, shoulders, and hamstrings.

Start lying on the floor with your lower arms level, ensuring that your elbows are adjusted straightforwardly under your shoulders.

Draw in your center and raise your body off the floor, keeping your lower arms on the floor and your body in an orderly fashion from head to feet. Keep your abs drawn in and do whatever it takes not to allow your hips to rise or drop. Rather than 8 to 12 reps, hold for 30 seconds. If it hurts your lower back or turns out to be excessively troublesome, place your knees down on the ground.

MODIFIED PUSH-UP

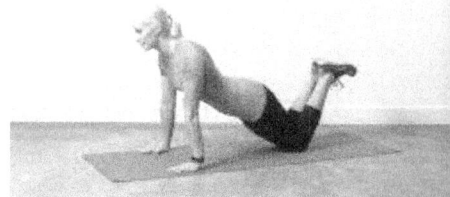

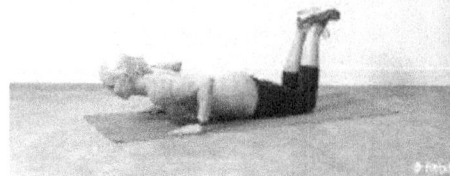

If you have trouble doing regular push-ups effectively, you can always switch to modified push-ups. It works on your upper body.

Start in a bowing situation on a tangle with hands beneath shoulders and knees behind hips, so the back is calculated and long.

Fold toes under, fix abs, and twist elbows to bring down the chest toward the floor. Keep your view before your fingertips, so your neck remains long.

Press chest rears up to the beginning position.

BIRD DOG

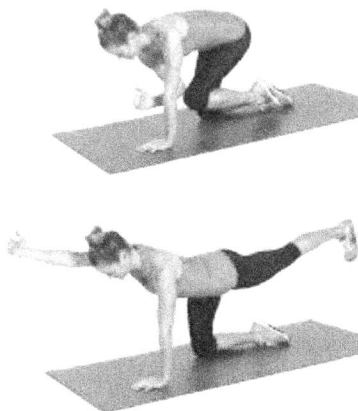

It is a simple exercise that improves stability and reduces lower back pain. It also helps to maintain proper posture.

Kneel on the ground on all fours.

Stand at one arm long, draw in the abs, and stretch the opposite leg long behind you.

Repeat 8 to multiple times and then switch sides.

SHOULDER OVERHEAD PRESS

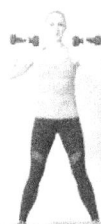

Start with feet hip-distance apart. Bring elbows out to the side, making a goal-line position with arms, hand weights are along the edge of the head, and abs are tight.

Press free weights gradually up until arms are straight. Gradually return to the initial point. Whenever wanted, you can likewise do this activity situated in a seat.

CHEST FLY

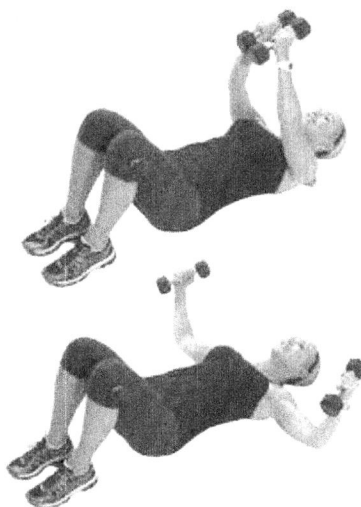

Hold a couple of hand weights carefully shrouded and place your shoulder bones and head on top of the ball with the remainder of your body in a tabletop position.

The feet should be hip-distance apart. Raise free weights together straight over the chest, palms looking in. Gradually lower your arms out to the side with a slight twist in your elbow, until elbows are about chest level.

Lie on your back with twisted knees hip-distance apart, and feet level

Crush glutes and lift hips off the tangle into a scaffold. Lower and lift the hips for 8-12 reps, then repeat on the opposite side.

BENT-OVER ROW

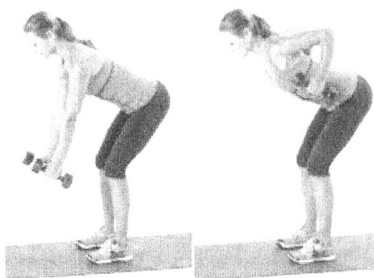

The composition is exceptionally significant with the twisted around the column, and the most ideal approach to guarantee you don't get messy is to pick the perfect measure of weight. Slow, controlled developments are definitely more incentive than snapping up an enormous weight and contorting everywhere in the shop.

When you have your hand weight stacked, remain with your feet shoulder-width apart.

Twist your knees and lean forward from the midsection.

Your knees should be twisted. However, your back stays straight, with your neck by your spine. Get the bar with your hands (palms-down), only more extensive than shoulder-width apart, and let it hang with your arms straight.

Support your center and crush your shoulders together to push the load up until it contacts your sternum. At that point, gradually drop it back down once more. There's one rep. With a lightweight, go for four arrangements of eight to 10 reps.

BASIC ABS

Indeed, there are various layers of muscles (in addition to delicate tissue, nerves, and veins) that make up the full stomach wall. Also, even though you can't see or truly feel them all, they're truly significant for keeping your whole body solid and stable.

There are various types of abs exercises.

ABDOMINAL HOLD

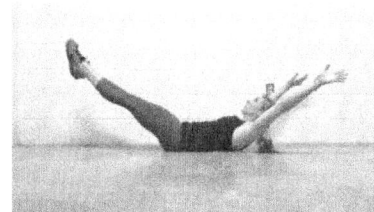

Sit tall on the edge of a solid seat (or step with four risers) and spot your hands on the edge with your fingers highlighting your knees.

Fix your abs and carry your toes 2 to 4 inches off the floor. Lift your butt off the seat. Hold this situation; however long you can — focus on 5 to 10 seconds. Let yourself down and repeat. Proceed for 1 minute.

THE SIDE CRUNCH

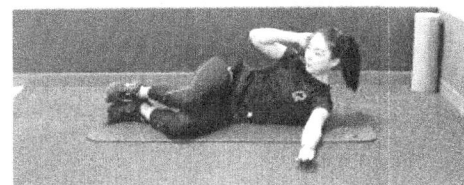

Bow on the floor and lean right over to your right side, putting your right palm on the floor. Keeping your weight-adjusted, gradually broaden your left leg and point your toes. Place your left hand above your head, guiding your elbow to the roof. Then, gradually lift your leg to hip height as you expand your arm over your leg, with your palm looking forward. Put your hand over while bringing the left half of your ribs to stay near your hip.

Lower to your beginning position and repeat 6 to multiple times. Complete two arrangements of 6 to 8 reps, and afterward switch sides

STANDING CALF RAISE

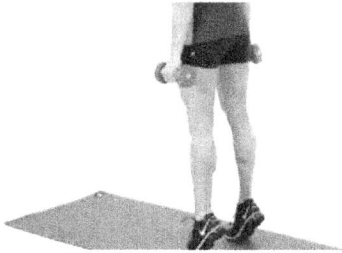

This exercise improves the mobility of your lower legs and feet and also improves your stability.

Here's how to perform it.

Hold a dumbbell in your left hand and place your right hand on something sturdy to give you balance.

When you are sure of your balance, lift your left foot off the floor with the dumbbell hanging at your side. Stand erect and move your weight so that you are almost standing on your toes.

Slowly return to the starting position. Do this 15 times before switching to the other leg and doing the same thing all over again.

SINGLE-LEG HAMSTRING BRIDGE

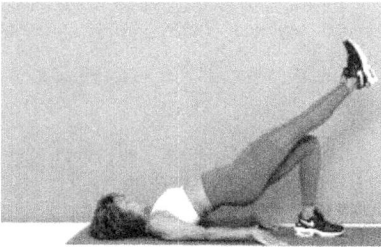

This move targets your glutes, quads, and hamstrings.

To do this:

Lie flat on your back.

Place your arms flat by your side and lift one leg straight.

Contract your glutes as you lift your hips into a bridge position with your arms still in place. Hold for about 2–3 seconds and drop your hips to the mat. Repeat about 10 times before switching your leg. Do the same again.

HOW TO OVERCOME DOWN MOMENTS

It really doesn't matter whether you are a newbie to intermittent fasting or you've been at it for a while. Each day you struggle to the finishing post, to the small window of time when you can eat but it seems that everywhere you look, people are eating delicious meals and sipping on full-fat flavored coffees. You find yourself resenting them while you sit and sip on a black coffee or a bottle of water, counting down the minutes and hours until you can eat again. Is that you? Most people who do on intermittent fast go through exactly the same thing but there is one way to get over it and that is to change your mindset and build up good healthy habits.

Many people who have tried dieting find themselves in a diet mindset – you are either on one or you aren't. You are either being good or you are cheating on your diet. And, it follows, that you are either losing weight or gaining it.

The same goes for intermittent fasting. You will, without a doubt, go at it with the same mindset – you'll reach your goal and then you'll work out how to maintain it. The biggest problem is that too many people see intermittent fasting as a temporary fix to the temporary problem of weight gain. The actual problem is in mindset. You must learn to see intermittent fasting as a permanent way of life and the only way to fix your mindset is to change it permanently. You need to shed the diet mindset and then you will start to see the results you want. You are no longer on a diet, there is no longer a point at which you stop. This is for life and the sooner you realize that, the easier it will become.

Now, this is the most important part of all. You will find yourself in another mindset – the 'can't' mindset. I can't eat until 6 pm. I can't eat when everyone else is eating. I can't add cream and sugar to my coffee. Instead of focusing on enjoying your lifestyle, you will be focusing on what you see as deprivation. Instead of thinking about what you can do, you constantly think about what you can't do. This is the mindset you need to shake off quickly because, until you do, you can't even enjoy intermittent fasting and, believe me, it is an enjoyable lifestyle.

Make that change and you'll find yourself cooking for your family without even thinking about whether you can eat or not.

How do you conquer the 'can't' mindset? How easy is it? Weight loss may be your goal, but intermittent fasting is about so much more. It's about cleansing your body and slowing the aging process. It's about improving your health and having more energy. It's about rediscovering yourself, the person that you are meant to be.

You need to understand that it has nothing to do with not being able to eat when you want; it's all about choosing not to. It's about choosing to understand that your body doesn't need that much food. It's about understanding that your body will benefit from you eating the right foods but giving your body a chance to recuperate and recover every day. It's about watching the fat melt away with just one simple change to your life. Where's the hardship in that? Where's the deprivation when you find yourself fitting into clothes you never thought you'd ever be able to wear again?

Are you ready to make a huge change in your life? Change your mindset and you'll be happier and healthier than you ever knew. And this all leads to something else – a change in your eating habits.

Because you can only eat during a certain window of time, you'll want to make the most of it. By feeding your body healthy nutritious and delicious foods, you won't want to go back to eating junk. Sure, you can 'treat' yourself occasionally, but I promise you this – after a while on intermittent fasting, once your body gets used to eating a healthier diet, you won't want those treats.

One more thing you need to understand – this won't happen overnight. You have to work at changing both your mindset and your habits so be patient and give yourself time.

PLAN FOR SUCCESS AND COMMIT TO YOURSELF

Once you are in a good rhythm with regard to your intermittent fasting, you will find it easy to work around your fasting and eating windows. At the very beginning of your journey, though, it is important to plan for success. Once you have selected a specific protocol to match your lifestyle, it is important to plan a month or so in advance to see if there are days when your chosen protocol may not work for you and plan around that.

While this may seem a small issue to be focusing on, it is actually extremely important. If you want to maintain consistency, the enemy of that is going to be issues that crop up that you haven't planned for. Similarly, consider what your family life looks like. Do you usually eat breakfast with your family in the morning? If so, you may need to explain to them that you are going to be embarking on a new lifestyle that will require you to skip breakfast. If they rely on you to make their breakfast, this is a good opportunity to change that. Cereals and toast are easy enough for most people to make on their own. If you feel that you may be tempted by being around your family when they are eating breakfast, turn their breakfast time into your exercise time.

Having plans for situations like this will help you avoid faltering on your intermittent fasting lifestyle. You will also feel more confident if you feel that you are in control of your lifestyle and that you are able to make good decisions on the spur of the moment because you have planned for them. A lot of these types of situations can be helped by sharing your plans with your family, close friends, and coworkers.

If you are specifically using intermittent fasting to lose weight, be sure to throw out your scale and whip out your measuring tape instead. In fact, in all weight loss endeavors, regardless of the method you are trying, you should never rely on a scale to determine your progress. The scale lies, perhaps unintentionally, but it does not tell you anything about what you really want to know. You want to know how much fat you have lost. When you weigh yourself, you include water and muscle? If you are increasing your water consumption for fasting, you are weighing all of that water, and if you are including muscle-toning, then you are also weighing additional muscle that you may have built during exercise.

SHARE YOUR PLANS

Your intermittent fasting lifestyle is a very personal choice, but it will have some impact on the lives of those around you. When you make the decision to embark on this journey, it is important to explain to those who are close to you exactly what you will be doing and why. Be prepared for some surprise or adverse reactions. Don't let this put you off; you have done your homework, and you can explain the science behind intermittent fasting to these people if necessary. Ultimately, this is your choice, and you only really need to share your plans so that others are able to support you if they so wish and not for their approval.

Your family will be the most impacted by your decision, but they will also likely receive the most benefit from your new lifestyle. Intermittent fasting will improve your mood and give you more energy. Its multiple health benefits should also be important to your family as they should want you to be as healthy as possible. Ideally, it would be beneficial to have your partner practice intermittent fasting with you as this will make things far easier at home. If they are not ready to try or are not interested in intermittent fasting, though, don't let this put you off. It is absolutely possible to still be successful in this new lifestyle without others in your home also embarking on it.

PLAN YOUR MEALS

By choosing intermittent fasting as a lifestyle, you have already taken a lot of pressure off yourself by structuring you're eating window and eliminating at least one meal. You can take this further and increase your chances of being successful by planning your meals and prepping your food beforehand. You don't have to plan your meals too far in advance— a week at a time is more than sufficient. If you have, for instance, decided to fast between Monday and Friday, set aside sometime on a Sunday afternoon for meal preparation for the week.

28 DAYS MEAL PLAN

28 DAYS	BREAKFAST	LUNCH	DINNER
Day 1	Breakfast Frittata	Quinoa and Scallops Salad	Chicken Wraps with Ricotta Cheese
Day 2	Intermittent Waffles	Avocado Stuffed with Tuna	Bacon and Egg Wraps with Salsa
Day 3	Pumpkin Pancakes	Cod Tacos with Salsa	Delicious Quinoa & Dried
Day 4	Buttermilk Pancakes	Dill Salmon Salad Wraps	Lettuce Fajita Meatball Wraps
Day 5	Ricotta Omelet with Swiss Chard	Cabbage and Prawn Wraps	Korean Beef and Onion Tacos
Day 6	Omelet with Goat Cheese and Herb	Tuna and Lettuce Wraps	Crunchy Chicken Egg Rolls
Day 7	Bacon and Zucchini Egg Breakfast	Tuna in Cucumber	Cheesy Sweet Potato and Bean Burritos
Day 8	Turkey and Scrambled Eggs Breakfast	Easy Lunch Salmon Steaks	Golden Chicken and Yogurt Taquitos

28 DAYS	BREAKFAST	LUNCH	DINNER
Day 9	Chia Breakfast Bowl	Cod Soup	Basil-Rubbed Pork Chops
Day 10	Cinnamon Roll Oatmeal	Shrimp Cocktail	Kalamata Parsley Tapenade and Salted Lamp Chops
Day 11	Breakfast Cereal	Squid and Shrimp Salad	Beef Tenderloin Steaks Wrapped with Bacon
Day 12	Best Intermittent Bread	Parsley Seafood Cocktail	Sausage, Beef and Chili Recipe
Day 13	Bread De Soul	Shrimp and Onion Ginger Dressing	Egg White Scramble with Cherry Tomatoes & Spinach
Day 14	Chia Seed Bread	Salmon and Cabbage Mix	Shrimp in Curry Sauce
Day 15	Special Intermittent Bread	Fruit Shrimp Soup	Tilapia with Olives & Tomato Sauce
Day 16	Intermittent Fluffy Cloud Bread	Buffalo Pizza Chicken	Lemon Garlic Shrimp
Day 17	Splendid Low-Carb Bread	Hot Chicken Meatballs	Baked Haddock
Day 18	Coconut Flour Almond Bread	Intermittent Chicken Enchiladas	Trout with Sauce
Day 19	Quick Low-Carb Bread Loaf	Home-Style Chicken Kebab	Roasted Salmon with Kimchi
Day 20	Intermittent Bakers Bread	Traditional Hungarian Gulyás	Parmesan Crusted Salmon
Day 21	Cheese Garlic Bread	Greek Chicken Stifado	Zoodles With White Clam Sauce
Day 22	Almond Flour Lemon Bread	Tangy Chicken with Scallions	Low Carb Oyster Recipe
Day 23	Seed and Nut Bread	Double Cheese Italian Chicken	Low Carb Soft Shell Crab
Day 24	Puri Bread	Middle Eastern Shish Kebab	Cheese and Seafood Stuffed Mushrooms
Day 25	Cranberry Bread	Capocollo and Garlic Chicken	Intermittent Salmon in Foil Packets with Pesto
Day 26	Avocado Salad Dish	Cheesy Mexican-Style Chicken	Simple Founder in Brown Butter Lemon Sauce
Day 27	Power Cream with Strawberry	Asian Saucy Chicken	Grilled Calamari
Day 28	Savory Intermittent Pancake	Duck Stew Olla Tapada	Souvlaki Spiced Salmon Bowls

CONCLUSION

These fasts can last anywhere from 8-20 hours, giving the body time to replenish its energy reserves. While intermittent fasting has been around for centuries, it's only recently become popular in Western countries because of its purported health benefits. I'm going to conclude by explaining the methodologies behind intermittent fasting for women over 50, as well as the potential benefits and drawbacks. But first: The benefits of intermittent fasting are countless. I can't list them all, but here's a synopsis of the ones I found interesting: 1) Since the body doesn't get enough time to replenish its energy reserves during normal eating, fasting helps you lose weight. 2) Intermittent fasting lowers the risk of disease, especially cancer and diabetes – this means it could aid your current health or even cure your illness. 3) Intermittent fasting can increase your testosterone levels (especially if you're overweight). 4) It's said that men can have sex more often while intermittent fasting, and you don't get any cramping because of low blood sugar levels. 5) Fasting can increase the body's resistance to oxidative stress (meaning you'll be healthier). 6) It can even help treat depression.

It's worth noting, however, that no conclusive evidence has been found to support the idea that intermittent fasting can cure cancer in humans or prevent it from occurring in the first place. A similar situation applies to diabetes – while it is believed that intermittent fasting could aid in curing diabetes, there is no sufficient evidence yet.

Clear benefits of intermittent fasting include weight loss and a lower risk of disease (especially cancer).

Athletes who train rigorously generally don't follow intermittent fasting, but that doesn't mean it's completely useless for men or women who work out regularly. Some athletes claim that intermittent fasting helps them maintain muscle mass while shedding fat.

Athletes who aren't looking to lose weight could use intermittent fasting as a way to fuel their workouts.

Intermittent fasting is often used by women who are trying to get pregnant. Since it suppresses normal ovulation, few eggs are released which makes it more difficult for the woman to conceive.

Not everyone agrees that intermittent fasting is effective for weight loss. Some argue that it doesn't translate into losing fat– the pounds just come from muscle mass instead (which isn't necessarily bad).

Intermittent fasting can be dangerous for women over 50 who experience periods of prolonged hunger.

This is because prolonged hunger can cause serious health problems, including high blood pressure, heart disease, stroke, diabetes and more. There's evidence to suggest that some women over 50 are at an increased risk of these conditions because of their tendency to snack during the day when they're feeling hungry. So how do you know if you should fast? Unfortunately, there's no easy way to tell if intermittent fasting is right for you before starting out. I've fasted many times without any adverse effects, but you could easily be allergic to one of the foods you're trying to eat and not even realize it. I think it's important for women over 50 who are planning to start an intermittent fasting regimen that they take a serious look at the evidence on this topic from a health standpoint. Personally, I prefer intermittent fasting in 8-hour intervals over 16:8. 8-hour periods give me more time to get done what I need to do, and I'm less likely to overeat afterward. However, it's not uncommon for women over 50 to experience a drop in their energy levels starting in the early afternoon. In this case, a 16:8 regimen might be advantageous. You should also consider your general health when it comes to intermittent fasting: If you have a low amount of body fat, or if you're overweight and want to lose weight, intermittent fasting could be right for you. If you're of normal weight and don't have any major health problems, intermittent fasting is still beneficial but not as much as it would be otherwise. You can always try the intermittent fasting and see if it works for you. If you don't feel well while you're on a fast, it's okay to break your fast and eat a meal. In fact, I would highly recommend doing this at least once during your first month of intermittent fasting. Break the fast with something that isn't too heavy, like oatmeal or fruit. This will give you a better idea of how your body is going to respond to future fast days. If you find that eating more frequently prevents overeating later in the day and if you feel better, then intermittent fasting might not be right for you. Does intermittent fasting harm the body? Some research suggests that periodic fasting could be beneficial for overall health. However, there's also evidence to suggest that it has harmful effects on the body. For example, a study from the University of Southern California found that intermittent fasting does not increase human longevity. The scientists who conducted the research said intermittent fasting may benefit some people by allowing them to lose weight and lower their cholesterol levels, but it won't lengthen their lifespan. Other studies in mice have shown that intermittent fasting can reduce longevity and increase the risk of disease. On top of this, if you're looking to get pregnant in the near future, intermittent fasting is probably not ideal for you since it suppresses natural ovulation. So, should you fast? There's no right or wrong answer here. **If you're a woman over 50, intermittent fasting is one of the best possible ways to improve your quality of life.**

You'll hear a lot about intermittent fasting these days and, if you're interested in living longer and healthier, it's worth taking some time to make sense of what it is.

Intermittent fasting is becoming more popular, but do you know what it is? So far, the benefits of intermittent fasting are well studied and widely accepted. Now that you're armed with all the information needed to better understand it.

Our metabolic rate, or resting metabolism, decreases with age. You'll burn fewer calories at rest as you get older, even if your diet and activity levels remain the same. This is why it's recommended that people over age 50 eat the same number of calories as younger adults, but spread over more meals. This helps your body stay in an anabolic state (meaning you build more muscle and burn more fat).

While your metabolic rate decreases with age, studies show that intermittent fasting can help keep it stable and even increase it during the fasting period, resulting in faster weight loss and a slimmer waist.

Research shows that not skipping breakfast or lunch can make us less likely to overeat at our next meal, burn more fat and calories throughout the day, and feel fuller for longer compared with people who skip breakfast or eat late in the day.

Another benefit of intermittent fasting may be that it helps your body to better digest food by boosting your digestive enzymes and decreasing levels of the stress hormone cortisol.

One study found that intermittent fasting changed gene expression in white fat cells. These are the fat cells that accumulate around our waist, hips and thighs. By increasing the number of good genes and reducing bad genes in these fat cells, intermittent fasting protects us from developing serious diseases such as type 2 diabetes, heart disease, stroke, and some cancers.

So why is eating less important for those over 50?

We also know that women over 50 tend to have a slower metabolism than men due to lower levels of testosterone (a hormone important for maintaining muscle mass). This means women's bodies burn fewer calories at rest than men's and, therefore, they need fewer calories for maintenance. As women age, their metabolic rate tends to decline even further.

Skipping meals is a poor way to lose weight and won't help you live longer. It can actually do the opposite by slowing your metabolism, which makes it harder to lose weight and more likely that you'll gain fat over time. In fact, eating too few calories has been shown to decrease life expectancy in animals and humans.

Your body needs the energy to run all aspects of your life, from breathing to thinking.

Made in the USA
Coppell, TX
09 November 2021